HEALTH

AND

HUMAN RIGHTS

a reader

edited by

Jonathan M. Mann, Sofla Gruskin,

Michael A. Grodin, George J. Annas

ROUTLEDGE
New York and London

Published in 1999 by
Routledge
29 West 35th Street
New York, NY 10001

Published in Great Britain in 1999 by
Routledge
11 New Fetter Lane
London EC4P 4EE

Copyright © 1999 by Routledge

Printed in the United States of America on acid-free paper
Design: Jack Donner

Library of Congress Cataloging-in-Publication Data

Health and human rights: a reader /
edited by Jonathan M. Mann, Sofia Gruskin, Michael A. Grodin,
and George J. Annas.

p.   cm.

Includes bibliographical references and index.
ISBN 0–415–92101–5 (hc.). — ISBN 0–415–92102–3 (pbk.)
1. Public health—Moral and ethical aspects.   2. Human rights—Health aspects.
3. Medical policy—Moral and ethical aspects.   4. Human experimentation
in medicine—Moral and ethical aspects.   5. Discrimination in health care.
I. Mann, Jonathan, Gruskin, S., Grodin, M., and Annas, G. J.

RA427.25.H42   1998
174'.2—dc21   98–20899
CIP

To all people

who promote and protect

human rights and health

throughout the world

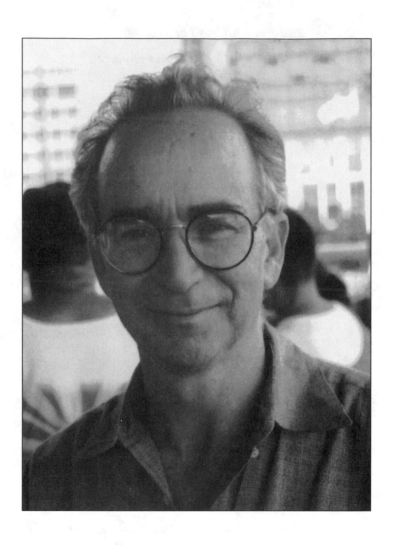

Dedication to Jonathan Mann

On September 2, 1998 Jonathan Mann was tragically killed in the crash of Swissair Flight 111. Jonathan was born in 1947, the year the Universal Declaration of Human Rights was being drafted—a document he treasured and dedicated his professional life to promoting. It is bitterly ironic that his life was cut short in the year we celebrate its fiftieth anniversary and that of the World Health Organization—one an emblem of human rights, the other of public health. Jonathan Mann and his wife, Mary Lou Clements-Mann, were on their way to Geneva, to the World Health Organization and to UNAIDS, to pursue work that had taken them all over the world. Mary Lou and Jonathan were bringing to Geneva their unique personal and professional partnership to support the global response to the AIDS pandemic. Mary Lou was bringing her scientific expertise, and Jonathan his vision of a world where HIV/AIDS would be recognized and responded to through a combined, largely expanded health, social and economic development strategy firmly grounded in human rights.

Jonathan had the charisma and the ability to reach through layers of bureaucracy and cynicism and to touch the hearts of people. He inspired people by challenging them. He challenged people in public health to recognize their dual responsibility, as agents of the state, to promote and protect not only health but also human rights. He challenged people in human rights to move beyond just criticizing health policy and government actions impacting on health after they had occurred, but to get involved from the beginning in helping to shape them. Out of this he catalyzed today's health and human rights movement.

Jonathan frequently reminded us that our work is possible because we stand on the shoulders of the giants—the giants in health and in human rights—who had preceded us. Jonathan believed deeply in the possibility of changing the world, of making it a better place. His life ended before he was fully able to play out his own role in doing so. We share his belief that the health and human rights movement has a collective responsibility to move this work forward as, to use Jonathan's words, "equal partners in the belief that the world can change." We will stand on his shoulders, even as we will deeply miss him.

Contents

Acknowledgments

We would like to thank our Routledge editor, Heidi Freund, for her commitment to the subject matter and for sharing our vision of the importance of the linkage between health and human rights. We would like to thank Albina du Boisrouvray for her lasting support. This book would not have been completed without the administrative and secretarial support of Jacoba von Gimborn, Marilyn Ricciardelli, Megan Bell, and Jen Zoble. Finally, we owe our sincere thanks to the many health and human rights students with whom we have had the privilege of teaching and learning over the past years.

Introduction

Jonathan M. Mann, Sofia Gruskin,
Michael A. Grodin, and George J. Annas

- *Discrimination against ethnic, religious, and racial minorities, as well as on account of gender, political opinion, or immigration status, compromises or threatens the health and well-being and, all too often, the very lives of millions. In its most extreme forms, prejudice or the devaluation of human beings because they are classified as "other" has led to apartheid, ethnic cleansing, and genocide. Discriminatory practices threaten physical and mental health and result in the denial of access to care, inappropriate therapies, or inferior care.*

- *Human rights violations exist in the design and implementation of health policies, to the detriment of health. For example, population policies have often failed to respect individual decision-making and informed choices. Promotion and protection of such human rights as education, information, privacy, and equal rights in marriage and divorce are necessary if women's health is to be protected.*

- *In the more than ninety civil and international conflicts currently raging across the globe, there is a stark connection between the disregard for human rights and the health and well-being of entire populations. Since the fall of the Berlin Wall, violent conflict has claimed the lives of more than four million people. In early 1997 alone, more than thirty-five million people became refugees or were internally displaced as a result of violent conflict and forced to live in conditions that contribute to disease, malnutrition, and early death.*

- *Respect for human rights in the context of HIV/AIDS, mental illness, and physical disability leads to markedly better prevention and treatment. Respect for the dignity and privacy of individuals can facilitate more sensitive and humane care. Stigmatization and discrimination thwart medical and public health efforts to help people with disease or disability.*

- *Conventional practices in biomedical and behavioral research often violate human rights. Contemporary medical research studies often lack adequate informed consent procedures and offer disproportionate risks in relationship to benefits. The medical research community continues to use disenfranchised and vulnerable populations for human experimentation at great detriment to their physical and mental health.*

Human rights and public health are two complementary approaches, and languages, to address and advance human well-being. The human rights approach seeks to describe—and then to promote and protect—the societal-level prerequisites for human well-being in which each individual can achieve his or her full potential.

Modern human rights is a civilizational achievement, a historic effort to identify and agree upon what governments should not do to people and what they should assure to all. Human rights are nonprovable statements that derive their legitimacy from having been developed, voted upon and adopted by the nations of the world and having been incorporated into the domain of international law; they do not achieve their status from divine inspiration or religion.

Health concerns the physical, mental, and social well-being of individuals. Public health can be defined as "ensuring the conditions in which people can be healthy." The core of public health knowledge, based on research and experience, is that a blend of individual and societal-level factors are involved in determining health status. For many, if not most people, the societal context is the major determinant of vulnerability to preventable disease, disability, and premature death.

The Universal Declaration of Human Rights—the cornerstone document of modern human rights—through its focus on the societal-level determinants of well-being addresses a panoply of public health issues and concerns, even though the word *health* itself appears only once in the document. The focus of the Universal Declaration on these societal-level health determinants provides public health with a framework, vocabulary, and guidance for analysis and direct response that may ultimately prove more useful to promote public health than frameworks inherited from biomedical and public health traditions.

From a human rights perspective, interest in health has primarily focused on governmental actions taken in the name of public health and their impact on the rights enshrined in international human rights law. Most actions taken in the name of public health are carried out under the aegis of governmental authority and responsibility. Most are actually performed by governmental agencies, and others are indirectly supported and organized by governmental funding and regulation. Recognition of the dependency of health on societal factors, and of the linkages between these factors and the fulfillment of human rights, provides a new approach to monitoring governmental responsibility and accountability for rights affecting health.

Public health deals with populations and prevention. Nonetheless, public health has generally ignored the societal roots of health in favor of interventions which operate farther downstream. Epidemiology, public health's major methodology, has contributed to this narrowed focus because it most often identifies individual risk behaviors in isolation from the critical societal context. Since the way in which a problem is defined determines what interventions seem reasonable, recognition of human rights will help to define the direction and nature of societal change needed to promote public health.

Both those actively engaged in public health and those in human rights recognize that discrimination and other violations of human rights directly impact on health and well-being, and that they must deal directly with the underlying societal issues that largely determine who lives and who dies, when, and of what.

Health and Human Rights is a reader of previously published leading articles. The articles selected provide a comprehensive introduction to the new and burgeoning field of human rights and health. There is a journal, *Health and Human Rights*, published by the François-Xavier Bagnoud Center for Health and Human Rights, but there are no books focusing on this new field. This book is written for health workers, human rights workers, and others interested in protecting and promoting human rights and health. It can also be used in courses on health and human rights and courses on human rights at the undergraduate and graduate levels, with particular emphasis on schools of law, public health, medicine, and nursing. The chapters are reprinted as they originally appeared. For consistency, all articles are referred to as chapters, misspellings have been silently corrected.

The text is divided into six sections. Introductions to each section written by the editors frame the nature, context, importance, and interrelationship of the articles in that section. Section I contains introductory essays on human rights and public health. Section II addresses the impact of health policies and programs on human rights, and Section III discusses the health impacts resulting from violations of human rights. Section IV explores the inextricable linkage between health and human rights. Section V focuses on medicine and human rights. Section VI identifies how to proceed from concept to action. Finally, appendices containing selected international human rights documents and resources are included.

PART I

Human Rights and Public Health

In exploring the connection between health and human rights, we propose three relationships, each of which focuses on an important aspect of this critical linkage. These relationships are outlined in broad terms in the first article in this section, "Health and Human Rights," the inaugural article of the journal *Health and Human Rights*. This article provides a framework and basis for considering the health and human rights nexus explored throughout this reader.

The first relationship, which can be diagrammed simply as H ——> HR concerns the potential impacts of health policies, programs, and practices on human rights. As described in Part II, recognition of the complementarity of public health goals and human rights norms can lead to more effective health policies and programs. The challenge is to negotiate the optimal balance between promoting and protecting public health and promoting and protecting human rights.

The second relationship, which can be diagrammed equally simply as H <—— HR, expresses the idea that violations or lack of fulfillment of any and all human rights have negative effects on physical, mental, and social well-being (health). This is true in peacetime and, of course, in times of conflict and extreme political repression. The articles in Part III explore this relationship.

The third relationship, which can be diagrammed as H <——> HR, conveys the idea of inextricable connection. The central idea of the health and human rights movement is that health and human rights act in synergy. Promoting and protecting health requires explicit and concrete efforts to promote and protect human rights and dignity, and greater fulfillment of human rights necessitates sound attention to health and to its societal determinants.

As an entry to the world of health and human rights thinking and action, the chapters in this section also include a primer on public health and one on human rights. These chapters are drawn from a manual intended for use by people in the fields of public health and human rights in order to provide sufficient knowledge of each field to facilitate a practical working relationship between them. Since this reader is intended for people interested in one or both of these domains, we hope that even those already familiar with either public health or human rights will read these introductory chapters, which set the stage for consideration of the complex and fascinating health and human rights paradigm.

Health and Human Rights 1.

Jonathan M. Mann, Lawrence Gostin, Sofia Gruskin,
Troyen Brennan, Zita Lazzarini, and Harvey Fineberg

Health and human rights have rarely been linked in an explicit manner. With few exceptions, notably involving access to health care, discussions about health have not included human rights considerations. Similarly, except when obvious damage to health is the primary manifestation of a human rights abuse, such as with torture, health perspectives have been generally absent from human rights discourse.

Explanations for the dearth of communication between the fields of health and human rights include differing philosophical perspectives, vocabularies, professional recruitment and training, societal roles, and methods of work. In addition, modern concepts of both health and human rights are complex and steadily evolving. On a practical level, health workers may wonder about the applicability or utility ("added value"), let alone necessity, of incorporating human rights perspectives into their work, and vice versa. In addition, despite pioneering work seeking to bridge this gap in bioethics,[1] jurisprudence,[2] and public health law,[3] a history of conflictual relationships between medicine and law, or between public health officials and civil liberties advocates, may contribute to anxiety and doubt about the potential for mutually beneficial collaboration.

Yet health and human rights are both powerful, modern approaches to defining and advancing human well-being. Attention to the intersection of health and human rights may provide practical benefits to those engaged in health or human rights work, may help reorient thinking about major global health challenges, and may contribute to broadening human rights thinking and practice. However, meaningful dialogue about interactions between health and human rights requires a common ground. To this end, following a brief overview of selected features of modern health and human rights, this chapter proposes a provisional, mutually accessible framework for

structuring discussions about research, promoting cross-disciplinary education, and exploring the potential for health and human rights collaboration.

MODERN CONCEPTS OF HEALTH

Modern concepts of health derive from two related although quite different
disciplines: medicine and public health. While medicine generally focuses on
the health of an individual, public health emphasizes the health of populations. To oversimplify, individual health has been the concern of medical and
other health care services, generally in the context of physical (and, to a lesser
extent, mental) illness and disability. In contrast, public health has been defined as "[ensuring] the conditions in which people can be healthy."[4] Thus,
public health has a distinct health-promoting goal and emphasizes prevention of disease, disability, and premature death.

Therefore, from a public health perspective, while the availability of
medical and other health care constitutes one of the essential conditions for
health, it is not synonymous with "health." Only a small fraction of the variance of health status among populations can reasonably be attributed to
health care; health care is necessary but clearly not sufficient for health.[5]

The most widely used modern definition of health was developed by the
World Health Organization (WHO): "Health is a state of complete physical, mental and social well-being and not merely the absence of disease or
infirmity."[6] Through this definition, WHO has helped to move health thinking beyond a limited, biomedical, and pathology-based perspective to the
more positive domain of "well-being." Also, by explicitly including the
mental and social dimensions of well-being, WHO radically expanded the
scope of health and, by extension, the roles and responsibilities of health
professionals and their relationship to the larger society.

The WHO definition also highlights the importance of health promotion,
defined as "the process of enabling people to increase control over, and to
improve, their health." To do so, "an individual or group must be able to
identify and realize aspirations, to satisfy needs, and to change or cope with
the environment."[7] The societal dimensions of this effort were emphasized
in the Declaration of Alma-Ata (1978), which described health as a "social
goal whose realization requires the action of many other social and economic
sectors in addition to the health sector."[8]

Thus, the modern concept of health includes yet goes beyond health care
to embrace the broader societal dimensions and context of individual and
population well-being. Perhaps the most far-reaching statement about the
expanded scope of health is contained in the preamble to the WHO Constitution, which declared that "the enjoyment of the highest attainable standard of health is one of the fundamental rights of every human being."[9]

MODERN HUMAN RIGHTS

The modern idea of human rights is similarly vibrant, hopeful, ambitious,
and complex. While there is a long history to human rights thinking, agree-

ment was reached that all people are "born free and equal in dignity and rights"[10] when the promotion of human rights was identified as a principal purpose of the United Nations in 1945.[11] Then, in 1948, the Universal Declaration of Human Rights was adopted as a universal or common standard of achievement for all peoples and all nations.

The preamble to the Universal Declaration proposes that human rights and dignity are self-evident, the "highest aspiration of the common people," and "the foundation of freedom, justice and peace." "Social progress and better standards of life in larger freedom," including the prevention of "barbarous acts which have outraged the conscience of mankind," and, broadly speaking, individual and collective well-being, are considered to depend upon the "promotion of universal respect for and observance of human rights."

Several fundamental characteristics of modern human rights include: they are rights of individuals; these rights inhere in individuals because they are human; they apply to all people around the world; and they principally involve the relationship between the state and the individual. The specific rights that form the corpus of human rights law are listed in several key documents. Foremost is the Universal Declaration of Human Rights (UDHR), which, along with the United Nations Charter (UN Charter), the International Covenant on Civil and Political Rights (ICCPR)—and its Optional Protocols—and the International Covenant on Economic, Social and Cultural Rights (ICESCR), constitute what is often called the "International Bill of Human Rights." The UDHR was drawn up to give more specific definition to the rights and freedoms referred to in the UN Charter. The ICCPR and the ICESCR further elaborate the content set out in the UDHR, as well as set out the conditions in which states can permissibly restrict rights.

Although the UDHR is not a legally binding document, nations (states) have endowed it with great legitimacy through their actions, including its legal and political invocation at the national and international levels. For example, portions of the UDHR are cited in numerous national constitutions, and governments often refer to the UDHR when accusing other governments of violating human rights. The Covenants are legally binding, but only on the states that have become parties to them. Parties to the Covenants accept certain procedures and responsibilities, including periodic submission of reports on their compliance with the substantive provisions of the texts.

Building upon this central core of documents, a large number of additional declarations and conventions have been adopted at the international and regional levels, focusing upon either specific populations (such as the International Convention on the Elimination of All Forms of Racial Discrimination, entered into force in 1969; the Convention on the Elimination of All Forms of Discrimination Against Women, 1981; the Convention on the Rights of the Child, 1989); or issues (such as the Convention Against Torture and Other Cruel, Inhuman or Degrading Treatment or Punishment, entered into force in 1987; the Declaration on the Elimination of All Forms of Intolerance and of Discrimination Based on Religion or Belief, 1981).

Since 1948, the promotion and protection of human rights have received increased attention from communities and nations around the world. While there are few legal sanctions to compel states to meet their human rights obligations, states are increasingly monitored for their compliance with human rights norms by other states, nongovernmental organizations, the media, and private individuals. The growing legitimacy of the human rights framework lies in the increasing application of human rights standards by a steadily widening range of actors in the world community. The awarding of the Nobel Peace Prize for human rights work to Amnesty International and to Ms. Rigoberta Menchu symbolizes this extraordinary level of contemporary interest and concern with human rights.

Since the late 1940s, human rights advocacy and related challenges have gradually extended the boundaries of the human rights movement in four related ways. First, the initial advocacy focus on civil and political rights and certain economic and social rights is expanding to include concerns about the environment and global socioeconomic development. For example, although the right to a "social and international order in which (human rights) can be fully realized" (UDHR, Article 28) invokes broad political issues at the global level, attention to this core concept as a right has grown only in recent years.

Second, while the grounding of human rights thinking and practice in law (at national and international levels) remains fundamental, wider social involvement and participation in human rights struggles is increasingly broadening the language and uses of human rights concepts.

Third, while human rights law primarily focuses on the relationship between individuals and states, awareness is increasing that other societal institutions and systems, such as transnational business, may strongly influence the capacity for realization of rights, yet they may elude state control. For example, exploitation of natural resources by business interests may seriously harm rights of local residents, yet the governmental capacity to protect human rights may be extremely limited, or at best indirect, through regulation of business practices and laws that offer the opportunity for redress. In addition, certain individual acts, such as rape, have not been a traditional concern of human rights law, except when resulting from systematic state policy (as alleged in Bosnia). However, it is increasingly evident that state policies impacting on the status and role of women may contribute importantly, even if indirectly, to a societal context that increases women's vulnerability to rape, even though the actual act may be individual, not state-sponsored.

Finally, the twin challenges of human rights promotion (hopefully preventing rights violations; analogous to health promotion to prevent disease) and protection (emphasizing accountability and redress for violations; analogous to medical care once disease has occurred) have often been approached separately. Initially, the United Nations system highlighted promotion of rights, and the nongovernmental human rights movement tended to stress protection of rights, often in response to horrific and systematic rights violations. More recently, both intergovernmental and nongovernmental agencies have recognized and responded to the fundamental interdependence of rights promotion and protection.

In summary, despite tremendous controversy, especially regarding the philosophical and cultural context of human rights as currently defined, a vocabulary and set of human rights norms are increasingly becoming part of community, national, and global life.

A PROVISIONAL FRAMEWORK: LINKAGES BETWEEN HEALTH AND HUMAN RIGHTS

The goal of linking health and human rights is to contribute to advancing human well-being beyond what could be achieved through an isolated health- or human rights-based approach. This chapter proposes a three-part framework for considering linkages between health and human rights; all are interconnected, and each has substantial practical consequences. The first two are already well documented, although requiring further elaboration, while the third represents a central hypothesis calling for substantial additional analysis and exploration.

First, the impact (positive and negative) of health policies, programs, and practices on human rights will be considered. This linkage will be illustrated by focusing on the use of state power in the context of public health.

The second relationship is based on the understanding that human rights violations have health impacts. It is proposed that all rights violations, particularly when severe, widespread, and sustained, engender important health effects, which must be recognized and assessed. This process engages health expertise and methodologies in helping to understand how well-being is affected by violations of human rights.

The third part of this framework is based on an overarching proposition: that promotion and protection of human rights and promotion and protection of health are fundamentally linked. Even more than the first two proposed relationships, this intrinsic linkage has strategic implications and potentially dramatic practical consequences for work in each domain.

The First Relationship:
The Impact of Health Policies, Programs and Practices on Human Rights

Around the world, health care is provided through many diverse public and private mechanisms. However, the responsibilities of public health are carried out in large measure through policies and programs promulgated, implemented, and enforced by, or with support from, the state. Therefore, this first linkage may be best explored by considering the impact of public health policies, programs, and practices on human rights.

The three central functions of public health are: assessing health needs and problems; developing policies designed to address priority health issues;

and assuring programs to implement strategic health goals.[12] Potential benefits to and burdens on human rights may occur in the pursuit of each of these major areas of public health responsibility.

For example, assessment involves collection of data on important health problems in a population. However, data are not collected on all possible health problems, nor does the selection of which issues to assess occur in a societal vacuum. Thus, a state's failure to recognize or acknowledge health problems that preferentially affect a marginalized or stigmatized group may violate the right to nondiscrimination by leading to neglect of necessary services, and in so doing, may adversely affect the realization of other rights, including the right to "security in the event of . . . sickness [or] disability" or to the "special care and assistance" to which mothers and children are entitled (UDHR, Article 25).

Once decisions about which problems to assess have been made, the methodology of data collection may create additional human rights burdens. Collecting information from individuals, such as whether they are infected with the human immunodeficiency virus (HIV), have breast cancer, or are genetically predisposed to heart disease, can clearly burden rights to security of person (associated with the concept of informed consent) and of arbitrary interference with privacy. In addition, the right of nondiscrimination may be threatened even by an apparently simple information-gathering exercise. For example, a health survey conducted via telephone, by excluding households without telephones (usually associated with lower socioeconomic status), may result in a biased assessment, which may in turn lead to policies or programs that fail to recognize or meet needs of the entire population. Also, personal health status or health behavior information (such as sexual orientation or history of drug use) has the potential for misuse by the state, whether directly or if it is made available to others, resulting in grievous harm to individuals and violations of many rights. Thus, misuse of information about HIV infection status has led to: restrictions of the right to work and to education; violations of the right to marry and found a family; attacks upon honor and reputation; limitations of freedom of movement; arbitrary detention or exile; and even cruel, inhuman, or degrading treatment.

The second major task of public health is to develop policies to prevent and control priority health problems. Important burdens on human rights may arise in the policy-development process. For example, if a government refuses to disclose the scientific basis of health policy or permit debate on its merits, or in other ways refuses to inform and involve the public in policy development, the rights to "seek, receive and impart information and ideas . . . regardless of frontiers" (UDHR, Article 19) and "to take part in the government . . . directly or through freely chosen representatives" (UDHR, Article 21) may be violated. Then, prioritization of health issues may result in discrimination against individuals, as when the major health problems of a population defined on the basis of sex, race, religion, or language are systematically given lower priority (e.g., sickle-cell disease in the United States, which affects primarily the African-American population; or, more globally, maternal mortality, breast cancer, and other health problems of women).

The third core function of public health, to assure services capable of realizing policy goals, is also closely linked with the right to nondiscrimination. When health and social services do not take logistic, financial, and sociocultural barriers to their access and enjoyment into account, intentional or unintentional discrimination may readily occur. For example, in clinics for maternal and child health, details such as hours of service, accessibility via public transportation and availability of day care may strongly and adversely influence service utilization.[13]

It is essential to recognize that in seeking to fulfill each of its core functions and responsibilities, public health may burden human rights. In the past, when restrictions on human rights were recognized, they were often simply justified as necessary to protect public health. Indeed, public health has a long tradition, anchored in the history of infectious disease control, of limiting the "rights of the few" for the "good of the many." Thus, coercive measures such as mandatory testing and treatment, quarantine and isolation are considered basic measures of traditional communicable disease control.[14]

The principle that certain rights must be restricted in order to protect the community is explicitly recognized in the International Bill of Human Rights: limitations are considered permissible to "(secure) due recognition and respect for the rights and freedoms of others and of meeting the just requirements of morality, public order and the general welfare in a democratic society" (UDHR, Article 29). However, the permissible restriction of rights is bound in several ways. First, certain rights (e.g., right to life, right to be free from torture) are considered inviolable under any circumstances. Restriction of other rights must be: in the interest of a legitimate objective; determined by law; imposed in the least intrusive means possible; not imposed arbitrarily; and strictly necessary in a "democratic society" to achieve its purposes.

Unfortunately, public health decisions to restrict human rights have frequently been made in an uncritical, unsystematic, and unscientific manner. Therefore, the prevailing assumption that public health, as articulated through specific policies and programs, is an unalloyed public good that does not require consideration of human rights norms must be challenged. For the present, it may be useful to adopt the maxim that health policies and programs should be considered discriminatory and burdensome on human rights until proven otherwise.

Yet this approach raises three related and vital questions. First, why should public health officials be concerned about burdening human rights? Second, to what extent is respect for human rights and dignity compatible with, or complementary to, public health goals? Finally, how can an optimal balance between public health goals and human rights norms be negotiated?

Justifying public health concern for human rights norms could be based on the primary value of promoting societal respect for human rights as well as on arguments of public health effectiveness. At least to the extent that public health goals are not seriously compromised by respect for human rights norms, public health, as a state function, is obligated to respect human rights and dignity.

The major argument for linking human rights and health promotion is described below. However, it is also important to recognize that contemporary thinking about optimal strategies for disease control has evolved; efforts to confront the most serious global health threats, including cancer, cardiovascular disease, and other chronic diseases, injuries, reproductive health, infectious diseases, and individual and collective violence increasingly emphasize the role of personal behavior within a broad social context. Thus, the traditional public health paradigm and strategies developed for diseases such as smallpox, often involving coercive approaches and activities that may have burdened human rights, are now understood to be less relevant today. For example, WHO's strategy for preventing spread of the human immunodeficiency virus (HIV) excludes classic practices such as isolation and quarantine (except under truly remarkable circumstances) and explicitly calls for supporting and preventing discrimination against HIV-infected people.

The idea that human rights and public health must inevitably conflict is increasingly tempered with awareness of their complementarity. Health policy-makers' and practitioners' lack of familiarity with modern human rights concepts and core documents complicates efforts to negotiate, in specific situations and different cultural contexts, the optimal balance between public health objectives and human rights norms. Similarly, human rights workers may choose not to confront health policies or programs, either to avoid seeming to undervalue community health or due to uncertainty about how and on what grounds to challenge public health officials. Recently, in the context of HIV/AIDS, new approaches have been developed, seeking to maximize realization of public health goals while simultaneously protecting and promoting human rights.[15] Yet HIV/AIDS is not unique; efforts to harmonize health and human rights goals are clearly possible in other areas. At present, an effort to identify human rights burdens created by public health policies, programs, and practices, followed by negotiation toward an optimal balance whenever public health and human rights goals appear to conflict, is a necessary minimum. An approach to realizing health objectives that simultaneously promotes—or at least respects—rights and dignity is clearly desirable.

The Second Relationship:
Health Impacts Resulting from Violations of Human Rights
Health impacts are obvious and inherent in the popular understanding of certain severe human rights violations, such as torture, imprisonment under inhumane conditions, summary execution, and "disappearances." For this reason, health experts concerned about human rights have increasingly

made their expertise available to help document such abuses.[16] Examples of this type of medical–human rights collaboration include: exhumation of mass graves to examine allegations of executions;[17] examination of torture victims;[18] and entry of health personnel into prisons to assess health status.[19]

However, health impacts of rights violations go beyond these issues in at least two ways. First, the duration and extent of health impacts resulting from severe abuses of rights and dignity remain generally underappreciated. Torture, imprisonment under inhumane conditions, or trauma associated with witnessing summary executions, torture, rape, or mistreatment of others have been shown to lead to severe, probably lifelong effects on physical, mental, and social well-being.[20] In addition, a more complete understanding of the negative health effects of torture must also include its broad influence on mental and social well-being; torture is often used as a political tool to discourage people from meaningful participation in or resistance to government.[21]

Second, and beyond these serious problems, it is increasingly evident that violations of many more, if not all, human rights have negative effects on health. For example, the right to information may be violated when cigarettes are marketed without governmental assurance that information regarding the harmful health effects of tobacco smoking will also be available. The health cost of this violation can be quantified through measures of tobacco-related preventable illness, disability, and premature death, including excess cancers, cardiovascular disease, and respiratory disease. Other violations of the right to information, with substantial health impacts, include governmental withholding of valid scientific health information about contraception or measures (e.g., condoms) to prevent infection with a fatal virus (HIV).

As another example, the enormous worldwide problem of occupation-related disease, disability, and death reflects violations of the right to work under "just and favorable conditions" (UDHR, Article 23). In this context, the World Bank's identification of increased educational attainment for women as a critical intervention for improving health status in developing countries powerfully expresses the pervasive impact of rights realization (in this case to education, and to nondiscrimination on the basis of sex) on population health status.[22]

A related, yet even more complex problem involves the potential health impact associated with violating individual and collective dignity. The Universal Declaration of Human Rights considers dignity, along with rights, to be inherent, inalienable, and universal. While important dignity-related health impacts may include such problems as the poor health status of many indigenous peoples, a coherent vocabulary and framework to characterize dignity and different forms of dignity violations are lacking. A taxonomy and an epidemiology of violations of dignity may uncover an enormous field of previously suspected, yet thus far unnamed and therefore undocumented damage to physical, mental, and social well-being.

Assessment of rights violations' health impacts is in its infancy. Progress will require: a more sophisticated capacity to document and assess rights violations; the application of medical, social science, and public health methodologies to identify and assess effects on physical, mental, and social well-being; and research to establish valid associations between rights violations and health impacts.

Identification of health impacts associated with violations of rights and dignity will benefit both health and human rights fields. Using rights violations as an entry point for recognition of health problems may help uncover previously unrecognized burdens on physical, mental or social well-being. From a human rights perspective, documentation of health impacts of rights violations may contribute to increased societal awareness of the importance of human rights promotion and protection.

The Third Relationship:

Health and Human Rights—Exploring an Inextricable Linkage

The proposal that promoting and protecting human rights is inextricably linked to the challenge of promoting and protecting health derives in part from recognition that health and human rights are complementary approaches to the central problem of defining and advancing human well-being. This fundamental connection leads beyond the single, albeit broad mention of health in the UDHR (Article 25) and the specific health-related responsibilities of states listed in Article 12 of the ICESCR, including: reducing stillbirth and infant mortality and promoting healthy child development; improving environmental and industrial hygiene; preventing, treating, and controlling epidemic, endemic, occupational and other diseases; and assuring medical care.

Modern concepts of health recognize that underlying "conditions" establish the foundation for realizing physical, mental, and social well-being. Given the importance of these conditions, it is remarkable how little priority has been given within health research to their precise identification and understanding of their modes of action, relative importance, and possible interactions.

The most widely accepted analysis focuses on socioeconomic status; the positive relationship between higher socioeconomic status and better health status is well documented.[23] Yet this analysis has at least three important limitations. First, it cannot adequately account for a growing number of discordant observations, such as: the increased longevity of married Canadian men and women compared with their single (widowed, divorced, never married) counterparts;[24] health status differences between minority and majority populations which persist even when traditional measures of socioeconomic status are considered;[25] or reports of differential marital, economic, and educational outcomes among obese women, compared with nonobese women.[26]

A second problem lies in the definition of poverty and its relationship to health status. Clearly, poverty may have different health meanings; for example, distinctions between the health-related meaning of absolute poverty and relative poverty have been proposed.[27]

A third, practical difficulty is that the socioeconomic paradigm creates an overwhelming challenge for which health workers are neither trained nor equipped to deal. Therefore, the identification of socioeconomic status as the "essential condition" for good health paradoxically may encourage complacency, apathy, and even policy and programmatic paralysis.

However, alternative or supplementary approaches are emerging about the nature of the "essential conditions" for health. For example, the Ottawa Charter for Health Promotion (1986) went beyond poverty to propose that "the fundamental conditions and resources for health are peace, shelter, education, food, income, a stable eco-system, sustainable resources, social justice and equity."[28]

Experience with the global epidemic of HIV/AIDS suggests a further analytic approach, using a rights analysis.[29] For example, married, monogamous women in East Africa have been documented to be infected with HIV.[30] Although these women know about HIV and condoms are accessible in the marketplace, their risk factor is their inability to control their husbands' sexual behavior or to refuse unprotected or unwanted sexual intercourse. Refusal may result in physical harm, or in divorce, the equivalent of social and economic death for the woman. Therefore, women's vulnerability to HIV is now recognized to be integrally connected with discrimination and unequal rights, involving property, marriage, divorce, and inheritance. The success of condom promotion for HIV prevention in this population is inherently limited in the absence of legal and societal changes which, by promoting and protecting women's rights, would strengthen their ability to negotiate sexual practice and protect themselves from HIV infection.[31]

More broadly, the evolving HIV/AIDS pandemic has shown a consistent pattern through which discrimination, marginalization, stigmatization, and, more generally, a lack of respect for the human rights and dignity of individuals and groups heighten their vulnerability to becoming exposed to HIV.[32] In this regard, HIV/AIDS may be illustrative of a more general phenomenon in which individual and population vulnerability to disease, disability, and premature death is linked to the status of respect for human rights and dignity.

Further exploration of the conceptual and practical dimensions of this relationship is required. For example, epidemiologically identified clusters of preventable disease, excess disability, and premature death could be analyzed to discover the specific limitations or violations of human rights and dignity that are involved. Similarly, a broad analysis of the human rights dimensions of major health problems such as cancer, cardiovascular disease, and injuries should be developed. The hypothesis that promotion and protection of rights and health are inextricably linked requires much creative exploration and rigorous evaluation.

The concept of an inextricable relationship between health and human rights also has enormous potential practical consequences. For example, health professionals could consider using the International Bill of Human Rights as a coherent guide for assessing health status of individuals or populations; the extent to which human rights are realized may represent a better and more comprehensive index of well-being than traditional health status indicators. Health professionals would also have to consider their responsibility not only to respect human rights in developing policies, programs, and practices, but to contribute actively from their position as health workers to improving societal realization of rights. Health workers have long acknowledged the societal roots of health status; the human rights linkage may help health professionals engage in specific and concrete ways with the full range of those working to promote and protect human rights and dignity in each society.

From the perspective of human rights, health experts and expertise may contribute usefully to societal recognition of the benefits and costs associated with realizing, or failing to respect, human rights and dignity. This can be accomplished without seeking to justify human rights and dignity on health grounds (or for any pragmatic purposes). Rather, collaboration with health experts can help give voice to the pervasive and serious impact on health associated with lack of respect for rights and dignity. In addition, the right to health can be developed and made meaningful only through dialogue between health and human rights disciplines. Finally, the importance of health as a precondition for the capacity to realize and enjoy human rights and dignity must be appreciated. For example, poor nutritional status of children can contribute subtly yet importantly to limiting realization of the right to education; in general, people who are healthy may be best equipped to participate fully and benefit optimally from the protections and opportunities inherent in the International Bill of Human Rights.

CONCLUSION

Thus far, different philosophical and historical roots, disciplinary differences in language and approach, and practical barriers to collaboration impede recognition of important linkages between health and human rights. The mutually enriching combination of research, education, and field experience will advance understanding and catalyze further action around human rights and health. Exploration of the intersection of health and human rights may help revitalize the health field as well as contribute to broadening human rights thinking and practice. The health and human rights perspective offers new avenues for understanding and advancing human well-being in the modern world.

REFERENCES

1. D. E. Beauchamp, "Injury, Community and the Republic," *Law, Medicine and Health Care* 17, no. 1 (Spring 1989): 42–49; Ronald Bayer, Arthur Caplan, and

Norman Daniels, eds., *In Search of Equity: Health Needs and The Health Care System,* Hastings Center Series in Ethics (New York: Plenum Press, 1983).

2. Ronald Dworkin, *Taking Rights Seriously* (Cambridge: Harvard University Press, 1978).

3. Scott Burris, "Rationality Review and the Politics of Public Health," *Villanova Law Review* 34 (1989): 1933; Lawrence Gostin, "The Interconnected Epidemics of Drug Dependency and AIDS," *Harvard Civil Rights-Civil Liberties Law Review* 26, no. 1 (Winter 1991): 113–184.

4. Institute of Medicine, *Future of Public Health* (Washington, DC: National Academy Press, 1988).

5. The International Bank for Reconstruction and Development, *World Development Report 1993: Investing in Health* (New York: Oxford University Press, 1993).

6. World Health Organization, *Constitution,* in *Basic Documents,* 36th ed. (Geneva: WHO, 1986).

7. *Ottawa Charter for Health Promotion,* presented at first International Conference on Health Promotion (Ottawa: November 21, 1986).

8. *Declaration of Alma-Ata,* "Health for All" Series no. 1 (Geneva: WHO, September 12, 1978).

9. WHO, *Constitution* (see note 6).

10. *Universal Declaration of Human Rights,* adopted and proclaimed by UN General Assembly Resolution 217A(III) (December 10, 1948).

11. *United Nations Charter,* signed at San Francisco, June 26, 1945, entered into force on October 24, 1945.

12. WHO, *Constitution* (see note 6).

13. Emily Friedman, "Money Isn't Everything," *Journal of the American Medical Association* 271, 19 (1994): 1535–1538.

14. American Public Health Association, *Control of Communicable Disease in Man,* 15th ed. (Washington, DC: APHA, 1990).

15. International Federation of Red Cross and Red Crescent Societies, *AIDS, Health and Human Rights: A Manual* (chapters 2, 3, and 5 this volume).

16. H. J. Geiger and R. M. Cook-Deegan, "The Role of Physicians in Conflicts and Humanitarian Crises: Case Studies from the Field Missions of Physicians for Human Rights, 1988–1993," *Journal of the American Medical Association* 270 (1993): 616–620.

17. Physicians for Human Rights, *Final Report of UN Commission of Experts.* UN document #S/1994/674 (May 27, 1994).

18. R. F. Mollica and Y. Caspi-Yavin, "Measuring Torture and Torture-Related Syndromes," *Psychological Assessment* 3, 4 (1991): 1–7.

19. Timothy Harding, "Prevention of Torture and Inhuman or Degrading Treatment: Medical Implications of a New European Convention," *Lancet* 1 (1989): 1191–1194.

20. Anne E. Goldfield, Richard F. Mollica, Barbara H. Pesavento et al., "The Physical and Psychological Sequelae of Torture: Symptomatology and Diagnosis," *Journal of the American Medical Association* 259, 18 (1988): 2725–2730.

21. Metin Basoglu, "Prevention of Torture and Care of Survivors: An Integrated Approach," *Journal of the American Medical Association* 270, 5 (1993): 607.

22. *IBRD, World Development Report 1993* (see note 5).

23. D. B. Dutton and S. Levine, "Overview, Methodological Critique, and Reformulation," in J. P. Bunker, D. S. Gomby, and B. H. Kehrer, eds., *Pathways to Health. The Role of Social Factors* (Menlo Park, CA: Henry J. Kaiser Family Foundation), 1989.

24. J. Epp, *Achieving Health for All: A Framework for Health Promotion* (Ottawa: Health and Welfare Canada, 1986).

25. K. C. Schoendorf, C. J. Hogue, J. C. Kleinman, and D. Rowley, "Mortality Among Infants of Black as Compared with White College-Educated Parents," *New England Journal of Medicine* 326 (1992): 1522–1526.

26. S. Gortmaker, A. Must, J. M. Perrin et al., "Social and Economic Consequences of Overweight in Adolescence and Young Adulthood," *New England Journal of Medicine* 329 (1993): 1008–1012.

27. Ichiro Kawachi et al., "Income Inequality and Life Expectancy: Theory, Research and Policy," *Society and Health Working Paper Series* May 1994, no. 94–2 (Boston: The Health Institute, New England Medical Center and Harvard School of Public Health, 1994).

28. *Ottawa Charter* (see note 7).

29. Global AIDS Policy Coalition, "Towards a New Health Strategy for AIDS: A Report of the Global AIDS Policy Coalition" (Cambridge, MA: Global AIDS Policy Coalition, 1993).

30. Said H. Kapiga et al., "Risk Factors for HIV Infection among Women in Dar-es-Salaam, Tanzania" *Journal of Acquired Immune Deficiency Syndromes* 7, 3 (1994): 301–309.

31. Jacques du Guerny and Elisabeth Sjoberg, "Interrelationship Between Gender Relations and the HIV/AIDS Epidemic: Some Considerations for Policies and Programmes," *AIDS* 7 (1993): 1027–1034.

32. Global AIDS Policy Coalition, "Towards a New Health Strategy for AIDS" (see note 29); Jonathan M. Mann, Daniel J. M. Tarantola, and Thomas W. Netter, *AIDS in the World* (Cambridge: Harvard University Press, 1992).

Human Rights: An Introduction 2.

International Federation of Red Cross and Red Crescent Societies and François-Xavier Bagnoud Center for Health and Human Rights

There is no more vibrant, hope-filled, and complex idea alive in the world today than human rights and dignity for all. The struggle to achieve universal support for the idea that "all human beings are born free and equal in rights and dignity" has been long and difficult.[1]

This chapter reviews the main human rights principles and practices from a global perspective. It includes a description of:

- The foundation of human rights
- The system, including key documents and institutions that have been developed to promote and protect these rights
- The main categories of human rights
- The mechanisms for monitoring, responding to, and redressing human rights violations
- The concepts of discrimination and equal opportunity
- The interaction between human rights and health

FOUNDATION OF HUMAN RIGHTS

The basic features of human rights can be summarized in six points.

First, people have rights simply because they are human. As such, they are entitled to lead a human and dignified life. Human rights seek to ensure the conditions that make life as humane as possible and enable people to live together in harmony and mutual respect.

Second, human rights are universal, applying equally to all people around the world, regardless of who they are or where they live. Human rights are sometimes elaborated upon at a regional or national level, taking into account the specific circumstances and cultural backgrounds of various geographic areas. Therefore, in some parts of the world, regional human rights law provides a lesser standard of protection than is required by universal human rights law.

Third, following the principle that "all human beings are born free and equal in rights and dignity," *human rights treat all people as equal.* It does not require that all people should be treated the same or regarded as the same but requires that people should be treated equally and given equal opportunity. Human rights respect variations in human cultures and also recognize that people are different in race, color, sex, language, religion, political or other opinion, national or social origin, property, and birth or other status. Nevertheless, concerning their rights and dignity, people are all the same. Thus, governments are expected to provide equal and effective human rights protection tailored to all, regardless of differences. Additional attention should be provided to meet the specific needs of persons who are in a vulnerable position in society (e.g., women, children, disabled persons, racial minorities, stateless persons, and prisoners).

Fourth, these rights are primarily the rights of individuals. Human rights address directly the relationship between governments and individuals. Every human being has a claim upon his or her society or government, arising as a matter of right, not as a result of privilege or special favor. Societies and governments are obligated to the greatest extent possible to address and satisfy the claims resulting from these rights.

Fifth, human rights encompass the fundamental principles of humanity. Some rights, such as the right to life, freedom from slavery, and freedom from torture, are absolute. They cannot be interfered with under any circumstances (see the box on the following page). However, for the other human rights, international law allows—under exceptional circumstances—interference with their exercise or enjoyment. Interference with the enjoyment or exercise of a human right is justified only if and when a number of stringent criteria are met.

Sixth, the promotion and protection of human rights is not bounded by the frontiers of national states. Human rights hold each nation responsible for respecting and promoting human rights. Individuals, nations, and the community of states have a responsibility to uphold and to be concerned about human rights across borders in any place and at any time.

THE FRAMEWORK: DOCUMENTS AND INSTITUTIONS

The importance of human rights became widely recognized after the atrocities of the Second World War. The promotion of human rights became a core objective of the United Nations (UN) when it was founded in 1945. *Then, in 1948, the UN General Assembly adopted the Universal Declaration of Human Rights,* a document setting out a list of basic rights as "a common standard of achievement for all peoples and all nations." This declaration is the fundamental document of modern human rights (appendix A).[2]

Subsequently, *the UN developed two key international treaties: the International Covenant on Civil and Political Rights and the International*

Covenant on Economic, Social and Cultural Rights. Together with the Universal Declaration, they constitute the International Bill of Human Rights, the framework for modern human rights thinking and practice.[3]

As mentioned above, the UN Charter established general obligations that apply to all of its member states, including respect for human rights and dignity. Under the auspices of the UN, more than twenty multilateral human rights treaties have been formulated. These treaties (such as the two international covenants mentioned above) create legally binding obligations on the nations that have endorsed them. In addition, there are many international declarations, resolutions, and recommendations about international human rights that, although not strictly binding in a legal sense, provide broadly recognized norms.

Respect for and observance of human rights and dignity are not solely the responsibility of the UN, but are also the concern of regional organizations, national governments and nongovernmental organizations. On a regional level, the Council of Europe, the Organization of American States and the Organization of African Unity have formulated their own human rights documents. These regional documents elaborate on and detail some of the rights enshrined in the UN documents, while focusing special attention on the cultural and legal features of the region concerned. In addition, each of these regions has organizations authorized to receive and respond to inquiries and complaints about alleged human rights violations.

HUMAN RIGHTS RESTRICTIONS AND VIOLATIONS
Terminology Is Important

There are situations and times when a state may restrict human rights. Such a *restriction* is not termed a violation when it is justifiable and is done legitimately by the state. In contrast, unjustifiable, illegitimate restrictions are human rights *violations.*

Several other terms are used to mean "restriction of rights," such as *interference, limitation, encroachment, and infringement.*

A word with a specific use is *derogation.* This term is used when human rights are restricted during a crisis. For example, in a public emergency, a situation "threatening the life of a nation," such as civil war or epidemic disease, international human rights law permits a state to take measures "derogating" from certain human rights obligations. However, even in this context the derogation is acceptable only to the extent that the measures are not inconsistent with the state's other obligations under international law.

Nonfulfillment is another term used to describe a state's failure to comply with a human rights obligation. For example, a state that fails to establish a health care system or that establishes a health care system that meets the needs only of specific population groups fails to fulfill its obligations stemming from the right to health.

The ways in which national legislation has recognized human rights differ from country to country. In addition to endorsing international and regional human rights documents, some governments have adopted special human rights charters, included a human rights section in their constitution or have fostered human rights on a national level in other ways. However, national human rights legislation should be consistent with international human rights law.

Predictably, conflicts arise between governments and their citizens and among citizens claiming their rights. First, there is often disagreement about the content of these rights and the priorities among them when these rights are—or appear to be—in conflict. Second, in many countries there have been critical differences regarding the priority given to civil and political rights or to economic, social, and cultural rights. These groups of rights have sometimes been perceived to be in opposition. Third, tension arises among concepts of rights that are widely endorsed in different cultures and nations. This is particularly evident in the emphasis given to a particular right or set of rights and in balancing the interests of individuals and larger communities.

Nongovernmental organizations, operating on local, national, regional, and international levels, play a crucial role in promoting and protecting human rights and dignity. They have been particularly successful in advocating and monitoring human rights compliance and in developing new initiatives to strengthen the human rights system. For example:

- Amnesty International has a prisoner-focused mandate. It monitors human rights violations, writes reports, and lobbies governments at national and international levels.

- The International Federation of Red Cross and Red Crescent Societies can use its ideological basis, the Fundamental Principles and International Humanitarian Law, to defend human rights. The federation has focused its work on the rights to health and to education.

- The International Commission of Jurists is an international organization of jurists primarily concerned with promoting the rules of law and independence of the judiciary, and, more generally, the protection and promotion of human rights.

In summary, human rights have been defined through international, regional, and national mechanisms (universal declaration, covenants, treaties, and constitutions).

- Thus, a wide range of international human rights standards have been advanced, which have the status of international minimum norms.

- Human rights treaties are voluntary agreements among states to respect individual rights and to allow the rights of their own citizens to be considered (to varying degrees) a legitimate concern of others.

- Human rights should not be considered simply as a rigid list of static norms and standards, but rather a discipline that is constantly evolving.

- While human rights norms are established in the first instance at the international level, vitally important human rights documents are developed and work is carried out at regional and national levels by official and nongovernmental agencies and organizations. Together, these represent the dynamic world of modern human rights.

CATEGORIES OF HUMAN RIGHTS

Historically, the rights described in human rights documents are commonly divided into two categories: civil and political rights, and economic, social, and cultural rights.

- *Civil and political rights* include the rights to life, liberty, security of persons, freedom of movement, and the right not to be subjected to torture or to cruel, inhumane, or degrading treatment or punishment, or to arbitrary arrest and detention.
- *Economic, social, and cultural rights* include the rights to the highest attainable standard of health, to work, to social security, to adequate food, to clothing and housing, to education, and to enjoy the benefits of scientific progress and its application.

National obligations differ somewhat for these two categories of rights. Civil and political rights must be guaranteed immediately, whereas governmental obligation for economic, social, and cultural rights involves action to ensure that these rights are progressively realized.

In addition to these two basic recognized categories of rights, a third category of rights, known as *solidarity rights*, should be mentioned. These rights, which have not yet been generally recognized at the international level as legally enforceable, urge solidarity with the less privileged in order to rectify the unequal distribution of resources and to prevent and respond to human suffering. This category of rights includes the rights to development, to peace, to the equal enjoyment of the common heritage of humankind, and to an unpolluted natural environment.

While different categories of human rights can be identified, they are all interdependent and interrelated. The inseparable relationship between the various human rights was clearly stated and repeated at the 1993 UN International Human Rights Conference in Vienna.

MONITORING, RESPONDING TO, AND REDRESSING VIOLATIONS

States must not violate human rights. This also implies that states should be held accountable when individuals are unduly prevented from enjoying and exercising their human rights. As with any other wrongful act for which states bear responsibility, individuals can ask for redress at a local level; for example, by submitting a petition, filing a complaint, or starting legal procedures. In addition, an international human rights protection system ("machinery") has been created with both proactive and response capacities.

It monitors and assesses compliance with human rights, interacts with national systems that protect human rights and provides remedies to persons whose rights have been violated.

Monitoring of human rights engages UN bodies, and regional, national, and community official and nongovernmental agencies and organizations.

There are various levels of possible enforcement to secure compliance with human rights obligations. The need to enforce human rights and remedy their abuses highlights the potential conflict between the universality of these rights and national sovereignty. Viewed in a simple way, human rights restrict the freedom of countries to act "as they please" toward individuals within their borders. *Human rights make states accountable for the way they act, or fail to act.* Seen from this perspective, the sovereignty of states is not absolute. However, the extent to which individuals can enjoy and exercise their human rights depends first on national legislation and national institutions. As a rule, international human rights bodies are only permitted to review complaints (for countries that have accepted the individual complaint procedure) provided that all national remedies have first been exhausted. This is an important barrier and deterrent to many individuals who might wish to file a complaint with an international human rights body.

Under some treaties, states are obliged to submit periodic reports to the treaty monitoring body, detailing the measures the country has taken to promote and protect human rights. These reports are reviewed (along with additional information supplied by NGOs). States that are not in full compliance may then be requested to make certain changes. There is also an individual complaint procedure under the International Covenant on Civil and Political Rights. However, much of the work to protect human rights involves diplomatic persuasion, public exposure, and criticism. Nongovernmental organizations alert the public, stimulate public opinion, and "embarrass" the government by publicizing its human rights violations. Public opinion—and negative publicity in the national and international press—has been a major influence in some countries. Finally, rarely and in the extreme, imposition of trade and diplomatic sanctions or the collective use of armed force could be invoked.

DISCRIMINATION AND EQUAL OPPORTUNITY

The prohibition of discrimination is closely linked to the principle that "all human beings are born free and equal in rights and dignity." All people should be treated equally and given equal opportunity. *In international human rights terms, discrimination is a breach of a human rights obligation.*

The prohibition of discrimination is not restricted to ensuring equal protection before the law, but encompasses all kinds of discrimination, such as that related to housing or employment.

Treating people equally does not necessarily mean that people should be treated the same. *The term* discrimination *is used whenever people are treated adversely, either by treating them differently where they should be treated the same or by treating them the same where they should be treated differently.*

For example, both women and men have the right to vote. Therefore, if women cannot vote while men can vote, this is discriminatory because women would be treated adversely without justification. However, if young children are not allowed to vote while adults can vote, this difference is not discriminatory. Although they are treated differently, it is justified by a realistic and rational assessment of children's intellectual and social maturity. The main feature of discrimination is the irrelevance of the criteria used to differentiate between people.

Throughout history, people have attached negative connotations to others they perceive as inferior. Thus, typical characteristics resulting in discrimination include sex (notably, being a woman), race, ethnicity, religion, social origin, sexual orientation, and disability. Even states that have developed nondiscriminatory laws may not include certain categories of people. As an example, discrimination on grounds of sexual orientation is prohibited in only a few countries. In general, the people who are discriminated against are those who do not have the same characteristics as the dominant groups in the society. In addition, those who discriminate are often, although not always, in a better socioeconomic position, whereas the people discriminated against are usually socially and economically disadvantaged and marginalized. Thus, discrimination frequently reinforces societal inequalities, denying equal opportunities to persons such as women, people of color, immigrants, homosexuals, and disabled persons.

Finally, the groups most discriminated against tend to have diminished capacities to claim their rights or to remedy discrimination when it occurs.

HEALTH: A HUMAN RIGHTS ISSUE

The enjoyment and exercise of all human rights affect the health of individuals. This is especially evident when considering the modern definition of health as "a state of complete physical, mental and social well-being, not merely the absence of disease or infirmity."[4]

The right to health is expressed in the International Bill of Human Rights as "the right to the highest attainable standard of physical and mental health."[5] This right imposes a duty upon states to promote and protect the health of individuals and the community, including a responsibility to promote and protect health and ensure quality health care.

> The monitoring of human rights is vital, and enforcement is complex. Nations that routinely violate rights may be least likely to allow open reporting about the state of rights, while citizens of nations with full access to legal and other remedies to seek redress may be able to complain more openly about injustices perpetrated by their governments.

   States are required to provide resources for health promotion and disease prevention along with an adequate health care system. Health policy should be directed to the needs of all, avoiding any form of discrimination.

   In addition, public health is understood to represent such an important public interest that its protection and promotion can be a permissible reason for the restriction of some human rights. Yet restriction of human rights is usually a last resort. Using public health as a reason to restrict human rights requires great care; a list of stringent criteria needs to be met before the restriction can be considered just. For example, the restriction must be prescribed by law and applied in a nondiscriminatory manner and only when no less intrusive means are available to protect the public health. In order to assess if restricting a human right for reasons of public health is "necessary" and "proportional," it is essential that people experienced in human rights law and public health work closely together.

REFERENCES

   1. Article 1, *Universal Declaration of Human Rights* (1948).
   2. Preamble, *Universal Declaration of Human Rights*.
   3. *The International Bill of Human Rights* also includes the first Optional Protocol to the *International Covenant on Civil and Political Rights*.
   4. Preamble to the Constitution of the World Health Organization (WHO).
   5. See Appendix B, article 12, of the *International Covenant on Economic, Social and Cultural Rights*.

Public Health: An Introduction   3.

International Federation of Red Cross and
Red Crescent Societies and François-Xavier Bagnoud
Center for Health and Human Rights

Like human rights, public health involves a series of core concepts and a language to describe these central ideas and practices.

THE CONCEPT OF "PUBLIC HEALTH"

For many people, the history of public health is the history of infectious disease control, peopled with illustrious names like Pasteur, Jenner, and Koch. The term "public health" is exemplified by the eradication of small-pox, the "sanitary revolution" that established and applied the principles of modern hygiene, and dramatic progress made against historical scourges like tetanus, typhoid, poliomyelitis, diphtheria, and tuberculosis. Yet public health goes far beyond traditional infectious disease control.

> *Public Health* can be defined as "what we as a society do collectively to ensure the conditions in which people can be healthy" (Institute of Medicine, 1988, USA). *Each part of this definition is important.*

First, it is clear that public health deals with *society*: groups of people and actions affecting many people. For example, the addition of fluoride to water supplies in order to prevent childhood dental caries is a broad public health measure, affecting everyone who drinks the water. The procedure is designed to achieve a collective good (less tooth decay, and better dental health). This action will not guarantee every individual freedom from dental caries, but it will reduce the overall amount of caries occurring in the population. Public health actions seek to promote the health of the community.

Next, it is essential to identify the conditions required for people to be healthy. First, however, the definition of "health" needs to be recalled.

> The World Health Organization has defined "health" as "a state of complete physical, mental, and social well-being, not merely the absence of disease or infirmity."

The modern view of health is broad. It goes beyond individual diseases or viruses and includes all of the aspects of life that can affect our physical, mental, or social well-being.

Clearly, there are many underlying conditions that can influence a person's well-being. Such conditions include:

- access to medical services
- the physical environment
- the biological environment
- the social environment

Of these, the major determinant of population health status is societal.

In summary, public health works to ensure that the underlying conditions needed for physical, mental, or social well-being are provided to all people in society.

HEALTH PROMOTION AND DISEASE PREVENTION

Promoting health (physical, mental, and social well-being) involves three levels of prevention.

- *Primary prevention is "pure" prevention, or preventing the health problem from occurring at all.* Examples include: preventing lung cancer through avoidance of tobacco smoking; preventing polio by vaccinating children with a polio vaccine; or preventing rickets by ensuring an adequate intake of vitamin D. This is clearly the ideal (and usually the most cost-effective) approach. While primary prevention can be accomplished in several ways, education and active participation of people are essential. Primary prevention is often referred to as health promotion, the process of "enabling people to increase control over, and to improve their health."[1]

- In many cases, despite efforts at primary prevention, a health condition occurs (for example, high blood pressure). *Secondary prevention involves prompt detection and successful management or treatment of the health condition so as to avoid actual damage to the person's health.* For example, early detection and treatment of high blood pressure can prevent the strokes or kidney damage which result from uncontrolled hypertension.

- Finally, if primary prevention and secondary prevention have both failed or are not possible, and a person's health has already been damaged, *tertiary prevention seeks to limit the impairment, increase the quality of life and prolong life.* Examples include: providing emergency care for victims of automobile crashes; rehabilitative services to help maximize activity and independence after a stroke or heart attack; or hospice care to ensure a higher quality of life for terminally ill people.

In general, in order to achieve its goals, modern public health efforts tend to focus on primary prevention and, to a lesser extent, on secondary or tertiary prevention approaches.

PUBLIC HEALTH IN PRACTICE

How is public health work—concerned with "collective" action and the health of populations—carried out? Its specific domain is public, at the community, national, or global level. It therefore relies upon measures directed to small or large groups of people, rather than dealing separately with each individual. For all these reasons, a substantial portion of public health work is carried out by governmental or official agencies. However, in some countries, an important amount of public health work is provided by religious and other nongovernmental institutions.

The work of public health agencies can be summarized under three headings: *assessment, policy development,* and the *assurance of services.*

- *Assessment* means collecting and analyzing data in order to identify and understand the major health problems facing a community.
- *Policy development* establishes goals, sets priorities, and develops strategies to address health problems.
- *Assurance of services* involves the design, implementation, and evaluation of programs to address priority health problems in the community.

To assess health status, develop policy, and assure services, public health needs to collect information about populations. The science of epidemiology studies the distribution and determinants of health-related states and events in populations, with the goal of providing critical information for control of health problems.

For example, epidemiological study discovered the relationship between cigarette smoking and lung cancer, between inadequate vitamin A intake and acute respiratory disease in children, and between certain behaviors (smoking, sedentary living and diet) and heart disease and between bottle feeding and infant mortality in developing countries. The power of epidemiological analysis was also demonstrated in the HIV/AIDS epidemic. Several years before the virus of AIDS (HIV) was discovered, epidemiologists identified the behaviors ("risk factors") that spread the virus from person to person. Based on this information, health officials were able to formulate rational prevention strategies and programs.

In public health, knowledge serves a purpose: the promotion of health and the prevention of disease. Public health is an applied activity.

PUBLIC HEALTH AND HUMAN BEHAVIOR

While the history of public health was closely related to the control of infectious disease epidemics, modern public health is challenged mainly by problems resulting from human behavior, both individual and collective. *The major causes of death in the modern world involve to a substantial extent human behavior.* For example, many cancers are related to personal habits (tobacco, diet) or occupation. Heart disease is closely related to behaviors (diet, exercise, smoking, or stress). Even more obviously, sexually transmitted diseases (including HIV/AIDS), unwanted pregnancies, and sexual violence are health problems resulting from behavior. Environmental pollution is also largely a product of individual and collective behaviors (economic activities, use of automobiles, or chemical waste disposal).

PUBLIC HEALTH: FROM "ACCIDENTS" TO "INJURY CONTROL"

The history of the public health response to "accidents" provides a good picture of the evolution and power of public health principles and practice.

Until fairly recently, such events as automobile accidents, household fires, or drownings were simply considered "accidents." In other words, they were seen as unpredictable events occurring without warning. No one knew how common such accidents really were.

Then, epidemiological studies discovered two key facts: first, accidents are fairly predictable and are not really random events. For this reason, the name was changed from *accidents* (implying unpredictability) to *injuries* (implying an ability to predict, prevent, and control the problem). Second, injuries were found to be a major cause of hospitalization, disability and death in industrialized and developing countries.

Once the problem of injuries was recognized and scientifically studied, specific prevention interventions could be rationally designed, implemented, and evaluated. For example, burns could be prevented by changes in stove location or design, automobile seat belts could protect passengers from injury, and childproof caps on bottles of medication and household chemicals could prevent poisoning of children. These strategies have proven their effectiveness.

The basic strategies of injury prevention can be illustrated using the example of motor vehicle injuries. The ultimate and optimal goal (primary prevention) is to prevent automobile crashes in the first place. One approach is to modify human behavior, either through information and education (for example, education on safe driving) or through laws or other requirements (for example, severe penalties for speeding or driving while intoxicated). Another approach is to modify the environment (for example, creating safer roads with improved lighting, traffic signals, and separation of traffic flow).

When primary prevention fails, public health efforts can also help reduce the severity of the injury which will occur to automobile occupants in a crash (e.g., by requiring the use of seat belts). Finally, when a person is injured in an automobile crash, emergency medical services (tertiary prevention) may be lifesaving.

Finally, as more research was conducted on injuries, the stigmatizing, victim-blaming concept of an "accident-prone" personality was discredited. Rather than blaming the person, public health efforts to prevent automobile injuries shifted to the risk environment and the role of poverty and other societal conditions in creating the conditions in which accidents were more frequent.

In summary, due to public health studies, injuries (a major cause of death among young people worldwide) changed from being an invisible issue considered a matter of "chance" or "fate" to an important public health responsibility.

Perhaps because human behavior is the most complex challenge imaginable, public health has often neglected the behavioral dimension of health. For example, traditional public health programs designed to control sexually transmitted disease tended to focus on diagnosis and treatment, rather than on sexual behavior itself. Similarly, family planning programs emphasized making a range of safe and acceptable contraceptive options available (an extremely worthy objective), yet they also generally avoided discussions of sexuality.

Since efforts to modify human behavior are complex and difficult, many prefer to seek an environmental, technical, or engineering solution to public health problems. However, the major lesson from public health experience is that a combined strategy, using multiple approaches, generally works better than any single intervention. Indeed, precise identification of which factor, or combination of interventions, made the critical difference for improving health in a community is frequently difficult to determine.

Finally, while recognizing a legacy of neglect of human behavior in traditional public health, modern public health is working to correct this situation by emphasizing the critical importance of behavior for health.

In 1978, the International Conference on Primary Health Care, held in Alma-Ata, declared that primary health care (PHC) is the key to attaining the goal of health for all by the year 2000.

Primary health care is based on practical, scientifically sound, and socially acceptable methods and technology. It should be made universally accessible to individuals and families in their community through their full participation and at an affordable cost on a continuing basis. Primary health care takes place at the first contact between individuals and the national health system, as close as possible to where people live and work. It is the first element in a continuing health care process and forms an integral part of the country's health system.

Initially, the Declaration of Alma-Ata defined eight elements of PHC. Not all these elements are present in every PHC program. They should be encouraged in every community striving toward health for all. These elements are:

- education concerning prevailing health problems and the methods of preventing and controlling them
- promotion of food supply and proper nutrition
- an adequate supply of safe water and basic sanitation
- maternal and child health care, including family planning
- immunization against major infectious diseases
- prevention and control of locally endemic diseases
- appropriate treatment of common diseases and injuries
- provision of essential drugs

Additional elements have been included since 1978:

- mental health and dental health
- accident prevention

PUBLIC HEALTH: IN SOCIETY

Public health seeks to influence the societal conditions in which people can be healthy. This work necessarily leads far beyond ensuring access to medical care. It includes efforts to ensure societal opportunities (such as education), a healthful environment (including housing, nutrition, and workplace safety) and prevention of threats to mental or social well-being (such as violence or persecution).

It should be clear, therefore, that discussions of public health must always consider the societal context, including its economic and political dimensions. Increasing attention is now being paid to community responsibility and participation in ensuring the conditions in which people can be healthy. The historic International Conference at Alma-Ata in 1978 established the basis for primary health care (see box on p. 33). Primary health care, a concept applicable to all communities and nations, requires that people become directly involved, as active participants, in promoting their health and preventing disease. Thus, public attitudes and the viewpoint of political leaders are critical for public health. The Declaration of Alma-Ata, urging all countries to develop a system of primary health care, calls for local participation, participatory decision-making and constant involvement of community-based organizations in all health matters.

Economic conditions clearly constrain the potential for primary, secondary, and tertiary prevention. The ability of countries to promote health and prevent disease will be strongly influenced by societal resources, societal priorities, and commitment to health. Unfortunately, even within the resources devoted to health, many countries still spend too much on treatment of disease (tertiary prevention), often including expensive, high-technology interventions, rather than focusing on primary prevention for all the people.

In addition, while many studies have shown that socioeconomic status is a powerful determinant and predictor of health status, poverty is only part of an explanation for ill health, disability, and premature death. *There is increasing evidence that the level of respect for human rights and dignity independently and decisively influences health status.*

In summary, modern public health considers health in its broadest dimensions. Starting with a history of epidemic control, the modern public health movement is increasingly engaged in efforts to transform society in order to ensure the conditions in which people—all people—can be healthy.

The goals of public health, and the specific means it employs to reach these goals, inevitably bring public health into contact with human rights. The next section explores the several dimensions of this necessary and fundamental dialogue between public health and human rights.

REFERENCE

1. Ottawa Charter for Health Promotion, 1986.

PART II

The Impact of Health Policies and Programs on Human Rights

Discussions about human rights in the context of public health have nearly always been sparked by a collision in which public health advocates undertake action in a manner that seems to threaten or violate human rights, and human rights advocates respond. Individuals working in health and in human rights have inherited a tradition of conflictual relations, where each has believed that it is on the opposing sides and that the other will infringe upon its domain. It is often assumed, for example, that human rights will interfere with good public health work, or that public health will unnecessarily and wantonly trample upon human rights. Perhaps for this reason human rights have rarely been explicitly considered in the design and implementation of public health policies and programs.

When the public's health is threatened, crucial issues of safety and security come to the fore. Accordingly, from the outset, human rights law has recognized public health protection as a societal good that can, under certain limited circumstances, be invoked by governmental authorities to legitimately restrict some human rights. In this respect, public health is representative of a category of issues, such as national security and public emergency, where restrictions on the rights of individuals and population groups are permissible. Thus, for example, the International Covenant on Civil and Political Rights specifically mentions public health as a valid justification for restricting such rights as freedom of movement and expression, and rights to assembly and association.

It became evident to public health workers early in the HIV/AIDS pandemic that when the human rights of people infected with HIV/AIDS with AIDS were violated, public health goals were compromised. Likewise, as the severity and sheer number of violations committed by governments in the name of protecting the public from HIV/AIDS became more apparent, human rights advocates increasingly recognized the need to question restrictions justified as necessary for public health. The first chapter, by George Annas on AIDS and tuberculosis control, uses case examples drawn from the United States and Cuba to demonstrate the very real impacts that health policies and programs can have on human rights. While a number of contemporary health issues could have been used to illustrate this point, governmental actions justified as necessary for the public's health in the context of both TB and HIV/AIDS have most clearly challenged ideas and approaches to disease control and, in turn, to what constitutes a legitimate restriction on rights.

The advent of HIV/AIDS and the health and human rights challenges it helped uncover have highlighted the need for processes and methods that ensure careful attention to human rights in the design and implementation of public health policies and programs. The other two chapters in this section, by the International Federation of Red Cross and Red Crescent Societies and the François-Xavier Bagnoud Center, and Lawrence Gostin and Jonathan Mann, are critical efforts to bridge public health and human rights. Both chapters reflect the same goal and propose methods to negotiate (rather than dictate from either perspective) an optimal balance between accomplishment of public health objectives and respecting (and not violating) human rights. For practical purposes, both start from a simple premise: that we consider all public health policies, programs, and practices to be violative of human rights until proven otherwise. This is a challenge to public health to examine, proactively, the human rights burdens that may often inadvertently result from well-intended public health measures, and to work to eliminate or reduce them. Likewise, this is a challenge to human rights advocates to assume greater responsibility for helping to prevent violations before they occur, and not just to respond to them after they occur.

There is a need for genuine collaboration and open communication between the public health community and the human rights community. This is a substantial challenge, and one that requires careful attention to often unspoken assumptions and differences in attitude and language; it truly requires a transdisciplinary effort. Practical experience with negotiating optimal dual achievements is needed, so that a process for working through even apparently unresolvable areas of conflict can be developed. Ultimately, the common goal of human well-being—through both public health and human rights strategies—will lead us forward.

The Impact of Health Policies 4.
on Human Rights:
AIDS and TB Control

George J. Annas

AIDS and TB (tuberculosis) have become the two primary examples that critics of a public health vision that takes human rights seriously have used to argue that putting rights first promotes contagion and death.[1] This view, however, finds little support in fact, and contemporary public health officials mostly have concluded that taking human rights seriously is a necessary component of an effective public health strategy.

Ideas govern actions in both private and public realms, and language molds ideas. This is easy to see in the global context of the cold war, where a U.S. policy based on containment and deterrence led to the development of a vast nuclear weapons arsenal, an unsustainable arms race, and the ultimate destabilization of many of the world's countries. Not only did U.S. nuclear policy spawn its own peculiar strategies (such as mutually assured destruction), it also created new phrases to manage its discourse, such as "windows of vulnerability," "collateral damage," "surgical strikes," and "crisis management," all used to make nuclear war seem clean and controllable.[2] Metaphors matter; they make all the difference whether, in adopting a global AIDS strategy, nations adopt the war-containment or escalation discourse (the "war on AIDS" strategy), in which control is viewed as an end in itself and the infected body becomes a battlefield, or the human rights discourse, in which our collective futures and the values of human flourishing and the right to humane treatment are paramount.

In this chapter I examine the destructiveness of a militarized HIV containment strategy as pursued at a U.S. military base in Cuba, and a human-rights-based public health strategy, currently being pursued in response to the TB epidemic in the United States. The purpose is to expose the power of discourse models to affect the choices public health officials make, and how these choices affect both the lives of real people and the global course of the AIDS and TB epidemics, and thus all of our futures.

HAITIAN REFUGEES AT GUANTÁNAMO

After the military overthrow of President Jean-Bertrand Aristide in September 1991, human rights violations by the Haitian military, including murder, torture, and arbitrary arrest, prompted approximately 40,000 Haitians to flee their country. Approximately 10,500 such refugees were found to have a "credible fear" of return and have been granted admission into the United States; about 25,000 others were returned to Haiti. In the fall of 1991 the U.S. Immigration and Naturalization Service began testing "screened in" refugees for HIV, and in February 1992 those testing positive were interviewed and required to meet a higher standard to establish that they had a "well-founded fear" of persecution. The Immigration and Naturalization Service denied requests by the refugees' attorneys to be present at these interviews.

Haitians interdicted on the high seas were taken to the U.S. naval base at Guantánamo Bay for processing. "Screened out" refugees are not entitled to appeal or to legal representation under the Constitution. But when "screened in," the Haitians' fundamental legal and human rights status was changed vis-à-vis the United States government. Those HIV-positive refugees who successfully completed the interview were housed at a separate facility at Guantánamo Bay, Camp Bulkeley. In a lawsuit brought on behalf of the HIV detainees, Judge Sterling Johnson Jr. of the U.S. District Court described this camp as follows when it housed approximately two hundred HIV-positive Haitian refugees:

> They live in camps surrounded by razor barbed wire. They tie plastic garbage bags to the sides of the building to keep the rain out. They sleep on cots and hang sheets to create some semblance of privacy. They are guarded by the military and are not permitted to leave the camp, except under military escort. The Haitian detainees have been subjected to pre-dawn military sweeps as they sleep by as many as 400 soldiers dressed in full riot gear. They are confined like prisoners and are subject to detention in the brig without hearing for camp rule infractions.[3]

Although the military physicians were capable of providing general medical care to the Haitian detainees at Guantánamo, the facilities were inadequate to provide medical care to detainees with HIV infection and AIDS. The physicians themselves first raised this issue in May 1992, requesting that specific HIV-positive patients be evacuated to the United States because adequate medical care could not be provided for them at Guantánamo. Some of these requests were denied by the Immigration and Naturalization Service. At the trial, the United States conceded that the medical facilities at Guantánamo were insufficient to treat patients with AIDS "under the medical care standard applicable within the United States itself." Judge

Johnson himself described what the Immigration and Naturalization Service euphemistically called a humanitarian camp as "nothing more than an HIV prison camp."

The judge was asked to find that the medical conditions in the camp violated the U.S. constitutional due process requirement that the government provide its prisoners with adequate medical care and safe conditions—an issue that had not been raised in previous cases involving the Haitian refugees. Although American citizens still have no explicit right to health care, since 1976 American prisoners have been entitled to protection under the Eighth Amendment of the U.S. Constitution (which forbids cruel and unusual punishment) from "deliberate indifference to serious medical needs."[4] Judge Johnson found that "deliberate indifference" included "denial or delay of detainees' access to medical care, interfering with treatment once prescribed, [and] lack of response to detainees' medical needs."

Closely related to the issue of adequate medical care was the prospect of detaining the HIV-positive Haitians at Guantánamo indefinitely. Judge Johnson found that the detention was not due to any act committed by the Haitians, but to government actions. For example, 115 Haitians who had met the well-founded-fear standard had been detained for almost two years, with no indication of when, if ever, they would be released (although they had been told that they could be there for ten to twenty years or until a cure for AIDS was found). At the time of the judge's final decision in June 1993, there were 158 refugees in the camp: 143 HIV-positive adults, 2 HIV-negative adults, and 13 children who had not been tested. The court concluded, in terms that invoke universal human rights:

> [The] detained Haitians are neither criminals nor national security risks. Some are pregnant women and others are children. Simply put, they are merely the unfortunate victims of a fatal disease. . . . Where detention no longer serves a legitimate purpose, the detainees must be released. The Haitian camp at Guantánamo is the only known refugee camp in the world composed entirely of HIV positive refugees. The Haitians' plight is a tragedy of immense proportion and their continued detainment is totally unacceptable to this Court.[5]

The judge ruled that the attorney general had kept the Haitians in detention "solely because they are Haitian and have tested HIV-positive." Federal regulations do not permit medical status and HIV infection to be used as criteria for continued detention, and Congress had not provided for mandatory exclusion of persons with HIV infection from either "parole [the means by which interdicted aliens who are screened in are brought to the United States in order to pursue their asylum claims] or the grant of asylum in the United States." Under these circumstances, the judge concluded, further imprisonment of the HIV-positive Haitians "serves no purpose other than to punish them for being sick."

Judge Johnson permanently enjoined the processing of Haitians with "well-founded fear"; held unlawful the attorney general's denial of parole to the screened-in Haitians; and ordered that the screened-in HIV-positive Haitians "be immediately released (to anywhere but Haiti) from . . . detention." The Clinton administration announced it would comply with the court's order and the 158 Haitians held at Camp Bulkeley were almost immediately released and entered the United States.[5] Once the refugees were in the U.S., a number of organizations, including the New York's Haitian Women's Project and the Haitian Centers Council, helped the refugees make contact with friends and relatives, and obtained housing and Medicaid for them. About 60 percent of the HIV-positive refugees wound up in New York, and most of the rest in Miami and Boston.[6] New York, which invited the HIV-positive Haitians to live there, is also the primary site of the resurgence of multi-drug-resistant tuberculosis.[7]

TUBERCULOSIS CONTROL

In their history of tuberculosis, *The White Plague,* Renée and Jean Dubos note that the first national movement to control tuberculosis in the United States came from the Medico-Legal Society of the City of New York, a group of lawyers, scientists, and physicians devoted to solving social problems.[8] At a meeting in 1900 to organize an American congress on tuberculosis, the group drafted legislation designed to prevent the spread of the disease. Even though almost every state in the United States eventually passed tuberculosis control laws, it was not the passage of legislation, or even the development of effective treatment, that led to the decline of tuberculosis in the United States, but improvement in living conditions. The decline in the disease was so impressive that by the 1980s predictions were made that tuberculosis would soon be eradicated in the United States. With the increasing incidence of tuberculosis and the rise of multi-drug-resistant tuberculosis, especially among those with HIV infection, that optimism has disappeared.[9]

The inherent governmental power to act to protect the public's health and safety is referred to as the police power, and in the United States it resides in the individual states. In most of the rest of the world this power resides at the national level. This is why public health issues have almost always been dealt with at the state level in the United States, with state departments of public health taking the lead. And the states' powers are broad. When, for example, the states' power to permit local communities to require vaccination against smallpox was challenged at the beginning of the century, the U.S. Supreme Court ruled in *Jacobson v. Massachusetts* that "the safety and the health of the people of Massachusetts are, in the first instance, for the Commonwealth to guard and protect. They are matters that do not ordinarily concern the national government." Using military metaphors, the Court ruled as a general matter that "upon the principle of self-defense, of paramount necessity, a community has the right to protect itself against an epidemic of disease which threatens the safety of its members."[10] Actions designed to contain an epidemic will be upheld as constitutional as long as they are not arbitrary or unreasonable and are rationally related to the goal of protecting the public's health. A responsible public health approach to infectious epidemics requires surveillance, reporting, intervention, and the education of health professionals. All four must be coordinated or their efficacy will drastically decrease. But an effective public health strategy does not require a military response or the trampling of basic human rights.

States have the legal authority to identify infectious diseases through screening programs, and they have the legal authority to require physicians and others to report the names of persons with infectious diseases to the state. Screening and reporting are legitimate public health methods designed to protect the health and safety of citizens. Steps must, of course, be taken to protect the confidentiality of medical records and reports so that only public health officials with a legitimate need to know the identity of individual patients (such as officials responsible for monitoring or contact tracing) have access to their names.[11] More difficult human rights questions are raised by treatment of disease. Although involuntary confinement should be used only as a last resort, its availability as a legal option merits discussion because it illustrates both the broad scope of the states' public health powers, and ways to restrain it.

QUARANTINE

Many court cases, including *Jacobson*, provide legal authority for states to enact and enforce statutes that permit the confinement (at home, in a hospital room, or at a special facility or residence) of a patient with active tuberculosis who is a danger to others. If a state wishes to deprive such patients of their liberty on the grounds that they are a danger to others, however, the patients are now entitled to considerably more due process than they would have had at the beginning of the century.

The closest legal analogy is provided by court cases that have reviewed the constitutionality of state statutes permitting the involuntary commitment of mental patients on the basis that they have a disease that causes them to be dangerous. The Supreme Court has held, for example, that illness alone is an insufficient justification for confinement, if the patient is "dangerous to no one and can live safely in freedom."[12] Nor is "mere public intolerance or animosity" sufficient "constitutionally [to] justify the deprivation of a person's physical liberty." The Court has repeatedly held that "civil commitment for any purpose constitutes a significant deprivation of liberty that requires due process protection." For example, the minimal standard of proof that the state must meet to commit a person involuntarily to a facility is that there is "clear and convincing evidence" of his or her dangerousness (this is less stringent than the criminal standard "beyond a reasonable doubt," but more so than the usual civil standard of "preponderance of the evidence").[13]

The following due process rights, outlined by a West Virginia court in a case that involved the involuntary commitment of a patient with tuberculosis for treatment, are likely to be found constitutionally required by most U.S. courts (and should be required in all cases):

> (1) an adequate written notice detailing the grounds and underlying facts on which commitment is sought; (2) the right to counsel and, if indigent, the right to appointed counsel; (3) the right to be present, to cross-examine, to confront and to present witnesses; (4) the standard of proof by clear, cogent and convincing evidence; and (5) the right to a verbatim transcript of the proceedings for purposes of appeal.[14]

Although these safeguards may seem impressive, in fact the only issues likely to concern a judge in a tuberculosis (or HIV) commitment proceeding are two factual ones: does the person have active tuberculosis, and does the person present a danger of spreading it to others? Since it is unlikely that any case will be brought by public health officials when the diagnosis is in doubt, the primary issues will be the danger the patient presents to others and the existence of less restrictive alternatives to confinement that might protect the public equally well.

Under these circumstances, the burden of involuntary confinement falls most heavily on the homeless and those who live in crowded, inadequate housing, because they have no place to "confine themselves" during treatment for active tuberculosis. Since the rationale for involuntary commitment is danger to others based on the contagiousness of the patient's disease, under existing state statutes (written before multi-drug-resistant tuberculosis was identified as dangerous to the public) patients have a right to be released when their tuberculosis is no longer communicable and they are therefore no longer a danger to others.

The possibility of acquiring and spreading multi-drug-resistant tuberculosis poses a particularly difficult problem. Even though not currently a danger to others, the patient whose tuberculosis is inactive but not yet cured might be a danger in the future if a treatment regimen that will ultimately cure the patient is not followed and if, instead, the patient takes drugs in such a way as to transform his or her tuberculosis into a multi-drug-resistant variety, which later becomes active and communicable. Because clear and convincing evidence is required to prove dangerousness, the fact that a person might be a risk to others in the future is insufficient reason alone, under current laws, for confinement until cure.

DIRECTLY OBSERVED THERAPY

Current discussion is properly focused not on quarantine, but on less intrusive interventions such as routine and universal directly observed therapy. This mode of treatment delivery is now considered the standard of care by many commentators, but controversy remains. Although the data are incomplete, it appears that in the United States more than 80 percent of all tuberculosis patients between 1976 and 1990 completed twelve continuous months of drug therapy.[15] The completion figure is much lower for New York, but it is still a majority. There is an understandable egalitarian desire to try to treat everyone the same by subjecting everyone to directly observed therapy. There is, however, insufficient justification for requiring this annoying and inconvenient mode of treatment for those patients who pose virtually no risk of not taking their tuberculosis medications and thus pose no public health risk.

This is not a matter of conflict between public health and civil rights. It is a matter of common sense. As the Duboses rightly observed, measures to prevent the spread of tuberculosis generally do not require legal compulsion because they "have acquired the compelling strength of common sense." Requiring all persons to undergo directly observed therapy because it is necessary for some is wasteful, inefficient, and gratuitously annoying, as well as undercutting legitimate concern to individualize treatment and use the least restrictive and intrusive public health interventions. Moreover, in many if not most cases, reasonable discharge planning (including housing for the homeless) and counseling will greatly improve voluntary compliance. Of course, it can be difficult to accurately predict compliance for some patients, and individualized case management strategies and monitoring will be necessary.

Directly observed therapy is, of course, clearly preferable to quarantine, and efforts to deliver therapy on an outpatient basis should be diligently and imaginatively tried before involuntary confinement is contemplated. Both of these legal interventions, however, concentrate on the victims of societal neglect, rather than on the real sources of the new tuberculosis epidemic. This is understandable, because poverty is a much more difficult problem to address, but the evidence from the history of tuberculosis is that controlling tuberculosis depends much more on the general standard of living than on specific medical or legal interventions.

AIDS AND HUMAN RIGHTS

The reactions of both individuals and governments to people with HIV infection and AIDS have not, as one would expect in a "war," always been benign, and challenging discriminatory actions in court has become almost commonplace in the United States. Such challenges have been largely successful and helped prod the U.S. Congress to pass the Americans with Disabilities Act, which applies to virtually all diseases and handicaps. The AIDS epidemic has also prompted renewed interest in human rights with regard to health, especially in the international arena. There has, for example, been wide support in the public health community for unrestricted international travel by people with AIDS (or HIV infection), and discrimination on the basis of disease has been denounced. This was symbolized by the decision to move the 1992 World AIDS Conference out of the United States to protest U.S. immigration policy toward people with HIV infection.

Judge Johnson was correct in saying that Guantánamo had the only refugee prison camp exclusively for HIV-positive persons, but he had only to look more closely at Cuba itself to find the world's only facility where HIV-positive citizens are placed in mandatory quarantine. Located in a suburb of Havana, Cuba's main quarantine facility is largely fenced in and is composed of barracks housing hundreds of people.[16] Since inspectors from other nations have not been permitted to report on conditions in the quarantine facility, it is difficult to know how much better or worse they are than those at Guantánamo. We do know, however, that the liberty of those living there is extremely restricted and that they are separated from their families.[17] Unlike the United States, however, Cuba has no constitution guaranteeing individual rights and no independent court system to which the inmates in the Cuban facility can appeal for release.

As the United States and other countries become more and more concerned with immigration problems, it is likely that more draconian steps will be taken to restrict immigration worldwide. In the United States, for example, Congress voted in 1993 to ban immigration by those infected with HIV, and this bill was signed into law by President Clinton. The justification used was twofold: there is the cost of caring for those with HIV infection and AIDS, and there is the risk of spreading HIV to others. Both are legitimate areas of concern. But here the military metaphor of containment and defense counsels one action (barring entry) while the future-oriented human rights metaphor counsels another (building a world community).

The cost of caring for immigrants with HIV infection should be viewed in the same manner as the cost of caring for patients with any other expensive illness (including, in appropriate circumstances, requiring people to demonstrate sufficient ability to pay for their care). Likewise, the risk of spreading infection is a legitimate public health concern—one that justifies, for example, confining patients with active tuberculosis who refuse to cooperate with treatment and voluntary measures of infection control. But to avoid violations of human rights, the risk of a person's spreading the disease in question must be real, and its assessment must not be based primarily on irrational fear or prejudice.

Discrimination based solely on disease status has not yet received sufficient attention as a human rights violation. When governments sponsor such discrimination, the courts can help by speaking clearly and strongly in support of fundamental human rights. When discrimination also adversely affects medical care, physicians and lawyers should work together to defend and promote the interests of the sick, both in their own countries and internationally.[18] Using military metaphors in medicine and public health is ultimately destructive. Future-oriented views of a flourishing international community based on human rights provides a much more constructive model and the AIDS epidemic is helping the law and all of us to move, albeit painfully slowly, beyond the military metaphor and toward a sustainable international community.

REFERENCES

1. This chapter is adapted from G. J. Annas, "Control of Tuberculosis: The Law and the Public's Health," *New England Journal of Medicine* 328 (1998) 585–588, and G. J. Annas, "Detention of HIV-Positive Haitians at Guantánamo: Human Rights and Medical Care," *New England Journal of Medicine* 329 (1993): 589–592.

2. B. S. Klein, *Strategic Discourse and its Alternatives* (New York: Center on Violence and Human Survival, John Jay College of Criminal Justice, City University of New York, 1992).

3. *Haitian Centers Council v. Sale,* 823 F. Supp. 1028 (E.D.N.Y. 1993).

4. *Estelle v. Gamble,* 429 U.S. 97 (1976).

5. 823 F. Supp. 1028 (see note 3).

6. T. L. Friedman, "U.S. to Release 158 Haitian Detainees," *New York Times,* June 10, 1993, p. A12.

7. Personal communication with Dr. Marie Pierre-Louis of the Haitian Centers Council (Aug. 5, 1997). A number of these refugees still have a precarious legal status, according to Betty Williams, chair of the Quaker Friends HIV Residence. About half have received asylum. Shortly after my first account of the conditions at Guantánamo was published in 1993, Paul Farmer replied that I had under-estimated the lack of treatment there. See Paul Farmer, *The Uses of Haiti* (Monroe, ME: Common Courage Press, 1994), p. 295. Since I had no firsthand knowledge, but relied on court documents, he may well be correct, and I offer no excuses for U.S. actions regarding the HIV-positive refugees.

8. Renée Dubos and Jean Dubos, *The White Plague: Tuberculosis, Man, and Society* (Boston: Little, Brown, 1952).

9. B. R. Bloom, C. J. L. Murray, "Tuberculosis: Commentary on a Reemergent Killer," *Science* 257 (1992): 1055–1064; see also, WHO Global Surveillance Monitoring Project, "Assessment of Worldwide Tuberculosis Control," *Lancet* 350 (1997): 624–629.

10. *Jacobson v. Massachusetts,* 197 U.S. 11 (1904).

11. *Whalen v. Roe,* 429 U.S. 589 (1977).

12. *O'Connor v. Donaldson,* 422 U.S. 563 (1975).

13. *Addington v. Texas,* 441 U.S. 418 (1979).

14. *Greene v. Edwards,* 263 S. E.2d 661 (W.Va. 1980).

15. Bloom (see note 9).

16. R. Bayer and C. Healton, "Controlling AIDS in Cuba: The Logic of Quarantine," *New England Journal of Medicine* 320 (1989): 1022–1024; and see C. Burr, "Assessing Cuba's Approach to Contain AIDS and HIV, *Lancet* 350 (1997): 647 ("Based on the statistics [Cuba's AIDS policy] is the most successful AIDS program in the world." Nonetheless, the current "boom in sex tourism" has turned past success into a "desperate situation").

17. R. Bayer, "End the Quarantine at Guantánamo," *Washington Post,* January 12, 1993, p. A17.

18. M. A. Grodin, G. J. Annas, and L. H. Glantz, "Medicine and Human Rights: A Proposal for International Action," *Hastings Center Report* 23, 4 (1993): 4–12; and J. M. Mann, "We Are All Berliners: Notes from the Ninth International Conference on AIDS," *American Journal of Public Health* 83 (1993): 10–11.

5. The Public Health— Human Rights Dialogue

International Federation of Red Cross
and Red Crescent Societies and François-Xavier
Bagnoud Center for Health and Human Rights

Public health and human rights can be considered as two different, often complementary and occasionally conflicting ways of looking at the world. Even when they address similar or even identical problems, their language and underlying assumptions may differ. Consequently, to achieve useful and constructive dialogue and action it is important to bridge these worlds with understanding and sensitivity to each discipline's language and perspectives.

INDIVIDUALS AND SOCIETY

Public health is *concerned with promoting and protecting health—in other words, physical, mental, and social well-being—and with preventing or reducing morbidity (illness, disability, or suffering) and premature mortality.* A fundamental yet often unstated assumption is that public health seeks the greatest good for the greatest number of people.

Human rights are concerned with promoting and protecting the well-being of individuals by ensuring respect for individual rights and dignity. A central concern in human rights is the ethical principle of autonomy. It is therefore inevitable that some tension will emerge between public health and human rights perspectives and approaches to promoting human well-being. For example:

- At times, an individual may be considered dangerous for the health of the larger group. (e.g., a person with tuberculosis can infect contacts; the intoxicated driver may cause automobile crashes that endanger others). The public health response to these situations has often been to constrain the individual in order to protect the group.
- Certain public health measures, proposed on the basis of excellent scientific data (e.g., adding iodine to table salt to prevent iodine deficiency and

cretinism), may limit or eliminate individual choice and also have some side effects and costs.

- Some measures may be recommended or required by public health authorities based on their known effectiveness in reducing risks of morbidity or death to the individual (e.g., requiring motorcycle riders to wear helmets reduces head injury and deaths). In these cases, individual behavior is constrained; the public good involves maintaining productive life-years and limiting the financial costs (which the group will ultimately pay) for expensive trauma care or rehabilitation after a motorcycle-related head injury.

Before proceeding with how the public health and human rights perspectives can be integrated and developed together, it is crucial to note an important similarity: *Human rights and public health have increasingly recognized the vital role of the societal environment to both health and the realization of human rights.*

Even while many individuals do what they can to be healthy (for example, eating well and avoiding tobacco smoking), their health will be strongly influenced by a polluted environment, dangerous work conditions or lack of safe drinking water. Similarly, the freedom to make one's own decisions depends on conditions such as having a sufficient income, a place to live, and good health. In turn, these factors are heavily influenced by whether or not an individual belongs to a group that suffers discrimination. Thus, the relationship between the individual and the society is more complex than it may initially appear.

In spite of the importance attached to individual rights, situations arise in which it is considered legitimate to limit certain individual rights to achieve a broader public good. This public good is described in general terms in the International Covenant on Civil and Political Rights. The public good takes precedence over individual rights

- to secure due recognition and respect for the rights and freedoms of others
- to meet the just requirements of morality, public order, and the general welfare
- in time of emergency, where there are threats to the vital interests of the nation

Given the importance of health, it is not surprising that public health is considered a valid reason for limiting rights under some circumstances.

However, any limitation of individual rights is a serious issue, regardless of the apparent importance of the public good involved. *When a government limits the exercise or enjoyment of a right, this action must be a last resort, and can be permitted only when several specific and stringent conditions are met.*

- The goal of limiting rights may not be contrary to the purposes and principles of the United Nations Charter.

- The limitation must be justified by the protection of a legitimate goal such as national security, public safety, protection of public health or public order.
- Limitations can be allowed only in a democratic society which presumes a participatory decision process and capacity for redress.
- A right may be restricted only if the limitation is provided for by law.
- The limitation of rights must be strictly necessary in order to achieve the public good, which must be carefully assessed on a case-by-case basis.
- The limitation of individual rights must be proportional to the public interest and its objective (the so-called proportionality test).
- The limitation must be the least intrusive and least restrictive measure available which will accomplish the public health goal.
- The limitation of rights must not be applied in a discriminatory manner.

This chapter is based on the idea that despite their different approaches, assumptions, and language, public health and human rights goals and work can be complementary and mutually supportive. Promoting public health can contribute positively to human rights objectives, and vice versa. Society will be best served by maximal realization of both human rights and public health goals. Nevertheless, a systematic approach is clearly needed to explore and negotiate the potential tensions between human rights and public health policies, programs, and practices. The following presents a clear and consistent method to achieve this goal.

A FRAMEWORK FOR NEGOTIATION: HUMAN RIGHTS AND PUBLIC HEALTH

Beyond Negotiation: Complementary Goals

The mutual interdependence of public health and human rights is becoming increasingly clear. Substantial progress in resolving public health problems will require improvements in respect for human rights and dignity. Similarly, improvements in health create conditions which favor the full enjoyment of human rights and dignity.

For example, educational attainment for women is now considered to be one of the most important measures to improve health in developing countries. But increasing women's access to education will also from a human rights perspective, promote their right to education and reduce gender discrimination.

Once the synergy between public health and human rights is recognized, the next step is to coordinate action toward the common goal, taking full advantage of different skills, strategies, and spheres of influence. For example, health officials and experts could testify about the health benefits of education, or the negative effects on health created by discrimination against women. The credibility of health professionals and their specific technical knowledge may strengthen efforts to increase educational access for women. Similarly, health goals may be advanced when the influence and prestige of legal and human rights workers are focused on a specific health issue, such as access to health services, or the need to provide accurate and complete information about health risks associated with tobacco use.

When Public Health Goals and Human Rights Norms Appear to Conflict

A systematic approach is needed to identify, understand and negotiate the human rights impact of public health policies, programs, and practices.[1] *A public health policy or program that protects and promotes human rights, while still achieving its public health goal, is better than a policy or program of equal effectiveness that burdens or limits human rights.*

In a schematic manner, the central problem of negotiation can be depicted in a 2 x 2 diagram. One side of the diagram shows public health quality, and the other side shows human rights quality. Each side is divided into positive qualities (public health high quality or high respect for human rights and dignity) and negative qualities (low public health quality or low respect for human rights and dignity); see below.

The goal is to achieve the best possible harmonization of public health goals and respect for human rights and dignity. On the 2 x 2 table, this means approaching the upper right quadrant, which means high public health quality plus high human rights quality (point 3, sector A).

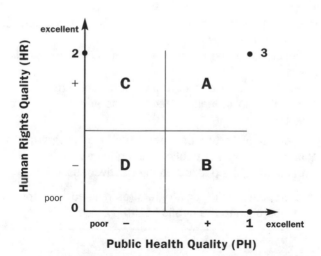

Sector explanation:
A: best case
B: need to improve HR quality
C: need to improve PH quality
D: worst case, need to improve
   both PH and HR quality

Points explanation:
0: poor quality
1: ideal PH quality
2: ideal HR quality
3: ideal PH + HR quality

This process requires dialogue and collaboration between public health and human rights workers. This simple framework is used by applying a four-step approach, based on four key questions detailed below.

FOUR-STEP IMPACT ASSESSMENT

Public Health and Human Rights

1. To what extent does the proposed policy or program represent "good public health"? In other words, where would you locate the proposed policy or program along the bottom line of the 2 x 2 table, from "poor public health" (point 0) to ideal public health (point 1)?

2. Is the proposed policy or program respectful and protective of human rights? In other words, where would you locate the proposed policy or program along the vertical line of the 2 x 2 table, from "poor" human rights quality (point 0) to ideal human rights quality (point 2)?

3. How can we achieve the best possible combination of public health and human rights quality (toward point 3)?

    3.1 How serious is the public health problem?

    3.2 Is the proposed response likely to be effective?

    3.3 What are the severity, scope and duration of the burdens on human rights resulting from the proposed policy or program?

    3.4 To what extent is the proposed policy or program restrictive and intrusive?

    3.5 Is the proposed policy or program overinclusive (too broad) or underinclusive (too narrow)?

    3.6 What procedural safeguards are included in the proposed policy or program?

    3.7 Will the proposed policy or program be periodically reviewed to assess both its public health effectiveness and its impact on human rights?

Identify specific changes to the proposed policy or program that increase its human rights and/or public health quality while maintaining (or even strengthening) its public health effectiveness.

4. Finally, does the proposed policy or program (as revised) still appear to be the optimal approach to the public health problem?

---

1. To what extent does the proposed policy or program represent "good public health?"

In other words, where would you locate the proposed policy or program along the bottom line of the 2 x 2 table, from poor public health (point 0) to ideal public health (point 1)?

To answer this question,

- The health problem as well as the public health goal, objectives, and strategy must be clearly described.
- A determination must be made about whether the public health objective is compelling.
- The likely effectiveness and feasibility of the policy or program, in relation to its costs, must be carefully examined.
- Only the health benefits, risk, and harms are considered at this step, not the human rights impact. For example, if an HIV testing policy is proposed, to whom will it apply, and what are the public health benefits and risks for participants? In addition, who will be ineligible (excluded from) the program?

Finally, locate the proposed public health policy or program along the line from poor (point 0) to ideal (point 1) public health quality, based on answers to these questions. Place a mark at the point you have selected.

2. Is the proposed policy or program respectful and protective of human rights?

In other words, where would you locate the proposed policy or program along the vertical line of the 2 x 2 table, from poor human rights quality (point 0) to ideal human rights quality (point 2).

To do this, you must describe the potential benefits for human rights and the potential burdens on human rights which will occur as a result of the policy or program.

- What specific rights will be burdened by the policy or program? For example, in an HIV testing program, are a person's rights to security and freedom from arbitrary interference with privacy respected? Will the results of the HIV test lead to discrimination, arbitrary detention, or a limitation in freedom of movement?
- To ensure that the full range of potential burdens on human rights is identified, each of the rights listed in the consolidated list should be considered.
- For each human right which may be violated, assess the *severity/invasiveness* of the rights violation and its *frequency, scope,* and *duration.*
- In addition to considering burdens on each specific right, the potential for discrimination to be caused by the proposed policy or program must always be carefully examined.

Finally, locate the proposed policy or program along the vertical line from poor (point 0) to ideal (point 2) human rights quality. Place a mark at the point you have selected.

3. How can we achieve the best possible balance between protecting public health and protecting and promoting human rights and dignity?

The goal is to realize a given public health objective and at the same time to minimize, to the greatest extent possible, the burdens on human rights resulting from the proposed public health policy, program, and practices. In other words, following the diagram, we are seeking to move the proposed policy or program as far into sector A of the diagram as possible. To do this, first locate the proposed policy or program by finding the intersection of the two points you have marked.

In each case, the goal will be to determine how the point of intersection (the balance between PH and HR quality) can be moved into sector A (high PH quality and high HR quality). In example 1, below, this will require both improving PH quality and improving HR quality; in example 2, it is the HR quality that requires attention.

To improve HR quality, consider how the burden on each specific right affected by the proposed policy or program can be reduced. For example, mandatory HIV testing (which burdens an individual's right to integrity and informed consent) can be changed to voluntary testing, or a program that excludes women (violating the right to nondiscrimination) can be broadened to include women.

To consider how to improve PH and HR quality, a review of the following seven questions may be useful:

3.1 How serious is the public health problem?

What is its nature, severity, extent, and future potential if not controlled? Is there a compelling public health need to respond?

3.2 Is the proposed response likely to be effective?

How confident are you that the proposed policy or program will achieve the public health goal or objective?

3.3 What are the severity, scope, and duration of the burdens on human rights resulting from the proposed policy or program?

How serious, widespread, and prolonged are the potential burdens on human rights?

3.4 To what extent is the proposed policy or program restrictive and intrusive?

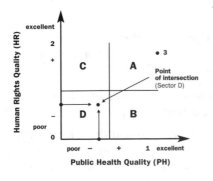
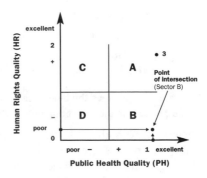

3.5 Is the proposed policy or program overinclusive (too broad) or under inclusive (too narrow)?

Does the policy or program reach too many people (e.g., testing for everybody and not, as a priority, only the groups who have risk behaviors) or too few people (e.g., education offered only for prostitutes and not for their clients)?

3.6 What procedural safeguards are included in the proposed policy or program?

Procedural protections may include providing information and opportunities for hearing and appeal.

3.7 Will the proposed policy or program be periodically reviewed to assess both its public health effectiveness and its impact on human rights?

Since responses continue to evolve, as does the epidemic itself, regular assessment is necessary to establish and maintain policy/program fidelity to the public health goals for which they were implemented, while assuring their continuing compatibility with human rights standards.

Now, identify specific changes to the proposed policy or program that can increase its human rights and/or public health quality. (Actually, in many cases, this analysis reveals weaknesses or flaws in the initial public health strategy.)

4. Finally, does the proposed policy or program (as revised) still appear to be the optimal approach to the public health problem?

The process of analysis may reveal or suggest creative, alternative policy and/or programmatic approaches which are both more respectful of human rights and more effective in achieving public health goals.

In summary, this assessment process ensures that public health and human rights goals are optimally realized and that conflicts are negotiated rationally, in a climate of mutual understanding and respect.

ACKNOWLEDGMENTS

This approach is based on the "Public Health/Human Rights Impact Assessment Instrument" developed by Jonathan Mann and colleagues at the François-Xavier Bagnoud Center for Health and Human Rights at the Harvard School of Public Health.

6. Toward the Development of a Human Rights Impact Assessment for the Formulation and Evaluation of Public Health Policies

Lawrence Gostin and Jonathan Mann

Public health policies are sometimes formulated without careful consideration of the goals of the policy, whether the means adopted will achieve
those goals, and whether intended health benefits outweigh financial and
human rights burdens. In particular, public health policies are seldom crafted
with attention to their impact on human rights or the norms of international
human rights law.[1] Implementing public health policies without seriously
considering their human rights dimension may harm the people affected and
render the policy ineffective or detrimental.[2]

The absence of careful thought about the human rights implications of
health policies is not surprising: few public health officials are familiar with
human rights doctrines, and even those who are may lack the skills and
knowledge to assess a policy from a human rights perspective. At the same
time, the human rights community has rarely written or litigated in the area
of public health.[3] Even so fundamental a human rights concept as the right
to health has not been operationally defined, and no organized body of
jurisprudence exists to describe the parameters of that right.[4] The absence
of an analytic tool that public health and human rights experts can apply
to assess systematically the impact of public health policies on human
rights has impeded development of collaborative scholarship and action in
the fields of human rights and public health.

This chapter proposes a human rights impact assessment—an instrument
to help evaluate the effects of public health policies on human rights and
dignity. The basic steps outlined in this assessment tool may help those
working in the public health domain to develop effective strategies that
respect human rights. The human rights impact assessment should also assist
human rights organizations and community-based groups in arguing for

incorporation of human rights standards into public health thinking and policies. To illustrate the human rights impact assessment, this article draws on recent experience with sexually transmitted diseases (STDs),[5] human immunodeficiency virus (HIV) infection,[6] and tuberculosis (TB).[7]

BACKGROUND: NOTE ON FACT-FINDING

Assessment is one of the primary functions of public health. Careful gathering of all relevant information, provided through the perspectives of various disciplines (e.g., epidemiology, virology, medicine, nursing, social services) is a fundamental prerequisite for effective public policy development. Assessments of the human rights dimensions of policy likewise require rigorous and impartial fact-finding.

Institutions that seek to justify public health strategies (such as ministries of health, environment, or justice) may present seemingly credible arguments based on "hard evidence." However, a set of "facts" presented by the government may be incomplete or biased. Proper fact-finding requires broad-based consultation with international agencies, nonprofit organizations, public health or other professional associations, community-based or advocacy groups, and community leaders, who can provide invaluable perspective regarding how health policies affect human rights in their communities.[8] Discussions with individuals affected by the policy, and their advocates, are particularly important. When consulting these sources, special efforts should be made to gather material representing all viewpoints, to ensure a balanced picture.

HUMAN RIGHTS IMPACT ASSESSMENT

The assessment involves a series of questions designed to balance the public health benefits of a policy against its human rights burdens.

Step I: Clarify the Public Health Purpose

A clear understanding of the public health purpose to be achieved is essential. Government has a responsibility to articulate this public health purpose. Claims, for instance, that the objective is to combat tuberculosis, AIDS, or some other prevalent disease are too vague and overbroad. A precise conceptualization of purpose will more likely lead to sound, properly conceived policies. Examples of narrowly defined public health goals include (1) prevention of HIV transmission through blood and blood products (through donor deferral, HIV screening, and heat treatment of blood products for people with hemophilia) or (2) prevention of tuberculosis transmission (by assuring compliance with treatment through directly monitored therapy).

Clearly articulated goals help to identify the true purpose of the intervention, facilitate public understanding and debate around legitimate health purposes, and reveal prejudice, stereotypical attitudes, or irrational fear.

Step II: Evaluate Likely Policy Effectiveness

Existence of a valid—even compelling—public health objective does not justify a policy. Public officials have the burden of showing that the means used are reasonably likely to achieve the stated purpose.

Step II requires an honest, rigorous investigation into a policy's potential effectiveness. This requires a careful and impartial examination of the facts and expert opinion, as well as consultation with the groups affected.

It may be argued that certain public health decisions must be made in an emergency, precluding deliberative reasoning and assessment of scientific evidence. Public health necessity, however, does not absolve the actor from basing judgments on all available data. Public health emergencies, like other urgent situations, require rapid and rigorous assessment of the available data.[9]

Several questions may help guide further thinking about the potential effectiveness of a proposed public health policy. The following are examples that have been selected from screening programs for STDs, HIV, and mycobacterium tuberculosis.

Is the Screening Program Appropriate and Accurate?

No screening test is 100 percent sensitive (meaning that all people with the condition have a positive test) and 100 percent specific (meaning that all people without the condition have a negative test). In addition to the inherent characteristics of testing methods, there are several important sources of potential problems: (1) human error, including improper manufacture or storage of laboratory reagents; (2) biological characteristics of the condition (i.e., for HIV infection, there is a several weeks' long "window" between infection and appearance of detectable antibodies); and (3) epidemiological characteristics, such as the prevalence of the condition in the population to be tested. Generally, given imperfect specificity of the test itself, the lower the prevalence of the infection in the population, the smaller the probability that a positive test accurately indicates that the person has the condition of interest. Therefore, screening low-prevalence populations leads to substantial potential for false-positive tests. The technical capability of the test cannot be separated from the specific context in which it is used.

Is the Intervention Likely to Be Effective?

The fact that a government establishes an aggressive program for screening, partner notification, or isolation does not necessarily mean it is "doing something" about the problem. The real issue is whether the policy leads to effective action.

With regard to screening programs, it is important to determine the marginal value of any test results. That is, given what is already known about the patient or population, does the test yield new, useful information? More important, does the policy respond effectively to that information?

If a government, for example, conducts a widespread screening program for STDs in acute care hospitals, prisons, or brothels in order to prevent transmission, the policy must be examined carefully to see whether it succeeds in achieving its objective. If the program is not also designed to provide prevention services (such as education and counseling) or if there is no follow-up with treatment, the program will have identified cases of infection but failed to intervene effectively. Screening, then, emerges as a constructive policy only if the information is demonstrably used for public health benefit.

It is sometimes misguidedly stated that gathering information about health status in a population is always beneficial. While screening can provide useful data, its validity or generalizability may be biased or flawed. A more reliable understanding of disease prevalence in a population can be obtained through epidemiological research methods.

Is There a Better Approach?

The proposed policy should be compared with alternatives. Certainly, exploration of a wide range of more humane policies brings with it a fresh perspective. Consider an example involving commercial sex workers and people who have multiple sex partners. Coercive or punitive interventions alienate these communities, even driving them away from health care providers and counselors who can help alter their high-risk behaviors. Instead of punitive measures, health officials could attempt to empower those women who may be impoverished, in abusive relationships, and unable to refuse sexual intercourse or demand that their partners use a condom. At the same time, public officials might work to meet employment, housing, health, and social needs of women to promote a lifestyle that respects their dignity as individuals and does not exploit them.[10]

Public policy development provides an avenue for improving community health. A hasty decision to pursue comprehensive programs of screening, contact tracing, or coercive measures imposes more than financial and human rights burdens, as there are also opportunity costs. That is, devoting resources to one policy or service costs a government the opportunity to introduce other, potentially more effective policies or services. The global community cannot afford to forgo cost-effective measures that prevent disease and promote access to care.

In sum, a thoughtful exploration of these questions can benefit both public health and human rights: Is the form of intervention appropriate and accurate? Is the intervention likely to lead to effective action? Is a particular policy as effective as other feasible options?

Step III: Determine Whether the Public Health Policy Is Well-Targeted

Well-conceived policies target the population in need. Ideally, public health strategies are tailored for those who will benefit from them. Thus, every policy creates a class of people to whom the policy applies and a class to whom it does not. For example, screening policies may target a specific group such as homeless persons, drug users, foreigners, commercial sex workers, or prisoners. A policy of isolating all persons with TB who do not complete the full course of treatment may primarily affect poor persons who have inadequate access to health care services. A policy that appears neutral may, in fact, disproportionately impact certain groups in society. Recognizing that all policies create classifications that may discriminate against disfavored people is crucial. This awareness sensitizes the public health community to human rights concerns and helps to ensure that classifications are strictly related to public health needs. Policies that target individuals because of their race, sex, religion, national origin, sexual orientation, economic status, disability, or homeless status often stem from invidious stereotypes.

Sound public health policies must avoid both under- and overinclusiveness.[11] A policy is underinclusive when it reaches some, but not all, of the persons it ought to reach. By itself, underinclusiveness is not necessarily a problem; a government may use its limited resources to address part of a public health problem. For example, a government's provision of disease prevention and treatment services (e.g., safe sex education, condom distribution, and health care) may be targeted to street children, but not to school-children or adults. The underinclusiveness of this policy does not necessarily reflect discrimination; it may simply indicate that particular country's public health problems and priorities.

This form of permissible underinclusion is shown in Diagram 1. Population A represents all adolescents at risk for STDs and unwanted pregnancies who could benefit from sex education and counseling. Population B represents all adolescents in institutional settings, such as prisons, foster homes, and mental hospitals (including both institutionalized adolescents and those in schools and the wider community). The proposed public health policy would provide comprehensive sex education and condom distribution to Population B only; this policy is based on the assumption that parents of all other adolescents will provide them with appropriate information, and when resources become available, the health education program will be extended. While this approach is not ideal, it does not necessarily raise fundamental problems of invidious underinclusion.[12]

However, certain underinclusive policies may mask discrimination—such as when a government uses coercive powers to target politically powerless and vulnerable groups, but not others that engage in similar behavior. The government is not obliged to devise policies that address the entire population with the potential to transmit disease. It may, instead, choose to address a public health problem one step at a time. However, if the subpopulation targeted for coercion or punishment is chosen for reasons not directly related to public health, the underinclusion is impermissible.

Diagram 2 illustrates such impermissible underinclusion. Population A includes all persons diagnosed with active tuberculosis. Those persons who are included in Population A (but not B) are mostly middle- to upper-income

Diagram 1: Permissible Underinclusion

Proposed policy: Provide comprehensive sex education
and condom distribution only to population B

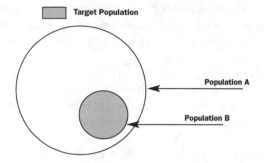

Population A = All adolescents at risk for STDs and unwanted pregnancies who could benefit from sex education and counseling

Population B = All adolescents in institutional settings such as prisons, foster homes, and mental hospitals

individuals in the dominant ethnic community. Population B includes all homeless persons diagnosed with active tuberculosis, and is composed solely of people in the lowest socioeconomic class, over 90 percent of whom are members of ethnic minorities. A policy of isolation during the active phase of the disease and directly observed therapy during the entire course of the treatment is invidious if applied only to Population B, because it makes prejudicial, unsupported assumptions about persons in the two populations. Public health officials assume that persons in Population A will remain

Diagram 2: Impermissible Underinclusion

Proposed policy: Isolation during the active phase of tuberculosis and directly observed therapy during the entire course of the treatment of persons in population B.

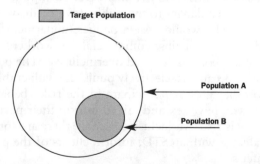

Population A = All persons diagnosed with active tuberculosis

Population B = All persons without a permanent address diagnosed with active tuberculosis voluntarily isolated in their homes during the active phase and can be trusted to take the full course of their medication. Officials also assume that persons in Population B will not voluntarily remain isolated, will fail to complete the full course of the medication and will knowingly remain in crowded areas, exposing others to infection. These assumptions are based, in part, upon generalizations about populations that separate individuals by their socio-economic class and race.

Even if the government policies are offering beneficial services rather than coercion, they still may be impermissibly underinclusive. For example, providing health care services to, or running clinical trials for, men but not women may reflect society's neglect of women rather than legitimate public health priorities.

Overinclusiveness occurs when a policy extends to more people than necessary to achieve its objective. Overinclusiveness may not be cost-effective, as when counseling all persons entering acute-care hospitals about HIV infection.

However, overinclusiveness with regard to a coercive power is almost always unacceptable. Impermissibly overinclusive policies impose compulsory measures on groups *assumed* to be at high risk of transmitting disease; however, many individuals in the group pose no risk at all to the public. Compulsory measures that apply to all homosexuals, commercial sex workers, intravenous drug users, or foreigners from countries with high rates of HIV stem from the erroneous belief that all members of the group will engage in unprotected sex or needle-sharing. Diagram 3 (p. 61), based upon the quarantine of HIV-infected persons in Cuba, illustrates such overinclusion. Population A includes all persons infected with HIV in Cuba. Population B represents HIV-infected persons who engage in high-risk behavior. The quarantine policy targets all individuals in Population A, even though only a small percentage of this population is likely to transmit infection. While the policy may be effective as a public health measure, it deprives many people of liberty who pose no risk to society.

Policies may be both under- and overinclusive. Such policies affect individuals who do not pose a danger to the public (overinclusiveness), yet fail to include individuals who would pose a danger (underinclusiveness). For example, criminal penalties against commercial sex workers but not their male agents or clients is both under- and overinclusive. The policy is suspiciously underinclusive because it selectively punishes a vulnerable population when at least two other groups participate in the risky behavior. (It also excludes all others who have sex and fail to inform their partners of their infection.) The policy is also overinclusive because there are some sex workers who are not infected with an STD, inform clients of the potential risks and/or practice safer sex.

Diagram 4 (p. 62) provides another illustration of over- and underinclusion. Population A represents all foreigners entering the country. Population B represents all foreigners entering the country from Region X. Population C

Diagram 3: Overinclusion

Proposed policy: Quarantine of HIV-positive persons in the country

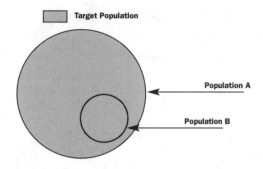

Population A = All persons with HIV in the country

Population B = All persons with HIV who engage in high-risk behavior

represents all foreigners entering the country from Region X who would engage in high-risk behavior. Population D represents all foreigners entering the country from outside Region X who would engage in high-risk behavior. The proposed policy of screening and excluding those who test positive for HIV infection is targeted to Population B only (foreigners from Region X). Such a policy is overly broad because, while some infected individuals in Population B may engage in high-risk behaviors, many group members are not infected, and many infected people will act responsibly. At the same time, the policy does not apply to foreigners outside of Region X, even though many of them are infected with HIV and may engage in high-risk behavior.[13]

Step IV: Examine Each Policy for Possible Human Rights Burdens
Having considered several important dimensions of public health policy making, it is now possible to examine the human rights impact of a proposed policy. The human rights impact assessment involves a meticulous balancing of the potential benefits to the health of the community with the human rights repercussions of the policy. Human rights burdens may outweigh even a well-designed policy. Identifying all potential infringements on human rights and evaluating those likely to occur will contribute to sound government action.

The International Bill of Human Rights may be considered the source of basic human rights.[14] These documents list and describe human rights, recognize duties of individuals to the community, create nonderogable rights that may not be infringed even in times of public emergency, and provide criteria for the limitation of other rights.[15]

Certain human rights are so essential to the dignity and well-being of people that they are considered absolute. These rights must never be

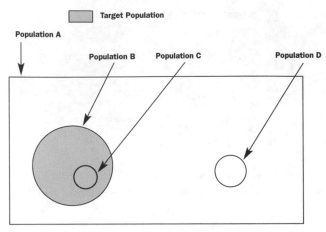

DIAGRAM 4: UNDER- AND OVERINCLUSION
Proposed policy: Quarantine of HIV-positive persons in the country

Population A = All foreigners entering the country
Population B = All foreigners from region X
Population C = All foreigners from region X with high-risk behaviors
Population D = All foreigners from outside region X with high-risk behaviors

infringed, even if the country is in a declared state of public emergency and the public health need is extraordinarily strong. Nonderogable rights include freedom from discrimination; the right to life; freedom from torture and from cruel, inhuman, or degrading treatment or punishment; freedom from slavery or involuntary servitude; freedom from imprisonment for failure to fulfill contractual obligations; freedom from retroactivity for criminal offenses; the right to recognition as a person before the law; and freedom of thought, conscience, and religion.[17] Thus, from this perspective, the public health benefits of policies that burden nonderogable human rights never outweigh the intrusion on human rights. In short, the fact that a policy improves public health does not justify any possible means to achieve that end.

Other rights may be restricted in certain situations. Article 29 of the Universal Declaration of Human Rights states that limitations of these rights must be "determined by law solely for the purpose of securing due recognition and respect for the rights and freedoms of others and of meeting the just requirements of morality, public order and the general welfare in a democratic society." Generally speaking, restrictions on human rights must be (1) *prescribed by law in a democratic society*—the restriction on rights must be based upon the thoughtful consideration of the legislature—and (2) *necessary to protect a valued social goal*—the legislature must be promoting a compelling public interest such as safety or health. Restricting human rights is not to be taken lightly. Indeed, in most cases coercive or punitive policies will harm, not enhance, the health of the public.

Civil and political rights that may be infringed if necessary to protect a valued social goal include: the right to liberty and security of person; freedom from arbitrary arrest, detention, or exile; freedom of movement; freedom from arbitrary interference with privacy, family, home and correspondence; the right to peaceful assembly and association; and freedom of opinion and expression, including the right to seek, receive, and impart information. Minor infringements on human rights may be justified when the public health interest is compelling and there is no other way to achieve the objective. For example, requiring the immunization of a population by means of a safe and effective vaccine may undermine the right to security of person, but the substantial reduction in morbidity and mortality may justify the intervention.

Economic, cultural, and social rights do not have the same standing in international law as civil and political rights.[16] Rights afforded in the International Covenant on Economic, Social and Cultural Rights (ICESCR) include the right to work (Article 6), to social security (Article 9), to an adequate standard of living including adequate food, clothing and housing (Article 11), to the enjoyment of the highest attainable standard of physical and mental health (Article 12), to education (Article 13), and to enjoyment of the benefits of scientific progress and its applications (Article 15). Economic, social, and cultural rights are not immediately enforceable, and the United Nations Committee on Economic, Social and Cultural Rights does not have power to require compliance. However, Article 2 of the ICESCR imposes an obligation on state parties to take steps, individually and through international assistance and cooperation, especially economic and technical, to the maximum of its available resources, with a view to progressive realization of these rights.

How can a human rights burden created by a public health policy be measured? Four factors may be considered: (1) the nature of the human right, (2) the invasiveness of the intervention, (3) the frequency and scope of the infringement, and (4) its duration.

Policies that adversely affect fundamental rights and freedoms create significant burdens on human rights. A decision to imprison, isolate, or otherwise restrict the liberty of a person substantially impacts the person's life. In contrast, while partner notification requirements potentially infringe on privacy, this type of invasion is usually less grave than a deprivation of liberty.

The second factor involves the degree of intrusion on a particular right. Neither liberty nor privacy is an absolute right. All societies tolerate some incursions on these rights, such as limitations on individual liberty where its exercise would interfere with the fundamental rights of others, or disclosure of private information when strict confidentiality would pose an imminent danger to another person.[18] However, the burdens (harms) from public health measures that intrude on either right may well outweigh their potential benefits.

For example, a government's decision to record the names of individuals with certain diseases and to grant public access to the information seriously intrudes on privacy rights of the infected individuals. Similarly, prohibiting all women with HIV infection from bearing children based on the risk of perinatal HIV transmission fundamentally burdens privacy in the context of reproductive decision-making.

A third question asks whether the restriction of rights applies to a few people or to an entire group or population. A decision to isolate an individual with active, contagious tuberculosis is clearly justified. However, a policy that quarantines a large population of persons infected with tuberculosis substantially burdens human rights. The Cuban government, for example, has sought to reduce the transmission of HIV in its population by screening and isolating all Cubans returning from abroad. The government might plausibly argue that it would achieve a compelling public health objective, but the gravity and scope of the human rights burdens are prohibitive.[19]

Fourth, the duration of a human rights burden must be considered. Isolating a person infected with tuberculosis during the active stage of the disease is a necessary, short-term intervention. However, isolating a person with HIV infection is almost always inappropriate; it raises the prospect of indefinite duration, since the person remains potentially infectious to others for his or her lifetime.[20]

Finally, legal and ethical standards strongly suggest that public health programs incorporate the principle of informed consent.[21] This doctrine is most clearly applicable to biomedical research, but may also include other health programs including testing and treatment. Principle I of the Nuremberg Code[22] provides the definition of consent from which subsequent international ethical guidelines are derivative:[23]

> The voluntary consent of the human subject is absolutely essential. This means that the person involved should have legal capacity to give consent; should be so situated as to be able to exercise free power of choice, without the intervention of any element of force, fraud, deceit, duress, overreaching or other ulterior form of constraint or coercion; and should have sufficient knowledge and comprehension of the elements of the subject matter involved as to enable him to make an understanding and enlightened decision.

Thus, the consent of the human subject to research must be legally competent, voluntary, informed, and comprehending.[23] Article 7 of the International Covenant on Civil and Political Rights prohibits medical or scientific experimentation without the person's free consent.

The grounds for extending the principle of informed consent to treatment and the exercise of other public health powers is found in Article 9 of the International Covenant of Civil and Political Rights, which guarantees the right to security of person. Security of person may be taken to mean that persons have a right to determine for themselves how they will be treated.

Respect for personal autonomy underlies the doctrine of informed consent. The principle of autonomy requires that every competent human being has the right to make decisions regarding his or her health and well-being.[25]

The concept of informed consent is critically important to maintaining sound public health practice. Consent should be viewed as more of a process of communication and interaction with the patient than a stark legal requirement. The process of consent provides the opportunity to counsel and educate while it preserves the integrity of health professionals and the dignity of the patient.

Human rights experts and nongovernmental organizations may invaluably assist those trying to evaluate a public health policy's impact on human rights and to enforce international legal protections. Establishing networks of experts in human rights and public health can facilitate constructive discussions. This can only lead to greater respect for human rights in policy development, implementation, and enforcement.

Step V: Determine Whether the Policy Is the Least Restrictive
Alternative That Can Achieve the Public Health Objective

The human rights impact assessment suggests a balance between the burdens and public health benefits of a policy. In general, broad or intrusive human rights violations are seldom, if ever, warranted. At the extreme, a public health approach that uses an effective means to achieve a compelling public health objective may sometimes warrant a limitation of human rights. In contrast, a dubiously useful government policy deserves less weight in the balance.

A vital step in the human rights impact assessment is the examination of alternative policies that burden human rights to a lesser extent, while still protecting the health of the community. The principle of the least restrictive alternative seeks the policy that is least intrusive while achieving the public health objective as well or better than the policy under consideration. The human rights community should insist that governments find alternatives that achieve the public health goal without unduly violating rights and dignity.

Public health officials sometimes misunderstand the principle of the least restrictive alternative. The principle does not require governments to adopt ineffective policies or to forgo effective policies. Rather, it proposes selective implementation of programs that are human-rights-sensitive as well as equally or more effective in achieving a valuable public health goal. On rare occasions, less intrusive alternatives are also less effective, and the principle of the least restrictive alternative does not require their adoption.

To determine the least restrictive alternative, noncoercive approaches should first be considered. If noncoercive approaches are insufficient, gradual exploration of more intrusive measures are permissible where clearly necessary. For example, if the provision of service or benefits programs (e.g., counseling, education and treatment) do not adequately protect public health, more restrictive policies may be warranted.

Governments sometimes feel public pressure to respond to an urgent public health concern with restrictive or punitive measures. For example, public opinion may blame foreigners, drug users, homosexuals, sex workers, or other disenfranchised populations for the health threat. A searching examination of a range of less restrictive alternatives can uncover policies that not only defend the rights of the individual, but also are more worthwhile for the population as a whole.

Intense conflicts between public health and human rights occasionally arise, with members of the public or politicians claiming that it is necessary to "get tough" on persons who transmit disease. Actually, public health and human rights are usually in harmony: promotion of human rights is most protective of health, and the best health strategies are respectful of the inherent dignity of the person. An overly coercive policy may discourage persons at risk from coming forward for testing, counseling, or treatment. Health care professionals then lose contact with persons likely to spread disease, ultimately causing greater harm to the public. Moreover, public health and human rights goals are usually synergistic; protecting human rights encourages cooperation and a shared vision of the need for safer behaviors and thereby promotes public health.

In order to explore further the concept of the least restrictive alternative, consider the case of a large city seeking to slow the spread of multi-drug-resistant tuberculosis. Public opinion may call for civil commitment or court-ordered, directly observed therapy for all people with active TB. However, offering persons with tuberculosis incentives and services such as travel allowances, food, shelter, and child care may be more effective in helping them complete the full course of their medication than compulsory treatment or commitment.[26]

Step VI: If a Coercive Public Health Measure Is Truly the Most Effective, Least Restrictive Alternative, Base It on the Significant-Risk Standard

After analyzing a range of policies, the health authority may conclude that a coercive approach is the most effective, least restrictive alternative. In this case, it should make an *individual determination* that the person poses a *significant risk* to the public.[27] The significant-risk standard permits coercive measures only to avert likely harm to the health or safety of others. The determination of significant risk requires public health inquiry. The intent is to replace decisions based on irrational fear, speculation, stereotypes, or pernicious mythologies with reasoned, scientifically valid judgments.

Significant risk must be determined on a case-by-case basis by means of fact-specific, individual inquiries. Blanket rules or generalizations about a class of persons do not suffice.

For infectious diseases such as HIV/AIDS or tuberculosis, the significant-risk standard is based upon four factors: (1) nature of the risk (i.e., mode of transmission), (2) probability of the risk (i.e., how likely it is that the transmission will occur), (3) severity of harm (i.e., the harm to the person if the infection were transmitted), and (4) duration of the risk (i.e., the length of time the person is infectious).

As for the nature of the risk, public health interventions must be based on epidemiologically supported modes of transmission. For example, epidemiological evidence shows that the major routes of HIV transmission involve sexual intercourse and sharing contaminated drug injection equipment. Exclusion of HIV-infected children from school, for example, based on the fear of biting, spitting, or rough play in sports activities would not meet the significant-risk test. Similarly, the possibility that people infected with HIV who handle food may bleed into it, or that airline pilots might have a sudden onset of AIDS dementia, is so low that it does not justify depriving a class of individuals of their rights and livelihood.

The risk to the public must be *probable*, not merely speculative or remote. Theoretically, for example, a person could transmit HIV by biting. But the actual risk is extremely low (approaching zero). To bring criminal charges for this behavior lacks a public health justification. The *harm* that results if the infection is transmitted must be substantial. However, even potential harms of great severity (e.g., HIV infection) do not justify coercion if the probability of transmission is exceedingly low. The significant-risk requirement holds that even though a disease can be serious or fatal, restrictions on individuals lack justification unless a reasonable probability of transmission exists. For example, some parents of schoolchildren have difficulty comprehending why officials can exclude children infested with head lice from school, but not those infected with HIV. The significant-risk standard is met in the former case because of the very high probability that other children will contract lice. In contrast, the risk of contracting HIV in that setting is highly remote.

Finally, regarding duration of risk, the person must be *currently contagious*. The significant-risk standard allows coercion only during the period that the person poses a risk to the public. As soon as the risk subsides, the justification for coercion similarly subsides.

Step VII: If a Coercive Measure Is Truly Necessary to Avert a Significant Risk, Guarantee Fair Procedures to Persons Affected

The fact that officials do not intend a public health intervention to be punitive would not alter the reality that it restricts personal liberty. International human rights standards require that governments provide a fair public hearing before they deprive persons of liberty, freedom of movement, or other fundamental rights.

Examples of this process are well described in the mental health context. The United Nations Principles for the Protection of Persons with Mental Illness and for the Improvement of Mental Health Care require procedural safeguards ("due process") prior to civil commitment.[28] As in the mental health setting, public health policies that deprive people of liberty in order to protect the public must guarantee procedural justice.

The natural-justice principle, as construed by the European Court of Human Rights, requires a hearing by a dispassionate decision-maker who is separate from the executive branch and the parties to the case.[29] Thus, an independent court or tribunal must adjudicate the dispute. The person whose liberty is threatened is entitled to advance notice of the hearing, representation, and an opportunity to present evidence.

Procedural safeguards are not merely formalistic. The aim is to ensure a more accurate fact-finding process and greater equity and fairness to individuals who face a loss of liberty. Hearings give public health officials the opportunity to review their general approach to the health problem as well as the human rights impact in an individual case.

A government that deprives an individual of liberty or other rights must provide a fair and public hearing. These substantive and procedural requirements of human rights help ensure that governments demonstrate the genuine necessity of compulsory measures to protect the community and preserve justice for the individual.

CONCLUSION

Public health programs that respect human rights will encourage individuals and communities to trust, and cooperate with, public health authorities. Promotion of human rights, particularly among previously disenfranchised groups, increases their ability to protect their own health. Finally, the right to health is a basic human right, related to and dependent on many other human rights. The Human Rights Impact Assessment described in this chapter provides a tool to achieve the best possible public health outcomes while protecting the human rights of individuals and populations.

ACKNOWLEDGMENTS

The Human Rights Impact Assessment evolved from work by a group of friends and colleagues working at the Harvard School of Public Health, including Dr. Katarina Tomasevski, Ms. Zita Lazzarini and Ms. Sofia Gruskin, in addition to the authors. The goal of the Human Rights Impact Assessment is to provide public health practitioners, human rights advocates, community workers, and others interested in health policy with a systematic approach to exploring the human rights dimensions of public health policies, practices, resource allocation decisions, and programs. The authors warmly acknowledge the expert assistance of Jean C. Allison in the conceptualization of this chapter, particularly the diagrams.

REFERENCES

1. Public health policies are often crafted in the absence of clear rules of domestic law. See Institute of Medicine, *The Future of Public Health*, (Washington, DC: National Academy Press, 1988); L. Gostin, "The Future of Public Health Law," *American Journal of Law and Medicine* 12 (1987): 461–490.
2. There does exist an influential and growing literature that uses the disciplines of

the philosophy of law and biomedical ethics for the evaluation of health policies. Influential jurisprudential analyses include those by Ronald Dworkin in his classic book *Taking Rights Seriously* (Cambridge, MA: Harvard University Press, 1977), and in his more recent analysis of death and dying in *The Law's Empire* (New York: Oxford University Press, 1993). See also, John Rawls, *A Theory of Justice* (Cambridge, MA: Harvard University Press, 1971). Some authors treat biomedical ethics and human rights as if they were the same subject. See Eugene B. Brody, *Biomedical Technology and Human Rights* (Paris: UNESCO, 1993). However, examination of health policy from a jurisprudential or ethical perspective, while important, is not a substitute for a human rights analysis. The human rights perspective is unique because it is based upon an organized set of internationally recognized and enforceable legal standards. See Philip Alston, ed., *The United Nations and Human Rights: A Critical Appraisal* (Oxford: Clarendon Press, 1992).

3. Major texts on human rights barely discuss the application of international law to public health. See, e.g., Frank Newman and David Weissbrodt *International Human Rights* (Cincinnati: Anderson Publishing Co., 1990). However, several excellent reports on the human rights impact of HIV infection have appeared. See Paul Sieghart, *AIDS and Human Rights* (London: British Medical Foundation, 1989); K. Tomasevski, S. Gruskin, Z. Lazzarini, and A. Hendriks, "AIDS and Human Rights," in J. Mann, D.J.M. Tarantola, T. W. Netter, eds., *AIDS in the World 1992* (Cambridge: Harvard University Press, 1992) pp. 537–573; "Rights and Humanity," The Rights and Humanity Declaration and Charter on HIV and AIDS, The Hague, 1992.

4. A notable exception appears in V. Leary, "The Right to Health," *Health and Human Rights* 1 (1994): 28. See Committee on Economic, Social and Cultural Rights, Ninth Session, 22 November–10 December 1993, *Implementation of the International Covenant on Economic, Social and Cultural Rights: Day of General Discussion on the Right to Health* (6 December 1993), E/C.12/1993/WP.27.

5. See, e.g. Allan Brandt, *No Magic Bullet: A Social History of Venereal Disease in the United States Since 1880*, rev. ed. (New York: Oxford University Press, 1987).

6. See, e.g., Ronald Bayer, *Private Acts, Social Consequences: AIDS and the Politics of Public Health* (New Brunswick, NJ: Rutgers University Press, 1991).

7. See, e.g., Sheila M. Rothman, *Living in the Shadow of Death: Tuberculosis and the Social Experience of Illness in American History* (New York: Basic Books, 1994).

8. See, e.g., Human Rights Watch, *World Report 1994* (New York: Human Rights Watch, 1994); Amnesty International, *Report 1993* (London: Amnesty International, 1993); Physicians for Human Rights, *Landmines: A Deadly Legacy* (New York: Human Rights Watch, 1993); Human Rights Watch and the American Civil Liberties Union, *Human Rights Violations in the United States* (New York: Human Rights Watch and the American Civil Liberties Union, 1993).

9. Elaine Scarry, *Thinking in an Emergency* (Cambridge: Harvard University Press, 1993).

10. J. Hauserman, *Ethical and Social Aspects of AIDS in Africa* (London: Commonwealth Secretariat, 1990).

11. The concept of under- and overbreadth is frequently used in equal protection analysis in the United States when the government infringes a fundamental right (such as the right to travel) or sets up a class based on race or some other suspect class. See, generally, Laurence Tribe, *American Constitutional Law*, 2nd ed. (Mineola, NY: Foundation Press, 1988), pp. 1446–1451.

12. Under certain circumstances, however, the policy might deprive noninstitutionalized adolescents of the right to education or the right to health. If these adolescents were at significant risk of contracting STDs or producing unwanted pregnancies and the government systematically denied them the education necessary to avoid these harms, telling arguments could be made under the International Covenant of Economic, Social and Cultural Rights.

13. L. Gostin, P. Cleary, K. Mayer, et al., "Screening and Exclusion of International Travelers and Immigrants for Public Health Purposes: An Evaluation of United States Policy," *New England Journal of Medicine* 322 (1990): 1743–1746.

14. The International Bill of Human Rights consists of the Universal Declaration of Human Rights (UDHR), the International Covenant of Civil and Political Rights (ICCPR), the International Covenant of Economic, Social and Cultural Rights (ICESCR) and the Optional Protocol to the International Covenant on Civil and Political Rights.

15. Article 29 of the Universal Declaration of Human Rights declares, "Everyone has duties to the community in which alone the free and full development of his personality is possible."

16. Article 4(2) of the International Covenant on Civil and Political Rights permits no derogation from Articles 6, 7, 8 (paras. 1 and 2), 11, 15, 16, and 18 even in cases of declared national emergencies.

17. P. Alston, "The Committee on Economic, Social and Cultural Rights." In *The United Nations and Human Rights: A Critical Appraisal* (Oxford: Clarendon Press, 1992), pp. 471–508.

18. E. M. Ankrah and L. O. Gostin, "Ethical and Legal Considerations of the HIV Epidemic in Africa," in *AIDS in Africa*, M. Essex, S. Mboup, P. J. Kanki, M. R. Kalengay, eds. (New York: Raven Press, 1994), pp. 547–558.

19. R. Bayer and C. Healton," Controlling AIDS in Cuba: the Logic of Quarantine," *New England Journal of Medicine* 320 (1989): 1022.

20. Wendy E. Parmet, "AIDS and Quarantine: The Revival of an Archaic Doctrine," *Hofstra Law Review* 14 (1985): 53–90.

21. R. R. Faden and T. L. Beauchamp, *A History and Theory of Informed Consent* (New York: Oxford University Press, 1986).

22. Nuremberg Code, 1947, *Trials of War Criminals Before the Nuremberg Military Tribunals Under Control Council Law No. 10*, vol. 2, pp. 181–182 (1949). The Nuremberg Code was part of the judgment reached by the Nuremberg Court in *United States v. Karl Brandt, et al.*, U.S. Adjutant General's Department, *Trials of War Criminals Under Control Council Law No. 10* (Oct. 1946–April 1949), vol. 2, *The Medical Case* (Washington DC: U.S. Government Printing Office, 1947) (Chapter 19, pp. 298–299 this volume).

23. See Declaration of Helsinki IV, I Basic Principles 9, 41st World Medical Assembly (1989); Council of International Organizations of Medical Sciences, International Guidelines for Ethical Review of Epidemiological Studies (Geneva: CIOMS, 1991).

24. Robert J. Levine, *Ethics and Regulation of Clinical Research* (New Haven: Yale University Press, 1988), pp. 98–99.

25. Arnold J. Rosoff, *Informed Consent: A Guide for Health Care Providers* (Rockville, MD: Aspen Publishers, 1981).

26. N. M. Dubler, R. Bayer, S. Landesman, and A. White, *The Tuberculosis Revival—Individual Rights and Societal Obligation in a Time of AIDS* (New York: United Hospital Fund, 1992).

27. This is similar to the standard used in the United States under the Americans with Disabilities Act. See L. Gostin, "Impact of the ADA on the Health Care System,"

in *Implementing the Americans with Disabilities Act: Rights and Responsibilities of All Americans*, L. Gostin and H. Beyer, eds. (Baltimore: Brookes Publishing, 1993), pp. 175–186.

28. United Nations, Principles for the Protection of Persons with Mental Illness and for the Improvement of Mental Health Care, G.A. Res. 119, U.N. GAOR, 46th Sess, Supp. No. 49, Annex, U.N. Doc. A/46/49 (1991), pp. 188–192.

29. *X v. United Kingdom*, European Court of Human Rights, judgment given November 5, 1981. See *Publications of the European Court of Human Rights, Series B: Pleadings, Oral Arguments and Documents*, vol. 41, 1980–82, Case of *X v. the United Kingdom*, Council of Europe, 1985.

PART III

Health Impacts Resulting from Violations of Human Rights

When health is understood to include physical, mental, and social well-being, it seems reasonable that the violation of any human right would impact adversely on health. Consider, for example, the right to rest and leisure, a right that when first considered might seem unnecessary or even frivolous. Yet even brief reflection on the physical and mental health effects of denying an individual rest or leisure clarifies why realization of this right is necessary for human well-being. As another example, consider the impact on health of violations of the right to association. The connection of this right with public health is extraordinarily powerful, for this right deals directly with the ability of individuals and communities to meet and to discuss issues relevant to public health. Imagine the world of family planning or HIV/AIDS education if diverse and active nongovernmental organizations were not allowed to exist!

The impacts on health of a human rights violation can be both obvious and subtle. For example, torture is a violation that causes immediate and direct harm to health. Yet only recently has the full measure of the effects of torture begun to be recognized, including the lifelong injury to the victim, the effects on the health of families and of entire communities, and the trans-generational damage. The process of documenting evidence of health impacts resulting from violations of human rights must therefore be thorough and thoughtful.

This is where the work of health professionals and that of human rights professionals come together. Health professionals can contribute the skills necessary to document and measure the health effects of a violation, while those working in human rights can provide the context necessary to understand the complexity of the violation and to ascertain whether the information can be used to monitor and ensure government accountability. This joint approach is necessary if proper attention is to be given to the health conse-quences of human rights violations. Only when health impacts are described, measured, and named as violations can the full extent of this relationship between health and human rights be realized.

In this section, we have drawn a somewhat artificial distinction between "conflict" and "peacetime" settings. Of the six chapters chosen to illustrate various aspects of the health impacts of human rights violations, the first three are most concerned with settings of conflict, and the last three are most relevant in times of peace. The reason for this separation is primarily to give recognition to alternative international legal structures applicable to the health and human rights paradigm. Human rights law is relevant in times of peace and of conflict, but it is most directly useful in times of peace. In con-trast, while stemming from similar underlying values, international humani-tarian law (e.g., the Geneva Conventions, the "laws of war") is specifically tailored to settings of conflict, speaking as it does about matters such as pro-tection of civilian noncombatants and cultural landmarks.

The first chapter, by Alain Destexhe, provides an historical overview of the role of humanitarianism and places in context current concerns about the actual benefits and harms to affected populations resulting from humanitar-ian aid. The chapter by Alicia Ely Yamin focuses on the International Crimi-nal Tribunal for the former Yugoslavia in order to explore application of the methods of human rights and of public health to the search for justice and truth. The Cécile Marotte and Hervé Rakoto Razafimbahiny chapter uses Haiti as a case example to provide a practical description of documentation undertaken by health professionals on the health effects of human rights vi-olations, and discusses the limitations of such an approach for the effective rehabilitation of the individuals concerned.

The three peacetime chapters draw attention to the variety and range of health issues that result from human rights violations occurring in our every-day lives. We begin with an chapter by Aart Hendriks that considers the impact of differentiation and discrimination on the rights and health of disabled persons. Then, using a human rights analysis, the Center for Economic and Social Rights describes the effects on the health of indigenous populations and on the environment of untreated toxic waste released by transnational corporations into the Ecuadorian Amazon. Finally, the chap-ter by Lynn Freedman, drawn from the introduction to a human rights report, illustrates the severe impact that violations of the right to informa-tion can have on women's health and women's lives.

From Solferino to Sarajevo   7.

Alain Destexhe

Politicians, soldiers, diplomats, intellectuals, and artists all belong to the cult of humanitarianism, which, following the proclaimed end of ideologies, is being gradually exalted into a new utopia. However, behind this consensual façade, while public aid has become an important element of the Western response to contemporary tragedies, numerous voices are questioning the role of humanitarian aid in conflict situtations. Could it be but a cover for political impotence? Does it needlessly draw out conflicts at the cost of thousands of additional victims? Other, older questions reemerged on the occasion of the Somalia intervention: are these "new barbarians" truly capable of governing themselves? Would it not be better to leave them to their wretched fate (to their "savagery"), or to place their country under international trusteeship in their best interest?

None of these questions is really new, even if media infatuation with humanitarian action and the emerging international context have renewed their poignancy. Humanitarian agents who act in conflicts, thereby changing their course, or who confront governments and ruthless totalitarian parties have always faced a recurring question: how to help the victims without playing into the hands of the oppressors? Or, in the words of W. Shawcross, how to nourish the victims without overfeeding the executioners? How to keep humanitarian aid from contributing to aggravation of the victims' fate rather than to their relief?

Using a few historical anchors, this chapter seeks to examine how humanitarian action responds to those questions.

BEFORE THE RED CROSS

Before the creation of the Red Cross, a specific international humanitarian framework did not exist. With a few exceptions, humanitarian aid was limited to a nation's own territory and, sometimes, to its colonies. During the eighteenth and nineteenth centuries, nonetheless, numerous wars and natural disasters led to a combination of private and public efforts to assist victims.

The modern concept of humanity emerged from the philosophers of the Enlightenment, who stated that all men are equal in rights and members of a universal community. Humanitarianism thus became the modern, rational form of charity and justice. In the eighteenth century, in his *Memorandum for Perpetual Peace in Europe*, Abbot Saint-Pierre proposed the creation of an organization of united nations. As for the "savage peoples," it was the "philanthropic mission" of enlightened men to bring them out of darkness. By the next century, however, this generous conception of the Enlightenment had become tainted with racism; for Jules Ferry, "the superior races have the right and duty to civilize the inferior races."[1] The colonial conquest was to be carried out under the banner of humanitarianism and civilization.

While dominated by the surge of nationalism, the international order of the nineteenth century witnessed the birth of a legal category that infringed on the principle of sovereignty: "humanitarian intervention." At the time of the Concert of Europe, sovereign states felt offended when Europeans or certain communities were threatened. At that time, legal interventions against "governments that violate the rights of humanity through excessive injustice and cruelty . . . in defiance of the laws of civilization" were considered legitimate when "the general interest of humanity is jeopardized by barbarians or a despotic government." The legal framework for these interventions was relatively well defined: the reality needed to be particularly atrocious, the strict objective of the intervention had to be to end the suffering of the victims, and it needed to be carried out on behalf of the international community. The humanitarian motive then justified the exception to the principle of sovereignty.[2]

This discourse, while tainted with racist statements, is somewhat similar to that used recently to justify intervention in Somalia. Today, of course, such interventions are no longer driven by powerful political or economic interests. The West would rather forget that Africa exists, and nobody pretends any longer to "civilize barbarians." Nevertheless, when directed toward peoples considered inferior, humanitarianism elevated to the rank of ideology reveals its profound ambivalence:

> In the humanitarian relation, the power one holds over the other is absolute. It is this which allows the immediate transformation of the life machine into a death machine, and vice versa. . . . For the master, the punishment is inseparable from the gift. The providential function of the humanitarian ideology is profoundly ambiguous, as only Providence, as its name indicates, has the transcendental power to feed and to kill, to lose and to save, to starve and to nurse, to destroy and to uplift.[3]

In the nineteenth century, with its faith in continued progress and the blessings of economic liberalism, the terrible Irish famine (1845–1850) occurred. The dominant ideology of the era further aggravated the fate of the victims: the liberal discourse was put forward, in total good faith, to justify the refusal to act; food should not be distributed to the hungry, since this would disturb the free play of the market, whereas it was thought the market would soon end the disaster thanks to the simple mechanism of supply and demand! The scarce relief offered to the hungry was construed as the main problem. This ideology overlooked the simple fact that human response to tragedy cannot wait for supply-and-demand adjustments to occur. During the famine, more than a million Irish died of starvation, and another million emigrated to the United States. Adam Smith's liberalism offered no relief to the hungry.

The press played only a marginal role in the famine. However, newspaper circulation exploded in the second half of the nineteenth century, and the invention of the telegraph enabled editorial offices and war correspondents to be in touch. Circa 1885, Gustave Moynier, president of the Red Cross, wrote: "Every day now, we know what happens in the entire world; information on any war development travels at the speed of lightning . . . bringing those dying on the battlefield under the eyes of the readers."[4] The Crimean War saw the emergence of a troublesome but inseparable couple: the press and humanitarian aid. Thanks to newspaper coverage, the British public discovered the sad fate of its soldiers: for each soldier killed by bullets, seven perished due to illness (especially cholera). In the hospitals, mortality reached 39 percent per month. The government was forced to take energetic measures aimed at fighting the epidemics. During the last six months of the campaign, after the French government had imposed rigorous censorship of the press, mortality among French soldiers became ten times higher than for British soldiers, even though both groups lived under the same conditions.

THE RED CROSS AND THE DILEMMAS OF NEUTRALITY

In 1859, having arrived almost by chance on the battlefields of Solferino, where Napoleon III was confronting the Austrians, Henry Dunant proceeded to define the principles of an institution that outlived him. The first Geneva Convention and the creation of the Red Cross constitute a landmark in the history of humanitarian action. First, the principle of neutrality was inscribed in an international convention with wide recognition. Second, the Geneva Committee gradually became an impartial organ universally recognized as such. Finally, the Red Cross underwent an extraordinary expansion and, with its three components—national Red Cross offices, the International Federation of Red Cross and Red Crescent Societies (FRC/RCS), and above all, the International Committee (ICRC) in Geneva—it constitutes today the oldest humanitarian movement in the world.

Neutrality was not invented by Dunant. Since ancient times there have been numerous examples of neutral conduct in conflicts, and of bilateral agreements aimed at respecting civilians, the injured, and prisoners. The genius of Dunant, however, was in stating this principle in a convention that he hoped would be, and which ended up being, universal. The four Geneva Conventions, signed in 1949, have been ratified by over 170 countries—the quasi-totality of nations. The Red Cross stands for charity supported by law and for the will to force belligerents to respect, even in the heart of war, certain elementary rules with regard to the injured, prisoners, and civilians.

Despite such undeniable progress, the principles of the Red Cross have from the beginning raised questions that remain relevant today. What does neutrality mean if these principles apply only to battles between European armies and become null and void when white men attack "barbarian peoples" in the name of civilization? In the Sudan in 1898, thirty years after signing the first Geneva Convention, the British did nothing to help fifteen thousand wounded Sudanese, abandoning them after the battle of Omdurman. And what does neutrality mean in the face of a war of aggression or a systematic genocide like that which happened in Armenia? Chateaubriand had already remarked on this: "When the warring parties are unequal in power, this neutrality is nothing but a derision, an act of hostility toward the weaker party and of complicity with the stronger one. It would be better to join forces with the oppressor against the oppressed, because then at least hypocrisy would not be added to injustice."

Moreover, even though the Red Cross is a private institution, it has always put itself in the hands of states, if only to allow for the enforcement of humanitarian law. Consequently, it has had to remain silent so as not to embarrass signatory states. Discretion has been the hallmark of the "Red Cross spirit." And in their respective countries, the Red Cross Societies, far from being apolitical or neutral, have in fact become devoted auxiliaries to the government.

The Red Cross developed at the time of triumphant liberalism. With Lenin, and even more so with Hitler, it was confronted with régimes that rejected the values upon which it was founded. Between respect for its principles and preserving the universality of the movement, the Red Cross has always chosen universalism because it was convinced—and not without reason—that this was the only way to continue to act as a neutral intermediary in the heart of conflict. It never burned its bridges, neither with Lenin, nor with Mussolini, nor with Nazi Germany, even when Jews were thrown out of the German Red Cross.

Thus it was confrontation with the "final solution" that clearly showed the limits of humanitarian action. Like the Allies, the Vatican, and others, the Red Cross knew of the terrible reality of Nazi extermination camps. Today it is reproached for not having denounced their existence and for its silence in the face of the largest genocide of the twentieth century. What is worse, it sought, despite everything, to help the deportees by giving German authorities care packages for the Jewish camp prisoners. Whatever the reasons brought forward to justify this silence, this chapter remains the darkest of the Red Cross's history—especially because it obscured ICRC's role in other areas, such as with prisoners of war and search agencies. Later organizations such as Médecins Sans Frontières (MSF) drew on this lesson: The inhuman is not to be humanized, it is to be denounced and opposed. For them, speaking out will occupy a central place, side by side with action.

1945–1979: THE REVOLUTION AGAINST HUMANITARIAN ACTION

The period 1945 to 1979 marked the intellectual discrediting of humanitarian action. Similar to British liberals in the last century who viewed free market mechanisms as the remedy for the Irish famine, progressive intellectuals, for whom one was either the oppressor or the oppressed, affirmed that all energy must be devoted to the world revolution. From the perspective of the Manichean confrontation that divided the world, humanitarian aid was considered at best a waste of time. In *Esprit*, Bertrand d'Atorg criticized Camus's *The Plague*: "The ethics of the Red Cross are solely valid in a world where violence against mankind comes only from eruptions, floods, crickets or rats. And not from men." Sartre, in *Les temps modernes*, gave Camus a final blow: "We are closer to Madame Boucicaut and the giving of alms."[5] Neither the drama of East Pakistan nor that of Biafra—the latter the first televised famine in history (1968–1970)—succeeded in shaking these certainties. The democratic opposition of the Awami League in Bangladesh and the Ojukwu régime in Biafra certainly did not incarnate the "forces of progress."

The Biafra crisis was a milestone in the evolution of the humanitarian movement. On one hand, it once again underscored the limits of the Red Cross approach. Despite the force of its neutrality, the Red Cross did not manage to obtain an agreement between the two parties to allow passage of food to the encircled Biafran enclave. It was a group of churches that ultimately decided, against the objections of Nigeria and the Red Cross, to launch an airlift to help secessionist Biafra in defiance of Nigerian sovereignty. In doing so, these precursors of MSF invented the modern concept of humanitarian intervention.

The Western powers played the humanitarian card without looking for a political solution. France, for example, openly encouraged Biafra's secession without recognizing the Ojukwu government or supplying the arms needed to compete with Lagos. One major, perverse consequence was that Biafra quickly understood that images of Biafran children remained its best weapon to bring about international mobilization. Ultimately, humanitarian aid, derisive given the magnitude of the disaster, maintained the illusion of international commitment—the world was convinced that it flew to the rescue of Biafra. Already, TV images were stronger than reality.

1979–1989: THE ZENITH OF THE "WITHOUT BORDERS" MOVEMENT

In the late 1970s and early 1980s, with the combined effects of the work of Solzhenitsyn, the invasion of Afghanistan, developments in Vietnam (including the drama of the boat people), and the discovery of the crimes of the Khmer Rouge, a veritable intellectual turnabout took place. The great cause of the 1980s became the fight against totalitarianism. The dynamic of democracy versus totalitarianism supplanted the antagonism between capitalism and socialism. Guerrilla forces lent themselves very well to the actions of organizations "without borders," by intervening secretly in most conflicts in defiance of international law and haughty sovereignties. Unlike the Red Cross, they were not founded on humanitarian law but on public opinion, which they wanted to be their witness.

Since the majority of great causes in the 1980s were linked to the advance of Soviet allies in the Third World, humanitarian aid became, consciously or not, an important instrument of the antitotalitarian struggle. Therefore, humanitarian action took place either in countries in which the Cold War was fought by proxy and in which only organizations "without borders" could penetrate, or at the borders of these countries in refugee camps that also then served as sanctuaries for guerrilla fighters.[6] More than 90 percent of refugees in this period fled from régimes allied with the Soviet Union. The United Nations High Commissioner for Refugees became one of the most important agencies of the humanitarian aid system, and the image of refugees "who vote with their feet" acquired a positive connotation.[7]

The greatest catastrophe of this period, the Ethiopian famine, again underscored the limits of humanitarian aid. In Colonel Mengistu's Ethiopia, international aid meant to relieve the famine was used—directly or indirectly—to finance massive displacement of peoples from the north to the south; humanitarian organizations were used as bait to attract starving farmers who were then deported to the south. Thousands of human lives were saved, but the entire international system was used, often with the support of the UN, for the execution of a project aimed at crushing the Ethiopian peasantry. Relief agencies found themselves caught in a now classic dilemma—to remain silent at the risk of becoming the accomplice of an inhuman process in which they were one of the cogs, or to speak out at the risk of expulsion and abandonment of those they had come to save. By seeing only the malnourished children in the dispensaries, and not recognizing that the entire system of international relief had been placed in the service of a project that flagrantly violated the most elementary of human principles, humanitarian organizations unwittingly were condemned to support this process.[8]

BOSNIA: HUMANITARIAN AID TURNED AGAINST THE VICTIMS?

The end of Soviet Communism and the evolution of international relations have profoundly changed the work of humanitarian organizations. The image of the refugee is now a negative one; the UN as well as certain states have turned humanitarian aid into a powerful tool of their diplomacy. Blue helmets, once ordered to keep the peace, now intervene with a humanitarian mandate, erasing the points of reference needed by belligerents and perpetuating uncertainty as to the real intentions of the parties involved.[9]

More troublesome, progress that had been made in the preceding period could now be turned against the victims. At the end of the 1970s, when victims finally ceased to be viewed as oppressed people waiting to be liberated (or as "collateral damage" of the revolution in progress), humanity no doubt made a small step forward. The Nicaraguan farmer fleeing Sandinista authoritarianism was finally put on equal footing with the Salvadoran peasant living in fear of the death squads; there were no more good and bad deaths, only victims worthy of compassion. The theme "all victims are equal" gave birth to an "ethic of emergency" that gradually imposed itself on the humanitarian movement. But it was too quickly forgotten that values flouted during the cold war coincided with those imposed by *realpolitik*: this ethic of indignation furnished a powerful tool for dismantling the logic of totalitarianism and denouncing the crimes of Soviet lackeys. From Afghanistan to Angola, from Nicaragua to Cambodia, no major Western power limited itself to the humanitarian realm to combat the Soviets, Cubans, or Vietnamese: political or military action was the principle element of a strategy of containment in which humanitarian action played only a modest role.

In the former Yugoslavia, this ethic of emergency turned against the Bosnians—they were no longer citizens fighting for values, but victims to be fed. They were not granted the right to decide whether they preferred weapons to defend themselves or humanitarian aid—it was decided for them. Humanitarian relief was the only somewhat consistent response by Europe to Serb aggression. It was a clear windfall for the aggressor, particularly in view of the fact that the humanitarian apparatus, in its laudable endeavors to protect the population, accelerated the process of ethnic cleansing. The blue helmets, symbols of international impotence in the field, became a cover for refusal to take any military action which could endanger them.

This is not meant to belittle the efforts, courage and devotion of all those (e.g., the Federation of Red Cross and Red Crescent Societies, ICRC, NGOs, blue helmets) who have earnestly sought to help people, but rather to note that humanitarian aid, as official policy, has ultimately encouraged and favored aggression. Moreover, it has contributed to public opinion resigning itself to a "tribal" reading of conflicts. The result is well known: hundreds of thousands of dead and injured, and four million displaced individuals and families. In the process, the European unification process was threatened, the new world order buried, and the essence of law ridiculed. "We wanted law without force, we got force without law."[10]

Today, the gap is immense between the principles and values posted on every street corner and the actions undertaken to defend them. As a result, societies end up congratulating themselves on the progress of a mythical right of interference, all the while tolerating ethnic cleansing. Apartheid, dismantled in South Africa, has been restored within Europe's borders with the blessing and encouragement of the UN.

Yesterday as today, humanitarian aid represents human nobility when it seeks to help the victims, then recognizes as human beings those who aspire to their own destinies. When, in the name of humanitarian aid, the international community prevents people from defending themselves, when it attempts to feed them almost against their will, it burdens them even more and becomes an accomplice to the crime of nonassistance to an endangered person.[11] Or in other words, to pass food through the window without evicting the killer from the house is not a humanitarian gesture.

In a peculiar swing of the pendulum of history, in the quarrel that opposed Sartre and his followers to Camus, it would probably be admitted today that the former were right. Camus, for whom revolt constituted the very meaning of life, "the refusal to be treated as object," might agree. But he would add: "Human solidarity is founded on the movement of revolt, which in turn finds its only legitimation in this complicity. Thus, we can rightfully say that any revolt that allows itself to destroy this solidarity by this very fact loses the name of revolt and consents to murder." We are there. In Bosnia, a perverse conception of humanitarian aid has triumphed over politics. And it is not certain that this will be to the benefit of the victims.

REFERENCES

1. Jules Ferry, quoted in Raoul Girardet, *Le nationalisme français* (Paris: Points Seuil, 1983).

2. Rougier states: "To the sovereignty of a government capable of disregarding the human rights of its citizens is substituted a foreign sovereignty to carry out this neglected task, annul the vitiated deed, or prevent future defaults." A. Rougier, *La Théorie de l'intervention d'humanité* (Paris: RGDIP, 1910).

3. H. Béji, "Le patrimoine de la cruauté," *Le Débat* 73 (1993).

4. Gustave Moynier, *Les causes du succès de la Croix-Rouge* (Paris: Académie des sciences morales et politiques, 1899).

5. *Editor's note:* Madame Boucicaut was a prominent personality of the nineteenth century who personified a charitable, perhaps condescending, attitude toward the poor and the sick.

6. J. C. Rufin, *Le piège: Quand l'aide humanitaire remplace la guerre* (Paris: Pluriel, 1993).

7. F. Jean, "Le fantôme des réfugiés," *Esprit*, Dec. 1992; and F. Jean, "Réfugiés de guerre: Un défi pour l'Occident," *Politique internationale* 60 (1993).

8. F. Jean, "Du Bon Usage de la famine," *Médecins Sans Frontières*, 1986; and see also J. Clay and B. Holcomb, "Politics and Famine in Ethiopia," Cultural Survival, report no. 20 (Cambridge, MA: November 1995). See also "West's Live Aid Digs Graves in Ethiopia," *The Wall Street Journal*, June 24, 1986; "Does Helping Really Help?" *Newsweek*, December 21, 1987.

9. R. Brauman, "Contre l'humanitarisme," *Esprit*, Oct. 1991; A. Destexhe, *L'humanitaire impossible ou deux siècles d'ambiguïté* (Paris: Armand Colin, 1993).

10. J. F. Deniau in *Le Monde*.

11. On different occasions, the Bosnian rulers stated that if they had to choose between humanitarian aid and weapons (or simply lifting the embargo), they would prefer the latter.

Ethnic Cleansing and Other Lies: 8.
Combining Health and Human Rights
in the Search for Truth and Justice
in the Former Yugoslavia

Alicia Ely Yamin

> I refuse to accept the idea that mankind is so tragically bound to the starless
> midnight of racism and war that the bright daybreak of peace and brotherhood
> can never become a reality. . . . I believe that even amid today's mortar bursts
> and whining bullets, there is still hope for a brighter tomorrow. I believe that
> wounded justice, lying prostrate on the blood-flowing streets of our nations, can
> be lifted from this dust of shame to reign supreme among the children of man.
>
> —Martin Luther King Jr.

In embracing the idea that human beings possess inalienable rights by virtue
of their unique capacities of reason and conscience, international human
rights instruments reflect a rationalist and fundamentally modernist philosophy.[1] Indeed, human rights may be the last modernist social movement in
an increasingly postmodern world in which post–cold war promises of a new
world order have too often become phantasmagoric refractions of night-
marish disorder and mass dystopias. Part, if not the core, of the modernist
underpinnings of human rights is an unwavering belief in the existence of an
ascertainable truth that cannot be decoupled from justice.

Even though the world has been hearing and seeing images of the practice of "ethnic cleansing" for nearly five years, nowhere more than in the
former Yugoslavia is there a greater challenge to the possibility for uncovering or constructing a just truth, let alone one that can coexist with peace.[2]
Along with ground combat, a war of words and information has been and
continues to be waged in that region, through which stories, histories, and
myths have been conflated, intertwined, and fragmented. This has left many
analysts and observers to wonder whether the world is caught in a dialectic
of enlightenment and denial—a labyrinth of mirrors—in which the revela-
tion of enlightenment itself becomes myth.[3]

Establishment of the International Criminal Tribunal for the former Yugoslavia reflects the human rights movement's commitment to the idea that not only can there not be justice without truth, but also that notions of justice must inform the process of extracting truth from the many stories, myths, and lies that have been told about ethnic cleansing. The way in which the tribunal conducts its work will be critical not only to revealing that truth—or, more accurately, the many truths—but also to legitimating the premises upon which international humanitarian and human rights law rests.

As a field emerging from its own social movement, public health shares the human rights movement's faith in the possibility of progressive improvement of the human condition. As a field drawing together various medical and scientific disciplines, public health brings to bear pragmatic strategies for identification and characterization of truth. This chapter argues that infusing the normative analysis of human rights with the practical, quantitative methods of public health can potentially provide the most powerful mechanism for establishing truth and concomitant accountability for ethnic cleansing. But just as claims to truth asserted by human rights principles remain in the realm of empty rumor without the substantive evidence that public health can provide, the methods of public health require the framework of human rights (in which the premises of ethnic cleansing are construed as pathological) in order to fulfill their underlying promise.

In the context of the tribunal's work, this chapter suggests that there are three dimensions to the relation between public health and human rights in the construction of truth. First, most attention has been paid to the use of clinical and forensic evidence in documenting abuses, in showing whether something—something awful labeled ethnic cleansing and now being denied and covered up—actually occurred. Second, public health has a larger role to play in the tribunal's work, in that its methodology can show us what happened and what ethnic cleansing means. Specifically, epidemiology—with its strategies for systematic collection, consolidation, and evaluation of relevant data—can help define a given violation as a crime cognizable under international humanitarian law, as well as the nature and scope of the harm ensuing from that crime. Third, using the normative understanding of the human condition provided by human rights, public health methods can be used to answer the largest question of all: how could the ethnic cleansing have occurred? In so doing, the combination of human rights concepts and public health tools may point us toward comprehending the premises of ethnic cleansing in the former Yugoslavia and ethnic strife in general.

DISCOVERING TRUTHS

For the first time since the Nuremberg and Far East trials following World War II, in February 1993 the United Nations Security Council agreed to establish an international tribunal to investigate and prosecute war crimes committed in the former Yugoslavia; the tribunal's statute was adopted in May of that year.[4] Significantly, the tribunal was established not pursuant to a separate convention but directly under Chapter VII of the United Nations Charter which is also used to authorize peacekeeping missions. Consequently, the tribunal's creation was not a question of voluntary accession to jurisdiction but rather part of charter-based law. Further, the connection between accountability and justice, on one hand, and peace and international stability, on the other, was established from the outset. In fact, the Secretary General's report, adopted by the Security Council together with the tribunal's statute, announced as its purpose, to "contribute to the restoration and maintenance of peace."[5] By characterizing the tribunal in this way, the Security Council explicitly rejected the view that attempting to hold violators of international humanitarian law individually accountable might intensify the fighting of warring factions. Indeed, the Secretary General's report implicitly accepts the notion that accountability may act as a deterrent even in ongoing conflict.[6]

That twofold purpose—the retributive justice notion of accountability and punishment, together with the deterrence of future international outlaws—has been keenly reflected in the documentation work that public health professionals have already contributed to the work of the tribunal. Physicians and forensic professionals have been devoted largely to gathering evidence of human rights violations and in pointing out the differences between international human rights and humanitarian law, as codified in international human rights instruments and the 1949 Geneva Conventions respectively, and the practice of ethnic cleansing, as evidenced by battered bodies and broken corpses. In short, health professionals have been summoned to the former Yugoslavia to provide the basis—both through forensic and clinical examinations—upon which to choose between two competing truths: either to confirm or to deny the claims of ethnic cleansing. The forensic or clinical evidence is either found or is not. The focus is always on the study of concrete, *observable* evidence and irrefutable facts.

Forensic Evidence

To this day, thousands of people remain missing or unaccounted for around the former UN "safe haven" of Srebrenica in eastern Bosnia, overtaken by Bosnian Serb forces in July 1995, as well as in other parts of Bosnia-Herzegovina. Indeed, the practice of ethnic cleansing in the former Yugoslavia has, according to conservative estimates, resulted in several thousand disappeared people.[7] Forced disappearance is perhaps the ultimate eradication of truth, in that it simultaneously negates both the life and death of a human being, thereby denying relatives and friends of the disappeared even the possibility for grief.[8] In the face of this phenomenon, forensics has proven one of the most effective means of recuperating the truths eradicated by disappearances. As a forensic anthropologist noted: "When we put the bones together, it's a person with a story to tell, no longer a jumble of bones. . . . Our mission is to get the truth."[9] Indeed, excavation of mass graves by international teams of forensic anthropologists and pathologists, who meticulously reconstruct shattered bones and skulls and record marks left by massacres, has already provided invaluable evidence for the tribunal.[10]

Investigation of mass graves usually involves fastidious removal of small and fragile items such as teeth, bullets, and scraps of cloth from the bodies. When excavations are done properly, these clues can identify the types of victims: elderly, women, children, or infants. This evidence can also determine the cause of death, or at least indicate whether the victims died in combat, which is often the allegation of accused perpetrators.[11] Careful documentation of execution-style bullet wounds and bodies lined up in mass graves provides evidence of systematic murder that is impossible to refute. Analyzing the remains of plants and insects found in the graves then helps to establish a time of death.

Other forensic work must be performed in a laboratory, where the skeleton is examined and any dental and medical X rays taken before death can be compared with those taken after death. DNA is then placed under a microscope for more precise personal identification. Discussing this innovative work, pathologist Dr. Robert Kirschner, who has led teams of pathologists in Rwanda and the former Yugoslavia on behalf of the Boston-based nongovernmental organization Physicians for Human Rights (PHR), explains that until forensic work was introduced, virtually all human rights work "involved witness statement and testimony [that,] while powerful, are subject to another person saying 'it didn't happen that way' or 'this person isn't telling the truth.' What we showed . . . is that you could provide physical, irrefutable evidence of what has happened to someone."[12]

In practice, what happens is that witnesses identify the site of a potential mass grave and pathologists, archaeologists and anthropologists proceed to exhume bodies. For example, Kirschner, and Kari Hannibal of PHR recount the story of the Vukovar excavation in Croatia:

> When Vukovar was under siege by Serbian forces, it was agreed that some 420 Croatian patients at the hospital would be evacuated to Croatian-held territory. . . . Witnesses saw the patients being taken away from the hospital by Serbian soldiers and transported to a garage in Ovcara where they were beaten. They also saw vans loaded with about 20 patients each being driven away from the garage and returning 15 to 20 minutes later empty. Investigators of the fate of patients at this hospital had a list of 180 Croatian patients and 30 staff members who were in the hospital at the time and who were unaccounted for.[13]

Kirschner and Hannibal go on to detail how a preliminary investigation of the gravesite in December 1992 determined that a mass execution had taken place, with up to two hundred bodies buried there: "The pattern of spent metal casings of machine gun bullets and the location of the bodies revealed how the executions had been carried out."[14] Over the course of the next three years, PHR sent (and will continue to send) teams of forensic scientists to the Croatian site to excavate the grave and to identify the victims as patients from the Vukovar hospital.

A great risk to forensic work in particular is the destruction of the evidence. For example, as in many conflicts, after the existence of a particular concentration camp or mass grave became known to international investigators, those responsible have attempted to destroy the evidence. The Vukovar gravesite was first discovered in October 1992; the site was guarded initially by Russian soldiers attached to the United Nations Protection Forces, and subsequently by soldiers from the Implementation Forces.[15] Kirschner recalls an unfortunate incident in Bosnia in 1993: "After much touch-and-go negotiation between the warring factions, the UN had received approval for the exhumation ... which is in UN-controlled territory but surrounded by Serbian strongholds. The digging never began. At the last minute, the Serbian government pulled back on the agreement and threatened physical force if we continued ... so we couldn't do that exhumation."[16] The converse of that danger, however, is that this truth-finding is indeed the most objective work that health professionals can perform because the truth is literally evidenced by bones and bodies. That is, once access has been provided, forensic documentation can provide evidence of an abuse or atrocity.

Clinical Documentation

Not all medical documentation done on behalf of the tribunal, or independently by NGOs, has been forensic. Indeed, the ability of medical professionals to provide virtually irrefutable indicia of violations that have resulted from ethnic cleansing has been widely espoused in the former Yugoslavia. For example, Jeffrey Sonis and Thomas Crane argue that physicians are "uniquely capable of collecting physical evidence of abuse through physical examination, laboratory testing, and collection of specimens for pathological examination. Physical evidence of abuse is much harder to refute than even the best verbal testimony."[17] Again, there is the sense that clinical documentation provides *objective* truth in the midst of the difficult and controversial situations in which abuses of human rights occur.

A prominent example of the use of clinical documentation in conflict in the former Yugoslavia exists in the important recognition of rape as a crime of war. An enormous amount of energy has been devoted to documentation of rape in the Bosnian Serb concentration camps. Swiss and Giller have noted that, in conjunction with this effort, health professionals are in a "unique position to recognize and document individual incidents of rape in war [and it is] important for health workers to be aware of common physical findings following rape, such as signs of violence to the genitalia ... bruising on the arms and chest, and other evidence of the use of force."[18] Thus, physicians and health professionals more broadly can bring to bear their experience in diagnosis to provide evidence that is more compelling than anecdotal accounts traditionally used by human rights fact-finders attesting that abuses such as rape occurred.

With respect to rape in particular, Swiss and Giller argue that methods developed in criminal prosecutions in the United States can be used to provide the same sort of irrefutable evidence of violations as the forensic work provides of murder:

> In countries at war, for women who are able to seek gynecologic help within a day or two of being raped (although most do not or are not able to), sperm collected from the genital tract could be dried on a microscope slide and stored for later analysis. For those women who become pregnant as a result of rape, placental tissue (following abortions or delivery) could be frozen and preserved for future testing. . . . Matching of DNA or human lymphocyte antigen protein markers from such specimens can help determine paternity even many years later, using blood samples or hair follicles from the alleged perpetrator.[19]

While perhaps somewhat utopian in their assessment of the resources and abilities of health workers to operate in times and zones of conflict, Swiss and Giller make it clear that medical documentation of the immediate physical sequelae of rape can be an important part of documenting one form of violation that has constituted a method of ethnic cleansing in the former Yugoslavia.

In sum, the focus of the health work done during the conflict and immediate after the conflict in the former Yugoslavia has been devoted to the question of whether alleged abuses such as murder and rape actually occurred and, in practice, to substantiating the instances in which they did occur. Inherently ex post facto, this documentation work has the dual aim of providing a basis for accountability and justice and of deterring others who believe that such atrocities can go undetected. Indeed, the theory behind much forensic work is that even when physicians or health professionals cannot heal, they must maintain respect for the dead in order to have respect for the living. In both the documentation of deaths through forensic evidence and the documentation of clinical sequelae of aspects of ethnic cleansing, finding "the truth" has been constructed as a matter of choosing between dichotomous realities.

DEFINING TRUTHS

As critical as the forensic and clinical documentation of abuses are to the work of the tribunal, documentation cannot tell the whole story of what happened in the former Yugoslavia or of the policy known euphemistically as ethnic cleansing. That is, in addition to uncovering the manifestations of the abuses, there is a need to interpret the meaning of that physical evidence. A Bosnian friend of mine who worked as an emergency medicine doctor with the Institute of Public Health in Sarajevo while it was under siege asks me often, "Why do they call it ethnic cleansing? What Karadzic, Mladic, Milosevic did—that was genocide."[20] Language is the medium through which reality is created. Far from being a semantic matter, what an act or event is called determines *what it is*. The corollary of that insight is that one who has the power to name what an act or event is has the power to define it. Thus, there is a need both to define the nature of the injury manifested most immediately in certain physical sequelae and to define the crime within the framework of international human rights and humanitarian law.

The practice of ethnic cleansing, while ill-defined by the media and in general discourse, has generally been deemed by scholars and commentators to include harassment, discrimination, beatings, torture, summary executions, expulsion, forced crossing of the lines between combatants, intimidation, destruction of secular and religious property, mass and systematic rape, arbitrary arrests and executions, deliberate military attacks on civilians and civilian property, use of siege, and cutting off essential supplies destined for civilian populations.[21] But ethnic cleansing is not a cognizable act or event under international law. Theodor Meron writes, "Many of these methods [of ethnic cleansing] considered in isolation, constitute a war crime or a grave breach. Considered as a cluster of violations, these practices also constitute crimes against humanity and perhaps also crimes under the Genocide Convention."[22]

Although what I suggest is clearly a less neutral role for public health professionals than the recording of sequelae of abuses, I argue that the way violations of human dignity are prosecuted through the intricate maze of international norms and procedures makes it imperative that public health tools be summoned to define certain critical factors: first, the crime with which the perpetrators are charged, and second, the nature of the violation of human dignity that underlies the crime. That is, viewing the health consequences of ethnic cleansing as pathology permits the use of epidemiology to quantify the occurrence of that pathology in a systematic fashion, a method less subject to political manipulation than anecdotal argument.[23] Moreover, the ability of public health strategies—as opposed to pure clinical practice—to take into account the psychosocial and explicitly societal dimensions of the pathologies induced by ethnic cleansing are indispensable to an understanding of the nature of the injury, as well as to facilitate healing.

Defining the Crime

The tribunal's jurisdiction includes war crimes, crimes against humanity, and genocide (which is often construed as a particular form of crime against humanity). The importance of how a crime is defined cannot be overestimated because of the constraints on situations in which perpetrators can be held accountable, where jurisdiction can be established, and where the precedential value of a culpability finding can be determined.[24] In the first instance, war crimes, which are governed by humanitarian law, apply principally to international wars. For example, the 1907 Fourth Hague Convention, which provided the basis for the post–World War II prosecutions, and the "grave breaches" provisions of the Geneva Conventions and of Protocol I apply only to international conflicts between sovereign states.[25] By enumerating the offenses of grave breaches of the Geneva Conventions and the violations of the laws or customs of war, in Articles II and III of the tribunal's statute, the Security Council implicitly characterized at least part of the conflict in the former Yugoslavia as international.

Although the morality and even the health consequences of the actions may be the same, it is nevertheless critical from a legal standpoint to understand the significance of the distinction.[26] Grave breaches and crimes against humanity give rise to so-called universal jurisdiction, which permits any state to prosecute a suspect.[27] Moreover, violations committed before or after the full-scale conflict are not subject to the "grave breaches" provisions or to international humanitarian law at all and would have to be prosecuted as crimes against humanity in order to give rise to universal jurisdiction. Given the impossibility of apprehending and prosecuting all of the perpetrators of ethnic cleansing, it is clearly desirable to characterize the charges as those giving rise to universal jurisdiction.[28]

Furthermore, assuming that the facts support such prosecution, there is tremendous precedential as well as symbolic value to demonstrating that acts implicated in ethnic cleansing constitute "crimes against humanity"—and, as such, affront and threaten human dignity everywhere, as opposed to being just isolated abuses or breaches of the laws and customs of war. Indeed, in consideration of their special significance, crimes against humanity are considered *jus cogens*, or peremptory norms, of international law.[29] "Crimes against humanity" were first defined in Article VI of the Nuremberg Charter as "murder, extermination, enslavement, deportation and other inhumane acts committed against any civilian population, before or during war, or persecution on political, racial or religious grounds . . . whether or not in violation of the domestic law of the country where perpetrated."[30] Article V of the tribunal's statute explicitly adds imprisonment, torture, and rape. The Nuremberg jurisprudence suggests that war crimes, if committed in a widespread, systematic manner on political, racial, or religious grounds, may also amount to crimes against humanity.[31] Conversely however, proof of systematic governmental planning of alleged acts has been deemed a necessary element of crimes against humanity, which therefore makes them more difficult to establish than war crimes.[32] Meron observes, "The acquisition of facts supporting policy planning, mass character and command responsibility may present evidentiary hurdles to possible prosecutions [for crimes against humanity]."[33]

Thus, returning to the example of rape, the second dimension of the truth-seeking collaboration between public health and human rights involves a determination of whether the rapes were carried out as individual acts, war crimes, or even as part of a systematic policy of ethnic cleansing that would give rise to culpability for crimes against humanity. Rape was neither mentioned in the Nuremberg Charter nor prosecuted in Nuremberg as a war crime under customary international law.[34] Nevertheless, rape was prosecuted in Tokyo as a war crime and, even more to the point, the International Committee of the Red Cross has specifically declared that the grave breach of "willfully causing great suffering or serious injury to body or health" under Article 147 of the Fourth Geneva Convention covers rape.[35] Meron suggests that in addition to evidence of rape as a war crime, rape could be prosecuted as a crime against humanity: "That the practice of rape has been deliberate, massive and egregious, particularly in Bosnia-Herzegovina, is amply demonstrated. . . . The Special Rapporteur appointed by the UN Commission on Human Rights, Tadeusz Mazowiecki, noted the role of rape as a method of ethnic cleansing 'intended to humiliate, shame, degrade and terrify the entire ethnic group.'"[36]

Yet, precisely because evidence of the systematic use of rape as a method of ethnic cleansing has been widely disputed, it is essential for the legitimacy of the prosecutions to use the methods of epidemiology to establish the true dimensions of the practice. Swiss and Giller note that "when the media first focused attention on the rapes in Bosnia, published estimates of the number of rape survivors fluctuated widely from 10,000 to 60,000. In most instances there appeared to be no method for arriving at the stated figures. . . . Unsubstantiated claims risk creating questions about the credibility of the numbers themselves and the scale of human rights violations against women in general."[37] It is essential for the legitimacy of the tribunal's prosecutions as well as for the development of a body of internal criminal law that the truth—meaning valid numbers—be ascertained amidst the propaganda for which rape statistics have been used in the former Yugoslavia.[38]

The use of epidemiological methods to document the distribution of disease and identify clusters of unusual data are uniquely useful in establishing the extent and scale of rape—or any other abuse that is part of ethnic cleansing—as either a series of individual events or as a crime against humanity. Swiss and Giller argue that "using a public health approach, medical personnel can help provide evidence of the scale of these abuses."[39] For example, based on the use of epidemiological methods and statistical modeling, Swiss and Giller estimate that "based on the assumption that one percent of acts of unprotected intercourse result in pregnancy, the identification of 119 pregnancies, therefore, represents some 11,900 rapes."[40] As opposed to human rights workers, who are unaccustomed to (and even uncomfortable with) quantifying violations, public health professionals are uniquely attuned to the need to consider bias in reporting, selection, and diagnostic criteria and to keep in mind strict definitional standards in order to establish valid statistical conclusions.[41] For example, Swiss and Giller detect a general problem of underreporting coupled with potential overreporting by women who had suffered multiple rapes.[42] They clarify that "the goal is not to come up with an exact number, which is impossible, but rather to use medical data to suggest a scale of violations that cannot be determined from individual testimonies alone."[43] That is, evidence of a systematic pattern—which is the critical factor in determining whether rape constituted part of a crime against humanity—is revealed more by the magnitude and extent of violations than by precise figures.

Genocide is even more difficult to prove than the general category of crimes against humanity because it involves the intent to destroy in whole or in part a national, ethnic, racial, or religious group *as such*.[44] That is, even the mass scale of violations is insufficient to demonstrate genocide; the calculated intent to destroy an ethnic or religious group as such must be proven. The Genocide Convention, which is incorporated into and expanded upon in Article IV of the tribunal's statute, defines this to include "killing members of the group . . . causing serious bodily or mental harm to members of the group," and "deliberately inflicting on the group conditions of life calculated to bring about its physical destruction in whole or in part."[45] Meron argues that "The violence in the former Yugoslavia targeted against religious or ethnic groups, especially in cases of mass killing or ethnic cleansing, gives rise to a strong case for genocide."[46] Nevertheless, given the unparalleled gravity of the charge of genocide, it becomes even more essential for the legitimacy of the tribunal's process as well as the substantive human rights law of the Genocide Convention that allegations of genocide be substantiated as credibly and thoroughly as possible.

Again, it is the tools of epidemiology that can be used to interpret the numbers and the distribution of killings based upon the forensic evidence and witness testimonies in order to demonstrate the calculated attempt to destroy an ethnic group as such. Indeed, as "the study of the distribution and determinants of disease frequency in human populations," epidemiology is based on the premise that human pathology does not occur at random, and that pathologies have both causal and preventative factors that are discernible through systematic investigation of different populations or subpopulations in different places or at different times.[47] Thus, public health methodology can be used to place a framework of interpretation around the evidence provided by witness testimonies and forensic work, which only offer evidence that the killings had occurred.

Defining the Harm

If public health methods can be used to ascertain and document the scale of atrocities involved in ethnic cleansing in order to demonstrate a systematic aspect of their commission, the same skills can be used to probe more deeply into the nature of the harm. In this view, both the immediate physical sequelae of ethnic cleansing and its long-term health consequences constitute violations of dignity and rights. As opposed to clinical recording of sequelae, a public health perspective can bring to bear an understanding of the impact of the cluster of violations known as ethnic cleansing on the individual over the long term as well as on communities.

The population-based effects of war crimes, and ethnic cleansing in particular, have received little attention by either the human rights or the medical communities. For example, with respect to rape, Swiss and Giller note, "Despite the fact that rape has always been part of war, little is known about its scale, the circumstances that provoke or aggravate it, or how to prevent it. We know even less about how women heal after the trauma of rape in war and how rape affects the communities in which they live."[48] Clearly, much of the analysis needs to be contextual and sensitive to the relation between perpetrators and victims. For instance, Swiss and Giller have documented how in the former Yugoslavia "dozens of testimonies have revealed that many women knew the names of and often knew personally, the men who raped them."[49] But once again, the methods of public health are ideally suited to attempt to systematically consider and compare across situations how rape in war disrupts—and indeed is used in ethnic cleansing to disrupt—not only individual but also social and community bonds.[50] Thus, the harm done by rape goes far beyond the bruising, lacerations, and other physical sequelae—the victim's entire affective universe can be destroyed. Public health studies in combination with the framework of human rights might be used to redefine the nature of victimization in terms of the family and community, which in turn can create new, nonbiomedical paradigms for treatment and healing.[51]

Such an analysis is equally applicable to the psychiatric health consequences of ethnic cleansing. For example, Weine and colleagues argue that "the psychiatric sequelae of ethnic cleansing include not only traumatic stress symptoms but also responses to the mutilation of identity and core relationships."[52] Mollica and Caspi-Yavin are even more explicit:

> The outer and inner worlds of many of these survivors of genocidal trauma have been shattered. Mass destruction of a community that historically took pride in being a good example of coexistence and tolerance of ethnic and religious differences—a multiethnic community—leaves the individual bereft of a sense of identity and belonging.[53]

It is significant that the terms Mollica and Caspi-Yavin employ suggest that the full nature of the health effects of ethnic cleansing are not easily translated into the biomedical lexicon.

An immediate implication of this insight is that while public health professionals, through use of longitudinal and community-based studies as well as empirical evaluations of torture and rape, can potentially improve understanding of how ethnic cleansing assaults the physical, mental, and social well-being of the individual and the community, that understanding must be mediated through a conceptual framework external to the methods of medicine and perhaps to conventional public health.[54] The normative understanding of human dignity that infuses human rights calls for justice and truth as part of any healing process and would preclude, for example, any strategy that reduces the trauma to affected individuals to biochemical imbalances treatable simply with medication. Indeed, part of the collaboration of public health and human rights in identifying and characterizing the nature of the harm and encoding potential modes of treatment must include examination of the impotence of each to grapple with the meaning of the implications of ethnic cleansing in isolation from the other.

In sum, as Meron argues, "the character and systematic nature of some of the atrocities [in the former Yugoslavia], especially mass murder and ethnic cleansing, make it imperative that appropriate prosecution be based on crimes against humanity and that a precedent be established."[55] As crucial as the clinical and forensic documentation of events or actions is to building cases, it can only begin to tell the story of what happened. But in combination with testimonies and circumstantial evidence, public health expertise in quantification of information can provide invaluable support in proving the scale and systematic nature of certain abuses, such as rape, and thereby defining for the international community, as well as for the tribunal, the nature of the crime that occurred. Moreover, the delineation of immediate health consequences diagnosed by forensic and clinical examinations is just the beginning of determining the nature of the underlying injury to human dignity. Public health methods, designed and implemented through the lens of the core principles of human rights, can and must be used not only to determine truth in the dichotomous sense of whether an event or crime occurred, but also to define the extent of the harm caused from a legal as well as a bio-psycho-social standpoint.

CONSTRUCTING TRUTHS

Even if all of the perpetrators of crimes against humanity and genocide were miraculously indicted, tried, and convicted, the larger question about how the ethnic cleansing could have occurred would remain unanswered. Indeed, the single most enduring and damaging myth that needs to be shattered by the tribunal's prosecutions is that the ethnic cleansing was an inevitable result of ancient hatreds. There are two pieces to this myth: first, that there are qualities inherent to Serbs, Muslims and Croats that made the ethnic nationalisms inevitable; and second, that because of these essential qualities, there is a collective guilt on the part of entire ethnic groups. By contrast, in positing that all individuals are endowed with faculties of reason and conscience, human rights norms reflect a definition of humanity that rejects this collective essentialism and demands individual accountability for the exercise or nonexercise of those faculties.

Thus, if the second dimension of truth-seeking involves defining the nature of the harm in order to place it within a legal framework of human rights and humanitarian law, the third dimension is about defining the nature of identity. Here, instead of a legal framework into which acts of ethnic cleansing can be placed, human rights norms provide an even more fundamental philosophical framework that determines questions about the very nature of accountability and identity. Once again, epidemiology can be used to systematize risk factors for ethnic conflict in a far more powerful way than simply debating sociological or historical theories. Moreover, public health perspectives more generally can change the paradigm of the inevitable misfortune of ethnic cleansing as a simple population exchange gone awry, by thematizing issues of identity formation and the premises used to construct a regime of truth. This is, however, the most politicized and difficult of roles for public health professionals to play in conjunction with the tribunal's work precisely because of the invisibility of this truth, the creation of which is indistinguishable from the formation of identity itself. Indeed, far from the micro-level focus on objective data, public health tools would be engaged in the transformation of consciousness, in constructing a truth that conforms to human rights principles of dignity.

Individualizing Guilt and Examining Dehumanization

As Justice Jackson stated at the Nuremberg Tribunal fifty years ago, "Crimes against international law are committed by men, not by abstract entities, and only by punishing individuals who commit such crimes can the provisions of international law be enforced."[56] By prosecuting individuals in the former Yugoslavia, the International Criminal Tribunal can once again convey the message that individuals must be held accountable for their actions. To a régime of liberal justice, the importance of establishing individual accountability for actions cannot be overstated. Hannah Arendt reminds us that "where all are guilty, no one is."[57] While Arendt was writing about racism, the same reasoning applies even more strongly to ethnicity in the former Yugoslavia: "The real rift between black and white is not healed by being translated into an even less reconcilable conflict between collective innocence and collective guilt."[58] The converse of the understanding that individuals are capable of rational choice and consciousness is the recognition that "ethnic groups" do not possess agency and "ethnic groups" do not commit war crimes or genocide.

Merely the act of prosecuting individuals encodes the understanding that not every Serb was a camp commander, just as not every Croat was a member of the Ustashe. As David Rieff says, "Wars are no simpler than individuals.... Many Serbs behaved loyally and honorably toward their Muslim and Croat friends."[59] Moreover, individual prosecution of the leaders and orchestraters focuses attention not only on the crimes committed—for example, on that portion of the violence committed by Bosnian Serbs against Muslims—but also on the rights of the Serbs themselves. Article 7 of the Universal Declaration of Human Rights states: "All are equal before the law and are entitled without any discrimination to equal protection of the law. All are entitled to equal protection against any discrimination in violation of this Declaration *and against any incitement to such discrimination"* (emphasis added). [60] The orders issued by Bosnian Serb commanders to the Serbs leaving Sarajevo suburbs to burn and loot as they go is an ongoing violation of this right, in turn reflecting a persistent attempt to undermine the possibility for a human rights consciousness in the former Yugoslavia.

If individuals and not peoples commit acts of barbarism, public health can help document the ways in which elite orchestraters coerce the participation of individuals in the violence of ethnic cleansing. For example, Alain Destexhe, former secretary-general of Médecins Sans Frontières, used public health methodology implicitly to analyze the genocide in Rwanda. In the context of Rwanda, Destexhe argued persuasively that "a prerequisite of genocide is effective organization."[61] The same applies to ethnic cleansing in general. Rieff carefully explains how the ethnic cleansing was orchestrated and conducted in Bosnia:

> One common method used was for a group of Serb fighters to enter a village, go to a Serb house, and order the man living there to come to the house of his Muslim neighbor. As the other villagers watched he was marched over and the Muslim brought out. Then the Serb would be handed a Kalashnikov assault rifle or a knife—knives were better—and ordered to kill the Muslim. If he did so, he had taken that step across the line the Chetniks had been aiming for. But if he refused as many did, the solution was simple. You shot him on the spot. Then you repeated the process with the next Serb house-holder.[62]

Rieff observes that it rarely took more than three households before a Serb who had witnessed the previous interactions agreed to participate.

Once an individual crossed that line—performing the irrevocable act of killing another human being and renouncing aspiration to membership in civilized society—inhibition against the next killing was diminished. Thus, loss of the perpetrator's individual identity is dialectically connected to the capacity to dehumanize the victim.[64] Indeed, the sociologist Herbert Kelman defines dehumanization as the denial of identity and community: "To accord a person identity is to perceive him as an individual, independent and distinguishable from others, capable of making choices. To accord a person community is to perceive him—along with with one's self—as part of an interconnected network of individuals, who recognize each other's individuality and respect each other's rights."[65] The mechanisms of this process of dehumanization remain little understood and largely relegated to the work of social scientists.

While some work has been done by the medical profession on the psychological dimensions of torture, public health has largely eschewed serious investigation of the mechanisms and modes of collective violence.[66] Despite the fact that dehumanization has clear health consequences and occurs at societal levels, the implicit notions of dignity and identity that underlie theories of dehumanization have not been easily incorporated into the traditional concepts or the largely biomedical vocabulary of mainstream public health. It is therefore essential to combine public health with the tools and framework of human rights in order to harness the power of systematic investigation that public health methods bring to bear to the question of how ethnic cleansing could occur.

Identity Formation

Individualizing the guilt for atrocities of ethnic cleansing and demonstrating that the crimes were not committed spontaneously constitute the first steps toward attacking the myth of the inevitability of ethnic cleansing. In the context of the truth-seeking roles of both human rights and public health, the study of dehumanization—or the destruction of identity—must be coupled with study of the formation of identity in order to fully grasp the interaction between structures of thought and action, between human consciousness and human agency. The argument that has been and continues to be widely circulated is "that Yugoslavia had been an impossible idea from the beginning, that Croats [and Muslims] were so different from Serbs that the two peoples had never had any business living together in the same country in the first place."[67] Given this understanding of reality, ethnic cleansing—which by its very definition encodes a model of multiethnicity as somehow dirty and corrupted—becomes understandable as a distorted and violent manifestation of a population exchange that could not, and indeed perhaps ought not, be prevented. However, public health methods combined with human rights principles can change the truth paradigm from one of historic inevitability to one of societal pathology.

Rieff argues that establishing the conflict as an inexorable truth was itself an integral part of the strategy of Radovan Karadzic, the Bosnian Serb leader:

> In Karadzic's formulation, Serbian-ness, Croatian-ness, and Muslim-ness were essences—unchanging and immutable.... The savagery of the war he had unleashed made what otherwise might have appeared to be his mad ideas convincing to people; and more than that, made them appear to have been confirmed by their experience. The fact that they had had these experiences because of plans conceived of by Karadzic, Milosevic, and their colleagues did not alter the fact that people were now likely to feel in their guts that they had been true all along.[68]

Thus, at the time Karadzic first started spouting hate propaganda, it was widely perceived as a complete lie, but five years later it had in a sense become "the truth." Rieff argues persuasively that "ethnic nationalism was no more inevitable in the former Yugoslavia than Hitlerism had been inevitable in Germany in the 1930s. It was one possibility—inevitable only in the sense that everything that happens is inevitable in hindsight."[69] Vlado Koprivica, a Serb who decided to stay in Vogosca after its return to Bosnian authority, anecdotally confirms Rieff's analysis, observing to Western journalists, "We could have lived together for a thousand years. There was never a problem. My neighbor across the hall was a Muslim, and both my neighbors upstairs were Muslim. We were like a family."[70] Thus, the establishment of the truth of ethnic cleansing manifested the Bosnian Serbs' power far more than any military victory possibly could.

But if the so-called truths of ethnic essentialism have been used to prop up fascist ideologies, an alternative human-rights-based truth can be used to question those social and moral judgments and to unmask those power structures. The tribalism argument presents a threat to the most fundamental tenets of human rights.[71] Human rights principles teach us that we not only are determined by a multiplicity of different social and cultural factors, but also possess autonomous reason that allows us to be free, self-defining subjects, whose essence is drawn from a universal capacity for reason and not from any ethnic—or racial or religious—mask we may wear.[72] Indeed, freedom, rationality, and autonomy constitute our basic meta- and infrapolitical understandings of what it means to be human in a human rights framework, which then allow us to define permissible understandings of human society and politics.

If, given this human rights premise, ethnic conflict and strife is reimagined as societal pathology and authentic multiculturalism is viewed as a condition of societal health, the tools of epidemiology can be brought to bear to identify risk factors that might predispose (but not predetermine) ethnic nationalisms. Descriptive epidemiology, concerned with the study of which populations develop a pathology and how the frequency of such a pathology varies over time, could be critically useful in diagnosing risk factors for ethnic conflict. Information about different characteristics of populations can be used to formulate epidemiological hypotheses about the causal and preventative factors of ethnic violence, hypotheses that concur with existing knowledge (developed through the social sciences) about its occurrence.

In *Epidemiology in Medicine*, Charles Hennekens and Julie Buring note, "For any public health problem, the first step in the search for possible solutions is to formulate a reasonable and testable hypothesis."[73] The commonly used methods of hypothesis formulation about disease etiology could usefully systematize the outbreaks of ethnic violence in a way social science tools alone are not equipped to do. Moreover, public health professionals are far more familiar with developing the kind of multifactoral and longitudinal analysis of problems required for an etiology of ethnic cleansing than are traditional human rights professionals. A multilevel analysis that considers global, national, and institutional as well as communal and individual factors would be essential to deciphering the different and contextualized roles of, for example: economic collapse, rising nationalisms, control and use of media to disseminate propaganda messages, public espousal of nostalgic or distorted views of the past, and grossly uneven development (e.g., urban versus rural, as well as amongst different regions). The goal is not to perform a regression analysis of these sorts of variables, but to begin to seriously investigate how they interact to produce different outcomes. The existence of "preexisting cleavages" or a "plural society" has too often been the end instead of the beginning of an analysis of social and structural factors in the causation of ethnic conflict.[74]

While this third aspect of truth construction in particular potentially subjects the use of public health methods to some of the same vulnerabilities and abuses as the "softer" social sciences or traditional modes of human rights, it is a misreading of the nature both of truth and of power to expect public health professionals simply to act as neutral, objective truth finders in evaluating the meaning or underlying causes of ethnic cleansing. The construction of the truth of "ethnic cleansing's inevitability" is closely associated with the construction (and destruction) of identity, and is itself an exercise of power that is being implicitly challenged by the tribunal's individual prosecutions and the fundamental principles underlying the régime of international human rights law. Human rights norms are as prescriptive as they are descriptive and suggest that certain claims to truth are simply incompatible with the notion that human beings are born free and equal in dignity and rights.

CONCLUSION

To use the term "ethnic cleansing" to describe what has happened over the past five years in the former Yugoslavia obfuscates more than it reveals. In its ambiguity, ethnic cleansing does not indicate whether the practice involved merely population movement or violent atrocities and human rights abuses. In its vagueness, the term does not clarify the nature and implications of the human rights or humanitarian law violations involved. Finally, in its usage and premises, it implies a view of society in which multiethnicity is conceived of as impure—literally uncleansed—and in so doing challenges the most fundamental tenets of human rights. In this chapter, I have argued for a multivalent collaboration between public health and human rights professionals to begin to unravel the underlying truths of the ethnic cleansing in the former Yugoslavia.

I have suggested that in addition to the crucial work of forensic and clinical experts reporting evidence of sequelae of conflict and abuses, health professionals have a role to play in interpretation of that evidence as well. That is, in addition to the truths that can be discovered by unearthing mass graves and recording physical consequences, there are truths to be defined and constructed. Public health methodology can be brought to bear to define both the nature of the crimes committed and the nature of the harms ensuing from those crimes. Moreover, public health tools can help create and reinforce conceptions of individual responsibility and identity formation that refute the premises of ethnic cleansing, and that are essential to the future of the tribunal and to international human rights law in general.

This three-pronged approach to the role of public health methods—diagnosing whether there is a problem, evaluating and interpreting what constitutes the problem, and deciphering the etiology of how the problem could have occurred—is critical to the success of the tribunal's work in establishing a just truth. Public health deals with facts and attempts to build theories around them, while human rights announces general, universal principles and attempts to apply them to facts. Each is indispensable to the other in the search for truth and justice in the former Yugoslavia. If the tribunal fails in its mission, it will be a failure for the prospects of peace in the former Yugoslavia and for an international order based on notions of justice and individual rights.

Clearly, this chapter constitutes only the beginning of a provisional framework of how human rights and public health can be combined in the work of the tribunal and, more generally, in the quest for truth in the midst of catastrophic human rights and public health atrocities. With more considered examination, some critical understanding—and, dare I say, even prevention—of the gross human rights violations involved in ethnic cleansing campaigns might become possible. It is worth remembering that a final disillusioning truth brought to light by the war in the former Yugoslavia is the shattering of the self-excusing myth about the Holocaust: that if the world had seen what went on in the Nazi death camps, we would have intervened. In the former Yugoslavia, the world looked on and did nothing as hundreds and thousands of people died often anguished deaths. Establishment of the tribunal should not, indeed must not, constitute a coverup for the truth about and accountability for the international community's past and current role in the former Yugoslavia.[75]

REFERENCES

1. For example, Article 1 of the Universal Declaration of Human Rights states: "All human beings are born free and equal in dignity and rights. *They are endowed with reason and conscience and should act towards one another in a spirit of brotherhood*" (emphasis added). Universal Declaration of Human Rights, Article 1, G.A. Res. 217A (III), U.N. GAOR Res.71, U.N. Doc. A/810 (1948).
2. See note 20 and accompanying text for the definition of ethnic cleansing.
3. For example, the journalist P. Maass recently wrote: "Since leaving Bosnia, I have often been asked the same questions: Did you visit those camps? Were they really so bad? I still find it hard to believe that Americans and Western Europeans are confused about Bosnia and, in particular, about the camps. Yes, I visited them, and yes, they were as bad as you could imagine. Didn't you see the images on television? Don't you believe what you saw? Do you give any credence to the word of Radovan Karadzic, the indicted Bosnian Serb leader, who said the news photographs were fakes?" (P. Maass, "Bosnia's Ground Zero," *Vanity Fair*, March 1996, p. 199). For a spectrum of different views on the difficulty of establishing truth in this conflict, see, e.g., D. Binder, "Anatomy of a Massacre," *Foreign Policy* (Winter 1994–95): 97 (discussing inability to establish responsibility of either Serb or Muslims for mortar shell bombing of Sarajevo market on February 5, 1994); N. Belloff, "Memorandum on Goldstone Tribunal," America Online, Feb. 6, 1996 (arguing illegitimacy and bias of tribunal); and see generally D. Rieff, *Slaughterhouse: Bosnia and the Failure of the West* (Touchstone Books, 1996).
4. Security Council Resolution 808, UN Doc. S/25704, 3 May 1993. Note that the International Criminal Tribunal for Rwanda was established pursuant to a Security Council resolution in November 1994 and began work on June 26, 1995. Security Council Resolution 955, 3,453rd meeting, UN Doc. S/Res/955, 8 November 1994.

5. Report of the Secretary General Pursuant to Paragraph 2 of Security Council Resolution 808, UN Doc. S/25704, 3 May 1993 (hereafter "Report of the Secretary General").

6. "Dispensing International Justice: The Yugoslav and Rwandan Criminal Tribunals," *Interights Bulletin* 39 (Summer 1995).

7. M. O'Connor, "Harvesting Evidence in Bosnia's Killing Fields," *New York Times*, April 7, 1996, Section 4, p. 1. The estimates are between three thousand and eight thousand men were executed at sites surrounding Srebrenica.

8. For an excellent discussion of documenting forced disappearances as human rights violations, see J. Mendez and J. M. Vivanco, "Disappearances and the Inter-American Court of Human Rights: Reflections on a Litigation Experience," *Hamline Law Review* 13 (1990): 507.

9. E. Kaban, "PHR CM," America Online: Reuters, Aug. 11, 1995. For similar aspects of the Rwandan experience, see also "Hundreds of Bodies Are Unearthed at Rwandan Site," *Boston Globe,* Feb. 17, 1996, p. 6; J. McKinley, "From a Grave in Rwanda, Hundreds of Dead Tell Their Tale," *New York Times*, Feb. 16, 1996, p. A3.

10. In fact, evidence of the mass graves at Vukovar in Croatia, which was presented to the War Crimes Commission by Physicians for Human Rights in 1993, probably played a significant role in the vote by the Security Council to create the tribunal. See notes 13–15, and accompanying text.

11. The Rwandan situation provides perhaps even more vivid examples of how this evidence can be used to refute allegations of combat. For example, a lack of machete wounds on the upper extremities and hands indicated to Rwandan and international investigators that there had been no self-defense initiated or possible. Also, the cutting of victims' Achilles tendons indicates a pattern of hobbling victims so that they could not escape before they were hacked to death. See, e.g., Kaban (see note 9).

12. See R. Kirschner and K. Hannibal, "The Application of Forensic Sciences to Human Rights Investigations," *International Journal of Medicine and Law* 13 (1994): 451, 455; "Grim Remains," *University of Chicago Magazine,* Feb. 1994, p. 14.

13. Kirschner and Hannibal, pp. 458–459 (see note 12).

14. Ibid.

15. Similarly, a more recent *New York Times* article from 1995 states: "Near Pudin Han [in Bosnia] is a site outside a cave that has human bones poking up out of a large circular depression. Another site, known as Crvena Zemlja, or red earth, has already given up bones and clothing. Here in Prhovo, now a vacant ruin perched on a hillside … a man who witnessed a mass killing led [Bosnian government] authorities to a spot where officials believe dozens of victims of the massacre lie buried. … 'In Prhovo we have a list of 53 people we believe are buried in the plot of land at the entrance of the village,' said the officer in charge of locating the mass graves, who asked to remain unidentified." C. Hedges, "Bosnia Begins the Grim Search for Muslim Victims of the War," *New York Times*, Sept. 26, 1995, p. A1.

16. "Grim Remains," p. 1 (see note 12).

17. J. Sonis and T. Crane, "Family Physicians and Human Rights: A Case Example from Former Yugoslavia," *Family Medicine* 27 (1995): 242, 246.

18. S. Swiss and J. Giller, "Rape as a Crime of War: A Medical Perspective," *Journal of the American Medical Association* 270 (1993): 612–613.

19. Ibid., pp. 613–614.

20. Conversations with Nedim Jaganjac, MPH candidate, Harvard School of Public Health (Oct. 1995–Mar. 1996).

21. T. Meron, "The Case for War Crimes Trials in the Former Yugoslavia," *Foreign Affairs* (Summer 1993): 132. See also generally T. Meron, *Human Rights and Humanitarian Norms as Customary Law* (New York: Clarendon Press/Oxford University Press, 1989), pp. 41–76.

22. Meron, p. 132 (see note 21). "War crimes" are governed by international humanitarian law as codified principally in the four 1949 Geneva Conventions and the two Additional Protocols of 1977, which over 150 and 100 states, respectively (including the former Yugoslavia in both instances) have ratified. "Grave breaches" refer to breaches of certain fundamental guarantees of respect for the person. Article 147 of the Fourth Geneva Convention lists the following among acts considered to be "grave breaches": willful killing, torture or inhuman treatment, willfully causing great suffering or serious injury to body or health, unlawful deportation or transfer, unlawful confinement, depriving a protected person of the right of a fair and regular trial, the taking of hostages, and extensive destruction and appropriation of property not justified by military necessity and carried out unlawfully and wantonly. See also "grave breaches" provisions in Protocol Additional to the Geneva Conventions of 12 August 1949, and Relating to the Protection of Victims of International Armed Conflicts and Protocol Additional to the Geneva Conventions of 12 August 1949, and Relating to the Protection of Victims of Non-International Armed Conflicts, opened for signature Dec. 12 1977, 1125 UNTS 609, reprinted in 16 ILM at 1442 (hereinafter "Protocol I" and "Protocol II," respectively). The "Genocide Convention" refers to the United Nations Convention on the Prevention and Punishment of Genocide, which is a human rights convention governing the actions of states during both peace and wartime. UNGA Res., 260A (III) 9 December 1948, entered into force 12 January 1951 (hereinafter the "Genocide Convention").

23. See C. Hennekens and J. Buring, *Epidemiology in Medicine* (Boston: Little, Brown and Co., 1987), p. 54: "A prerequisite for any epidemiologic investigation is the ability to quantify the occurrence of disease."

24. Meron argues: "There is a distinct advantage in being able to prosecute offenders for the crime of genocide or other crimes against humanity, or even both. . . . Some killings and other violations might fall outside the specific offenses of the crime of genocide and crimes against humanity because of either definitional difficulties or a failure to satisfy the burden of proof." Theodore Meron, "International Criminalization of Internal Atrocities," *American Journal of International Law* 89 (1995): 554, 558.

25. UN Doc. S/25704 Annex (1993); see also J. O'Brien, "The International Tribunal for Violations of International Humanitarian Law in the Former Yugoslavia," *American Journal of International Law* 87 (1983): 639, 647.

26. Universal jurisdiction means that any country has jurisdiction to arrest and prosecute suspected perpetrators. See discussion in T. Meron, "The Case for War Crimes Trials" (see note 21), pp. 127–128. Thus, for example, the perpetrators of even the grossest atrocities in Rwanda cannot be prosecuted for grave breaches or war crimes, but only for the crime of genocide, which is much more difficult to establish, and for crimes against humanity. See notes 44–46, and accompanying text.

27. In contrast, violations of common Article III and Additional Protocol II of the Geneva Conventions, which apply to internal conflicts, are subject to universal jurisdiction. See Restatement Third of the Foreign Relations Law of the United

States, section 402, 404 (1987); T. Meron, "International Criminalization of Internal Atrocities" (see note 24), 568–569.

28. Note that Article V of the tribunal's statute may imply that crimes against humanity can be committed during peace as well as during armed conflicts. However, the tribunal's only statute has jurisdiction over such crimes only when committed in international or internal armed conflicts. Report of the Secretary General (see note 2), paragraph 47.

29. In international law, *jus cogens* refers to a norm "accepted and recognized by the international community of states as a whole as a norm from which no derogation is permitted and which can be modified only by a subsequent norm of general international law having the same character." Article 53, Vienna Convention on the Law of Treaties, 1155 UNTS 331, UN Doc. A/Conf. 39/27 (1969).

30. Agreement for the Prosecution and Punishment of the Major War Criminals of European Axis, Charter of the International Military Tribunal, Article VI (c), Aug 8, 1945, Stat. 1544, 82 UNTS 279, reprinted in *American Journal of International Law* 39 (1945): 257 (hereinafter "Nuremberg Charter").

31. T. Meron, "The Case for War Crimes Trials in the Former Yugoslavia" (see note 21), p. 130.

32. Ibid.

33. Ibid.

34. At the end of World War II, the Allies' Control Council Law No. 10 expanded the formulation of crimes against humanity by including rape among the prohibitions listed in Article II (1)(c) and did away with the jurisdictional distinction between war crimes and crimes against peace. See T. Meron, "War Crimes in Yugoslavia and the Development of International Law," *American Journal of International Law* 88 (1994): 78.

35. International Committee of the Red Cross, Aide-Mémoires Dec. 3, 1992; T. Meron, "Rape as a Crime Under International Humanitarian Law," *American Journal of International Law* 87 (1993): 424, 426.

36. T. Mazowiecki, Report on the Situation of Human Rrights in the Territory of the Former Yugoslavia, UN Doc. A/48/92-S/25341, Annex, at 20, 57 (1993); T. Meron, "Rape" (see note 35), p. 425.

37. S. Swiss and J. Giller (see note 18), p. 613.

38. "Because the use of rape statistics for propaganda purposes is common during war, documenting rape—already difficult during peacetime—is even more challenging in the midst of war." S. Swiss and J. Giller (see note 18), p. 613.

39. Ibid.

40. Ibid.

41. For example, does a gang rape constitute a single rape or multiple rapes?

42. S. Swiss and J. Giller (see note 18), p. 613.

43. Ibid.

44. The crime of genocide is not based on a link to war and is thus equally applicable in times of peace.

45. Genocide Convention (see note 22); Report of the Secretary General (see note 2), paragraph 46.

46. T. Meron, "The Case for War Crimes Trials" (see note 21), p. 130.

47. C. Hennekens and J. Buring (see note 23), p. 3.

48. S. Swiss and J. Giller (see note 18), p. 612.

49. Ibid., p. 613.

50. Ibid., p. 614.

51. Ibid.: "Community-based interventions that are sensitive to the local context and methods of healing may be the best approach to treating the wounds of rape in many situations."

52. S. Weine, D. Becker, T. McGlashan et al., "Psychiatric Consequences of Ethnic Cleansing: Clinical Assessments and Trauma Testimonies of Newly Resettled Bosnian refugees," *American Journal of Psychology* 152: 536, 543.

53. Ibid., p. 536.

54. See, e.g., R. Mollica and Y. Caspi-Yavin, "Measuring Torture and Torture-Related Symptoms," *Psychological Assessment: Journal of Consulting and Clinical Psychology* 3 (1991): 581.

55. T. Meron, "The Case for War Crimes Trials" (see note 21), p. 130.

56. Trial of the Major War Criminals Before the International Military Tribunal, Nuremberg, 14 November 1945–1 October 1946, 1 Official Documents 223 (1947), cited in T. Meron, "International Criminalization of Internal Atrocities" (see note 27), p. 562.

57. H. Arendt, *On Violence* (London: Harcourt Brace and Co., 1969).

58. Ibid.

59. D. Rieff (see note 3), p. 90.

60. Universal Declaration of Human Rights, Article 7.

61. A. Destexhe details how in the case of Rwanda: "True to form, the Rwandan genocide was thoroughly planned in advance. Ethnic identity cards introduced by the Belgians in the 1930s allowed the militias to select their victims easily. They quickly set up roadblocks and checked everyone who passed. In addition, the militia leaders in every area organized the systematic elimination of the Tutsis by assigning them to groups of ten families and allocating a militia member to each group. Lists of people to be killed were already in circulation before [then President] Habyarimana's death." A. Destexhe, "The Third Genocide," *Foreign Policy* (Winter 1994–95): 8.

62. D. Rieff (see note 3), p. 111.

63. Ibid., p. 110.

64. See, e.g., discussion in H. Arendt (see note 57), p. 67.

65. H. Kelman, "Violence without Moral Restraint: Reflections on the Dehumanization of Victims and Victimizers," *Journal of Social Issues* 29, 48–49 (1973), cited in L. Kuper, *Genocide* (New Haven and London: Yale University Press, 1981), p. 87.

66. A notable exception is A. Zwi and A. Ugalde's "Toward an Epidemiology of Political Violence in the Third World," *Social Science and Medicine* 28: 633. Nevertheless, even this example is more suggestive than substantive.

67. D. Rieff (see note 3), pp. 62–63.

68. Ibid., p. 73.

69. Ibid., p. 111.

70. "Vogosca Stories," Bosnet Report, *Bosnet Digest*, Applicom, Feb. 29, 1996.

71. Analogies may be drawn to Rwanda, where the tribalism myth is perhaps even more entrenched. A. Destexhe notes how: "The ethnic problems (between Hutu and Tutsi) date only from the days of colonization. Indeed, it could be said that it is a purely artificial problem, dreamed up by the Germans who first colonized Rwanda, and reinforced by the Belgians who succeeded them." Destexhe documents how Tutsi cattle owners and Hutu farmers had been interdependent

and intermingled throughout the area, "where they spoke the same language, practiced the same religion, and shared the same culture and mythology. Thus, Hutus and Tutsis are not ethnically distinct groups and the physical stereotypes do not always hold true. Under certain circumstances, a Hutu could even become a Tutsi. . . . As for the children of Rwanda's intermarriages, they have always inherited their ethnic identities from their fathers." A. Destexhe (see note 61), pp. 5–6 .

72. See Universal Declaration of Human Rights, Article 1.

73. For example, three commonly used methods are: the "method of difference," which involves looking at different disease frequencies in different sets of circumstances; the "method of agreement," which involves identifying a single factor that is common to a number of situations in which a given disease occurs with high frequency; and the "method of concomitant variation," which involves looking at circumstances in which the frequency of a factor varies in proportion to the frequency of disease. C. Hennekens and J. Buring (see note 23), p. 112.

74. See, e.g., A. Destexhe, (see note 61); compare L. Kuper (see note 65), p. 57.

75. See D. Rieff, "The Institution That Saw No Evil," *New Republic*, Feb. 12, 1996, p. 19; see also generally D. Rieff (see note 3).

9. Haiti 1991–1994: The International Civilian Mission's Medical Unit

Cécile Marotte and Hervé Rakoto Razafimbahiny

> *Tout moun se moun.*
> (Every human being is a human being.)
> —Creole Haitian proverb

The experience of providing assistance to a population subjected to repression led the health care professionals who were members of the Medical Unit of the International Civilian Mission and the International Human Rights Observer in Haiti Mission to the following observations:

- Health care workers operating in a context of human rights violations must reexamine their usual approach to medical care.
- A broadened concept of human rights can lead to a new outlook and approaches to public health.

REPRESSION IN HAITI FROM 1991 TO 1994

Since becoming independent in 1804, Haiti has endured various forms of repression. Although more or less violent in nature, this repression has always been associated with the state government. The Duvaliers' thirty-year-long dictatorship (1957–1986) targeted intellectuals, bourgeois, and mulatto groups, and the black petty bourgeoisie. These people were forced into exile or killed, or they simply disappeared.

In contrast, the repression and human rights violations that occurred between 1991 and 1994 were of a different nature and against a different population. The de facto government, which came to power following the military coup that overthrew President Jean-Bertrand Aristide on September 30, 1991, involved ferocious repression and organized violence, carried out by the Haitian armed forces and by paramilitary groups connected to them.

They systematically targeted poor Haitians, a population that had always lived on the threshold of poverty, if not below it. This repression included damage or obliteration of the public health infrastructure and health care resources.

The consequences in human rights terms were tragic. Almost four thousand people were killed, and more than three hundred thousand people were internally displaced.[1] For political reasons, many were disappeared; others received gunshot or knife wounds; others, mostly women, were raped and sexually assaulted; and many others were victims of arbitrary arrest and cruel, inhuman, or degrading treatment. This stimulated a large number of people to seek refuge elsewhere, either across the land border with the Dominican Republic or across the sea, in most cases sailing to the United States, resulting in a "boat people" phenomenon that raised a whole new series of issues while influencing many of the subsequent U.S. policy decisions.

THE MEDICAL UNIT OF THE CIVILIAN MISSION: CREATION AND EVOLUTION

The human rights situation during this time was recognized internationally as disastrous. Immediately following the 1991 military coup, the Organization of American States (OAS) and the United Nations (UN) voted an embargo of Haiti, which resulted in civil unrest and economic devastation. One year later, acting upon a request from President Aristide, then in exile in the United States, these organizations decided to create an international human rights observer mission for Haiti. In February 1993, a civilian international human rights observer mission was organized (Mission Civile Internationale en Haïti, or Civilian Mission), involving approximately two hundred people. It was directed by OAS career diplomat Ambassador Colin Granderson, from Trinidad, and Ian Martin, a former secretary-general of Amnesty International, as head of its human rights division.

The Civilian Mission was active from February 1993 to February 1996, with two short interruptions due to an evacuation for safety reasons and an expulsion ordered by the de facto government.

From the start, the Civilian Mission was faced with victims of severe human rights violations, some of whom required immediate medical assistance, and for whom observation and documentation alone was inadequate. For the first time a medical unit for human rights (Medical Unit) was created within an OAS or UN mission and eventually an "active observation" response was implemented. The Medical Unit's principal objective was to facilitate access to health care for victims of severe human rights violations and to ensure their safety during medical treatment.

The Medical Unit's initial members were all physicians. From the start, the unit was faced with four urgent needs:

- To facilitate victims' access to medical care in Haiti's public hospitals and private clinics

- To ensure victims' safety in the context of continued human rights violations
- To intervene in prison settings—an innovation for Haiti—although obtaining access to the prisons was difficult
- To perform medical documentation of human rights violations

During 1993 and 1994, the Medical Unit experienced many obstacles and was faced with daily difficulties; therefore, three facts concerning its operation are of profound importance. First and most important is that the majority of the health care was provided by Haitian health care workers, most of whom worked in inadequate health care structures under extremely difficult conditions and at great personal risk. While the Medical Unit team and human rights observers witnessed some instances of refusal to observe medical ethics and to provide care for victims, the courage and dignity of Haitian health care workers (physicians as well as nurses) who assisted victims of human rights violations must be emphasized.

Second, an essential role was played by nonmedical personnel in facilitating access to health care for victims. Most of these workers were members of Haitian human rights organizations or other Civilian Mission observers, especially those working outside of the capital.

And third, the establishment of an emergency fund for victims by the Canadian Fund (a Canadian government project) helped support day-to-day field functioning, medical and surgical care, drugs, and medical supplies. This provided decisive help in many difficult situations, such as for the purchase of orthopedic equipment or obtaining therapeutic drugs for individual victims.

In early 1995, several elements helped strengthen the effect of the Medical Unit. Two physicians working with Médecins du Monde (MDM, Doctors of the World) joined the team. A human rights clinic in Port-au-Prince opened, which aimed to consolidate access to medical help for victims. A psychologist with ethnopsychiatric training—a practice that takes into account the psychological benefits that a population can achieve from traditional cultural therapeutic sources—was brought in. Up to this time psychological and psychiatric care for victims of human rights violations had not been considered.

THERAPEUTIC INTERVENTION AND THE BOUNDARIES OF DOCUMENTATION

Within the mandate of the Civilian Mission, therapeutic intervention initially consisted mainly of documenting—case by case—victims of repression who came of their own accord to register a complaint. This documentation was the primary objective of the Medical Unit during the program's early phase. In early 1993, medical evaluation was limited to short case summaries, primarily because the tense situation and fierce repression in the field made emergency assistance and the effort to ensure safety for victims and health care workers the Medical Unit's highest priority.

The Medical Unit sought to document the physical findings of severe human rights violations, including executions, bullet and knife wounds, torture, cruel, inhuman, and degrading treatment. For example, some victims, mainly women, had been threatened with or subjected to politically motivated sexual violence, including many cases of rape. This medical evaluation process was intended to back up the reports of the Civilian Mission with additional information before they were transmitted to the secretary-general of the OAS and the UN secretary-general.

Beginning in 1994, the first time the Civilian Mission returned to Haiti (following reinstatement of constitutional order), three factors contributed to the expansion of a more extensive and thorough documentation process. The Civilian Mission hoped to make up for lost time by adding a medical dimension to the evidence of human rights abuses. In addition, the victims were anxious to go beyond short-term medical care, to seek justice and to add meaning to their experience. Also, Haiti's National Truth and Justice Commission, which operated from March through October of 1996, asked for the Medical Unit's assistance in medical documentation.

In spite of the UN mandate, which initially limited their action, the Civilian Mission observers shifted toward "active observation"—in other words, intervention. It was recognized that the reality of medical problems resulting from human rights violations required health professionals to intervene and to establish links with existing public health and health care structures. In addition, health care workers tried to establish the extent to which reliance on traditional and cultural resources had been successful and what coping strategies victims had adopted in situations of destitution at every level—material, therapeutic, institutional, and symbolic. As time went on it became increasingly evident that many complaints could no longer be relieved by classical biomedical care, but required a revised therapeutic approach.

Altogether, approximately five thousand cases of severe human rights violations were documented by the Civilian Mission: five thousand stories of horror and irreversible physical and psychological damage.[2]

Of these five thousand cases, only nine hundred victims received assistance from the Medical Unit between 1993 and early 1996. Furthermore, even though most victims presented symptoms consistent with post-traumatic stress disorder, the belated introduction of psychological and psychiatric support meant that only eighty cases actually benefited from treatment of that condition.

LIMITATIONS

In part a result of the urgency of the situation, there was a lack of preparation, conceptualization, and definition of the Medical Unit's role within the scope of the Civilian Mission.

The Medical Unit was further hampered by the narrow interpretation given by the Civilian Mission's mandate. The Mission's headquarters wished to restrict the Medical Unit's role to documenting human rights abuses. Health workers involved with the Medical Unit felt that medical ethics demanded that this process be complemented by providing care whenever the situation called for medical assistance.

The Medical Unit was also confronted daily with difficulties in terms of confidentiality and liability. For example, many victims contacted the Medical Unit after being released from detention centers where they had been tortured. The Civilian Mission leadership sought to lessen the involvement of staff members from the Medical Unit in the follow-up for these cases. They said this was necessary both for security reasons and to maintain the strict neutrality of the health care providers. However, this approach conflicted with the Medical Unit's perspective, which called for immediate assistance. Even though the health care workers involved in the Medical Unit were experienced in humanitarian missions, they were often unaccustomed to the specific challenges associated with these forms of human rights violations. Human rights work requires expertise, gained through appropriate training and experience.

Some Medical Unit team members reacted in very different ways when faced with human rights victims, from acute emotional reactions to denial and systematic refusal to acknowledge the reality of long-term health consequences of repression. Cultural prejudice, fear of interaction, deadlocks, exacerbated power struggles, cultural differences, and culture shock—all these reactions were found in the people working on the team.

Medical Unit members were also faced with a major dilemma, which remains unresolved and is applicable to comparable situations in many parts of the world. This had to do with the possibility, once immediate safety is assured, of offering victims access to health care beyond the reach of most of the population. For example, should financial support be provided for a surgical procedure or for certain private consultations that are unavailable in the public health care sector? Humanitarian projects seeking to strengthen existing health care structures by introducing state-of-the-art techniques—CT scans, for example—may turn out to be useless in a society which lacks the necessary technological support. Such projects do not benefit the majority of the population, since most Haitians do not have access to even basic health structures.

EXCLUSION, DIGNITY, AND HUMAN RIGHTS

In the context of conventional therapeutic intervention, the Medical Unit was faced every day with the dramatic state of helplessness of most of the victims. These patients were without jobs or financial resources in most cases, and were often homeless. Some arrived at their medical consultations without having eaten for several days. Simple medical care was clearly not enough. Medical intervention along standard medical and psychotherapeutic lines was bound to fail to achieve classical, measurable results. The fact that human rights violations cause specific and severe disorders that sometimes irreversibly alter a victim's health had to be taken into account.

Indeed, this suffering, after being partially relieved by medical care, opened the door to another endemic source of suffering, not treatable with conventional medical and psychological approaches. The victims of torture and other human rights abuses were already societal victims—in other words, victims of stigmatization, discrimination, and violations of their personal dignity. The daily trauma to an individual caused by lack of respect for human rights has been referred to as "survival trauma" and should be distinguished from an exacerbated violation of such rights (e.g., torture). The victims' vulnerability is thus increased and must be examined in its context: these victims' usual, social living conditions entail daily violations of their rights. Therefore, the Medical Unit was seeking to assist a population already suffering from denial of its civil, economic, political, and social rights.

The root of a victim's vulnerability lies in the fact that he or she can never enjoy these rights while existing social and state structures remain unchanged. Care providers cannot provide medical and psychological care to victims of organized violence—who are already victims of human rights abuse—without an expanded understanding of what a victim is and the inherent and concurrent vulnerability that accompanies this status.

TOWARD A MULTIDISCIPLINARY AND GLOBAL APPROACH

This experience in Haiti prompted recognition of several key aspects regarding medical assistance for the victims of human rights abuses.

Human rights violations carried out against the Haitian population between 1991 and 1994 had a great impact on the health of the population—on an individual as well as a community level. Only nine hundred victims were evaluated and followed up during the Medical Unit's twenty-six-month-long mission. Many Haitians were killed, disappeared or became political refugees. Mental and physical consequences on countless other members of the population are documented, although a quantitative evaluation of the medical consequences of this repression is currently under way. There is a demonstrated need for long-term medical, psychological, and psychiatric follow-up.

Along with other health professionals, the authors are striving to create a Haitian Rehabilitation Center for Victims to continue the work initiated by the Haitian health professionals, Medical Unit members and MDM.

Beyond this conventional approach to health care, the painful realization of the shortcomings of our efforts led us to try to introduce a wider perspective to our work through contacts and conversations with several ministries, including those of health, justice, social affairs, and women's affairs, with Haitian human rights associations and with international organizations with interests in health and development such as WHO, UNICEF, and the European Union.

Our role as medical evaluators in collaboration with Haiti's National Truth and Justice Commission also involves a new dimension. As health care professionals, we must work jointly with human rights and legal professionals so that victims may be recognized as such, and assist them in their difficult search for justice and compensation.

We would also like to underline two particular roles that health care professionals can and must play. At a national level, health care workers help to protect and enhance human rights by familiarizing themselves with the International Bill of Human Rights and the Alma-Ata Declaration. By doing so, they can provide unique expertise in terms of human rights, and their privileged position in civilian society should enable them to exert a favorable influence, becoming important actors working toward change in society. Medical care specifically required in the context of human rights missions should be taught in universities, medical and nursing schools, and international research centers.

A second task and responsibility of heath workers is to distribute information and to share experience and knowledge. The same is true for UN agencies and other international organizations, specialized centers that care for victims, human rights organizations, nongovernmental humanitarian organizations, international medical associations, and research centers. This information could widen the international network of health care professionals interested in reflection and action upon health and human rights issues. It could also favorably affect certain political decisions made both at the national and international level in such institutions as the UN or the OAS, so that medical units could be included as a matter of course in other human rights missions.

CONCLUSION

The experience of health care professionals working for human rights in Haiti was unprecedented. It was unique because of the prevailing international context: this was the first time that two international organizations, the UN and the OAS, created a medical unit as part of a human rights mission. But more important, our experience in Haiti has shown that we have to go beyond traditional approaches in both human rights work and health work and that this particular setting called for a reexamination of the role of health care professionals in relation to human rights.

This dimension of the profound linkage between health and human rights not only is relevant to peacetime and traditional public health, but is vital to understanding and responding to conflicts and to situations that have thus far been characterized as humanitarian crises.

REFERENCES

1. Report of the National Truth and Justice Commission, September 1996.
2. Figures are confirmed by the reports and press releases of the International Civilian Mission and by the reports of the secretary-general of the UN on Haiti.

Disabled Persons and Their Right 10. to Equal Treatment: Allowing Differentiation While Ending Discrimination

Aart Hendriks

The relationship between public health professionals and disabled people is a rather ambivalent matter.[1] While disabled people are often dependent on services of individual care providers and public health institutions, these institutions, to become or remain integrated into society, have often enhanced the segregation of disabled people from mainstream society. Nowadays, persons with disabilities are increasingly turning toward a discipline that has almost systematically neglected their own interests: the law. Only recently have international human rights bodies paid attention to massive violations of disabled people's human rights.[2] In addition, all the past decade's studies indicate that disabled people are disproportionately represented among the poorest segments of society and lack equal opportunities to improve their living conditions.[3] Without an improvement of their basic rights, it seems unlikely that disabled people can break the vicious spiral of dependence, segregation, human rights violations, lack of opportunities, and poverty.

The silence of human rights scholars about disabled people's rights may be due to reluctance to embark on issues widely believed to pertain to medicine or public health combined with uncertainty about applicability of the basic principles of equality and nondiscrimination. One need not be a legal expert to understand that equality cannot be achieved merely by treating disabled and able-bodied persons identically in all situations, since in certain, specific circumstances these two groups of people must be treated differently. This raises the question of when differentiation, or a lack thereof, amounts to discrimination.

Disability-based discrimination means denying disabled people equal enjoyment and exercise of their rights. Recognition of the inherent equality of all human beings as well as the entitlement of each individual to all human rights form the core of human rights law. At the same time, selective denial of human rights to those with a history of disadvantage and vulner-ability perpetuates the deep-rooted patterns of discrimination that are at the heart of many human rights violations.

Essentially, discrimination means treating certain people less favorably than others. It usually reflects prejudice and misinformation, a rejection of human variety, and superiority toward those one considers "different." Discrimination typically, although not always, reflects power inequalities. Those who hold power seek to reinforce their position, to the detriment of all others.

When examining the root causes and expressions of discrimination, vari-ous forms of less favorable treatment can be distinguished, including direct and indirect discrimination[4] and intentional and unintentional dis-crimination.[5] There is even reverse discrimination, a term that some commentators reserve for positive- (or affirmative-) treatment programs.[6]

Disability-based discrimination results from either under- or overesti-mating the importance of human variation. We commonly perceive people whom we consider members of our own group as "the same" and "normal," whereas we regard all others as "different" and "abnormal." The genesis of disability-based discrimination goes back to the inability (or reluctance) of mainstream society to accommodate "different" people. Whereas disabili-ties are no longer associated with witchcraft, immorality, or possession by the devil or other evil spirits, societal views about disabilities continue to be negative.[7] This may not always be obvious, because laws and policies of the self-proclaimed civilized societies with respect to disabled persons commonly seek to rehabilitate or, when that is unfeasible, to financially compensate disabled people for their lack of productivity.[8] This approach is in fact inherently paternalistic and fails to represent disabled persons as human beings of equal worth and dignity. Hilary Astor was painfully right when she wrote that "society's expectations of people with disabilities are that they be dependent, unassuming and the grateful recipients of charitable assistance."[9]

Exploring the meaning of discrimination and difference in the context of disabled people requires dealing with principles of equality and nondiscrim-ination. Genuine equality implies a redistribution of resources and rights commensurate with the different needs of individuals.[10] To what degree, however, do human variations count as "differences" to the extent that they should be transformed into distinct entitlements? Further questions emerge, including: To what extent are disabilities a relevant criterion for differentiat-ing between people? To what extent are disabled people "the same" as able-bodied persons? What is the legal significance of the overlap between differ-ence and disadvantage? Does equality imply that all differences be duly respected, or does it require that certain differences be modified?

In this chapter I attempt to answer these questions in light of the inter-nationally recognized and newly emerging human rights standards. It is only during the past two decades that human rights acknowledged the importance of the integration of disabled people into society, notably in the context of work.[11] Recently, the scope of these standards was significantly expanded with adoption of the Standard Rules on the Equalization of Opportunities for Persons with Disabilities (Standard Rules)[12] and the General Comment on People with Disabilities (General Comment).[13] In this chapter I pay special attention to the implications of these new documents for the position of disabled persons under international human rights law.

EQUALITY AND NONDISCRIMINATION

Unfortunately, in common language as well as in scholarly papers and official documents, the terms *equality* and *nondiscrimination* are often used interchangeably.[14] This represents a deep-rooted misunderstanding of the meaning of each concept, leading to frequent conceptual confusion.

In ethics, equality is founded upon the idea that all persons are of equal value and importance. An equal society is understood to mean a society in which all are equally able to participate. Pursuant to the ethical principle of equality, each person is entitled to and should be afforded equal respect, concern, and protection.[15] Equalization (or the enhancement of equality) should not be construed to deny human variety. The ethical principle of justice implies that people with different needs are treated differently commensurate with their difference.[16] By way of contrast, equality requires that human varieties that are unnecessary and avoidable, and considered unfair, unjust, and unacceptable, be rectified.[17] These latter differences I will call *inequalities*.

In law, equality entails the entitlement of each individual to all human rights. Furthermore, human rights law assumes that all humans possess equal dignity, irrespective of individual or social variations. Besides that, equality entitles each person to equal membership in society.[18] In international human rights law, equality is founded upon two complementary principles: nondiscrimination and dignity.[19]

The principle of nondiscrimination seeks to ensure that all persons can equally enjoy and exercise all their rights and freedoms. Discrimination occurs when some people are treated less favorably than others; it involves arbitrary denial or restriction of equal human rights. In other words, discrimination violates the principle of equality. Under international human rights law, one person may be treated less favorably than another "if the criteria for such differentiation are *reasonable and objective* and if the aim is to achieve a purpose which is *legitimate*" (emphasis added).[20] These criteria were originally developed by the European Court of Human Rights in the so-called Belgian Linguistic case:

> The principle of equality of treatment is violated if the distinction has no objective and reasonable justification. The existence of such a justification must be assessed in relation to the aim and effects of the measure under consideration, regard being had to the principles which normally prevail in democratic societies. A difference of treatment in the exercise of a right laid

down in the Convention must not only pursue a legitimate aim: Article 14 is likewise violated when it is clearly established that there is no reasonable relationship of proportionality between the means employed and the aim sought to be realized.[21]

Respect for dignity, being the other component through which equality manifests itself, implies respecting humanity in all its variations. As human beings we are all, in the words of the Universal Declaration of Human Rights, "born free and equal in dignity and rights" (Article 1). Individual and group variations should therefore be duly respected in the way society treats its members, unless it concerns unacceptable differences. The latter differences, termed "inequalities," should be the target of comprehensive antidiscrimination and social justice policies.

FORMAL AND MATERIAL EQUALITY

Both ethics and law can play an important role in ameliorating the individual, social, economic, political, and legal conditions of disadvantaged and vulnerable groups, such as disabled people. Equality not only implies preventing discrimination (e.g., the protection of individuals against unfavorable treatment by introducing antidiscrimination laws), but also remedying discrimination against groups suffering discrimination in society (e.g., by introducing social justice programs to alleviate or compensate for disadvantages).[22] Active promotion of equality thus goes further than mere prohibition of less favorable treatment of individuals or groups. The extent to which one expects society—and particularly the state—to undertake positive (affirmative) action to enhance genuine equality very much depends on the notion one holds about equality and the enforceability of social rights.

Legal commentators commonly distinguish between two different forms of equality. First, there is the formal notion of equality. Formal equality means equality in the form of the law. It requires that the law treat persons similarly who are situated alike.[23] The formal equality discourse builds on one of the ideas of the Greek philosopher Aristotle, who said that "things that are alike should be treated alike, whereas things that are unalike should be treated unalike in proportion to their unalikeness."[24] More recently, this notion of formal equality became associated with classical liberalism. This political philosophy presumes that individuals are free to compete with each other and that all can make their own choices, a view that entails some unrealistic assumptions about individual autonomy and rationality. Individual and social disparities and their impact on free competition are largely neglected. With respect to the role of equality, the main concern of classical liberals is to ensure that distinctions made between individuals are in proportion to their unalikeness. This implies that the role of equality is confined to prohibiting less favorable treatment of those individuals who are similarly situated as others are, and to bestowing individuals with identical civil and political rights.

Critique of the formal notion of equality was expressed by such diverse theorists as Rousseau,[25] Hegel[26] and Marx[27] and is also echoed in the work of most feminist legal commentators.[28] Although adversaries of formal equality discourse do not advocate similar alternatives, they all claim that the rules of the market cannot be relied upon to enhance justice and equality, that the market players are not necessarily similarly situated and that formal equality fails to correct structural inequalities. Moreover, these critics assert that the market tends to favor the advantaged and to oppress those with a history of disadvantage and vulnerability.[29] Therefore, the "similarly situated" test became—at least in literature—increasingly rejected, because it relies on a notion of comparability that is alien to most real-life situations. In addition, the "similarly situated" test, in combination with the rules defining the burden of proof, makes it particularly difficult for members of disadvantaged and vulnerable groups to complain about adverse or adverse impact treatment. Racial, religious, national or sexual minorities as well as women and people with disabilities experience social, physical, and legal barriers to societal integration that their counterparts (dominant racial, religious, national and sexual groups, men, and able-bodied persons) may never face. For example, able-bodied persons will never be excluded from the bulk of social activities, nor will they ever feel the embarassment and humiliation of having to perform sheltered labor specially devised for people with disabilities.

The notion of material, or substantial, equality emerged in response to the "sameness of treatment" doctrine. Material equality encompasses both formal equality and economic, social and cultural equality.[30] As such, the notion of material equality acknowledges the importance of both personal and environmental barriers that inhibit the equal participation of certain members of groups in society.[31] In order to overcome these barriers, mechanisms that directly or indirectly discriminate against people should be prohibited, while respecting other individual or group differences unless these distinctions cause or reflect unacceptable differences ("inequalities"). In the material equality perspective, society is obliged to modify those differences that deny or impair the right of each individual to be an equal member of society. The design of positive- (affirmative-) action programs may be required to achieve real equality in situations where some are less advantaged or more vulnerable than others.[32]

Both in international legal literature and in the case law of the international courts the notion of material equality is gaining support.[33] Recognition of the material equality perspective dates back to jurisprudence of the Permanent Court of International Justice, the predecessor of the International Court of Justice. In the case of the German settlers in Poland (1923) the court stated that: "there must be equality in fact as well as ostensible legal equality in the sense of the absence of discrimination in the words of the law."[34] In the case of the minority schools in Albania (1935) the court elaborated on this formulation—in this case, by explicitly recognizing the importance of different treatment in order to achieve equality: "It is perhaps not easy to define the distinction between the notions of equality in fact and equality in law; nevertheless, it may be said that the former notion excludes the idea of a merely formal equality." It finally concluded that: "Equality in law precludes discrimination of any kind; whereas equality in fact may involve the necessity of different treatment in order to attain a result which establishes an equilibrium between different situations."[35]

After World War II, the dichotomy between formal and material equality was further elaborated upon. Within the United Nations (UN), the representative of Ukraine (at that time, the Ukrainian SSR) emphasized the importance of material equality with regard to the nondiscrimination provisions enshrined in the International Covenant on Economic, Social and Cultural Rights (ICESCR). The committee in charge of the preparations of this Covenant was, according to the Ukrainian representative, "elaborating principles of *de jure* equality; from those principles would arise the de facto equalization of human rights. It would be wrong to confuse those two concepts . . . equality of rights went further than mere nondiscrimination; it implied the existence of positive rights in all the spheres dealt with in the draft Covenant [on Economic, Social and Cultural Rights]."[36]

Similar concerns were expressed during elaboration of the International Covenant on Civil and Political Rights (ICCPR). For example, when the draft Article 26 of the ICCPR was discussed by the UN General Assembly, there were objections that this clause might be held to mean that the law should be the same for everybody, perhaps precluding introduction of legal provisions protecting such groups as minors and people with learning disabilities. In reply to such concerns, it was explained that this provision was intended to ensure equality, not identical treatment, and would not prohibit reasonable differentiation between individuals or groups of individuals on grounds that were relevant and material.[37]

The importance of different treatment to achieve equality became recognized in more recent human rights documents, notably as a means to combat gender and racial discrimination. Whereas admissibility of positive action programs remained implicit in the International Bill of Rights,[38] subsequently adopted human rights documents delineate temporary special benefits to guarantee "full and equal enjoyment of human rights and fundamental freedoms."[39]

Support for the material equality perspective can also be deduced from statements of the UN Human Rights Committee. In its famous General Comment No. 18 on nondiscrimination, the Committee held that: "The enjoyment of rights and freedoms on an equal footing, however, does not mean *identical* treatment in every instance" (emphasis added). And further on: "The Committee also wishes to point out that the principle of equality sometimes requires States parties to take affirmative action in order to diminish or eliminate conditions which cause or help to perpetuate discrimination prohibited by the Covenant."[40]

Recognition of material equality has steadily gained support in the European region. By 1963, the Court of Justice of the European Community seemed to opt for the material equality perspective. For example, in the case of *Italy v. Commission,* the court stated that prohibited discrimination consists not only in treating similar situations differently but also in treating different situations identically.[41] In its further case law, the court failed, however, to elaborate on this decision.[42] Instead, it focused on the distinction between direct and indirect discrimination.[43] Indirect discrimination essentially refers to situations in which similar treatment has an adverse effect on certain groups of persons. Whereas prohibition of indirect discrimination does not always go as far as the material equality approach, it should be noted that prohibition of indirect discrimination—and thus rejection of the "sameness of treatment" concept of equality—forms an explicit recognition of the shortcomings of formal equality discourse.[44]

As for the Council of Europe, reference should be made to the case law of the European Court and the European Commission of Human Rights. Despite the accessory nature of the antidiscrimination provision in the European Convention on Human Rights (ECHR),[45] and notwithstanding the fact that the indirect discrimination does not figure in the jurisprudence of the ECHR, the meaning both bodies attach to Article 14 of the convention goes slightly further than the promotion of formal equality.[46]

Concerning recognition of the material equality perspective on a national level, reference should be made to the *Andrews v. Law Society of British Columbia* case in Canada.[47] McIntyre deliberated in the case as follows:

> To approach the ideal of full equality before and under the law ... the main consideration must be the impact of the law on the individual or the group concerned. Recognizing that there will always be an infinite variety of personal characteristics, capacities, entitlements and merits among those subject to the law, there must be accorded, as nearly as may be possible, an equality of benefits and protection and no more of the restrictions, penalties or burdens imposed upon one than the other.[48]

Also in other Canadian Charter cases, the Supreme Court of Canada adopted the material equality discourse.[49] According to these cases, courts should take into account the history of groups and their respective vulnerability in the face of laws and legal changes.[50]

Recognition of material equality is also firmly rooted in the Australian jurisdiction. The three most prominent federal laws created to protect and promote the rights of disadvantaged and vulnerable groups—the Racial Discrimination Act (1975), the Sex Discrimination Act (1984), and the Disability Discrimination Act (1992)—each explicitly allows governments to enact "special measures" in favor of less advantaged groups in order to attain genuine equality. In a number of cases, members of dominant groups filed complaints asserting that they were being discriminated against by positive-action measures. The Australian courts repeatedly held that special and preferential treatment may be justified to achieve equal opportunities for various groups.[51]

EQUAL RIGHTS AND NONDISCRIMINATION—
TOWARD A RIGHT TO REASONABLE ACCOMMODATION

The notion of material equality was warmly embraced by the disability rights movement, which emerged during the 1960s. Awareness rose that disabled persons had little to gain from the "sameness of treatment" concept as long as a range of environmental barriers existed to prevent their societal integration. Frustrated with the social welfare approach, disabled people began claiming the right, instead of the privilege, to full participation and equality with others.

An important first step in global recognition of the equal rights of disabled persons was the World Programme of Action Concerning Disabled Persons (WPA). In this program, adopted without a vote by the UN General Assembly in 1982, the principle of equal rights is described as the following:

> The principle of equal rights for the disabled and non-disabled implies that the needs of each and every individual are of equal importance, that these needs must be made the basis for the planning of societies, and that resources must be employed in such a way as to ensure, for every individual, equal opportunity for participation.[52]

Referencing ideas underlying the discourse of material equality, the focus in the equality debate herewith shifted from ensuring similar treatment to achieving equal outcomes. This view was reconfirmed in 1987 by the Global Meeting of Experts on Disability. This forum reaffirmed the principle that the law should take full account of the needs and rights of all population groups instead of advocating uniform treatment of all people.[53]

In both the Standard Rules and the General Comment, the adherence of the international community of states to the principle of material equality was—at least vis-à-vis disabled people—reinforced. In the introduction to the Standard Rules the principle of "equal rights" is described as implying: "that the needs of each and every individual are of equal importance, that those needs must be made the basis for the planning of societies and that all resources must be employed in such a way as to ensure that every individual has equal opportunities for participation."[54]

The General Comment explicitly refers to the wording of the equal rights provision in the WPA.[55] What is new about the General Comment is that it contains an all-embracing definition of discrimination on the grounds of disability that corresponds directly to a material interpretation of the principle of equality:

> For the purpose of the Covenant [ICESCR], "disability-based discrimination" may be defined as including any distinction, exclusion, restriction or preference or denial of reasonable accommodation based on disability which has the effect of nullifying or impairing the recognition, enjoyment or exercise of economic, social or cultural rights.[56]

It is particularly the latter requirement, the duty to make a "reasonable accommodation," that indicates overall recognition of the fundamental equality of disabled persons as human beings.[57] Modifications or adaptations that ensure societal participation of disabled persons are no longer considered a charitable goal, but a legally enforceable right.

Reasonable accommodation can be defined as "providing or modifying devices, services, or facilities, or changing practices or procedures in order to match a particular person with a particular program or activity."[58] In short, a reasonable accommodation is a modification or adjustment that allows a person with disabilities to participate in society on an equal footing with a nondisabled person. Examples of "reasonable accommodation" include installment of a wheelchair ramp and elevators for people with mobility impairments, the introduction of part-time work schedules for workers with impaired conditions, availability of readers for people with visual impairments, and sign translation for people with hearing impairments.

Not surprisingly, conceptualization of the entitlement to reasonable accommodation emerged in those Anglo-Saxon countries with a strong civil rights tradition, including Australia, Canada, and the United States.[59] In the United States, it emanated from jurisprudence relating to the antidiscrimination clause of the Rehabilitation Act (1973). The courts interpreted the meaning of section 504 broadly, not confined to "abstaining from unequal treatment" but rather giving disabled persons a right to require that action be taken to lift barriers obstructing their societal participation.[60] The courts thereby acknowledged that disabled people need a material interpretation of the principle of equality.

In many respects, recognition of this new right is a breakthrough. Martha McCluskey phrased it like this: "Reasonable accommodation goes beyond a simple equal treatment principle to require changes in some practices and structures to alleviate the disadvantageous effects of physical differences."[61]

Little by little, the duty to provide reasonable accommodation, as embodied in general or specific antidiscrimination provisions, is also gaining momentum in other jurisdictions.[62] After the General Comment on Persons with Disabilities is adopted, it is expected that more countries will give a material interpretation of their equal rights and antidiscrimination provisions.

DISABILITIES AND OTHER "DIFFERENCES"

It follows, then, that "equality" and "discrimination" are essentially relational concepts that make little sense without comparison. The same holds true for the concepts of "disability" and "difference" as well as "sameness"; all are social constructions and presuppose a relationship between people.[63] Since no human being is identical to another, our definition of difference depends on our point of comparison. Commonly, the labeling of people as "normal" or "different" follows the same pattern. It starts with determining what is "normal," usually the group that we belong to ourselves. Subsequently, we compare the "normal" with a counterexample, which we call "different"—or even "abnormal."[64] Whom we call "different" thus depends on whom we call "normal."

Differentiating between groups of people is a delicate issue. While it is true that able-bodied and disabled persons are at least in some respect different from each other, it should be acknowledged that there are other traits that could be used to distinguish people. Classifications based on individual qualities or group attributes may reinforce negative stereotyping that has been used to exclude members of disadvantaged and vulnerable groups from societal participation. In addition, labeling groups as "disabled" or "different" often reflects societal power structures and may exacerbate the societal position of members of less powerful groups.[65] Labeling people as "different" and perceiving oneself as the "norm" forces "others" to shoulder the burdens of their difference. In other words, these "different" persons are expected to adapt to the norms and standards of the "normal" society. In the case of disabled persons, one can wonder to what extent, if at all, it is fair and just that disabled persons should adapt to the norms and standards of the able-bodied mainstream.[66] Wouldn't it be more fair if society sought to accommodate the needs of disabled persons, instead of the other way around? From a perspective of material equality the latter option deserves careful attention.

It follows that distinguishing among people based on disability can be permitted only when the disability is crucially relevant in a given situation. It cannot be denied that some disabilities inhibit societal participation of the persons concerned. The extent to which disabled people are unable to perform or compete on an equal basis with their able-bodied counterparts should, however, be neither under- nor overestimated. Overestimation occurs when other negative criteria that are irrelevant in a given situation are attributed to a disabled person. Distinguishing between people based solely on disability, without objective justification, amounts to discrimination. Discrimination between an able-bodied person and a disabled person may also take place when differentiation takes place on a criterion other than physical or mental disability, but de facto results in the adverse treatment of persons with disabilities. For example, selecting people according to height or mobility may lead to the exclusion of large groups of people with physical disabilities. Similarly, selection of persons on the basis of mental health care consumption may be to the detriment of people with a history of mental disabilities. For situations in which such criteria are imposed without an objective justification, such as scientific evidence that such distinctions are in the interest of public safety, these criteria would amount to indirect discrimination toward disabled persons.

ADMISSIBLE AND INADMISSIBLE DIFFERENTIATION

The next issue we should address concerns whether to what extent "differences" between people should be reflected in the way we treat them. In other words, what weight should we attach to the features that show that we are all (slightly or enormously) different? The answer to this question depends on how relevant a feature is in a given situation. According to international human rights law, distinguishing between people with respect to individual and group features—such as race, sex, national or social origin, religion, political or other opinion—is, as a matter of principle, never allowed unless there is an objective justification to do so. Although disability-based discrimination[67] is as yet less firmly rooted in international human rights law than inter alia, gender and racial discrimination, there are reasons to believe that we can determine the (in)admissibility of differentiation on the grounds of disability analogous to other forms of prohibited discrimination.[68]

Pursuant to internationally recognized human rights standards, it is permitted to distinguish between people to the extent that such differentiation is commensurate with the degree in which people are different from each other. There are two exceptions to this rule: commensurate differentiation amounts to discrimination if (1) the persons involved are not "similarly situated" and the "commensurately different treatment form" would increase—instead of decrease—their inequality, and (2) the "commensurately different treatment form" would otherwise impair or deny the right to equality.

With respect to the first exception—which is primarily founded on a formal equality theory—it should be noted that the "similarly situated" test is everything but unproblematic. The "similarly situated" test confines the meaning of equality to requiring that only persons who are in a similar situation need to be treated equally. It has often been asserted by those who are critical of this test that it overlooks social and economic inequalities between (members of) groups. This challenges the overall legitimacy of this test, since it fails to rectify some of the main causes of societal injustice. In addition, it has been said that this test is too rigid and mechanical to handle the true complexity of equality.[69] In response, new theories on equality evolved in which the emphasis shifted from the starting situation to the very result of the "commensurately different (or similar) treatment form." It was felt that material equality requires not only that we should focus on the starting situation in which people find themselves ("similarly situated"), but that attention should notably be paid to the actual outcome of different (or identical) forms of treatment. The actual distribution of benefits should parallel the distribution of those attributes that are judged relevant.[70] The similarly situated test not only fails to question the relevance of individual qualities and group attributes; it ignores the outcome of different (or identical) forms of treatment. For this reason, the material equality approach uses the enhancement of equal rights as a yardstick against which to measure the (in)admissibility of different (and similar) forms of treatment.

It follows from both the formal and material equality discourses that different treatment is sometimes admissible but at other times inadmissible. Differentiation between disabled and able-bodied persons seems justifiable when a disability is crucially important to categorize or distinguish between

people. Having two legs, for example, is an absolute requirement for playing certain sports, as is the possession of some musical talent for being
admitted to a school of music, and good vision is necessary for becoming a
pilot. Where a disability is either irrelevant or when a physical or mental
limitation can easily be compensated by making a reasonable accommodation, it is—in principle—not allowed to be cause to differentiate between
disabled and nondisabled persons. In such situations, differentiation, as
well as the refusal to provide a reasonable accommodation, would amount
to discrimination.

Are there, however, situations in which differentiation between disabled
and nondisabled persons is required, even if the disability as such is irrelevant? According to the formal equality discourse, this will hardly ever be the
case. At best, differentiation can be "permitted" to serve a higher social
objective such as the enhancement of equality. The material equality
discourse has a slightly different approach. Given the importance this
discourse attaches to achieving genuine equality, a differentiation of treatment between disabled and able-bodied persons can be considered the most
suitable manner in which to attain equal rights. This will particularly be the
case when:

- differentiation is made between (members of) different groups to achieve
  equality in the context of a social policy (programs and measures designed
  to eliminate discrimination and to encourage un[der]represented groups to
  reach a situation in which they are more likely to compete with others on an
  equal basis)
- differentiation is made to achieve equality in the context of a preferential
  treatment program (e.g., measures taken in favor of disadvantaged and
  vulnerable groups to diminish or eliminate conditions that cause or help
  perpetuate discrimination against members of the target group)

The latter two policies are commonly referred to as positive-action
programs, with preferential-treatment programs being much more controversial than social policy measures.[71]

FROM FIGHTING DIFFERENTIATION TO FIGHTING DISCRIMINATION: SOME CONCLUDING REMARKS

From the above examination of the principles of equality and nondiscrimination in the context of disability issues it follows that differentiation is not
always necessarily wrong ("discrimination") and that identical treatment is
not always necessarily right ("equal"). The principles of equality and nondiscrimination seek to conserve human variety and to enhance the equality of
outcomes. Equality and nondiscrimination imply that unnecessary and
avoidable differences ("inequalities") should be prevented and, once they
have occurred, remedied. The latter can be achieved by a combination of
antidiscrimination measures aimed at the prohibition of adverse forms of
(similar and different) treatment and positive action measures aimed at the

promotion of equal rights of disadvantaged and vulnerable groups. The latter set of measures pertains to a differential- ("positive"-) treatment policy.

The implication of this analysis for the rights of disabled persons is twofold. First, it seems necessary to bestow on disabled people an enforceable entitlement to protection against direct and indirect forms of discrimination, as well as the denial of reasonable accommodation, by way of antidiscrimination legislation. Antidiscrimination provisions can be enshrined in both general and specific laws in which disability is explicitly mentioned as a prohibited ground of discrimination. Second, positive-action programs should be designed to rectify the historical subordination of disabled people to their able-bodied environment. Programs should be developed to fight the real causes of disadvantage and vulnerability and should take away all the environmental barriers (including negative attitudes) that inhibit disabled persons' enjoyment and exercise of equal rights. Differences should be fought to the extent that they reflect inequalities, whereas differences that reflect human variation should be carefully respected.

The enactment of both types of measures is in full conformity with the principles laid down in the Standard Rules and the General Comment. The international community of states no longer expects disabled persons to unconditionally conform to the norms and standards of "mainstream" environments. True respect for human diversity requires respect for mental and physical variation, and intolerance of mechanisms that discriminate against (groups of) persons on the basis of individual or group variations. It is to be hoped that these principles will be properly reflected in national policies and legislation.

REFERENCES

1. Pursuant to the International Classification of Impairments, Disabilities and Handicaps (ICIDH, 1980) a disability is "a restriction or lack (resulting from an impairment) of ability to perform an activity in the manner within the range considered normal for a human being." Despite widespread criticism against the individual outlook of the ICIDH typology, until today the ICIDH has been the sole authoritative international document to provide a comprehensive definition of disability. See A. Hendriks and T. Degener, "The Evolution of the European Perspective on Disability Legislation: From a Public Health to a Human Rights Approach," *European Journal of Health Law* 1, 4 (1994): 343–366.
2. L. Despouy, "Human Rights and Disability," final report by the special rapporteur of the Sub-Commission on Prevention of Discrimination and the Protection of Minorities, UN Doc. E/CN.4/Sub.2/1991/31, 12 July 1991.
3. See, e.g., OECD, "Employment Policies for People with Disabilities: Labour Market and Social Policy," occasional paper no. 8, OECD, Paris, 1992. For an in-depth study on the interrelationship between poverty and human rights, see L. Despouy, "The Realization of Economic, Social and Cultural Rights—Human Rights and Extreme Poverty," interim report by the special rapporteur of the Sub-Commission on Prevention of Discrimination and the Protection of Minorities, UN Doc. E/CN.4/Sub.2/1994/19, 10 June 1994.

4. In the United States, the terms *disparate* (direct) discrimination and *adverse impact* (indirect) discrimination are commonly used.

5. Besides these categories, a Canadian judge identified "systemic discrimination, adverse impact discrimination, constructive discrimination and perhaps others." *Toronto (City) Board of Education v. Quereshi* (1991), 14 C.H.R.R. D/243 at D/249.

6. A. H. Goldman, *Justice and Reverse Discrimination* (Princeton: Princeton University Press, 1979).

7. C. Barnes, *Disabled People in Britain and Discrimination* (London: Hurst and Company, 1991), pp. 12–13; Human Rights and Equal Opportunity Commission, *Human Rights and Mental Illness*, report of the National Inquiry into the Human Rights of People with Mental Illness (Canberra: Australian Government Publishing Service, 1993), pp. 38–39.

8. S. Klosse, *Menselijke schade: vergoeden of herstellen?* (Antwerpen/Apeldoorn: Maklu, 1989).

9. H. Astor, "Anti-Discrimination Legislation and Physical Discrimination: The Lessons of Experience," *Australian Law Journal* 64, 3, (1990): 113–128.

10. R. Wiggins, *Needs, Values, Truth* (Oxford: Basil Blackwell, 1991).

11. See, e.g., International Labour Organisation (ILO), Vocational Rehabilitation and Employment (Disabled Persons) Convention, 1983 (no. 159). Published in *International Labour Conventions and Recommendations 1919–1991*, 2 vols. (Geneva: ILO, 1992).

12. General Assembly of the UN, Resolution 48/96 (20 December 1993).

13. UN Committee on Economic, Social and Cultural Rights, General Comment on People with Disabilities (1994), UN Doc E/C.12/1994/WP.13, 1 December 1994.

14. E.g., in the drafting process of Articles 2 and 26 of the International Covenant on Civil and Political Rights, these concepts were regularly used without distinction. See B. G. Ramcharan, "Equality and Nondiscrimination" in L. Henkin, ed., *The International Bill of Rights—The Covenant on Civil and Political Rights* (New York: Columbia University Press, 1981), p. 251.

15. Cf. R. Dworkin, *Taking Rights Seriously* (London: Duckworth, 1977), p. 199.

16. Wiggins (see note 10).

17. Cf. M. Whitehead, *The Concepts and Principles of Equity and Health*, doc. no. EUR/ICP/RPD 414 (Copenhagen: WHO, Regional Office for Europe, 1990), p. 9.

18. D. C. Galloway, "Three Models of (In)Equality," *McGill Law Review* 68 (1993): 83.

19. Cf. address by the Swiss head of the Political Department at the opening of the World Conference to Combat Racism and Racial Discrimination on 14 August 1978, *Report of the World Conference to Combat Racism and Racial Discrimination*, UN Doc. A/CONF.92/40 Annex IC (1979).

20. Human Rights Committee, General Comment No. 18 (37), Non-discrimination, para. 12.

21. Belgian Linguistic case, 23 July 1968, Public. ECHR, Series A, no. 5–6.

22. Cf. J. Wilson on the purpose of subsection 15 (1) of the Canadian Charter of Human Rights and Freedoms in *R. v. Turpin*, [1989] 1 S.C.R. 1296 at 1333, 69 C.R. (3d) 97, 48 C.C.C. (3d) 8.

23. F. S. Royster Guano Co. v. Virginia, 253 U.S. 412 (1920).

24. Aristotle, *The Nicomachean Ethics* (Oxford: Oxford University Press, 1980), book V, III, 113a–113b (translated by D. Ross).

25. J. J. Rousseau, *Discours sur l'origine et les fondements de l'inégalité parmi les hommes* (Paris: Pléiade, 1964).

26. G.W.F. Hegel, *Grundlinien der Philosophie des Rechts* (Leipzig: G. Lasson, 1921).

27. K. Marx, "Das Kapital," in K. Marx and F. Engels, *Gesamelte Werke*, vol. 23 (Berlin: Dietz Verlag, 1978).

28. J. E. Goldschmidt and R. Holtmaat, *Vrouw en recht—trendrapport* DCE/STEO (The Hague: DCE/STEO, 1993), notably chapter 23 (pp. 441–464).

29. The political philosopher Michael Walzer studied this phenomenon extensively. He proposed a sharp line of distinction between the different spheres inherent in society. See M. Walzer, *Spheres of Justice: A Defence of Pluralism and Equality* (Oxford: Basil Blackwell, 1983).

30. E. W. Vierdag, "The Concept of Discrimination in International Law" (The Hague: Martinus Nijhoff, 1973), p. 3.

31. Lepofsky and Bickenbach distinguish the following environmental barriers: tangible structural barriers, intangible structural barriers, and attitudinal barriers. D. Lepofsky and Bickenbach, "Equality, Rights and the Physically Handicapped," in A. F. Bayefsky and M. Eberts, eds., *Equality Rights and the Canadian Charter of Rights and Freedoms* (Toronto: Carswell, 1985), p. 326.

32. Positive action programs seek to (temporarily) aid disadvantaged and vulnerable groups by giving them special treatment. These programs should facilitate the fair and equal distribution of benefits and burdens. J. E. Goldschmidt, "Staats— en bestuursrechtelijke aspecten van positieve actie," in B. P. Sloot, J. E. Goldschmidt, and W.J.P.M. Fase. eds., *Positieve discriminatie, preadviezen van de NJV* (Zwolle: W. E.J. Tjeenk Willink, 1989), p. 57–117.

33. T. Loenen, "Rethinking Sex Equality as a Human Right," *Netherlands Quarterly of Human Rights* 12, 3 (1994): 253–270.

34. Advisory Opinion of 10 September 1923 on German Settlers in Poland, PCIJ, Ser. B, no. 6.

35. Advisory Opinion of 6 April 1935 on the Minority Schools in Albania case, Ser. A/B, no. 64, p. 19.

36. Ukrainian SSR, UN Doc. A/C.3/SR.1183, 1962, para. 10.

37. 10 GAOR Annexes, UN Doc. A/2929, 1955, para. 179; Ramcharan (see note 14), p. 254.

38. Ramcharan (see note 14), pp. 259–261; Vierdag (see note 30), pp. 74–78.

39. E.g., Art. 2, para. 2, International Convention on the Elimination of Racial Discrimination, and Art. 4, Convention on the Elimination of All Forms of Discrimination Against Women.

40. Committee on Human Rights, General Comment No. 18, Non-Discrimination, UN Official Records, Suppl. No. 40 (A/45/40), pp. 173–175, paras. 8 and 10.

41. Case 13/63, *Italy v. Commission* [1963] ECR 31.

42. C.W.A. Timmerman, "Verboden discriminatie of (geboden) differentiatie," *SEW* 6 (1982): 444 ff.

43. See, e.g., case 170/84, *Bilka-Kaufhaus GmbH v. Weber von Harz* [1986] ECR 1607.

44. Goldschmidt and Holtmaat (see note 28), p. 511.

45. Article 14 does not prohibit discrimination in general, but only discrimination in relation to the rights and freedoms guaranteed by the convention. See Appl. 841078, *X v. Federal Republic of Germany*, D & R 1980; 18 at 220.

46. See P. van Dijk and G.J.H. van Hoof, "Theory and Practice of the European Convention on Human Rights," *Kluwer Law and Taxation Publishers* (Boston: Deventer, 1990), p. 539. See also Loenen (note 33), pp. 262–263.

47. See, e.g., M. Gold, "Comment: *Andrews v. Law Society of British Columbia,*" *McGill Law Journal* 34 (1989), pp. 1063–1079, and N. C. Shephard, "Recognition of the Disadvantaging of Women: The premise of *Andrews v. Law Society of British Columbia,*" *McGill Law Journal* 35 (1989), pp. 207–234. See also K. Mahoney, "The Constitutional Law of Equality in Canada," *New York University Journal of International Law and Politics* 24 (1992): 759–793.

48. *Andrews v. Law Society of British Columbia* [1989], 1 S.C.R. 143, 56 D.L.R. (4th) 1, 10 C.H.R.R. D/5719.

49. Mahoney (see note 47).

50. See, e.g., *R v. Keegstra* (1990), 3 S.C.R. 697, and *R v. Huttler* (1992), 1 S.C.R. 452.

51. *Gerhardy v. Brown,* CLR 1984–1985, 159: 70; *Proudfoot v. Human Rights and Equal Opportunity Commission,* ALR 1991, 100: 557. See A. Hendriks, "Vormt de AWGB een bedreiging voor vrouwengezondheidszorg?," *NJCM-Bulletin* 18, 8 (1993): 879–897.

52. General Assembly of the UN, Resolution 37/52, 3 December 1982, para. 25.

53. UN. Doc. CSDHA/DDP/GMA (1987), para. 31.

54. Standard Rules, para. 25.

55. General Comment, para. 17.

56. General Comment, para. 15.

57. The duty to provide "reasonable accommodation" is balanced by the proviso that such an accommodation is not required if it would cause "unjustifiable" or "undue hardship." See J. Cooper, "Overcoming Barriers to Employment: The Meaning of Reasonable Accommodation and Undue Hardship in the Americans with Disabilities Act," *University of Pennsylvania Law Review* 139 (1991): 1423–1436.

58. C. G. Bell and R. L. Burgdorf, *Accommodating the Spectrum of Individual Abilities: United States Commission on Civil Rights,* Publication No. 81 (Washington, DC, Clearinghouse, 1983), p. 122.

59. G. Quinn, M. McDonagh, and C. Kimber, *Disability Discrimination Law in the United States, Australia and Canada* (Dublin: Oak Tree Press, 1993).

60. Section 504 reads as follows: "No otherwise qualified handicapped individual . . . shall, solely by reason of his handicap, be excluded from participation in, be denied the benefits of, or be subjected to discrimination under any program or activity receiving federal financial assistance." See also the landmark case *Southeastern Community College v. Davis,* 422 U.S. 397 (1979), in which the Supreme Court held that educational institutions are obliged to make a reasonable accommodation.

61. M. McCluskey, "Rethinking Equality and Difference: Disability Discrimination in Public Transportation," *Yale Law Journal* 97 (1988): 867.

62. For the Netherlands, see, e.g., *Goldsteen v. Roeland,* 13 December 1991, RvdW 1992, 9. Finland and Sweden have introduced special laws bestowing disabled persons with a right to assistance: Service and Assistance for the Disabled Act (3 April 1987/380) and Act Concerning the Support and Service for Persons with Certain Functional Impairments (27 May 1993/SFS 1993:307).

63. According to Lisa Waddington, the current disability definitions locate the origins of these constructions in a series of artificial constraints that are imposed on a group of persons who consequently become labeled as disabled. See L. Waddington, "More Disabled Than Others: The Employment of Disabled Persons Within the European Community: An Analysis of Existing Measures and Proposals for the Development of an EC policy," doctoral thesis, University of Limburg, Maastricht, 1993, p. 12.

64. M. Minow, *Making All the Difference: Inclusion, Exclusion, and American Law*, Ithaca, N.Y.: Cornell University Press, 1991.
65. Cf. S.C. Ainlay, *The Dilemma of Difference: A Multidisciplinary View of Stigma* (New York: Plenum,1983). See also J. Goldschmidt, *We Need Different Stories* (Zwolle, W. E.J. Tjeenk Willink, 1993).
66. M. Oliver, "Discrimination, Disability and Social Policy," in M. Brenton and C. Jones (eds.), *Yearbook of Social Policy (1984–1985)* (London: Routledge and Kegan Paul, 1985), pp. 74–97.
67. The same holds true with respect to health-related discrimination. See J.M.V. Canada, Human Rights Committee, Com.559 11993, U.N. Doc CCPR/C/ 50/D/559/1993 (8 April 1994).
68. "Article 2 of the Universal Declaration of Human Rights, which provides that everyone is entitled to all the rights and freedoms set forth in this Declaration, without distinction of any kind, such as race, colour, sex, language, religion, political or other opinion, national or social origin, property, birth or other status, applies also to disabled persons." Sub-Commission on the Prevention of Discrimination and the Protection of Minorities, Resolution 1982/1 (7 September 1982). See also Resolution 1991/19 (28 August 1991).
69. J. McIntyre noted that "the [similarly situated] test cannot be accepted as a fixed rule or formula for the resolution of equality questions arising under the [Canadian] Charter. Consideration must be given to the content of the law, to its purpose, and its impact upon those to whom it applies, and also those whom it excludes from its application."
70. A. F. Bayefsky, "The Orientation of Section 15 of the Canadian Charter of Rights and Freedoms," in J. M. Weiler and R. M. Elliot, eds., *Litigating the Values of the Nation: The Canadian Charter of Rights and Freedoms* (Toronto: Carswell, 1986).
71. Hendriks (see note 51), pp. 888–890.

11. Rights Violations in the Ecuadorian Amazon: The Human Consequences of Oil Development

Center for Economic and Social Rights

The physical environment is one of the key determinants of human health. The human cost of environmental degradation has spurred a strong international movement to link environmental protection with human rights. This trend can be seen both in the growing awareness of the need for sustainable development and in the recent emergence of a new right—the right to a healthy environment. The 1972 Stockholm Declaration supported the view that the environment should be protected in order to ensure established rights, such as the rights to life, health, personal security, suitable work conditions, and private property, for current as well as future generations. The International Covenant on Economic, Social and Cultural Rights (ICESCR) recognizes the right of everyone to the enjoyment of the highest attainable standard of physical and mental health. In Article 12b, ICESCR states that "steps to be taken by the States Parties to the present Covenant to achieve the full realization of this right shall include those necessary for the improvement of all aspects of environmental and industrial hygiene." This study represents one of the first attempts to apply the rights to health and to a healthy environment in assessing the human consequences of a country's development policies.

The chapter provides a brief background of the economic, social, and political aspects of oil development in Ecuador; describes the health effects of crude oil's toxic constituents; details Ecuador's failure to protect the rights to health and to a healthy environment; and assesses the human rights implications of oil production in the Oriente.

BACKGROUND

The Oriente in Ecuador consists of more than forty million hectares of tropical rain forest lying at the headwaters of the Amazon river network. The region contains one of the most diverse collections of plant and animal life in the world, including a considerable number of endangered species. According to tropical biologist Norman Myers, the area "is surely the richest biotic zone on earth and deserves to rank as a kind of global epicentre of biodiversity."[1] The Oriente is also home to eight different indigenous peoples who have lived in the rain forest for thousands of years.

THE OIL BOOM IN THE ORIENTE

In 1967, a Texaco-Gulf consortium discovered a rich field of oil beneath the rain forest, leading to an oil boom that has permanently reshaped the region. While the state has retained dominion over all mineral rights, private companies have built and operated most of the oil infrastructure. The Oriente now houses a vast network of roads, pipelines, and oil facilities. Settlers attracted by the roads and encouraged by government land policies have entered in large numbers, clearing vast regions of the rain forest and displacing indigenous inhabitants. This process has contributed to a deforestation rate of almost a million acres a year in the Oriente, one of the highest rates in Latin America.[2] Half of the Oriente is currently slated for oil development, including the concessions offered in the seventh round of licensing in January 1994, which has almost doubled the amount of rain forest under development.[3]

Experts and observers have questioned the environmental soundness of practices and technologies used by Texaco and Petroecuador for oil exploration in the Oriente.[4] Exploration for crude oil has involved thousands of miles of trail clearing and hundreds of seismic detonations that have caused erosion of land and dispersion of wildlife. Each exploratory well that is drilled produces an average of 4,165 cubic meters of drilling wastes, containing a mixture of drilling muds (used as lubricants and sealants), petroleum, natural gas, and formation water from deep below the earth's surface (containing hydrocarbons, heavy metals, and high concentrations of salt). These wastes are deposited into open, unlined pits called waste pits or separation ponds, from which they are either directly discharged into the environment or leach out as the pits degrade or overflow from rainwater.[5]

The major release of contaminants begins at the point of production. In a recent case brought against Texaco for contaminating the Oriente, the International Water Tribunal declared that "insufficient and at most superficial measures were taken for retaining and minimalizing spillage of oil and contaminating substances and leakages from pits" leading to "deterioration in the quality of the river water which is essential for the sustainable livelihood of the local population."[6] Until 1992, oil operations in the Oriente produced 1.7 billion barrels of oil, 489 million barrels of formation water, and more than 355 trillion cubic feet of gas.[8]

As oil is extracted from the wells, it is pumped to separation stations, which separate oil from wastes that include formation water, oil remnants, gas, and toxic chemicals used in the extraction and separation stages.[8] Every day, existing stations discharge more than 4.3 million gallons of untreated toxic wastes (called produced water or toxic brine), which includes 2,100 to 4,200 gallons of oil, into waste pits. Virtually all of the waste eventually leaches from the pits into the environment. An additional 1,000 to 2,000 gallons of oil spill from the flowlines connecting the wells to the stations every two weeks.[9] Oil and chemicals are spilled from leaks in tanks and storage drums. Through 1989, the Ecuadorian government had reported thirty separate spills in the main trans-Ecuadorian pipeline, involving a total of almost 17 million gallons of crude oil far more than the 10.8 million gallons spilled in the Exxon *Valdez* disaster.[10] Overall, more than 30 billion gallons of toxic wastes and crude oil have been discharged into the land and waterways of the Oriente since 1972.[11]

ECONOMIC, SOCIAL, AND CULTURAL ASPECTS OF OIL DEVELOPMENT

Oil development has failed to improve Ecuador's economic situation. While the start of the oil boom corresponded to rapid increases in per capita income and gross national product, the national debt has risen from $200 million in 1970 to more than $12 billion today, forcing structural adjustments and cuts in social spending.[12] The impact on the poor majority is reflected in the rising poverty rate, from less than 50 percent in 1975 to 65 percent in 1992.[13] Moreover, the country's overwhelming dependence on oil revenues, accounting for roughly half of the national budget, has left it extremely vulnerable to oil price fluctuations. As international prices have slumped and reserves decline, Ecuador has sought to expand production in marginal oil fields and protected natural parks. At current production rates Ecuador's reserves will be depleted within fifteen years.[14]

A small segment of the population has disproportionately enjoyed the benefits of oil development; at the same time, few of the profits have been reinvested in the Oriente. The majority of the benefits have been captured by the elite and the military, while the urban poor, colonists, and indigenous groups have almost uniformly suffered worsening conditions.[15] Settlers drawn to the region by the promise of jobs and land now cluster in desperate and squalid oil towns, with little running water, in adequate sanitation and few basic health facilities. According to the World Bank, "Field visits to the urban areas of Napo province indicate that local public service levels and coverage in the region are in a calamitous condition."[16] A 1989 government study revealed that Shushufindi, a primary oil center that accounts for almost half of national production, lacked public sewers and provided electricity and water to only one in five hundred homes.[17]

The oil boom has most severely affected the indigenous population, which accounts for more than 40 percent of Ecuador's total population of 11 million. Eight different nations, each with a total population of between 100,000 and 250,000 people, inhabit the Oriente. The Quichua and Shuar account for the majority, with the rest divided among the Huaorani, the Secoya, the Siona, the Shiwiar, the Cofan, and the Achuar. These peoples have distinct cultures and traditions that are inextricably bound to the rain forest in which they have lived for thousands of years. Their economic and spiritual existence revolves around sustainable management of rain forest resources.

Despite an international trend towards legal recognition of indigenous rights and cultures, exemplified by the United Nations' International Decade of Indigenous Peoples (1995–2005), the government of Ecuador has refused to recognize indigenous ownership of lands and instead has encouraged a stream of immigration by granting title to any settler who clears and cultivates land. Since the discovery of huge oil fields beneath the rain forest, almost 250,000 settlers, mostly poor *campesinos,* have entered the Oriente through new oil roads, displacing indigenous residents from traditional areas and creating tension and occasional open conflict. In addition, contact with outsiders and the introduction of a cash economy have undermined traditional cultures and subjected indigenous peoples to discrimination. As one of Ecuador's foremost judges has noted, "Ecuador is a country characterized by deep racism against its own indigenous people. . . . This reality supersedes all constitutional declarations and international conventions on human rights, and there is constant discrimination and unequal application of the law."[18] These various factors have combined to drive some indigenous nations to the point of extinction.

HEALTH EFFECTS OF EXPOSURE TO CRUDE OIL

Crude oils are a mixture of a hundred or more hydrocarbons, sulfur compounds, and a range of metals and salts in smaller quantities.[15] In addition, a variety of other toxic pollutants are typically generated during oil drilling and production operations, including drilling fluids, drilling cuts, and treatment chemicals that contain heavy metals, strong acids, and concentrated salts.[20] These include polycylic aromatic hydrocarbon (PAH) compounds (e.g., benzo[*a*]pyrene) and volatile organic compounds (e.g., benzene and its derivatives), toxic, and carcinogenic substances that pose a threat to human health. Crude oil and its constituents enter the human body through three primary routes: (1) skin absorption, (2) ingestion of food and drink, and (3) inhalation of oil on dust or soot particles.

The fat solubility of most oil constituents allows them to be absorbed into and through the skin. Repeated or prolonged skin contact with crude oil has been reported to cause skin loss, dryness, cracking, changes in skin pigmentation, hyperkeratosis, pigmented plane warts, and eczematous reactions.[21] Limited evidence suggests that prolonged exposure to constituents of crude oil, such as benzo[*a*]pyrene and other hydrocarbons, can result in dermal neoplasms.[22]

Constituents of crude oil ingested in water or food, such as PAH compounds, have been linked to adverse health effects ranging from cancers to toxic effects on reproduction and cellular development.[23] The United States Environmental Protection Agency (EPA) estimates that exposure to a

PAH water concentration of 2.8 nanograms per liter corresponds to an upper-bound lifetime risk of cancer of one in one million.[24] This risk could be significantly increased through added skin and inhalation exposure.

Inhalation of high levels of crude oil fumes can lead to adverse effects on the nervous and respiratory systems, sometimes causing life-threatening chemical pneumonitis and other systemic effects.[25] In the Oriente, oil particulates have been emitted into the atmosphere from burning waste pits. These pits also contain drilling fluids with pentachlorophenols, which when burned are a formation pathway for tetrachlorodibenzo-dioxins.[26] In summary, substantial health effects from exposure to crude oil and associated toxic pollutants have been reported in the general environmental health literature.

In the Oriente, oil contamination allegedly damaged people's health, contaminated their water, and deprived them of fish, game, and crops. For example, the physician-director of the largest government hospital in Coca reported a rise in child mortality believed to be associated with drinking water contamination, a result of increased population density.[27] Other area health care providers have reported substantial apparent increases in birth defects and skin rashes. Studies and interviews cited in a report by the Natural Resources Defense Council found extremely high rates of child malnutrition in areas impacted by oil development.[28] As Robert Kennedy Jr. noted in his visit to the region:

> We met with the center's chief clinician and with the representatives of fourteen communities accounting for about 40,000 people from the Aguarico River basin. Each of them told the same story. Sick and deformed children, adults and children affected with skin rashes, headaches, dysentery and respiratory ailments, cattle dead with their stomachs rotted out, crops destroyed, animals gone from the forest and fish from the rivers and streams.[29]

A study of health effects from oil exposure was recently published by the Ecuadorian Union of Popular Health Promoters of the Amazon (UPPSAE).[30] That study examined 1,465 people in ten communities, of whom 1,077 resided in oil-contaminated areas and 388 were from noncontaminated areas. Those exposed to oil reported a higher occurrence of spontaneous abortion and elevated rates of fungal infection, dermatitis, headache, and nausea. Ten percent of the oil-exposed group surveyed were currently ill.

VIOLATIONS OF THE RIGHT TO A HEALTHY ENVIRONMENT

The recognition of a right to health dates to the Universal Declaration of Human Rights of 1948[31] and its two successor International Covenants of 1966.[32] However, while the right to health under the International Covenants includes a reference to environmental protection, the linkage of human rights to environmental concerns is relatively new. International treaties and national constitutions speak of rights to a "clean," "healthy," "decent," and/or "safe" environment, but no consensus yet exists as to the specific shape or meaning of such rights.

The 1972 Stockholm Declaration established a framework for this debate by recognizing that the environment is "essential to [human] well-being and to the enjoyment of basic human rights—even the right to life itself." In that declaration, the United Nations General Assembly unanimously endorsed the principle that "man has the fundamental right to freedom, equality and adequate conditions of life, in an environment of a quality that permits a life of dignity and well-being."[33] As this link between human welfare and environmental quality has become increasingly clear, national legislatures and international bodies have begun to develop a new standard to protect the environment for the benefit of human health: the right to a healthy environment. This right, which should not be confused with claims to protect the environment for its own sake, now appears in international declarations, regional covenants, and virtually every constitution revised or adopted in the last thirty years. In 1990, the UN General Assembly passed a resolution, echoing its earlier endorsement in the Stockholm Declaration, that "all individuals are entitled to live in an environment adequate for their health and well-being."[34] A similar principle was recognized in the 1992 Rio Declaration on Environment and Development, and in the World Charter for Nature. Regional treaties and declarations in the Americas, Africa, and Europe all recognize some form of the right to a healthy environment.[35]

Few attempts have been made to interpret in detail the rights to health or to a healthy environment; until uniform standards have been developed, violations must be judged on the basis of a minimum set of governmental duties necessary to make these rights meaningful.

The well-documented record of unsafe and unsanitary oil industry practices in the Oriente and the ostensible evidence and likelihood of oil-contamination-related health problems strongly suggest that the Ecuadorian government has failed to comply with the minimum duties associated with the right to a healthy environment, viz., (1) to take reasonable precautions to avoid contaminating the environment in a manner that threatens human health, (2) to regulate private actors effectively to prevent such contamination, and (3) to provide potential victims of contamination with judicial remedies, including access to information on oil development. Each of these three minimum duties is discussed below.

DIRECT CONTAMINATION

Under international and Ecuadorian law, the government is liable for any contamination caused by the state oil company, Petroecuador, in the Oriente. Since 1992, Petroecuador has owned and controlled almost all oil production in the Oriente. For the twenty preceding years, Petroecuador was part of a consortium whose operating partner, Texaco, released roughly 30 billion gallons of toxic wastes and 17 million gallons of crude oil into the environment. During this time, Petroecuador also operated its own facilities, accounting for roughly 11 percent of total production. The record shows that the state has been involved in the bulk of past contamination in the Oriente, and is responsible for nearly all ongoing contamination.

Reasonable precautions, such as safe disposal of toxic wastes, use of water-based instead of oil-based drilling muds, reinjection of produced waters deep into the ground, proper maintenance and monitoring of the pipelines and production facilities, and spill prevention and response measures, could have prevented much of the contamination and resulting health impacts.[36] Such measures would have added only a small percentage to overall production costs. Nevertheless, interviews with environmental and industry experts and recent field visits to Petroecuador facilities by environmental groups, independent observers and CESR confirm that Petroecuador still has not upgraded the equipment nor altered the environmentally dangerous practices inherited from Texaco.

INEFFECTIVE REGULATION

The government is responsible as well for contamination by private companies that results from ineffective regulation, as opposed to accidents or random acts. Although Ecuador's constitution calls for legislation to ensure the right to a contamination-free environment, the government has enacted a confusing and ambiguous set of laws with weak environmental provisions.[37]

Moreover, state agencies responsible for environmental protection have lacked the necessary resources, expertise, and political support to enforce their mandates. Interviews with independent industry experts, legal scholars, and environmentalists confirm the view that these agencies, in the words of one legal authority, "have functioned like silent spectators to the environmental problems of the country."[38]

Ecuador's three primary laws relevant to the environmental impact of petroleum development have done little to prevent oil-related contamination. The country's first petroleum law, adopted in 1971, included a provision requiring oil companies "to prevent pollution of the water, the atmosphere, and the land," but contained no specific standards to give the law substantive content.[39] This law was subsequently supplemented by a decree ordering companies "to prevent the escape and waste of hydrocarbons in order to avoid loss, damage and pollution."[40] A draft of the official audit criteria for measuring Texaco's environmental record, approved by the Ecuadorian government, Texaco, and Petroecuador, reported that due to the absence of standards, "no environmental compliance was necessary until August 19th, 1982."[41] This date merely refers to an amendment of the petroleum law stating that oil companies were to operate "in accordance with international practices in these matters." Specific environmental regulations for the oil industry were not passed until 1992.[42]

A second law, the 1976 Law of Prevention and Control of Environmental Contamination (LPCCA), has had no impact on oil operations in the Oriente.[43] Regulations interpreting this law were not elaborated until 1989, and then covered only water quality.[44] Moreover, neither the Ministry of

Health, charged under the LPCCA with ensuring the safety of Ecuador's water supplies, nor the Interinstitutional Committee for Environmental Protection, established as an enforcement agency under the LPCCA, has taken action to address the problem of contamination in the Oriente.[45]

The 1981 Law of Forestry and Conservation of Natural Areas and Wildlife, the third significant piece of legislation regulating oil development, was intended to protect certain areas designated as natural reserves and national parks. However, Petroecuador and private companies have circumvented the law's strict decree that natural areas must be "inalterably preserved," by interpreting the law to permit exploitation of subsurface minerals such as oil.[46] The constitution and the Law of Hydrocarbons grant the state control over all subsurface mineral rights within the country and leave it to the state oil company to exploit the oil either on its own or jointly with private companies.[47] Ecuador's courts have upheld this position, allowing oil companies to construct new roads and facilities and exploit oil in all of the protected areas with known deposits. Five of the six protected areas touching the Oriente are under some form of oil development.[48]

The lack of environmentally protective legislation is compounded by insufficient resources, expertise, and political support for the state environmental agencies charged with monitoring compliance with laws.[49] The main environmental agency, DINAMA, answers to the Ministry of Energy and Mines, which is also responsible for planning oil development policy. Not surprisingly, DINAMA has received little official support for conservation efforts. Since 1989, DINAMA's staff has been reduced from thirty-five to fourteen, only four of whom monitor the environmental impact of oil development.[50] According to DINAMA personnel, the agency now lacks the capacity even to review all the environmental impact statements received from oil companies, let alone to monitor compliance in the field.[51] To make matters worse, the current subsecretary for the environment, in charge of DINAMA, disavows any environmental problems within the oil industry, and challenges the need for independent studies or further investigation of oil damages in the Oriente.[52]

In 1992, the Ecuadorian Congress established a separate body, the Institute for Forestry, Natural Reserves and Wildlife (INEFAN), to manage and monitor activities in the protected areas. INEFAN has had some success in carrying out its mandate—challenging Petroecuador's illegal drilling in Cuyabeno Reserve, a protected area, and reserving a seat on its board for a representative of environmental organizations. But at the same time, INEFAN has permitted oil development in other protected areas such as Limoncocha and Yasuni National Parks. Also, staff members report that the agency lacks adequate resources to monitor oil companies effectively, and that its efforts have been hampered by the lack of government support.[53]

Finally, Petroecuador's internal environmental unit (UPA) lacks any independent authority to monitor industry practices. Experts generally agree that the UPA exists purely to boost Petroecuador's public image: the UPA has not acted to prevent Petroecuador's frequent violations of environmental laws.[54] In an interview with CESR and other environmental groups, UPA's current director dismissed reports of oil contamination and health problems by suggesting that the Oriente's inhabitants deliberately inflicted these harms on themselves to harass the oil companies.[55] The government plans to abolish or significantly reduce UPA in the near future.

LACK OF JUDICIAL REMEDIES AND INFORMATION

The right to a healthy environment requires Ecuador to provide citizens with access both to judicial remedies and to relevant information regarding oil contamination. However, Ecuador's judicial system provides no practical means to redress environmental harms, and private citizens have no standing to compel information from either state agencies or private companies.

Ecuador's tort system is inhospitable to environmental suits.[56] The civil code, relatively unchanged from laws introduced by the Spaniards in the seventeenth century, creates significant procedural barriers for potential plaintiffs. For example, courts lack jurisdiction over defendants with foreign domiciles, forcing Ecuadorian plaintiffs to sue foreign companies such as Texaco outside of Ecuador.[57] Plaintiffs may not join together to bring class-action environmental suits, rendering the costs to each individual plaintiff prohibitively expensive. Suits for personal damage may be brought only by those individuals directly affected; individuals may not represent a class of persons seeking compensation.[58] Also, compelled document production, an essential element of any suit against a major oil company, is extremely limited in Ecuador; plaintiffs may request only documents whose existence is known beforehand, and company refusal to produce such documents results only in a nominal fine.[59] In addition, plaintiffs may not call their own expert witnesses, but instead must rely on a court-appointed expert whom they may not cross-examine orally; most Ecuadorian experts in the oil industry and environmental science are affiliated with or dependent upon either the government or oil companies.[60] Finally, most judges are appointed by Congress for short, renewable terms, rendering them highly susceptible to political pressure, especially when dealing with an issue with broad national implications such as oil development. According to local lawyers and former judges, the corruption that accompanies such politicization has reached alarming proportions. In a speech given last year, Alejandro Ponce Martinez, a distinguished professor of law, observed that "corruption has reached absolutely unimaginable levels, judicial norms and principles lack effectiveness, and new problems facing the judicial system are avoided, hidden, not confronted, or completely ignored."[61] Ernesto Lopez Friere, Minister of the Tribunal of Constitutional Guarantees, concurred, recently stating that "according to the Constitution, there is an independent judiciary. In reality, it is weak, inefficient, vulnerable to political and economic pressure, lacking in human and economic resources, and characterized by a high level of corruption and ill-repute."[62]

As an alternative to the tort system, Ecuadorian lawyers have tried to sue the government before the Tribunal of Constitutional Guarantees (TCG). However, the TCG has limited ability to influence state agencies and has demonstrated susceptibility to oil industry pressures. In October 1990, one month after holding unanimously that plans by Petroecuador and Conoco to exploit oil in the Yasuni National Park violated Article 19(2) (the right to a contamination-free environment), the TCG abruptly reversed itself without explanation.[63] A judge subsequently revealed that the reversal had come in response to foreign oil companies' threats to freeze further investments in Ecuador. Jugo Ordenez, a judge on the Constitutional Tribunal, publicly described threats made to Ecuadorian officials by foreign oil companies intent on exploiting oil within the reserves. In a case brought two years later, the TCG again found violations of Article 19(2), this time based on drilling in the Cuyabeno.[64] However, because the TCG lacks a mechanism to enforce its decisions, the government has allowed this drilling in the Cuyabeno to continue. Following ten months with no compliance, Fundacion Natura brought another formal demand before the Tribunal, with no response yet given.[65]

Members of Ecuador's government have acknowledged that victims of oil contamination cannot receive justice from domestic courts. Not surprisingly, the government's Congressional Commission on Mining Affairs has publicly approved of recent cases brought against Texaco in United States federal courts by Ecuadorian plaintiffs, stating that "the Ecuadorian judicial system does not offer sufficient guarantees of justice to the petitioners."[66] As a judge on the TCG recently observed, "considering all the obstacles surrounding the Ecuadorian judiciary and taking into account that Amazonian peoples are among the most marginalized peoples in the country, there are no realistic possibilities to obtain a just and impartial decision in a lawsuit against Texaco [in Ecuador]."[67]

People affected by oil development are also severely handicapped by the lack of available information. While Ecuador requires oil companies to provide environmental impact statements to state environmental agencies, those agencies are not obliged to make their statements public. With no legal incentive to share information, agencies and oil companies have created a wall of secrecy around their operations, under the cloak of national security. Affected communities have no access to information regarding development plans, quantity and types of chemicals used and discharged during production, or potential health hazards from exposure to oil and related toxic waste. For example, the unprecedented two-year audit of Texaco's environmental damages, commissioned by Texaco and Petroecuador, has been withheld from private organizations.and communities in the Oriente.[68] Without such basic information, people are left ignorant of potential risks and cannot participate meaningfully in public policy or hold companies accountable for their actions.

All these obstacles to judicial remedies and access to information faced by Ecuadorian citizens are significantly compounded for indigenous peoples. In addition to widespread racism in Ecuadorian politics and society, indigenous peoples are politically, culturally, and logistically removed from the centers of decision-making power.

Ecuador's government has imposed significant harms on thousands of its citizens by failing to prevent, or provide remedies for, hazardous oil contamination in the Oriente. In view of this failure, even a conservative interpretation of the scope of Ecuador's legal obligations suggests that it has violated the rights to health and to a healthy environment under both international and constitutional law. The state oil company continues to place local communities at risk through irresponsible practices; environmental regulations and state protection agencies have proven incapable of or unwilling to monitor oil development effectively; and the state has left potential victims of toxic contamination ignorant of the risks and without legal redress, forcing them to seek relief in courts outside of Ecuador. While Ecuador's need to exploit natural resources for economic development is acknowledged, it cannot justify these violations of human rights.

CONCLUSION

Human rights can play an essential role in the search for solutions to these problems in the Oriente by mobilizing public and political pressure and by opening the possibility of legal avenues through which Ecuadorian citizens may take action against the state. However, human rights advocacy must be viewed as only one aspect of a broader struggle to protect the people and environment of the Ecuadorian Amazon.

Human rights' focus on the responsibility of state actors is less apparent today than it was fifty years ago, when sovereign states had near absolute power in the international legal system. The growing prominence of international law, and in particular of free trade arrangements like the General Agreement on Trade and Tarriffs and the North American Free Trade Agreement, has shifted significant power away from states to international regulatory and financial bodies, and to multinational corporations (MNCs). MNCs now exert tremendous power over human beings; the annual revenues of individual MNCs are often greater than the gross domestic product of developing countries. For example, Texaco's annual global earnings of about $40 billion dwarf Ecuador's $12 billion gross domestic product. As a result, the basic human rights goal of protecting human dignity is no longer adequately served through a focus limited to states and quasi-state actors (i.e., governments-in-exile, guerrilla movements).

The problems associated with Ecuador's oil development underscore the limitations of the current human rights framework. When the Texaco-Gulf consortium first discovered oil in the Oriente, the Ecuadorian government had neither the expertise nor the resources to develop it. As a result, the government relied wholly upon foreign companies to conduct exploration, build infrastructure, and extract the oil. Texaco has defended its technologies and practices as complying with Ecuador's environmental laws. However, placing full blame on the Ecuadorian government for failing to adopt and enforce stronger environmental regulations disregards the tremendous influence on national oil policy enjoyed by foreign companies such as Texaco.

In addition, exclusive focus on Ecuador's responsibility obscures the international community's critical influence on shaping the country's oil development policies. Like many other developing countries, Ecuador is caught in a financial vise in which it must weigh the costs of any added environmental measures against the need to maximize oil revenues to repay foreign debt. In 1991, more than one quarter of every dollar earned through exports went to repay foreign creditors. Rather than insist upon compliance with human rights or environmental norms as a condition for these enormous loans or for restructuring debt, these creditors have encouraged Ecuador's pursuit of higher oil revenues.

None of these factors can relieve Ecuador, or any sovereign state, of its fundamental obligation to protect human rights. At the same time, contribution to human rights violations in the Oriente by MNCs and the international community carries a corresponding responsibility to help resolve them.

Addressing the crisis in the Oriente should be a matter of vital interest to the entire international community. The recent Rio Conference and the World Conference on Human Rights underscore the growing importance and interdependence of human rights, environmental protection, and economic development. These concerns are joined in the debate over Ecuador's Amazon: promoting the human rights of the local population is essentially linked to protecting their environment. The outcome of the clash in the Oriente between shortsighted oil exploitation and human rights will provide a litmus test for the future direction of global development.

ACKNOWLEDGMENTS

CESR pays tribute to the people of the Oriente, who have sparked greater awareness of the need to develop natural resources in a manner supported by local communities and consistent with human rights. We wish to thank the John D. and Catherine T. MacArthur Foundation, Ping and Carol Ferry, and several other donors for their generous support. Our thanks to Lenore Azaroff, Anthony LaMontagne, Steve Kales, and Manuel Paillares for technical assistance. Special mention goes to Judith Kimerling, Adriana Fabra, Andy Ryan, Douglas Southgate, David Christiani, Debbie Loring, Matt Nimetz, Jonathan Mann, Paul Epstein, Oxfam America, Accion Ecologica, Fundacion Natura, Rainforest Action Network, Confederation of Indigenous Nationalities of Ecuador (CONAIE), Universidad Andina Simon Bolivar, Michael Ullman, Sarah Leah Whitson, Michael Eisner, and others who helped faciliate our work in Ecuador and the United States. We gratefully acknowledge the logistical assistance provided by the firm of Paul, Weiss, Rifkind, Wharton and Garrison and the Harvard Center for Population and Development Studies.

REFERENCES

1. N. Myers, *The Primary Source: Tropical Forests and Our Future* (New York: Norton, 1984).
2. J. Smith, "Problems Flow into Amazon," *L.A. Times*, Dec. 14, 1989; D. Jukofsky "Oil and Rainforest Mix," *American Forestry* 97 (1991): 48.
3. *Oil and Gas Journal*, February 7, 1994.
4. Interviews with and written materials from Judith Kimerling as well as interviews with Cornejo, Coello, Dávila, Southgate, Troya, and officials from Petroecuador, DINAMA, and private companies (Elf and Maxus).
5. J. Kimerling, "Disregarding Environmental Law: Petroleum Development in Protected Natural Areas and Indigenous Homelands in the Ecuadorian Amazon," *Hastings International and Comparative Law Review* 14 (1991): 849.
6. Ruling of the International Water Tribunal, reprinted in *La Campana Amazonia por la Vida*, 55–56.
7. M. Cornejo, "Explotacion de Petroleo en Ecuador" (unpublished document on file with CESR, 1993).
8. J. Kimerling with the Natural Resources Defense Council, *Amazon Crude* (Washington, DC: Natural Resources Defense Council, 1991).
9. J. Kimerling (see note 4) and interviews with Ministry of Energy and Mines and DINAMA.
10. See note 8.
11. Ministry of Energy and Mines, "I. Producciones de Petroleo, Agua de Formacion y Gas Natural," 1989.
12. World Bank, "Public Sector Finances: Reforms for Growth in the Era of Declining Oil Output," World Bank Discussion Papers, 1991.
13. D. Menacho, "La politica de la superlativa pobreza," *El Comercio*, Sept. 21, 1993, cited in Kimerling 1994.
14. Economist Intelligence Unit, *EIU Country Report, Fourth Quarter 1993, Ecuador.*
15. J. Hicks, H. Daly, S. Davis, and M. Lourdes, "Ecuador: Development Issues and Options for the Amazon Region," Report No. IDP-0054, Internal Discussion Paper: Latin America and the Caribbean Region, World Bank, 1990.
16. J. Hicks, "Ecuador's Amazon Region: Development Issues and Options," World Bank Discussion Papers, 1990.
17. DIGEMA 1989, cited in Kimerling (see note 8).
18. Unsworn declaration (1990) under penalty of perjury by Dr. Ernesto Lopez Freire, minister of the Tribunal of Constitutional Guarantees.
19. J. Green and M. W. Trett, Introduction to J. Green and M. W. Trett, eds., *The Fate and Effects of Oil in Freshwater* (London: Elsevier Applied Science, 1989), pp. 1–10.
20. J. C. Reis, "Coping with the Waste Stream from Drilling for Oil," *Mechanical Engineering*, 1992: 64–67.
21. J. F. Hansbrough, "Hydrocarbon Contact Injuries," *The Journal of Trauma* 253 (1985): 250–252.
22. IARC, *Monographs on the Evaluation of Carcinogenic Risks to Humans, Occupational Exposures in Petroleum Refining*, volume 45 (Geneva: World Health Organization, 1989).
23. U.S. Department of Health and Human Services, *Toxicological Profile for Polycyclic Aromatic Hydrocarbons (PAHs)* (Atlanta: USDHHS, 1993).
24. Ibid.

25. Canadian Center of Occupational Health and Safety (CCOHS), database print-outs (1983–92).
26. HBT AGRA Limited, "Final Assessment Criteria for an Environmental Evaluation of the Petroecuador Consortium Oil Fields" (unpublished document on file with CESR, 1992).
27. Interview with Dr. Ribadeniera.
28. See note 8.
29. R. Kennedy in Kimerling (see note 8), preface.
30. Unión de Promotores Populares de Salud de la Amazonía Ecuatoriana (UPPSAE), *Culturas Banadas en Petroleo: Diagnóstico de Salud Realizado por Promotores* (Quito: UPPSAE, 1993).
31. Universal Declaration of Human Rights, GA Res. 217A (III), UN Doc. A/810, at 71 (1948).
32. The International Covenant on Economic, Social and Cultural Rights (hereinafter ICESCR), GA Res. 2200 (XXI), 21 UN GAOR, Supp. (No. 16) 49, UN Doc. A/6316 (1966); The International Covenant on Civil and Political Rights, GA Res. 2200 (XXI), 21 UN GAOR, Supp. (No. 16) 52, UN Doc. A/6316 (1966).
33. Declaration of the United Nations Conference on the Human Environment (hereinafter Stockholm Declaration), princ. 1, UN Doc.A/Conf.48/14/Rev.1 (1972).
34. UNGA 1990. Res 45/94, UN Doc A/45/49; Draft United Nations Economic Commission for Europe Charter on Environmental Rights and Obligations, Experts Meeting of the ECE, princ. 1 (adopted Oct. 29–31, 1990).
35. African Charter of Human and Peoples Rights, art. 24, OAU Doc. CAB/LEG/67/3/Rev.5 (1981); Additional Protocol to the American Convention on Human Rights in the Area of Economic, Social and Cultural Rights (hereinafter Protocol of San Salvador), OASTS No. 69, art. 11 (1989)
36. Interviews with Dávila, Petroproducciones official, Cordero, Rosania, Kimerling, Southgate, Coello and Cornejo.
37. B. Real *Ecologia para lideres* (Quito: 1993); V. Serrano, *Ecologia y derecho* (Quito: 1988).
38. Real (see note 37).
39. Hydrocarbon Law (1971), Chap. III, art. 24(s) and (t).
40. R.O. 530, Ch VII, April 10, 1974.
41. HBT AGRA Limited, "Final Assessment Criteria for an Environmental Evaluation of the Petroecuador Consortium Oil Fields" (unpublished document on file with CESR, 1992).
42. Ministry of Energy and Mines, "The Environmental Regulations for Hydrocarbon Activities in Ecuador" (1992).
43. Supreme Decree 374, May 1976.
44. "Regulations for the Prevention and Control of Contamination Related to Water Resources," R.O. 204 (1989).
45. Interview with employees of IEOS, the agency responsible for water safety under the Ministry of Health, and with official from Petroproducciones.
46. Caso No. 338/89-7, *Corporacion para la Defense de Vida (CORDAVI) v. Petroecuador*, Ministro de Agricultura y Ganaderia, y Ministro de Energia y Minas (Tribunal de Garantias Constitucionales, Oct. 2, 1990, overturned Oct. 30, 1990).
47. Constitution, Art. 46(1); Law of Hydrocarbons, Decree No. 1459 (1971) (as revised, Chap I, arts. 1, 2).

48. J. Kimerling with Federacion de Comunas Union de Nativos de la Amazonia Ecuatoriana), *Crudo Amazonico* (Quito: 1993).
49. Interviews with de la Torre, Cornejo, and Troya.
50. Interviews with Cornejo, Troya, and DINAMA employees.
51. Interview with employees of DINAMA.
52. Interview with Solórzano.
53. Interview with Cordero and Rosania.
54. Interviews with Troya, Southgate, Cornejo, Coello, and Merino.
55. Interview with Maldonado (UPA).
56. Interviews with Kimerling, Perez, Troya, Real, and Merino.
57. Article 25, Ecuadorian Civil Procedure Code (CPC).
58. Articles 47, 78, CPC.
59. Articles 68–69 and 121–123, CPC.
60. Articles 254, 258, 261, and 267, CPC.
61. Speech given at seminar, "The Professional of the Twenty-first Century" (Quito, Oct. 18, 1993).
62. Lopez Declaration.
63. *CORDAVI v. Petroecuador.*
64. Case Nos. 377/90, 378/90, 379/90, 380/90 combined, *Fundacion Natura v. Petroecuador*, Ministry of Agriculture and Livestock, Ministry of Energy and Mines, and the Ecuadorian Institute of Hydraulic Resources, Resolution No. 230–92-CP (Tribunal of Constitutional Guarantees, Oct. 15, 1992).
65. Correspondence with Fundacion Natura; interview with Troya.
66. IPS, "Environment—Ecuador: Government Accused of Betraying the Amerindians," Jan. 14, 1994.
67. Lopez Declaration.
68. Service Lending Contract for the Environmental Audit of the CEPE-Texaco Consortium, April 15, 1992, art. 27.

Censorship and Manipulation 12.
of Family Planning Information:
An Issue of Human Rights
and Women's Health

Lynn P. Freedman

This chapter is a human rights report. It is a report about the ways that states censor, manipulate, and control information concerning reproduction and sexuality; it is about the effects of such actions on people's health and their humanity. The human rights violations reported here do not have the stomach-turning quality of a report on the torture of prisoners. They will not evoke the same horror as a report about the rape of women in war, nor fire the emotions of those who fight and risk their lives for journalistic freedom. Yet what we document here is a deprivation of human rights on a massive scale. It involves a fundamental assault on the personhood, the physical integrity and emotional well-being, of people from very different classes, cultures, and communities around the world. It reveals a range of ways in which people become the instruments or tools of state policies that deprive them of the knowledge and information necessary to make and implement decisions about their reproduction and to express their sexuality safely. It thus involves state control over some of the most basic elements of what it means to be human.

That we do not immediately recognize the state actions described here as human rights violations says much the way that we have been conditioned to think health, about women's reproduction, and about the concept of human rights itself. Unlike a classic human rights report documenting specific instances of horrific physical pain and bodily injury inflicted by government agents behind prison walls, here both the injury and the causality are harder to grasp.

The country reports presented in this chapter talk not so much about individual cases of death or disease as about health, primarily at the population or public health level, using the conventional language of demography and epidemiology. This has advantages and disadvantages. On the one hand, the language of statistics and science tends to disguise the human side of health: we talk about maternal mortality ratios, fertility rates, seroprevalence levels—yet do not hear the screams of a woman dying in childbirth, nor feel the desperation of a teenager frantically searching out a back-alley abortion, nor confront the devastation of whole communities stricken with HIV/AIDS. We lose the graphic shock value of a traditional human rights report that motivates action by appealing to the gut, to raw emotion.

On the other hand, by abstracting from the individual to look more broadly at the health of populations or segments of populations, we begin to allow a more complicated and more accurate picture of causality. We can link health not just to behavioral choices made by individuals or to their personal interaction with specific state actors, but also to much broader social, economic, and cultural forces. Conceptualizing reproductive health within its wider social context challenges traditional thinking about the role of information in reproductive health and clarifies the linkages between information and other aspects of health and human rights.

To appreciate the broader implications of the facts described in the country reports, we will need to go beyond formal legal argument and look critically at three features of this rocky terrain where women's reproduction, health, and human rights intersect. First, we need to consider the political dimensions of women's reproduction in order to understand how and why states attempt to manipulate family planning information in the first place and what is at stake when they do so.

Second, we need to question traditional modes of thinking about human rights, because they do not speak adequately to the problem we are facing. Censorship of information about reproductive and sexual health is not like torture, or repression of religious worship, or even violence against women. Our goal is not simply to eradicate the practice or prevent state intrusion on a basic freedom by rejecting any state involvement in the issue. Women need and want high-quality reproductive health services, and states are key to ensuring that they get them.

But health and health care are concepts that themselves must be subject to careful analysis, because health has become a politically powerful category. Thus the rhetoric of health, particularly women's health, has been used by forces as disparate as the "anti-choice" religious right, on the one hand, and population control advocates on the other, to promote and obscure their own agendas—agendas that in reality have precious little to do with health. This is not a new phenomenon: biomedical discourse and the models of health care associated with it have served historically to reinforce dominant ideological constructs about the proper role of women in the family and society. They have also stigmatized as unscientific, unhealthy, and sometimes even immoral, alternative approaches to understanding and delivering reproductive health care. Therefore, the third aspect that we must examine critically is how family planning information is sometimes used in the name of women's health to advance other social and political agendas.

But here again, we must be clear about the ultimate objective. The solution to the misuse of health information cannot be to do away with health policies and health care systems. Women need and want reproductive health services because they want—and have—a fundamental human right to live lives that are free from unnecessary physical and mental suffering, and that permit the exercise of fundamental freedoms.

That is why rights principles matter. The country reports in this chapter generally describe family planning information and barriers to its dissemination, and provide basic information about contraceptive use, and about fertility and mortality levels. But this is not a report about the promotion of family planning to control population growth, or to decrease infant mortality, or even to reduce maternal morbidity and mortality. Rather, it is about the role that information plays in ensuring that people can make and implement meaningful choices about their reproductive and sexual lives from within the families, communities, and states of which they are a vital part. At core, it is about the nature of women's lives and the conditions under which they struggle for basic freedom and dignity. Hence the need to begin with the emphatic statement: *This is a human rights report.*

DEFINING A HUMAN RIGHTS PERSPECTIVE

What does it mean to analyze policies and programs from a "human rights perspective"? That question can be answered in two distinctly different ways. First, human rights is a system of formal law codified primarily in covenants and conventions, but also found in doctrines of international customary law, that is, rules that are held to be binding on all states, even without explicit ratification. Challenging a specific law, such as a law censoring contraceptive information, through the formal human rights system requires familiar steps of legal analysis: accepted methods of interpretation are used to determine the reach of carefully worded legal rules and to apply them to the precise set of facts at issue, in order to hold a state legally accountable for obligations it has undertaken. The discussion of legal standards that follows shows how this kind of formal legal analysis applies to manipulation of family planning information. Such analysis is a critically important part of the effort to ensure universal respect for human rights.

But human rights is not just an exercise of legal formalism for lawyers and judges to undertake; it is also the legitimate territory of those who make political demands about basic justice—and it is to both of these complementary aspects of human rights work that we hope to speak. Thus, the second answer to the question of "what does it mean to take a 'human rights perspective'?" involves a rather different kind of analysis, which we develop in this chapter.

Here we begin by identifying basic principles found in human rights law, particularly as they apply to women's reproductive health and sexuality. Moving beyond the boundaries defined in (evolving) formal law, we use the principles of human rights as the lens through which to analyze the history of censorship laws, the conceptions of health that dominate official think-ing, the design and delivery of reproductive health care, and the role of infor-mation about contraception and abortion throughout. Even though formal human rights law is technically enforceable only against states, we use stan-dards of human rights to examine the actions of a wide range of actors, from families and community institutions to health care providers and develop-ment agencies.

Such a wide-ranging analysis serves several important purposes. First, it lays the groundwork for the evolution of formal law as states are increasingly held legally accountable for failure to prevent violations by nonstate actors within their jurisdiction.[1] Equally important, in the fields of population and family planning, international actors play a critical role in determining how health and development problems are conceptualized and how reproductive health care is delivered. These include multilateral development agencies, such as the United Nations Population Fund (UNFPA), the World Health Organi-zation (WHO), and the World Bank; bilateral aid agencies, most critically, the United States Agency for International Development (USAID); private corpo-rations, such as multinational pharmaceutical companies that develop and market contraceptives; nongovernmental organizations (NGOs), including major providers of family planning services, such as the International Planned Parenthood Federation (IPPF); and a large and complex establishment of population and family health researchers, analysts, and clinicians whose work profoundly influences policies and programs in this area.

While each of these actors has a different historical relationship to the development of policies and programs both generally and in particular coun-tries, many of them have officially in recent years stated that they will put respect for human rights among their highest priorities.[2] The Programme of Action of the United Nations International Conference on Population and Development (ICPD), initially drafted by the conference secretariat in the United Nations, and adopted after negotiation and revision by some 180 countries during the September 1994 Cairo conference, also states emphat-ically that the protection and exercise of human rights must be among the primary principles shaping population and development policies.[3]

We must take these commitments seriously. We must begin to do the hard work of defining what a commitment to human rights means in practice in the health and population fields, and developing standards—even if they are not now enforceable in formal law—that can guide the actions of the many different kinds of actors who influence women's reproductive health and rights. Such standards are now beginning to develop as human rights, repro-ductive health, and women's rights advocates from different political, economic, and cultural settings around the world articulate perspectives that emerge from their own experiences in these fields.[4] This chapter contributes to that effort by exploring how health and human rights concerns come together around the specific issue of the use of information about reproductive and sexual health.

Reproductive and Sexual Rights as Human Rights

The human rights system is premised on fundamental and universal values of human dignity and social justice. These are articulated as principles of, *inter alia*, "life, liberty and security of the person"; equality or nondiscrimination; and "freedom of opinion and expression."[5] Such values and principles are the foundation on which to build an understanding of women's reproductive and sexual rights as human rights. By reproductive and sexual rights, we mean *constellations of legal and ethical principles that relate to an individual woman's ability to control what happens to her body and her person by protecting and respecting her ability to make and implement decisions about her reproduction and sexuality.*

This definition focuses not on the content of women's choices, but on the relationship between a woman's ability to make and carry out those choices, and her ability to maintain a sense of control over what happens in her life—what happens to both her physical body and her spiritual/emotional person. Stated in the negative, human dignity implies a right not to be alienated from one's own reproductive and sexual capacity; a right not to have one's reproductive and sexual capacity used as an instrument to serve the interests of other individuals, collectivities, or states without one's consent and without the opportunity to participate in the political processes by which such interests are defined.[6]

Such control over reproduction and sexuality is an essential element of human dignity. It therefore has intrinsic—and not merely instrumental—value: although control over reproduction and sexuality is certainly an essential precondition for women's ability to exercise other rights and to fulfill other basic needs, it is also a worthy and valuable end in its own right, and not merely a means to reach other ends. This distinction between intrinsic and instrumental value is an important one because if women's control over reproduction is regarded only as instrumental, as a means to other ends, then theoretically it becomes dispensable if other means are found to reach those ends. For example, if we were to value reproductive control simply because it enables women to be employed, then we could easily imagine a situation where legislation banning discrimination in employment and making child care and maternity leave available would make employment possible but still leave women wholly without control over their reproductive and sexual lives.

Our definition of reproductive and sexual rights links the sense of control and dignity with protection of a woman's decision-making in reproduction and sexuality. That ability includes both a right to *make* decisions (i.e., a recognition of women as full moral agents capable of making decisions about their own lives), and a right to *implement* decisions. The latter is particularly important in this field because it acknowledges that the abstract right to make a decision is meaningless if the conditions needed to carry it out do not exist. It is here that the human rights value of social justice has prime application.

Liberal social and economic theories that underlie traditional notions of rights in Western legal systems (and in initial interpretations of the international human rights system as well) conceptualize the holders of rights as atomistic individuals making isolated decisions in a theoretical world shaped largely by market forces. In contrast, our definition of reproductive and sexual rights attempts to reflect more accurately the realities of women's experience. It requires that women's lives be understood as deeply connected to the families, communities, and states of which they are a part, and as being constrained not so much by abstract market forces as by pervasive systems of economic, racial, and gender inequality—by poverty, racism, and patriarchy. Defining reproductive and sexual rights to include a right to implement decisions ties their implementation directly to the struggle for social justice, to the fight against inequality.[7]

WOMEN'S REPRODUCTIVE HEALTH IN CONTEXT

In the population and family planning fields, health is generally thought about in purely biological terms, as an objective, physical condition marked by identifiable disease processes. While health certainly has biological markers and objective measures, these are not simply the result of discrete biological processes. Rather, the biological events by which we routinely measure health status are produced, and conditioned by, complex webs of social and economic relationships that exist at and between all levels of social life. Far too often, poor health is linked to social systems in which those relationships are marked by deep and pervasive inequality based on gender, race, and class.[8] Inequality—imbalances in power and access to resources—makes the control of women's reproduction by others both more possible and more likely. At the same time, such external control of reproduction and sexuality—and thus of women and their place in society—reinforces systems of inequality.

This cycle of inequality and external control works through multiple mechanisms. It is perpetuated most directly through patriarchal family and community systems, characterized by gender inequality, that value women primarily for their service as wives and sexual partners to men and as producers and rearers of children. Control over women's reproduction and sexuality in this context is typically justified and maintained by cultural/religious systems that view the patriarchal order and its often brutal health consequences for women as "natural" and/or divinely ordained.[9] A woman's rebellion against her assignment to culturally defined roles of wife and mother, and her refusal to accept the limitations or the consequences of such roles, is thus construed not only as socially inappropriate behavior but as a challenge to the moral foundations of community and, often, nation.

Yet the conception of women as wives and mothers that animates a remarkably diverse range of ideological and cultural systems is rarely an accurate reflection of reality. To the contrary, virtually everywhere in the world, women are active and indispensable participants in formal and informal labor markets, in subsistence and export-oriented agriculture, and in home-based production. The conditions under which such labor is performed are increasingly a product of economic inequality between and within countries and of deepening poverty—conditions made even more desperate by economic crisis and structural adjustment programs. Although women's work and the social and economic forces that structure it are rarely recognized in health policies focusing on maternal/child health (MCH) and family planning,[10] in fact they profoundly influence women's physical, mental and emotional health—and thus their reproductive health as well.[11]

Patriarchal social structures that function in a climate of deepening poverty create a level of economic dependence and vulnerability that contributes directly to women's inability to assert control over their reproductive and sexual lives. The most obvious example is when women who have no skills or education or possibility of other employment are forced by economic conditions (and sometimes by their families) to survive by selling sexual services, often under conditions that amount to slavery.[12] Researchers have also documented subtler ways that economic crisis sharpens conflict within patriarchal families and communities, often leaving women physically and mentally damaged; they have found, for example, that economic crisis contributes to increases in domestic violence (including marital rape) and emotional breakdown.[13]

In many parts of the world, control over women's reproduction is a function not only of gender and class, but of race as well. We see this clearly in the United States, where, for example, pregnant drug addicts have been criminally prosecuted under laws prohibiting child abuse or prohibiting the delivery of narcotics to a minor. The public justification given for such prosecutions is invariably the protection of fetal health; but studies of physicians' decisions to test and report women for substance abuse, and of prosecutors' decisions to pursue these cases demonstrate that the laws are used selectively against black women.[14] In an insightful article analyzing such prosecutions, Dorothy Roberts has shown how these policies must be viewed in an historical perspective in which "Black motherhood" itself has been demeaned, devalued, and controlled—a symptom of the legacy of slavery and persistent racism in the United States.[15]

Our point here is not to catalogue and explain all the ways in which the international economic order, racism, or patriarchy influence women's health. Rather our point is that in any given place and time, women's health cannot ultimately be understood in a way that is detached and separated from these kinds of forces. Indeed, to theorize about the health effects of family planning strategies or contraceptive information programs in isolation from these economic and social forces potentially undermines precisely the goal it purports to promote: women's health and well-being.[14]

A human rights perspective requires a view of health that takes seriously its connections to social conditions such as poverty and discrimination. Where biomedical approaches link health primarily to individual characteristics (including characteristics such as socioeconomic status) and promote strategies for improving health that focus primarily on changing individual behavior, a human rights approach to health would acknowledge that ill health is socially produced *and* socially ameliorated. Therefore, while individuals can make decisions that influence their own personal health (and must be empowered to do so), those decisions are embedded in, and constrained by, social and economic systems that must also change if human rights, including a "right to the highest attainable standard of physical and mental health,"[17] are truly to be vindicated.

The Epidemiological Evidence Linking Reproduction and Sexuality to Health

There is now a large body of evidence demonstrating that high fertility has detrimental health consequences for women and children, and that use of contraception can substantially reduce the incidence of poor biological outcomes.[18]

Children's health has received the most attention. Studies show a clear association between birth spacing of at least three years and significant improvements in child survival. The effect is seen in the survival rates of both the child born at the beginning of the interval and the child born at the end of the interval. It is not clear exactly why this association exists—and several of the most obvious hypotheses are not borne out by the evidence[19]—but it is a statistically powerful association that is found consistently in studies from every part of the world. Although maternal age and birth order are also associated with child survival, spacing has, by a wide margin, the strongest effect.[20]

Women obviously care deeply about the survival of their children, but they are also concerned about the effects of contraception, pregnancy, and childbirth on their own health, a matter that has been given short shrift in traditional MCH and family planning programs.[21] In recent years, however, women's health for its own sake has begun to receive more serious attention, although we still know surprisingly little about the incidence and prevalence of morbidity (illness) associated with pregnancy and childbirth. Mortality has been more carefully studied.

Every year, approximately 500,000 women die in pregnancy and childbirth.[22] The vast majority of these deaths occur in developing countries, particularly where women lack access to the emergency medical care necessary to treat most obstetric complications.[23] Access to emergency obstetric care is the single most important reason why maternal mortality has virtually disappeared from industrialized countries, yet remains tragically high in many poor countries in the world.[24] But access to contraception is important as well: if a woman does not become pregnant she will not die in pregnancy or childbirth.[23] Indeed, it has been estimated that if all women who say they want no more children were able to avoid pregnancy (through access to family planning), then nearly 25 percent of all maternal deaths would be averted.[25]

It is also important to recognize that between 67,000 and 200,000 deaths each year result from unsafe, usually clandestine and illegal, abortions.[26] Yet where abortion is legal, and high-quality care is freely accessible, it is also extremely safe.[27] While access to contraceptives can substantially lower the number of unwanted pregnancies, it will not eliminate the need to make safe abortion services accessible to all women.[28]

In sum, pregnancy and childbirth can have serious negative health consequences, and contraception and safe abortion play an important role in reducing their incidence and impact. But quite independently of pregnancy and childbirth, sex itself can have serious health effects, the most obvious being sexually transmitted diseases (STDs). Promotion of contraceptives, especially condoms, has a crucial role in public health strategies to curb the spread of STDs.

Unlike maternal mortality, which is now a public health problem only in developing countries, STDs continue to ravage every part of the world. In 1990 alone, there were an estimated 250 million *new* cases of STDs and HIV, including 120 million of trichomoniasis, 25 million of gonorrhea, 20 million of genital herpes, 3.5 million of syphilis, 2.5 million of hepatitis B, 2 million of chancroid, and 1 million of HIV.[29] The health consequences of these infections, acccumulating at a rate of 250 million a year, are staggering. They include chronic abdominal pain in women, discomfort and possibly genital erosion and infertility in men and women, and pneumonia or blinding eye infections in infants infected at birth. AIDS has received the most attention, but STDs can lead to other fatal complications, including stillbirths, ectopic pregnancies and cervical cancer.[30]

Another serious health consequence of STDs is their effect on fertility. Infertility occurs most often when the Fallopian tubes are scarred by pelvic inflammatory disease (PID), often a result of gonorrhea and chlamydia infections. But STDs can also cause subfertility (e.g., miscarriages caused by syphilis) and infant mortality (e.g., from herpes or AIDS). In some parts of the world this has already resulted in fertility problems of massive proportions. In Gabon, for example, 32 percent of all couples are involuntarily childless; in the Congo and Zaire the proportion is 21 percent.[31] By comparison, in the United States, only 5 percent of all couples suffer from this problem.[32]

Even this quick review demonstrates the importance that wide access to contraception and abortion can have for women's health. But the use of contraceptives can entail many risks as well. Some of those risks are biological, as contraceptive methods have varying levels of morbidity and mortality associated with their use.[33]

For example, while oral contraceptives ("the pill") have been shown to protect against ovarian and endometrial cancer, their use has also been associated with increased risk of circulatory problems including heart attack and stroke. Long-acting contraceptives such as Norplant and Depo Provera can lead to menstrual irregularities with associated social and physical consequences. Intrauterine devices (IUDs), particularly if inserted under septic conditions, have been associated with increased rates of PID, sterility, and ectopic pregnancy.[34] Yet, overall, it is estimated that contraceptives prevent far more death, disability, and disease than they cause.[35]

The Role of Information at the Clinical Level

The epidemiological data recited above are critical pieces of information that must inform any responsible effort to deliver reproductive health care to women. At the same time, it is important to recognize the limitations of such data. Epidemiological research is used to quantify risk by examining correlations between "risk factors" (e.g., maternal age) and outcomes (e.g., maternal mortality) within a population as a whole. Such statistical correlations may be evidence of, but are not proof of, causation. Health professionals then translate epidemiological risk measurements into guidelines for counseling or treating individual patients. This is a process fraught with uncertainty because, while data can tell us which kinds of people are most likely to experience a given outcome, they cannot tell us whether a particular individual will experience that outcome.

Moreover, while such data can quantify the risk of an outcome, they cannot tell us what *value* to put on that risk, since this is only one of many factors that go into a woman's analysis of her own situation. Sandra Gifford, writing about the many ways that risk is understood and experienced in the case of benign breast disease (a risk factor for developing breast cancer), has described the patient's perception of risk as "lived risk."[36] The way the woman, processes, understands and acts on information that the clinician gives her about her statistical risk can be understood only within the wider circumstances of her life and her own personal experiences.

These different approaches to information about risk have obvious implications for reproductive health programs. For example, epidemiological studies tell us that, as a group, women in their 40s are at "high risk" for maternal mortality. A health provider with this information might therefore counsel a 41-year-old woman that it is "dangerous" for her to become pregnant, and so might advise her about the possible costs and benefits of different methods of avoiding pregnancy. The "high risk" woman must then weigh these specific health risks together with a whole spectrum of social risks that stem from her roles as a wife, sexual partner, and mother. For example, what consequences will the use of contraception have on relations (sexual and otherwise) with her husband? What consequences will having or not having an additional child have on her present economic circumstances, her future security, her status in her community, her power in her family?

In short, the information that a health provider can (indeed is obligated to) give to a client, based on data of the kind described in the previous section, is only one piece of the entire body of information that will go into the decision that a woman seeking health care is facing. Ultimately it is up to her to assess the entire circumstances of her life, and make a decision about how she wishes to manage her fertility. In this sense, reproductive health must be understood from a woman's point of view, with biological factors as only one element of reproductive health and well-being. Even if the decision a woman ultimately makes seems "wrong" or "incorrect" from the outsider perspective of a provider or policy-maker, human rights principles require that the health system respect her decision and, further, that it support and facilitate her right and ability to make and implement it.

The kind of technical information about contraception and abortion that is the subject of most of the country studies in this report is, therefore, only one factor relevant to health decision-making. Other relevant information is generated by the woman herself. As we discuss in more detail later, information and knowledge that women bring to contraceptive decision-making has far too often been demeaned and dismissed as rumor or "backward" superstition.[33] This includes information and knowledge about contraceptive side effects that may never have been investigated by clinical researchers or are not considered by clinicians to be important or meaningful.

Although we do not mean here to glorify without qualification all traditional beliefs about health—indeed some are truly dangerous and damaging—the dismissal of women's knowledge about their own bodies and their own lives results in health services that, far from enhancing women's dignity and self-respect, belittle and disempower them.[38] It is certainly true that contraception can give a woman control over her fertility and, with it, control over many aspects of her life. But this will be the case only if a woman has control over the decision to use the contraception. Forced on her in disregard of the wider circumstances of her life as she understands and lives them—even if forced on her with goodwill in an honest attempt to improve her health—contraception becomes not a liberating option, but one more weapon in the arsenal of policies and practices that deny her control over her body, her person, and her life.

The Role of Information at the Public Policy Level

How information will be exchanged and acted upon in a clinical setting where contraceptives are provided depends not just on the broader circumstances of an individual woman's life, but also on the broader public policy context within which health clinics operate. In many countries of the world today, policy-makers view the communication of information between provider and patient as one element in an overall "IEC strategy." IEC, an acronym for "information, education and communication," has been defined by UNFPA as "a comprehensive programming intervention—an integral part of a country development program, which aims at *achieving or consolidating behaviour or attitude changes in designated audiences*" (emphasis in original).[39] IEC strategies encompass everything from mass media advertising campaigns about the dangers of population growth, to soap operas with fertility regulation messages, to training programs that teach counselors in family planning clinics how to discuss contraceptive side effects in a sensitive and supportive manner.

The very notion of an IEC strategy designed by government officials for the explicit purpose of changing the behavior and attitudes of a selected group of people should give human rights advocates pause. The implications of IEC programs for human rights—implications that could be either positive or negative—will depend on the kind of change desired, the extent to which information is distorted or manipulated in order to elicit such changes, and the broader program of which the IEC strategy is a part. But one thing is certain: reproductive health information will never come in pristine packages of neutral, objective, comprehensive, and value-free facts, "free as the air for all to breathe." If we are to ensure that reproductive health information is used in defense and support of human rights, we will first need to understand the nature of the power that such information imparts to those who are positioned to control it.

In the sections that follow we explore that power first by reviewing some of the methods by which, and reasons why, states have censored and suppressed reproductive health information. We then examine the role that the delivery of reproductive health information plays in different types of contraceptive and health programs.

POLITICAL DIMENSIONS OF REPRODUCTIVE HEALTH INFORMATION: MODES OF STATE MANIPULATION

States generally explain or justify the manipulation of family planning information by reference to two goals: (1) enforcement of demographic targets (both anti-natalist and pro-natalist); and (2) enforcement of moral codes concerning sexuality and the "proper" role of women in society. Although these two goals often appear distinct, with one or the other generally dominating the public discourse about family planning, they are in fact deeply connected. Understanding those connections, and how they differ in various societies and change over time, will be crucial for understanding the implications that manipulation of information has for health and health services. It is also central to our analysis of the human rights implications.

A closer look at how demographic concerns and morality concerns have interacted historically in three distinctly different countries—the United States, Algeria, and Chile—elucidates some of these issues.

United States

In the United States, public battles over women's access to contraception and abortion, and information about them, have historically been waged around formal legislation and judicial attempts to enforce, interpret, or invalidate it. The opening salvo in what has been a one hundred and twenty-year-long struggle was the first federal law dealing with contraception, the 1873 Comstock Act, named for its primary author and most vigorous enforcer, Anthony Comstock. Backed by the Young Men's Christian Association (YMCA) and the powerful industrialists who sat on its board, Comstock led a crusade to "sanitize" American society by ridding it of any and every word, representation or object deemed to be "obscene, lewd, or lascivious." Chief among them was "any article or thing designed or intended for the prevention of conception or procuring abortion," which the Comstock laws explicitly banned from importation, from dissemination through the mail, and (in states that enacted "Little Comstock Acts") from actual use as well.[40]

By choosing "obscenity" as the legal rubric under which contraception and contraceptive information were criminalized, lawmakers defined the legal issue as state enforcement of morality. Yet it would be a mistake to think that the Comstock laws were simply a reflection of Victorian prudery or modesty, a squeamishness about discussion or depiction of sex. Banning not just public expression or dissemination of information about contraception, *but also contraception itself,* the Comstock laws reflected a revulsion at the very notion of sex for any purpose other than procreation, and a clear conviction that the purpose of women was to be wives to men and mothers to their children. A popular anti-abortion tract of the time expressed the prevailing view rather graphically:

> Sexual intercourse, unhallowed by the creation of a child, is lust . . . wife without children is a mere sewer to pass off the unfruitful and degraded passions and lust of one man.[41]

It is no accident that the public hysteria about sexuality stoked by the Comstock crusades followed the beginnings of the modern U.S. women's movement, which included among its central planks the advocacy of "voluntary motherhood" and, somewhat later, of contraception itself.[42] That the debate was over the *morality* of contraception and nonprocreative sex was an acknowledged fact, not hidden behind health or economic justifications as it sometimes is today. Indeed, the Comstock laws resulted in many thousands of arrests and prosecutions, as well as a series of very public show trials including that of Margaret Sanger, founder of Planned Parenthood, in which the obscene and immoral nature of birth control and information describing it was precisely the issue given to judges and juries to decide.[43]

But there were many subtexts here as well. The fifty years during which the Comstock laws enjoyed their most vigorous enforcement, from 1873 through World War I, was a time of great political ferment and social turmoil in the U.S. It was marked by growing labor unrest, the rise of socialist and anarchist movements, and an increasingly vocal feminist movement. The country's demographic landscape was changing quickly and dramatically as well. Huge waves of immigration, mostly from eastern and southern Europe, coincided with a steady decline in the fertility of white American women: from a fertility rate of 7.04 children per woman in 1800, it dropped to 4.24 in 1880, and to 3.6 in 1900.[44]

These demographic facts fueled widespread fears over what was known as "race suicide," a term popularized by one of the loudest voices of alarm, the President of the United States, Theodore Roosevelt. To Roosevelt it was clear just who was at fault for the unfolding suicide of the "Yankee" race:

women (specifically white, upper, and middle-class women), selfishly using birth control to shirk their primary duty, motherhood, were the major culprits responsible for the pending demise of the race, and thus the nation. In fiery speeches, he urged American women of his own class and culture to do their duty to God and country and, quite simply, have lots of children.[45]

Certainly both the "race suicide" alarmists and the vice squads of Anthony Comstock cloaked their condemnation of women's use of contraception and perceived abandonment of their obligations as wives and mothers, in the moral righteousness of Christianity and religious duty. But these forces had another powerful ally as well: the medical profession.

In the context of American history and its specific political and legal culture, science and scientific medicine had a legitimizing power that even religion did not possess. For science was both the symbol and the engine of progress. Purporting to be neutral, objective, and verifiable, the scientific method revealed truths of Nature that were unchallengeable; and behind them lay the immutable and divine order of things. Indeed, when it came to biology and the workings of the human body, one did not need to have a direct line to God to see and understand such natural and divine truths; one needed only to have the tools and training (and state-sanctioned professional license) of a medical doctor. In fact, the growing power of the medical profession was to have a profound and lasting influence on the course that laws regulating information about fertility would take.

In the United States of this period, particularly among the masses of poor and immigrant women, such information and knowledge was disseminated through the "popular health movements" as well as through the traditional routes, from mother to daughter and within communities of women. Care in pregnancy and childbirth was the domain of midwives and traditional practitioners. In the same period, professional physicians were lobbying vigorously for legislation that would enable them to assert their authority over health care through a state licensing system that would exclude those not trained in professional schools.

Much of this battle for control over health care was waged over the bodies of women, as the newly formed specialty of obstetrics and gynecology attempted to bring pregnancy and childbirth into their exclusive domain. In order for the medical profession to exercise its hegemony over issues surrounding women's reproduction and sexuality, it first had to discredit and destroy competitive sources of knowledge, information, and authority.[46] The Comstock laws, by criminalizing the dissemination of birth control and information about it—matters traditionally within the sphere of women, female midwives, and lay healers—put the power of the state behind this effort. The fact that the Comstock laws hinged on a government-sanctioned view of morality made them especially useful from the medical establishment's point of view, since one sure strategy for consolidating the authority of the medical profession was to conflate health and morality. As a leading historian of the American birth control movement put it,

> Doctors were the new ecclesiastics . . . For many doctors, playing churchmen
> merely required translation of ecclesiastical language into medical language.
> What had been sin became physically injurious.[47]

Sometimes the conflation of health and morality was unabashed; the comment of one Boston gynecologist, that condoms "degraded love and caused lesions," and that lesions were "'God's little allies' in promoting chastity,"[48] has a chillingly familiar ring in this era of HIV/ AIDS. However, the harshest words of condemnation were reserved for women. In 1871, the American Medical Association's Committee on Criminal Abortion wrote this description of the woman who has an abortion:

> She becomes unmindful of the course marked out for her by Providence, she
> overlooks the duties imposed on her by the marriage contract. She yields to the
> pleasures—but shrinks from the pains and responsibilities of maternity; and
> destitute of all delicacy and refinements, resigns herself, body and soul, into the
> hands of unscrupulous and wicked men. Let not the husband of such a wife
> flatter himself that he possesses her affection. Nor can she in turn ever merit
> even the respect of a virtuous husband. She sinks into old age like a withered
> tree, stripped of its foliage; with the stain of blood upon her soul, she dies
> without the hand of affection to smooth her pillow.[49]

In the last quarter of the nineteenth century, the weight of medical opinion and the medical establishment itself were publicly opposed to contraception and abortion. However, individual doctors were also among the most vocal public supporters of the birth control movement—and even went to jail for speaking and acting on their convictions. Indeed, it was ultimately through the prestige and respect that physicians had begun to enjoy that the first wedges were driven into the wall of obstruction presented by the Comstock laws. In a series of cases beginning with the 1918 decision in the prosecution of Margaret Sanger,[50] the courts carved out an exception to the obscenity law by which the dispensing of contraceptives for medical purposes by a licensed physician was deemed to fall outside the law's prohibition.[51] Thus, in some states, contraceptives became legal, but only if channeled through the special expertise of licensed physicians. The result was that contraceptive *information* became the possession—even the "right"—of doctors and was theirs to distribute as they, with their certified and "superior" understanding of biology and nature, thought proper—a view that, to this day, dominates both health services and judicial opinions concerning contraception and abortion.[52]

The role of the medical profession, and the medicalization of contraception generally, is a complex story that does not lend itself to easy generalization or grand conspiracy theories. But it is undeniable that the trend of professionalization and medicalization of reproductive health care (including contraception and abortion)—combined with the development of modern contraceptives (the pill and IUD)—meant that fertility regulation could become an element of public policy, including foreign policy, in a way that it had never been before. Although contraceptive methods have been employed by individuals and couples for centuries,[53] the mass production of the oral contraceptive pill changed the possibilities and even the interests (including private interests of multinational corporations) at stake.[54]

In the 1960s, the U.S. led a major campaign to slow population growth, primarily in developing countries, through the spread of contraceptives. Whatever the true intent of U.S. policy in this area, and whatever the range of motives driving individuals working within the family planning movement, the *perception* of contraception as the front line of international capitalism's imperialist advance deeply influenced (and continues to influence) public and private reactions to family planning information in developing countries. At the same time, within some developing countries (as in some countries of the north), internal political considerations helped to make government control over, and censorship of, contraceptive information the chosen policy. The history of Algeria's policy on contraceptives is a striking example.

Algeria

In 1962, Algeria gained independence from France after a long and bloody struggle in which an estimated 1.5 to 2 million Algerians were killed. From the very start, the new government took a clear and public stand on contraception and abortion. Formally retaining the French colonial law banning contraception information that had been in place since 1920,[55] the government actively maintained a policy prohibiting all contraception and abortion for any purpose, as well as the dissemination of any information about them. This total ban on all means to regulate fertility was given several official explanations.

First, as a forthrightly pro-natalist policy, the ban on contraception and contraceptive information was intended to encourage a high birthrate to replenish a population that had been decimated during the war for independence. Second, the notion of population control as a development policy was strongly associated with Western imperialist motives, precisely the forces from which Algeria had finally freed itself. The adoption of a militantly anti-contraceptive policy was, both symbolically and in actuality, an act of defiance against Western capitalist interests and models of development.

A pro-natalist stance also fitted conveniently with other aspects of government policy in the early years after independence. After one hundred and thirty years of colonial domination, independence brought with it a campaign for a return to "authentic" Algerian culture, a movement to recover a tradition that increasingly over the next ten years, in public discourse at least, came to be defined largely by interpretations of Islam. Central to those interpretations was a view of women as repositories of cultural identity; and central to upholding their function as keepers of the culture was women's performance in their roles as wives and mothers.[56]

In the first two decades following independence, a policy totally banning contraceptives and contraceptive information thus served multiple functions at once: (1) as a national population policy, it served to increase population and simultaneously to define socialist Algeria in opposition to the capitalist West; and (2) it enabled the government to assert and enforce a view of women's proper role in the new Algerian society, a view articulated largely in terms of religion and morality. But, from a human rights perspective, it is critical to recognize an additional motive behind the absolute censorship policies of the 1962–1973 period: the policy was deeply controlling of the lives of individual people.

In the years immediately following independence, several committees had been organized to analyze the impact of population growth and the desirability of family planning; each time they reached conclusions favoring access to contraception, or further investigation of the issue. In addition, a body of religious leaders had also studied the question and issued a *fatwa* stating that family planning was permitted under Islamic law. Yet, despite demands from individuals and recommendations from these expert commissions, the government steadfastly refused to permit mention of, or access to, contraception. In the view of one Algerian activist, the persistence of an absolute contraceptive censorship policy in the face of such demands can best be explained by the fact that the policy also served the interests of the new ruling class. In essence, it enabled them to consolidate their power by quashing the exercise of freedom by a newly independent people:

> At a time when the newly freed masses hoped to handle directly their future in all economic, political, and private respects, . . . the new [dominant] class had to strangle people's power: self-managed factories came first, they were converted into state owned national companies; then came the peasants: self-managed farms remained as the window of socialism in Algeria but they were emptied of all the content of self-management. . . . We had forced and fake elections. . . . We have a prominent police and many secret policies, concentration camps, and political prisoners. Under such circumstances, . . . personal freedom is a threat to the dominant class; this includes the people's demand for controlling their fecundity, the women's attempts to participate in the new liberated nation.

> Having lived in my country the very days and months after independence when the people actually thought they could grab their present and future life, when, for some months, they could think they were in power, they wanted to plan everything, to grab everything; it was not necessary to push them or induce them to plan their families, for example.

> [W]hen the illusion of having power over one's own future occurs, it should not necessarily be defined in terms of wage earnings. It is much more complicated, and human. People want to plan their families, for instance, when it means their lives have other possible ways in which to bloom—they do not want to plan for the sake of a dominant class which just does not want to share the cake with too many people.[57]

Ultimately, however, the censorship policy did not serve the interests of any segment of Algerian society. In the years between 1962 and 1985, Algeria experienced one of the highest population growth rates in the world. By 1986, population growth was deemed to be a serious threat to the country's (and the government's) future. The government did a complete reversal in its policy, enacting a series of anti-natalist measures. In the area of information, where before there had been total censorship, now there was a major media campaign to encourage families to limit their size to two children.

During the twenty-four-year period that the government officially maintained a pro-natalist policy, reproductive health services underwent a series of transitions. In the first decade of this period, from 1962 to 1973, there was one clinic in the entire country dispensing contraceptives (and that under the guise of scientific research). In 1973, responding to appallingly high maternal mortality and infant mortality rates, the government initiated a program of birth spacing as part of its MCH services. This program, responding to health needs, focused on the retraining of midwives, and the giving of client-oriented care.[58] Interestingly, in 1986, when the government announced its new anti-natalist policy and contraception took on a demographic rationale, family planning programs were removed from the health services and put into a new ministry that relied primarily on physicians and a medical model of service delivery.

Clearly, contraception is now more accessible to women in Algeria, and with contraception and lower fertility rates have come improvements in women's health. But from the point of view of women's human rights, this is only half a victory. Women are still regarded as tools of government policy—it is just that the government policy has been reversed. Women's duties to the nation and state are still defined by a government-imposed view of their role in maintaining cultural authenticity—it is just that the doctrine has been reinterpreted. Information and services are still manipulated by the state in an attempt to assure that people do what the government decides— it is just that the government has changed its decision.

Finally, the new contraceptive policy, which suddenly opened access to contraception and affirmatively promoted fertility limitation through government-sponsored information campaigns, has to be evaluated in light of the broader insecurity within which Algerian women exist—including a climate of fear and intimidation that makes impossible any robust discussion of women's reproductive rights and their roles in family and society. In 1984, three women were arrested and jailed without trial for seven months for having *discussed* among themselves the proposed new Family Law Code in which, among other things, women were stripped of legal personhood. Although the Algerian Constitution granted equal rights to all its citizens, the Family Code places women under the legal control of their male guardians— first their fathers and brothers, and then their husbands. In this respect, changes in policies concerning contraceptive information simply cannot be evaluated from a human rights perspective without situating such policies within the broader political conditions shaping the lives of women.

The specific expression of, and official justification for, contraceptive policies in Algeria over the last thirty years have been determined largely by its colonial past and then increasingly by the role that religion has played in public discourse and government policy-making. But government control over women's reproduction and sexuality—as a means through which to impose its will and deny people autonomy—is not a tactic reserved for "socialist" governments or Islamic countries. In recent years it has been used by a wide variety of governments including, in quite blatant ways, the Pinochet dictatorship in Chile.

Chile

In Chile, a public health system with high-quality MCH services was operating as early as the 1950s. In the 1960s, alarmed at the very high number of hospital admissions for complications of illegal abortions, the government added family planning services as a public health measure. In the period between 1964, when family planning began, and 1979, when a policy limiting access to contraceptives and contraceptive information went into effect, Chile experienced a dramatic decline in the percentage of obstetric hospitalizations due to abortion complications (from approximately 21 percent to 13 percent) and in overall maternal mortality (from approximately 117 to 24 maternal deaths per 100,000 live births).[59]

But after the military seized power in the early 1970s, family planning began to lose its importance as a health measure and acquired a new and dangerous role—it became identified as a threat to national security. In 1979, a new population policy was promulgated as part of the National Security Doctrine. Information about contraception was removed from the mass media. In schools, the sex education and family life curriculum was eliminated, and public discussion of the subject stopped.[60] In clinics, both information and education about contraception were suppressed; under the "Maternal and Prenatal Programme," contraception was dispensed only if specifically requested by the user. In the view of the military government, the admitted health benefits that contraception had for women and children did not outweigh two other supposed consequences which were deemed to be threats to the country's security: (1) it weakened the country by suppressing population growth; and (2) it enabled women to stray from their duties as wives and mothers.[61] General Pinochet himself, expressing his view of women's needs and desires, echoed the familiar refrain of motherhood as the natural, and only, role of women:

> A woman, once she becomes a mother, ceases to desire anything more in the material domain, looking for and finding in her own children the meaning of her life, her only treasure, and the goal of all her dreams.[62]

In Chile then, as in the U.S. and Algeria, pro-natalist demographic concerns interacted with official views of morality that were expressed in a romanticization of motherhood and an elaboration of women's duties as producers and rearers of children. The result was censorship policies that effectively

prevented women from taking, or maintaining, control over their reproductive and sexual lives. Such censorship was justified to the public through
official/legal interpretations of obscenity (the U.S.), of cultural authenticity
and religion (Algeria), or of national security (Chile).

These three countries are not unique in their attempts to transform state
control over contraception into state control over women.[63] In fact, in the
controversy surrounding the 1994 Cairo Population Conference we can see
a parallel dynamic emerging in the international arena as well. Although
many press accounts of ICPD focused on the controversy over specific
language regarding contraception and, especially, abortion, it is critical to
recognize that the opposition to the conference voiced by the Vatican, by Al-
Azhar University in Egypt (perhaps the leading center of Islamic studies), and
by countries purporting to represent or defend either Catholic or Islamic
traditions, did not stem from a simple opposition to contraception or abortion *per se*. Indeed, Al-Azhar itself, as well as many Muslim countries and
religious bodies, have officially sanctioned and even promoted contraception
and fertility regulation on religious grounds.[64] The vehemence of their
denunciation can be explained by the fact that, in the context of *this* conference and *this* Programme of Action, contraception and safe abortion were
associated with a women's health and human rights movement that
promoted access to contraception and safe abortion as part of a broader
reproductive health agenda. And that reproductive health agenda, grounded
in a respect for human rights, challenged traditional idealizations of womanhood and motherhood—and efforts to impose such "ideals" on women in
pursuit of a wide variety of political ends.

In short, the political alignment that formed in opposition to the ICPD
makes it clear that the social impact of access to contraception and abortion
is not determined simply by the biological fact that these measures can
prevent births; rather the actual impact is as much a function of the policy
and program "package" in which access to contraception and abortion is
wrapped. As we explore in the following section, these "packages" have
human rights dimensions as well.

THREE PARADIGMS OF CONTRACEPTIVE DELIVERY PROGRAMS: DEMOGRAPHIC, BIOMEDICAL, AND REPRODUCTIVE HEALTH

If withholding contraceptives and contraceptive information denies women
reproductive freedom, the opposite is not necessarily true: making contraceptives available does not automatically ensure that freedom, for contraceptive delivery programs contain both promise *and* peril for women. Their
promise lies in the fact that contraceptives help women to control the consequences of sexual encounters, including direct biological consequences such
as STDs and the morbidity and mortality associated with pregnancy, as well
as a whole host of psychological, social, and economic factors linked to
childbearing and sexuality. But there is peril lurking here too: just as states
and other agencies have used denial of contraceptives to control women's

lives, so they have, at times, manipulated the provision of contraceptives to control women's lives just as effectively.

It is this conundrum of promise and peril that requires us to break the mold of traditional human rights analysis when we look at contraceptive delivery programs. Our purpose is not to keep the state out of health programs in order to keep the state out of people's lives; rather, our objective is to encourage states and other relevant actors to provide contraceptives and reproductive health information in a way that vindicates rights, health, and the well-being of women and society.[65] That requires using human rights principles not just to identify violations, but also to build an affirmative program of reproductive health.

In considering countries with policies for the provision, rather than the denial, of contraceptives, the analytical challenge, then, is distinguishing between a program that imperils rights, health and well-being, and a program that promotes them. That task is complicated by the fact that contraceptive programs are almost always described by their architects as being designed to promote public health and welfare. Knowing the importance of contraceptives to reproductive health, what facts can help us analyze the human rights dimensions of such programs? Information—the ways it is offered, elicited, used, and/or manipulated in contraceptive delivery programs—can be used as a barometer of respect for human. rights more generally.

Although information is relevant to many different aspects of contraceptive programs, from the development of new technologies to the training of providers, we zero in on the one aspect that is perhaps most central to human rights—the decision-making of the individual woman. For analytic purposes, we identify three paradigms that have influenced contraceptive programs and which, in broad and somewhat oversimplified terms, trace the historical development of the international family planning movement. For each paradigm, we focus on how individual decision-making and the role of information are conceptualized.

Demographic Paradigm

The large-scale family planning programs found in much of the world today began in the 1960s and 1970s as population control programs, driven by an apocalyptic view of population growth as a "bomb" waiting to explode and, quite literally, destroy the world. In this scenario, family planning programs were seen as almost warlike operations. Even academic discourse in this era is marked by military metaphors: we find articles about family planning programs that are characterized as "battlefront reports," and the family planning movement itself as an "organized protest," a "large-scale action," "a crusade," a "Holy War," of "truly heroic proportions."[66] Following "contraceptive inundation" strategies, the aim was to deploy family planning programs across a country like a military operation. As the minister for Health and Family Planning in India explained the intention, "The net of family planning is being spread in every nook and corner of the country. No one can escape it."[67]

In this paradigm, shaped predominantly by demographers concerned in the first instance with population growth at the macro level, little regard is given to the right of individual women to make decisions about their reproduction and sexuality. In fact, the very act of decision-making itself receives scant attention, being viewed as an abstract, almost detached process. In an insightful article entitled "If All We Knew About Women Was What We Read in *Demography,* What Would We Know?" Susan Cotts Watkins reviews twenty-five years of this leading journal and demonstrates how unarticulated beliefs about women and about gender roles and gender differences have shaped the way that demographers understand the dynamics of population change. She concludes,

> If all we knew about women was what we read in the articles on fertility, marriage, and the family, we would conclude that women are primarily producers of children and of child services; that they produce with little assistance from men; that they are socially isolated from relatives and friends; and that their commitment to the production of children and child services is expected to be rather fragile.[68]

In short, the realities of women's lives as understood or experienced by them are either consciously avoided or simply ignored or forgotten. Watkins found that, although nearly half of all articles concerned either fertility and contraception or marriage and family, "a birth appears to result from an immaculate conception," sex is avoided or abstracted into euphemisms such as "exposure to intercourse," men are almost entirely absent from the picture, and issues of power are "almost completely ignored."[69]

Perhaps most importantly, women are conceptualized as "separate selves," as "autonomous and impervious to social influence."[70] As the social context of women's lives drops away, traditional sources of information recede from view. As Watkins puts it, demographers tend to pay attention only to individual women of reproductive age and forget about "Granny in the back bedroom" and her inevitable effect on younger women of the household. They ignore the importance of women's social networks in shaping the ways that women understand and make decisions about their sexuality and reproduction—and about their options for fertility control.

When it comes to family planning programs designed on the demographic model with population reduction as their primary goal, the only information that really matters is information that program planners can deploy in order to convince women to use contraception. In fact, when early strategies focusing on the supply side of contraceptive programs failed to yield sufficiently high levels of contraceptive prevalence, programs began to emphasize "demand creation" strategies. In their mildest form, such strategies are designed to create demand for contraceptives by showing people what is "good" for them; IEC programs typically stress the benefits of small families and the dangers of "over population" with the explicit purpose of influencing individuals to change their behavior.[71]

In their harsher forms, demand creation strategies employ incentives and disincentives to ensure that people come to "want" the contraception that family planning providers are pressured to give. Such incentive and disincentive programs slide progressively closer to outright coercion.[72] In the most extreme versions of such programs, information about contraception and its effects becomes entirely irrelevant, as family planning becomes solely an instrument used by the state to decrease population growth, disregarding individual choice, health, and well-being.

Biomedical Paradigm

The harsh and single-minded contraceptive programs that characterized aggressive population control campaigns often collapsed under their own weight. People simply were not willing to surrender control over their reproductive lives as easily as many population controllers had supposed. Ultimately policy-makers were forced to recognize the futility of contraceptive programs that offered no justification other than the theoretical argument that decreases in overall population growth, while requiring painful sacrifices from some people in the short-term, would confer benefits on society as a whole in the longterm. Such arguments rang particularly hollow when made by politicians and power-brokers of questionable legitimacy and dubious track records to start with.[73]

In the late 1970s and throughout the 1980s, and spurred in part by the need for more convincing arguments to sell contraceptive programs, demographers, epidemiologists, and health professionals began to demonstrate that birth limitation and birth spacing also had immediate health benefits for individuals. Although such arguments may have been used in many cases to make population control programs more palatable to a doubting and recalcitrant public, the potential health benefits associated with contraceptive use are real and indisputable. Thus, family planning has become an important—indeed, an *essential*—element of Primary Health Care,[74] of Child Survival programs,[75] and of Safe Motherhood programs.[76] These programs or campaigns, formulated in U.N. specialized agencies and adopted in multilateral government meetings and conferences, have had a major impact on the formulation of health policies and programs by governments at the national and local levels.

The strong epidemiological associations between contraceptive use and improved health mandate that contraceptives be made widely available. But through what kind of programs? When family planning programs are justified primarily as health programs, they are often designed using the biomedical model of health and health care associated with conventional Western medicine. In contrast to programs modeled on the demographic paradigm, contraceptive programs based on a biomedical paradigm purport to give decision-making at the individual level primary importance. But from a human rights perspective, we need to examine closely the way that the biomedical model conceptualizes what is happening at that individual level.

First, health itself is understood to be a function of individual biological processes. When contraceptive programs are viewed through this lens, then the questions surrounding contraceptive decision-making tend to be framed in terms of biological risks, which in turn are understood to be a function of an individual woman's physical characteristics. Thus, for example, in assessing an individual woman's risk of maternal mortality, a clinician is likely to look at factors such as age (is she over 40 or under 18?), parity (has she had less than one, or more than three children?), and health status (is she anemic, hypertensive, or diabetic?). Using such factors, the clinician comes to a judgment about the overall risk that childbearing presents to the woman's health and, on that basis, recommends a course of action with respect to contraceptive decision-making.

The problem with the biomedical model is *not* that such factors are counted in—they are clearly relevant to contraceptive decision-making. The problem is what factors are left out. In the early sections of this chapter, we argued that biological factors are embedded in and influenced by webs of social and economic relationships. For example, anemia, a risk factor for potentially fatal complications in childbirth, may be the result of malnutrition caused by gender systems that require women to eat last and therefore, under conditions of poverty, to eat least as well. Moreover, an anemic woman's chances of surviving complications during childbirth depend less on her anemia than on her access to emergency obstetric care to treat the complications.[77]

We also argued that, once a biological risk is identified, the question of what *value* to give that risk in the context of contraceptive decision-making is a judgment that cannot be detached from the wider circumstances of a woman's life. For example, childbearing is not simply a question of weighing biological risks and benefits; it is a complex social and economic undertaking that unavoidably affects multiple aspects of a woman's economic, social, sexual, and emotional life and the life of her family and community. Yet when contraceptive programs are structured by the biomedical paradigm, it is the physician's assessment of the biological risks, not the woman's assessment of the full range of issues, that typically shapes the question to be decided, the knowledge to be valued, and the information to be considered.

Elizabeth Fee and Nancy Krieger, critiquing biomedical approaches to HIV/AIDS policies and programs, described the resulting attitude toward knowledge and information:

The canons of scientific objectivity, as embraced by this model, tend to discount the views and experiences of patients, the "objects" of scientific research and medical practice. Only scientists and physicians are seen as possessing the expertise to define disease and frame research questions . . . This model assigns physicians the unique responsibility for conveying specific knowledge about disease to individual patients. . . . It regards the patients' beliefs as mere superstitions or misinformation that can be overcome with therapeutic doses of factual information. Subjectivity and culture—of science and health care professionals as well as their patients—are deemed irrelevant to "truth"; scientific knowledge is held to be outside the bounds of social context.[78]

Indeed, in the biomedical model, the patient's behavior itself is held to be "outside the bounds of social context." Privileging the health professional's conception of an individual's risks, policies and programs initiated at the public health level typically focus on convincing the individual to avoid such risks by changing his or her behavior, rather than by changing the environment that causes the risk to start with. At the clinical level, the doctor-patient relationship is the key dynamic. Again privileging the health professional's view of risk, the objective of the doctor-patient encounter is typically to obtain "compliance" with medical instructions or to obtain "informed consent" to the procedure or treatment the doctor recommends.

Biomedical discourse wraps this dynamic in an aura of neutrality and objectivity that tends to immunize it from scrutiny and criticism. Yet, just as Watkins uncovered the ways in which unarticulated gender assumptions shaped demographic programs, so scholars have convincingly demonstrated that assumptions about gender have always played a formative role in biomedical conceptions of the physical body and in the health policies and programs that derive from them.[79]

Our brief description of the history of the birth control movement in the United States hinted at the process through which biomedicine and its proponents were able (whether consciously or not) to use the medicalization of reproduction and the professionalization of reproductive health care to exercise control over women's lives. In that process, the medical monopolization of health information—a monopoly reinforced by the law and the courts—played a crucial role. Aided by its ability to control the terms under which knowledge and information are deemed relevant to health, biomedical practice now, as then, quietly absorbs the dominant ideologies of the society in which it prospers.

Thus, cloaked in the rhetoric of health, the aura of scientific neutrality, and the authority and status of professional physicians, contraceptive provision programs premised on a biomedical paradigm often end up importing the very same two concerns that animate contraceptive censorship policies: (1) demographic concerns; and (2) concerns about morality and the role of women in family and society. Sometimes the mixture of medicine, morality and politics is explicit, as in the controversy that surrounded and ultimately destroyed government-funded research studies of sexual behavior in the U.S.—studies deemed by many to be essential to efforts to control STDs, including HIV/AIDS.[80]

More often, the dynamic is a subtler one in which biomedical programs, outwardly described as health programs, ultimately are designed in ways that reinforce social goals that actually have the potential to detract from health as we have defined it. For example, we see contraceptive programs that purport to promote women's health, but in fact are driven by anti-natalist objectives; hence their success is evaluated not so much by changes in health status as by "couple years of protection" or births averted. Similarly, supposed health programs that condition access to contraception on a woman's marital status, her husband's permission, or the number of births she has already experienced ultimately take contraceptive decision-making out of the hands of women and deliver it into the hands of doctors and husbands, thereby reinforcing dominant views of morality and gender roles—and making women's attempt to reject such views a potentially dangerous undertaking.

Reproductive Health Paradigm

Influenced by women's health advocates and by the growing strength of women's movements more generally, contraceptive programs have increasingly come to be conceptualized as "reproductive health" programs. One widely accepted definition of reproductive health is:

> a condition in which the reproductive process is accomplished in a state of complete physical, mental and social well-being and is not merely the absence of disease or disorders of the reproductive process. Reproductive health, therefore, implies that people have the ability to reproduce, to regulate their fertility and to practice and enjoy sexual relationships. It further implies that reproduction is carried to a successful outcome through infant and child survival, growth and healthy development. It finally implies that women can go safely through pregnancy and childbirth, that fertility regulation can be achieved without health hazards and that people are safe in having sex.[81]

Clearly this is a definition of health that reaches deeper than its biomedical dimensions. Programs designed to promote reproductive health (defined in this way) are based on an understanding of reproduction and sexuality both as a key to women's empowerment and as the site, historically, of women's vulnerability. This gives human rights a very different role to play. In the demographic and biomedical paradigms, human rights are construed as a *limiting* principle: they define just how far policies or service providers can go on the continuum towards outright coercion, as they attempt to achieve abstract programmatic goals, such as lowering fertility rates or infant mortality rates. By contrast, in the reproductive health paradigm, human rights are a *formative* principle. The very purpose of a reproductive health program is to enable its clients to maintain control over their lives by enabling them to make and implement choices about their reproduction and sexuality in a safe and healthful manner.

In the reproductive health paradigm, as in the biomedical paradigm, decision-making at the individual level is key. But the conceptualization of the decision-making process and its implications is distinctly different. In the reproductive health paradigm, it is the woman's own perspective on reproduction and sexuality that frames the questions relevant to contraceptive deci-sion-making—and that ultimately determines the answers as well. Biological risks matter deeply; but so do the many other risks inherent in sexual rela-tionships and childbearing. Thus reproduction, while critical to biological health, is understood in its full social, economic and psychological context. And, as elaborated in the early sections of this chapter, that context is under-stood from the woman's perspective. Thus, where ethically sensitive biomed-ical programs champion informed *consent*, viewing women as the objects of medical practice, reproductive health programs champion informed *choice*, viewing women as the subjects and architects of health strategies.

In this paradigm, the universe of information relevant to reproductive health and to contraceptive decision-making is far broader than in the biomedical model. While the doctor-patient relationship is still necessarily a central one, information does not flow downhill on a one-way street, from doctor to patient. Rather, the information generated by the woman, derived from her own experience, is elicited and taken seriously, since it is that information that just as surely shapes her choices.

Though the individuality of each person is valued and respected in the reproductive health paradigm, women are not viewed as detached and autonomous selves, "impervious to social influence," as in the demographic paradigm. Nor are they viewed as abstract individuals "'free' to 'choose' health behaviors."[82] Instead, the reproductive health paradigm understands individual choices to be embedded in, and constrained by, social forces and conditions, including racism, poverty, and patriarchy.

Indeed, rather than ignore or obfuscate the influence of gender, as in the demographic and biomedical paradigms respectively, the reproductive health paradigm consciously seeks out and openly examines the gender dimen-sions of reproduction and sexuality. In the process, reproductive health and contraceptive decision-making are inextricably linked to a wider process in which women struggle to maintain their essential human dignity by demand-ing the right to maintain control over these most intimate and fundamental aspects of their lives.

CONCLUSION

This brings us full circle, to our first emphatic statement that this is a human rights report. In evaluating policies and programs related to reproductive health information, including the sometimes subtle differences among demo-graphic, biomedical, and reproductive health programs, the reference point—the value against which facts are judged—must be the basic notions of human dignity and social justice that we elaborated at the start. One essential element of that dignity and justice is the right of each individual to maintain an element of control over what happens to his or her body and person. For women, such control lies fundamentally in the ability to manage their own reproduction and sexuality; when that ability is wrested away, so is an essential element of what it means to be a full human being.

In the last century, contraception and abortion have been one key site of the struggle over reproduction and sexuality, for whoever controls access to contraception and abortion effectively owns the tools to control women's reproduction. And one key to controlling access to contraception and abortion is to control information about them and their uses. We have demonstrated that, depending on political and economic exigencies, information is sometimes manipulated to deny contraception, sometimes to impose it. Either way, such manipulation denies women the full exercise of their human rights.

In the controversy that has swirled around attempts to inject human rights into population and family health policies, women's demand for control over reproduction and sexuality as a basic human right has often been misrepresented by opponents as being individualistic, selfish, antisocial and even immoral. We reject that charge, not least because we reject its basic premise: that women cannot be trusted to make decisions that will be good for the families and societies in which they live; that what is "good" for a family, a community or even an individual woman's own health is something that must be determined by others who "know better" and then imposed on her. In fact, our contention is precisely the opposite: that women are committed, invested participants in family and society, who are entitled by virtue of their very humanity to participate in determining the role that childbearing and sexuality—that their own bodies and lives—will have in shaping those families and societies.

Trusting women means acknowledging their right to make decisions about reproduction and respecting their ability to do so. It also requires a commitment to ensuring that decision-making is based on full and appropriate information. That, in turn, will require changes in many levels of social life, from state policy, to health systems, to family and community dynamics. Traditional human rights law has been used most effectively at the first level, in addressing state policies, particularly censorship policies that inhibit the flow of information. But truly vindicating human rights in the area of reproduction will also require a long process of affirmative rebuilding of the health systems through which contraceptives and abortion services are delivered. The precise features of such health systems will differ from place to place, just as the substantive decisions that women make and the context in which they make them will differ. But everywhere, that process should be guided by an understanding of women's fundamental right to maintain control over what happens to them—to their bodies, their lives, their humanity—and the extraordinary power of information both to advance and to endanger that right.

NOTES

1. This obligation is explicit in the language of the Convention on the Elimination of All Forms of Discrimination Against Women, Art. 2(e), which requires States Parties "[t]o take all appropriate measures to eliminate discrimination against

women by any person, organization or enterprise." See also the International Covenant on Civil and Political Rights, Arts. 2 and 26, and decisions by the Human Rights Committee interpreting them.

2. See, e.g., International Planned Parenthood Federation, *Vision 2000: Strategic Plan* (1992).

3. A/CONF.171/13.

4. See S. Corrêa in collaboration with R. Reichmann, *Population and Reproductive Rights: Feminist Perspectives from the South* (New Delhi: Kali for Women and London: Zed Books, 1994); R. Petchesky and J. Weiner, "Global Feminist Perspectives on Reproductive Rights and Reproductive Health." Report on the Special Session held at the Fourth Interdisciplinary Conference on Women, Hunter College, New York (1990).

5. Universal Declaration of Human Rights. See, generally, R. J. Cook, *Women's Health and Human Rights* (Geneva: WHO, 1994).

6. See R. Petchesky. "The Body as Property: A Feminist Re-Vision," in F. Ginsburg and R. Rapp (eds.), *Conceiving the New World Order* (Berkeley, California: University of California Press, 1995).

7. For two excellent discussions of the issues involved in defining women's reproductive and sexual rights, see S. Corrêa and R. Petchesky, "Reproductive and Sexual Rights: A Feminist Perspective," in Sen, Germain and Chen (eds.), *Population Policies Reconsidered* (Cambridge, Massachusetts: Harvard University Press, 1994); and R. Dixon-Mueller, *Population Policy and Women's Rights* (Westport, CT: Praeger, 1993). I am indebted to both for clarifying my own thinking on this issue.

8. E.g., A. C. Laurell, "Social Analysis of Collective Health in Latin America," 28(11) *Social Science & Medicine* (1989), 1183–1191; E. Fee and N. Krieger, "Understanding AIDS: Historical Interpretations and the Limits of Biomedical Individualism," 83(10) *American Journal of Public Health* (1993) 1477–1486; L. Freedman and D. Maine, "Women's Mortality: A Legacy of Neglect," in Koblinsky, Timyan and Gay (eds.), *The Health of Women: A Global Perspective* (Boulder, CO: Westview Press, 1993).

9. Martin Luther, remarking on maternal mortality, expressed this view as well as anybody:
   "And even if [women] bear themselves weary—or ultimately bear themselves out—that does not hurt. Let them bear themselves out. This is the purpose for which they exist." Martin Luther, "The Estate of Marriage," (1552) in Vol. 45 of Luther's Works, *The Christian in Society II* (Philadelphia, PA: Muhlenberg Press, 1962), 46.

10. L. P. Freedman, "Women, Health, and Third World Debt: A Critique of Public Health Responses to Economic Crisis" (unpublished. 1990).

11. C. H. Browner, "Women, Household and Health in Latin America," 28(5) *Social Science & Medicine* (1989), 461–473; A. Raikes, "Women's Health in East Africa," 28(5) *Social Science & Medicine* (1989), 447–459; L. Beneria and M. Roldan, *The Crossroads of Class & Gender: Industrial Homework, Subcontracting and Household Dynamics in Mexico City* (Chicago, IL: University of Chicago Press, 1987); UNICEF, *The Invisible Adjustment: Poor Women and the Economic Crisis* (Santiago, Chile: UNICEF, 1988).

12. Asia Watch and Women's Rights Project, *A Modern Form of Slavery: Trafficking of Burmese Women and Girls into Brothels in Thailand* (New York: Human Rights Watch, 1993).

13. Commonwealth Secretariat, *Engendering Adjustment for the 1990s* (London: Commonwealth Secretariat, 1989); C. Barroso and T. Amado, "Impact of the Crisis on the Health of Poor Women: The Case of Brazil," in *The Invisible*

Adjustment (see note 11); C. Moser, "The Impact of Recession and Adjustment Policies at the Micro-level: Low Income Women and Their Households in Guayaquil, Ecuador," ibid.; Beneria and Roldan, note 11 above.

14. Chasnoff, Landress and Barrett, "The Prevalence of Illicit Drug or Alcohol Use During Pregnancy and Discrepancies in Mandatory Reporting in Pinellas County, Florida." 322 *New England Journal of Medicine* (1990), 1202; D. E. Roberts, "Punishing Drug Addicts who Have Babies: Women of Color, Equality, and the Right of Privacy," 104 *Harvard Law Review* (1991), 1419.

15. Roberts, ibid.

16. D. Maine, L. Freedman, F. Shaheed, and S. Frautschi, "Risk, Reproduction, and Rights: The Uses of Reproductive Health Data," in R. Cassen, ed., *Population and Development: Old Debates, New Conclusions* (Washington, DC: Overseas Development Council, 1994).

17. International Covenant on Economic, Social and Cultural Rights, Art. 12; See V. Leary, "The Right to Health in International Human Rights Law," 1 *Health and Human Rights* (1994), 24.

18. Far less attention has been given to the opposite problem: the health consequences of infertility and subfertility. Yet in societies where women are valued primarily for their ability to bear children, these conditions can be devastating.

19. D. Maine and R. McNamara, *Birth Spacing and Child Survival* (New York: Center for Population and Family Health, 1985).

20. The evidence is summarized in Maine and McNamara, ibid.

21. D. Maine and A. Rosenfield, "Maternal Mortality: A Neglected Tragedy: Where is the M in MCH?," 2 *The Lancet* (15 July 1985), 83–85.

22. C. AbouZahr and E. Royston, *Maternal Mortality: A Global Factbook* (Geneva: WHO, 1991).

23. This includes relatively simple technologies such as blood transfusions to treat hemorrhage, antibiotics to treat infections, and cesarean sections to treat obstructed labor.

24. D. Maine, *Safe Motherhood: Issues and Options* (New York: Center for Population and Family Health, 1991).

25. Ibid. Certain women are at higher risk for developing fatal complications: for example, women younger than 20 and older than 40, and women having a first birth or having a fourth or higher parity birth, have a statistically higher risk of complications than women between the ages of 20 and 40 having second or third births. It is important to make contraceptives available to these women and to give them appropriate information about all the risks involved. However, it is *not* appropriate to "target" such women for family planning. Although they have a higher *relative* risk, the largest number of deaths actually occurs among "low risk" women (women without these or other risk factors), because the vast majority of all pregnancies occur within that group. Therefore, even viewed solely as a public health problem of how to decrease maternal mortality in the population, making contraceptives widely available to *all* women is the measure best supported by the epidemiological evidence. Maine et al., (see note 16).

26. Estimates vary with the methodology used to calculate incidence. See WHO, *Mother-Baby Package: A Road Map for Implementation in Countries* (Geneva: WHO, 1994) (citing unpublished WHO estimates for the 67,000 figure) and United Nations, *The World's Women: Trends and Statistics, 1970–1990* (citing S. K. Henshaw, "Induced Abortion: A World Review, 1990", 22(2) *Family Planning Perspectives* [March/April 1990], 76–89, and the Health Statistics Data Base of WHO for the 200,000 figure).

27. Henshaw (see note 26).

28. There will always be a demand for safe abortion services because (1) all contraceptives have some failure rate, however small; (2) many women cannot or will not use contraceptives for a wide range of reasons; and (3) often women cannot control the circumstances in which sexual intercourse occurs and therefore are unable to prevent unwanted pregnancies.

29. WHO, "Sexually Transmitted Infections Increasing—250 million new infections annually," 152 *WHO Features* (Dec. 1990), 1–6.

30. Population Reports, "Controlling Sexually Transmitted Diseases," Series L, Number 9, June 1993.

31. A. Meheus, "Women's Health: Importance of Reproductive Tract Infections, Pelvic Inflammatory Disease and Cervical Cancer," in A. Germain et al. (eds.). *Reproductive Tract Infections* (New York: Plenum Press, 1992). Involuntary childlessness may be due to infertility, pregnancy wastage or infant or child mortality. Involuntary infertility related to chromosomal, congenital or endocrinological abnormalities in both men and women is estimated to affect 5 percent of all couples. The balance of involuntary childlessness in a given population can therefore be assumed to be caused by either acquired infertility (mostly due to infections), pregnancy wastage (often a result of malnutrition) or infant and child mortality.

32. J. R. Wilkie, "Involuntary Childlessness in the United States," 10(1) *Zeitschrift Fur Bevolkerungswissenschaft* (1984), 37–52.

33. S. Harlap, K. Kost and J. D. Forrest, *Preventing Pregnancy, Protecting Health: A New Look at Birth Control Choices in the United States* (New York: Alan Guttmacher Institute, 1991).

34. Hatcher et al., *Contraceptive Technology* (16th revised edition) (New York: Irvington, 1994).

35. Harlap et al. (see note 33 above).

36. S. Gifford, "The Meaning of Lumps: A Case Study of the Ambiguities of Risk," in C. R. James, R. Stall and S. M. Gifford (eds.), *Anthropology and Epidemiology: Interdisciplinary Approaches to the Study of Health and Disease* (Dordrecht: D. Reidel, 1986).

37. M. Nichter, "Modern Methods of Fertility Regulation: When and for Whom are they Appropriate?," in M. Nichter (ed.), *Anthropology and International Health* (Dordrecht, 1989).

38. A. Cornwall, "Building Bridges: Exploring Women's Knowledge in Rural Zimbabwe," in *Qualitative Research Methods Newsletter,* no. 6 (April 1994), Documentation Cell, Department of Health Services Studies, Tara Institute of Social Sciences, Bombay, India.

39. S. I. Cohen, *Developing Information, Education and Communications (IEC) Strategies for Population Programmes,* Technical Paper No. 1 (New York: UNFPA, 1994), 3.

40. The Comstock Act was officially entitled *An Act for the Suppression of Trade in, and Circulation of Obscene Literature and Articles of Immoral Use,* 17 Stat. Ch. 258, sec. 148 (1873).

41. Abbot Kinney, quoted in L. Gordon, *Woman's Body, Woman's Right* (New York: Penguin Books, 1990). 158.

42. Gordon, ibid.

43. E. Hovey, "Obscenity's Meaning, Smut-fighters, and Contraception: 1872–1936," 29 *San Diego Law Review* (1992), 13; M. A. Blanchard, "The American Urge to Censor: Freedom of Expression Versus the Desire to Sanitize Society—From Anthony Comstock to 2 Live Crew," 3 *William & Mary Law Review* (1992), 741. Margaret Sanger's was not the first such show trial. In

England. in a celebrated criminal trial in 1877, Annie Besant and Charles Brad-laugh were charged with "obscene libel" for having republished a pamphlet, *Fruits of Philosophy; or the Private Companion of Young Married Couples,* by an American, Charles Knowlton, advocating contraception within marriage. In the 1920s, Marie Stopes, who had opened the first birth control clinic in England, was a party in a series of sensational civil libel trials regarding the character of her book, *Married Love,* which advocated the use of contraception within marriage. See R. Manwell, *The Trial of Annie Besant and Charles Bradlaugh* (New York: Horizon Press, 1976) and M. Box (ed.), *Birth Control and Libel: The Trial of Marie Stopes* (New York: A. S. Barnes, 1967).

44. Gordon (see note 41).

45. Ibid.

46. B. Ehrenreich and D. English, *For Her Own Good: 150 Years of Experts' Advice to Women* (New York: Doubleday, 1978).

47. Gordon (see note 41), pp. 167–168.

48. Quoted in Gordon, ibid., at 168.

49. Atlee and O'Donnell, "Report of the Committee on Criminal Abortion," 22 *Transactions of the American Medical Association* (1871), 241, quoted in C Smith-Rosenberg, *Disorderly Conduct: Visions of Gender in Victorian America* (New York: Alfred A. Knopf, 1985), pp. 236–37.

50. *People v. Sanger,* 222 N.Y. 193 (1918).

51. Hovey (see note 43). Laws banning the use of contraception were not held to be unconstitutional until 1965 in *Griswold v. Connecticut,* 381 U.S. 479 (1965). Only in 1972 did the U.S. Supreme Court find a constitutional right of non-medical people to distribute contraceptive information to unmarried persons *Eisenstadt v. Baird,* 405 U.S. 438 (1972). In two subsequent cases the court specifically ruled that state laws prohibiting advertisement and display of contraceptives actually violated the constitutional guarantee of free speech. *Carey v. Population Services International.* 431 U.S. 678 (1977) and *Bolger v. Young Drug Products,* 463 U.S. 60 (1983).

52. See, e.g., *Roe v. Wade,* 410 U.S. 113 (1973) (finding a constitutional right to abortion under certain circumstances).

53. Gordon (see note 41).

54. Because of the way that pharmaceuticals are developed and marketed, and the way that testing, advertising, and distribution are regulated by the state, multinational corporations end up playing a huge role in the creation and dissemination of medical and technical information about contraceptives. Indeed, the history of the scientific and commercial development of oral contraceptives is itself an illuminating case study of issues in international economic development. See G. Gereffi, *The Pharmaceutical Industry and Dependency in the Third World* (Princeton: Princeton University Press, 1983).

55. In France, an explicit ban on contraceptive advertising was enacted in 1920 and interpreted by the French courts to include a ban on dissemination of contraceptive devices as well 12(1) *Bulletin des Lois* (1920), 3254). The French law then became part of the law governing French colonies in Africa. At independence, most former colonies passed "reception statutes" adopting the old legal codes; as in Algeria, specific laws were then retained, repealed, or modified as a new set of internal and external concerns came into play with the formation of new nation-states. Although in France itself the law was modified in 1967 and 1974 to permit distribution of contraceptives, in a number of Francophone African countries, the 1920 law prohibiting contraceptive information remains on the books to this day. A. Kader Boye, K. Hill, S. Isaacs and D. Gordis,

"Marriage Law and Practice in the Sahel," 22(6) *Studies in Family Planning* (1991), 343–349.

56. See, generally, V. Moghadam (ed.), *Identity Politics & Women: Cultural Reassertions and Feminisms in International Perspective* (Boulder, CO: Westview Press, 1994). In Algeria in the early years after independence, women were seen not only as wives and mothers, but also as freedom fighters who would help build the new Algeria. The 1962 constitution stated that Islam was the state religion. Over the next decade, the image of women as freedom fighters began to fade as the government increasingly used the language of Islam to legitimate policies that confined women to the traditional roles of wife and mother. M. A. Hélie-Lucas, "Women, Nationalism and Religion in the Algerian Struggle," reprinted in M. Badran and M. Cooke (eds.), *Opening the Gates: A Century of Arab Feminist Writing* (Bloomington: Indiana University Press, 1990).

57. M. A. Hélie-Lucas, "The Veiled Production: A Political and Feminist Approach to Women and Reproduction in Algeria after Independence: 1962–1982," Seminar on Women and Reproduction, 23–28 Oct. 1986, Stockholm, Sweden.

58. M. Ladjali, "Conception, Contraception: Do Algerian Women Really Have a Choice?" in M. Turshen (ed.), *Women and Health in Africa* (Trenton, NJ: Africa World Press, 1991).

59. Asociación Chilena de Protección de la Familia, "Actualización del Documento 'Evaluación de 10 Años de Planificación Familiar en Chile'" (unpublished, 1978) cited in D. Maine, *Family Planning: Its Impact on the Health of Women and Children* (New York: Center for Population and Family Health, 1981).

60. T. Valdes, J. Gysling, and M. C. Benavente, "Género y Políticas de Población en Chile" (Santiago: FLACSO, 1994).

61. Official policy was to sponsor and support programs that "dignify and encourage motherhood." United Nations, *World Population Policies*, Vol. 1 (1987).

62. Speech by Gen. Augusto Pinochet quoted in *De la Miel y los Implantes*, 177. See also X. Jiles, "Historia de las políticas de regulación de la fecundidad en Chile," in T. Valdes and M. Busto (eds.), *Sexualidad y Reproducción: Hacia la Construcción de Derechos* (Santiago, Chile: CORSAPS and FLACSO, 1994).

63. See, for example, Hanna Papanek's comparative examination of the anti-abortion movement in the U.S., *lebensraum* policies in Nazi Germany, and temporary marriage *(mut' a)* in Khomeini's Iran, in "The Ideal Woman and the Ideal Society: Control and Autonomy in the Construction of Identity," V. Moghadam (ed.), *Identity Politics & Women*, note 56 above.

64. See A. R. Omran, *Family Planning in the Legacy of Islam* (New York: Routledge, 1992).

65. The ICPD Programme of Action adopts this basic view of the objective of family planning programs: "The aim of family planning programmes must be to enable couples and individuals to decide freely and responsibly on the number and spacing of their children and to have the information and means to do so and to ensure informed choices and make available a full range of safe and effective methods" (para. 7.12).

66. This analysis of the military metaphors is taken from S. C. Watkins, "If All We Knew About Women Was What We Read in *Demography*, What Would We Know?" 30(4) *Demography* (1993), 551–557, 556.

67. *Swatantra Bharat*, 6 Aug. 1976, quoted in K. P. Bahadur, *Population Crisis in India* (New Delhi, India: National Publishing House, 1977), 167.

68. Watkins (see note 66), p. 553.

69. Ibid.

70. Ibid., p. 565.

71. Cohen (see note 39).

72. L. Freedman and S. Isaacs, "Human Rights and Reproductive Choice," 24(1) *Studies in Family Planning* (1993), 18–30.

73. Dixon-Mueller (see note 7); D. P. Warwick, *Bitter Pills: Population Policies and their Implementation in Eight Developing Countries* (Cambridge, UK: Cambridge University Press, 1982).

74. World Health Organization, *Primary Health Care*, Report of the International Conference on Primary Health Care, Alma-Ata, USSR (Geneva: WHO, 1978).

75. See, e.g., UNICEF, *Children and Development in the 1990s: A UNICEF Sourcebook*, prepared for the World Summit for Children, 29–30 Sept. 1990 (New York: UNICEF, 1990).

76. A. Starrs, *Preventing the Tragedy of Maternal Deaths: A Report on the International Safe Motherhood Conference*, Nairobi, Feb. 1987 (Washington, DC: World Bank, 1987).

77. Maine (see note 24).

78. Fee and Krieger (see note 8).

79. See, e.g., R. Hubbard, M. S. Henifin, and B. Fried (eds.), *Biological Woman—The Convenient Myth* (Cambridge, MA: Schenkman, 1982); V. Sapiro (ed.), *Women, Biology, and Public Policy* (Beverly Hills, CA: Sage, 1985).

80. E. O. Laumann, R. T. Michael, and J. H. Gagnon, "A Political History of the National Sex Survey of Adults," 26(1) *Family Planning Perspectives* (1994), 34–38.

81. M. F. Fathalla, "Reproductive Health: a Global Overview," 626 *Annals of the New York Academy of Sciences* (1991), 1–10.

82. As Fee and Krieger note, this is a view that biomedicine adopts from liberal political and economic theory: "It [biomedicine] treats people as consumers who make free choices in the marketplace of products and behaviors, and it generally ignores the role of industry, agribusiness, and government in structuring the array of risk factors that individuals are supposed to avoid (see note 8)" p. 1481.

PART IV

Exploring the Inextricable Linkage Between Health and Human Rights

The essence of the health and human rights linkage derives from the deep complementarity of the public health goal to ensure the conditions in which people can be healthy and the human rights goal of identifying, promoting, and protecting the societal determinants of human well-being. The articles presented in this section consider the larger societal determinants of health with specific attention to HIV/AIDS, gender, and sexuality.

From a public health perspective, human rights provides a framework for identifying the civil, political, economic, social, and cultural dimensions of life that are linked to, and may even be determinant of, health status. The methods and perspective of public health offer human rights new approaches for promoting the conditions necessary for human well-being. This conceptual linkage between health and human rights provides different ways to examine problems and conceive solutions.

To understand the ways in which human rights and public health are relevant to each other, the nature of the essential conditions for health must first be addressed. The chapter by Nancy Adler and colleagues poses the core problem: What are the so-called societal factors that determine, more than anything else, who lives, who dies, who is ill—of what and when? There is now overwhelming evidence that the major determinants of health status are societal, but the nature of these determinants remains vague. The extent to which socioeconomic status is a true explanation or merely a surrogate for other, less readily defined characteristics or societal features remains unclear.

The HIV/AIDS pandemic has provided sustained insight into the health and human rights connection. The chapter by Jonathan Mann presents the connections between vulnerability to HIV/AIDS and the status of respect for human rights and dignity, while the chapter by Jacques du Guerny and Elisabeth Sjöberg considers the specific influence of gender relations for the design of HIV/AIDS policies and programs. HIV/AIDS has posed a challenge to global society and ways of thinking, and has broadened understanding of the contribution of societal factors to vulnerability and to preventable disease, disability, and premature death. Early in the pandemic, the World Health Organization identified discrimination toward HIV-infected people and people with AIDS as counterproductive to public health efforts (see Part II), and preventing discrimination toward infected people therefore became an integral part of the global AIDS strategy. As the epidemic advanced, the contribution of societal factors to vulnerability to HIV infection and their connection to human rights became increasingly evident. This recognition has been incorporated into the strategic approach of the UNAIDS program (the Joint United Nations Programme on HIV/AIDS).

In recent decades, the collective work of women's health and women's human rights advocates pioneered the convergence of health and rights through the application of a gender perspective. The chapter by Rebecca Cook discusses the underlying social conditions and gender roles that compromise women's health and explains how human rights law can remove barriers to women's ability to achieve optimal health status. Lynn Freedman explores the linkages between the analytical tools of public health and the emerging theories of human rights. The application of these approaches to enhanced research and advocacy strategies is examined with a focus on women's reproductive health and reproductive rights. Finally, Alice Miller and colleagues propose that the health issues faced by lesbians are often inextricable from their most basic human rights, and that none of several movements, including those identified with human rights, women's rights, gay rights, women's health or lesbian health, has sufficiently taken into account the health and human rights paradigm. Their chapter then proposes the application of this paradigm as a way to move forward, thereby underscoring the opportunities provided by new thinking for new action.

Socioeconomic Status and Health: 13.
The Challenge of the Gradient

Nancy Adler, Thomas Boyce, Margaret A. Chesney,

Sheldon Cohen, Susan Folkman, Robert L. Kahn,

and S. Leonard Syme

Throughout history, socioeconomic status (SES) has been linked to health. Individuals higher in the social hierarchy typically enjoy better health than do those below; SES differences are found for rates of mortality and morbidity from almost every disease and condition (Antonovsky, 1967; Illsley and Baker, 1991). Despite recognition for decades of this fundamental association, the reasons for its existence remain largely obscure. Because SES is such a powerful risk factor, a search for other etiologic factors in disease endpoints is often regarded as suspect unless the influence of SES is controlled. As a result, SES has been almost universally relegated to the status of a control variable and has not been systematically studied as an important etiologic factor in its own right. As Marmot, Kogevinas, and Elston (1987) noted, it is generally included "with as much regularity but with as little thought as . . . gender" (p. 111).

Socioeconomic status is "a composite measure that typically incorporates economic status, measured by income; social status, measured by education; and work status, measured by occupation" (Dutton and Levine, 1989, p. 30). The three indicators are interrelated but not fully overlapping variables. Often researchers use one or another of the indicators as the measure of SES. The fact that associations between SES and health are found with each of the indicators suggests that a broader underlying dimension of social stratification or social ordering is the potent factor. In this article we consider SES effects broadly and examine studies using a variety of specific indicators.

Of those studies that have examined the health effects of SES, most have compared the health of individuals at the very bottom of the SES hierarchy either with those above the poverty level or with those at the top of the hierarchy (for reviews, see Antonovsky, 1967; Haan, Kaplan, and Syme, 1989). The effects of severe poverty on health may seem obvious through the impact of poor nutrition, crowded and unsanitary living conditions, and inadequate medical care. As important as these variables are, such an analysis underestimates the potent and pervasive effects of SES on biological outcomes. There is evidence that the association of SES and health occurs at every level of the SES hierarchy, not simply below the threshold of poverty. Not only do those in poverty have poorer health than those in more favored circumstances, but those at the highest level enjoy better health than do those just below (Adelstein, 1980; Kraus, Borhani, and Franti, 1980; Marmot, Smith et al., 1991; Marmot, Shipley, and Rose, 1984). This poses a challenge to understand the mechanisms by which SES affects health because factors associated with low SES are not likely to account for differences in health status at upper levels. Identifying factors that can account for the link to health all across the SES hierarchy may shed light on new mechanisms that have heretofore been ignored because of a focus on the more readily apparent correlates of poverty.

The goal of this chapter is threefold. First, we review evidence that the relationship of SES to health is not simply a threshold effect in which morbidity and mortality increase only at severe levels of deprivation, but is a graded relationship occurring at all levels within the spectrum of social position. Second, we begin the exploration of the gradient by considering factors that could account for this SES-health gradient. This exploration highlights the potential importance of psychosocial variables. Finally, we present a challenge to develop and apply new conceptual and statistical approaches to help understand the nature of the SES-health gradient.

EVIDENCE FOR THE GRADIENT

Although most studies of SES and health dichotomize individuals on SES or present a single correlation between gross levels of SES and a health outcome, some researchers have become aware of "finely stratified mortality differences running from the top to the bottom of the social hierarchy" (Smith and Egger, 1992, p. 1080). Figure 1 illustrates the findings of a representative subset of studies that have examined mortality rates for at least four levels of SES, and Figure 2 illustrates this for disease prevalence by SES. Because the SES indicators and the cutoff points used to define levels are not standardized, it is not possible to make direct comparisons across studies. However, these figures demonstrate that the SES differences in health occur at every level of SES, no matter what the SES indicator or cutoff point.

The most notable of the studies demonstrating the SES-health gradient is the Whitehall study of mortality (Marmot et al., 1984), which covered 17,350 British civil servants over a period of 10 years. The British civil service has ranked grades of employment. The lowest grade consists of unskilled workers (e.g., messengers). The next lowest consists of clerical workers, followed by the professional and executive levels, up to the top administrators. Relative risk of mortality over 10 years significantly increased as employment grade decreased. Compared to mortality risk of the

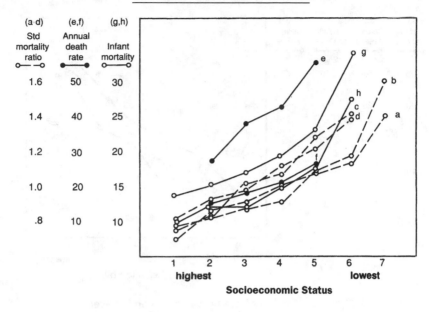

Figure 1. Mortality Rate by Socioeconomic Level

Note. (a) Standardized mortality ratio, observed to expected deaths (SMR) male (Kitagawa & Hauser, 1973). (b) SMR female (Kitagawa & Hauser, 1973). (c) SMR male (Adelstein, 1980). (d) SMR female (Adelstein, 1980). (e) Annual death rate per 1,000 (ADR) male (Feldman, Makuc, Kleinman, & Cornoni-Huntley, 1989). (f) ADR female (Feldman et al., 1989). (g) Infant mortality per 1,000 live births (IM) male (Susser, Watson, & Hopper, 1985). (h) IM female (Susser et al., 1985).

top administrators and controlling for age, relative risk of mortality was 1.6 for the professional-executive grades, 2.2 for the clerical grades, and 2.7 for the lowest grades. Because the sample was relatively homogeneous, with all sharing employment in the civil service and having access to nationalized health care, these differences in mortality are all the more striking.

Similar findings emerge from census data in the United Kingdom. Susser, Watson, and Hopper (1985) documented a gradient between five levels of occupational status and standardized mortality rates (SMR, the ratio of observed to expected deaths) in a range of diseases including malignant neoplasms, infectious and parasitic diseases, and diseases of the respiratory, digestive, and circulatory systems. Similarly, Adelstein (1980), using census data, found that SMRs for all causes of death decreased at each of six increasing levels of SES based on occupational status. The SES gradient emerged not only in SMRs but also in the prevalence rates for most, although not all, specific diseases.[1]

The SES-health gradient has been shown in U.S. studies as well.[2] For example, Kitagawa and Hauser (1973) found a graded relationship between mortality and years of education. The ratio of observed to expected deaths

Nancy Adler et al.

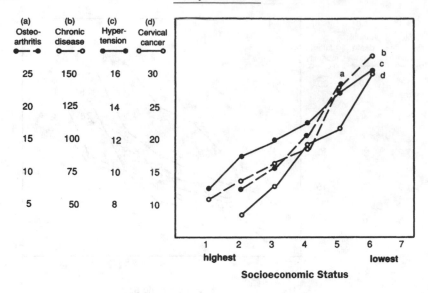

Figure 2. Morbidity Rate by Socioeconomic Level

Note. (a) Percent diagnosed osteoarthritis (Cunningham & Kelsey, 1984). (b) Relative prevalence of chronic disease (Townsend, 1974). (c) Prevalence of hypertension (Kraus, Borhani, & Franti, 1980). (d) Rate of cervical cancer per 100,000 (Devesa & Diamond, 1983).

within subgroups among white men ages 25 to 64 years was .70 for those with a college education or better, .85 for those with some college, .91 for high school graduates, 1.03 for those with some high school, 1.07 for those completing eight years of schooling, 1.13 for those with five to seven years of education, and 1.15 for those with four years or less. Comparable ratios for white women of this age were .78, .82, .87, .91, 1.08, 1.18, and 1.60 for each of the education levels. In brief, the more years of education, the lower is the ratio of observed to expected deaths. The gradient for both income and education also emerged in more recent analyses of a national sample reported by Pappas, Queen, Hadden, and Fisher (1993). Pappas et al. compared the degree of association of mortality with education and with income in their data, collected in 1986, with that in the data analyzed by Kitagawa and Hauser (1973), collected in 1960. In the 26 years between the two studies, death rates declined, but the decreases were greater in more versus less educated groups. The resulting SES health gradient was, thus, steeper in 1986 than it had been in 1960.

Socioeconomic status is also linked to prevalence and course of disease. Pincus, Callahan, and Burkhauser (1987) examined reports of health problems for individuals at four levels of educational attainment in a national sample and tested for a linear trend across educational levels. The frequency of 32 of 37 conditions assessed was greater the lower the educational level.

The individual conditions were grouped into eight disease categories, and differences by education were analyzed separately in each of three age groups: 18–44, 45–54, and 55–64 years. There was a significant linear trend for almost all of the diseases in all three groups. The only disease category that was unrelated to education in all age groups was neoplastic disease.[3] Among a group of patients with rheumatoid arthritis, Pincus and Callahan (1985) found that the lower a patient's educational level, the greater was the chance of subsequent mortality or major decline in functional capacity over a nine-year period, even when controls were entered for age, sex, smoking, functional status at baseline, treatments indicative of more severe disease, or duration of disease.

POSSIBLE MECHANISMS

Having reviewed substantial evidence for a graded association between socioeconomic position and health, we next examine three possible explanations for the basis of the association. First, the empirical link between SES and health might represent a spurious association, arising from the relationships of both SES and health outcomes to underlying, genetically based factors. For example, physical size or intellectual capacity might lead concurrently to lower social position and poorer health. This explanation is plausible but improbable. As noted in both the Whitehall I and Whitehall II studies (Marmot et al., 1984; Marmot et al., 1991), although job status is inversely related to physical height, the association between job status and health persists even after adjustments for height and body mass index. As noted by Kohn and Schooler (1978), intelligence and cognitive flexibility are important correlates of job status; but it is less clear, beyond the known relationship of mental retardation to greater disease risk, that intelligence in a normative population is reliably linked to health. Indeed, there is evidence that health behaviors such as compliance with medical advice are unrelated to intelligence or education (Becker, Drachman, and Kirscht, 1974; Stimson, 1974). A biologically driven predisposition to both lower SES and poorer health status appears unlikely, given the evidence at hand, to offer a sound explanation for the SES-health association. Furthermore, if genetic predispositions that we have not accounted for are involved in the SES-health link, they are very likely, as are most complex genetic influences, to become important only when environmental and behavioral factors impinge on them.

A second possible explanation for the SES-health gradient, known as the *drift hypothesis,* suggests that the association reflects the influence of illness on SES, rather than of SES on illness. There is evidence, for example, that individuals with schizophrenia follow a trajectory of descending socioeconomic resources as the natural history of their disease unfolds (Goldberg and Morrison, 1963). Nonetheless, two thorough recent reviews have concluded that, although some downward drift in social position accompanies poorer health status, the phenomenon is unlikely to play an important role in accounting for the SES-health relationship (Haan et al., 1989; Wilkinson, 1986). Deteriorating health status among older adults, which has been linked to educational levels, cannot logically affect past education (Haan et al., 1989). Furthermore, if illness principally influenced SES, then no association would be expected for family members when SES is determined by income or occupation of the head of the household, or for retired individuals for whom income is no longer dependent on health. However, such SES-health associations are generally as strong as those found for working heads of households.

Finally, the third explanation for the association is that SES affects biological functions that, in turn, influence health status. Surprisingly, we know little about how SES operates to influence biological functions that determine health status. Part of the problem may be the way in which SES is conceptualized and analyzed. It is usually treated as a main effect, operating independently of other variables to predict health. In reality, however, components of SES, including income, education, and occupation, shape one's life course and are enmeshed in key domains of life, including (a) the physical environment in which one lives and works and associated exposure to pathogens, carcinogens, and other environmental hazards; (b) the social environment and associated vulnerability to interpersonal aggression and violence as well as degree of access to social resources and supports; (c) socialization and experiences that influence psychological development and ongoing mood, affect, and cognition; and (d) health behaviors.

Within these domains, many specific candidate variables may contribute to the SES-health gradient. In this review we have selected those variables that could operate at the upper as well as at the lower end of the hierarchy, although the mechanisms or their relative impact may well differ at different levels. We have focused on variables for which there is empirical evidence of a linear relationship both with SES and with important health outcomes. This review is not exhaustive, but rather it is suggestive of the types of variables and approaches that can be taken to understanding the SES-health gradient. Elsewhere, we have considered the role of access to care in explaining the SES-health gradient and concluded that access alone could not explain the gradient (Adler, Boyce, Chesney, Folkman, and Syme, 1993). Here, we place particular emphasis on psychological and behavioral variables that have largely been overlooked because of the predominant focus on material aspects of SES differences.

Health Behaviors

Health risk behaviors such as cigarette smoking, physical inactivity, poor diet, and substance abuse are closely tied to both SES and health outcomes. Despite the close ties, the association of SES and health is reduced but not eliminated when these behaviors are statistically controlled (Marmot et al., 1984).

Smoking

Cigarette smoking is strongly linked to indexes of SES, including education, income, and employment status, and it is significantly associated with morbidity and mortality, particularly from cardiovascular disease and cancer (Adelstein, 1980; Centers for Disease Control, 1987; Devesa and Diamond, 1983; Escobedo, Anda, Smith, Remington, and Mast, 1990; Kraus et al., 1980; Marmot et al., 1991; Pugh, Power, Goldblatt, and Arber, 1991; Remington et al., 1985; Seccareccia, Menotti, and Prati, 1991; U.S. Department of Health, Education and Welfare, 1979; Winkleby, Fortmann, and Barrett, 1990). Smoking rates vary inversely with SES. In a U.S. community-based survey of 3,349 adults, approximately 41 percent of men with 12 years' education or less smoked, versus 30 percent of those with 13–15 years' education, 25 percent of those with 16 years' education, and 18 percent of those with more than 16 years' education. Comparable rates of smoking among women at each educational level were 36 percent, 24 percent, 15 percent, and 17 percent, respectively (Winkleby et al., 1990). A linear gradient between education and smoking prevalence was also shown in a community sample of middle-aged women: Forty-three percent of women with less than a high school education were current smokers, versus 30 percent of those with some college, 23 percent of those with a college degree, and 19 percent of those with advanced degrees. Additionally, among current smokers the number of cigarettes smoked was related to SES (Matthews, Kelsey, Meilahn, Kuller, and Wing, 1989).

Significant employment grade differences in smoking were found in the Whitehall II study, which examined a new cohort of 10,314 subjects from the British Civil Service beginning in 1985 (Marmot et al., 1991). Moving from the lowest to the highest employment grades, the prevalence of current smoking among men was 33.6 percent, 21.9 percent, 18.4 percent, 13.0 percent, 10.2 percent, and 8.3 percent, respectively. For women, the comparable figures were 27.5 percent, 22.7 percent, 20.3 percent, 15.2 percent, 11.6 percent, and 18.3 percent respectively. Social class differences in smoking are likely to continue because rates of smoking initiation are inversely related to SES and because rates of cessation are positively related to SES (Escobedo et al., 1990; Kaprio and Koskenvuo, 1988: Pugh et al., 1991).

Physical Activity

Involvement in physical activity has both a direct association with health outcomes and an indirect effect insofar as it is associated with obesity. Both lack of physical activity and obesity are positively associated with poor health outcomes (U.S. Department of Health and Human Services [DHHS], 1989; Bouchard, Shepard, Stephens, Sutton, and McPherson, 1990) and are inversely related to SES (Cauley, Donfield, LaPorte, and Warhaftig, 1991; Ford et al., 1991; Kahn, Williamson, and Stevens, 1991; Marmot et al., 1991; Sobel and Stunkard, 1989).

The association of both obesity and lack of physical activity with SES emerged in the Whitehall II study for men but less strongly for women. Among the men but not among the women, those at lower employment grades were significantly more likely to report getting no moderate to vigorous exercise. In a U.S. study, Ford et al. (1991) found an association of physical activity and SES in an urban community sample. Higher-SES women spent significantly more time than did their lower-SES counterparts in leisure-time, job-related, and household physical activity. The men showed qualitative differences in physical activity by SES: lower-SES men spent significantly more time doing household chores and walking, whereas higher SES men spent more time engaged in leisure physical activity.

Alcohol

Alcohol consumption shows a pattern opposite to that of smoking and other risk behaviors. Several studies (Cauley et al., 1991; Marmot et al., 1991; Matthews et al., 1989) have found a positive correlation of alcohol consumption with SES as measured by education or job status. The relationship between alcohol consumption and health outcomes, however, is not uniform across diseases. For example, although alcohol may increase risk of some cancers (e.g., cancer of the larynx) and alcohol abuse increases risk of cirrhosis of the liver, moderate levels of alcohol consumption are associated with lower risk for coronary heart disease, the leading cause of death for both men and women in the United States. In this context, the interpretation of alcohol intake as a risk factor is unclear.

Psychological Characteristics

There has been increasing evidence that psychological characteristics of the individual contribute to risk of morbidity and mortality. Of these variables, depression and hostility have shown the most consistent relationship with both SES and physical health outcomes.

Depression

Depression has been studied both as a pathological state of major depression and in terms of general depressive symptoms. Socioeconomic status is inversely related to both major depression and depressive symptoms. In a Canadian community sample, the prevalence of major depression was 1.9 percent, 4.5 percent, and 12.4 percent in high-, average-, and low-SES groups, respectively. Over 16 years, the inverse gradient repeated itself in annual incidence of new depression (Murphy et al., 1991). Kaplan, Roberts, Camacho, and Coyne (1987) found higher rates of new reports of depressive symptoms over a nine-year period among those lower in income and education.

Depression is linked to health outcomes, particularly coronary heart disease. Within a sample of patients with coronary artery disease, twice as many of those with a major depressive disorder experienced at least one major cardiac event (e.g., myocardial infarction [MI], bypass surgery) in the subsequent year compared with nondepressed patients (77.8 percent vs. 34.9 percent, $p < .02$: Carney et al., 1988). In a meta-analysis of 15 studies of psychological predictors of coronary heart disease, depression was found to have a combined effect size of .21 ($p < .001$); the strongest association was with MI (combined effect size of .26, $p < .001$; Booth-Kewley and Friedman, 1987).

Hostility

Hostility—a disposition prone to anger; a cynical, distrusting view of others; and antagonistic behavior (Barefoot, Dodge, Peterson, Dahlstrom, and Williams, 1989)—also relates both to SES and to disease risk. For example, in a national sample in the United States, hostility was inversely related to five levels of education ($p < .001$), occupational status ($p < .001$), and income ($p < .003$; Barefoot et al., 1991). Similarly, Scherwitz, Perkins, Chesney, and Hughes (1991) found greater hostility among less educated than among more educated adults in four urban areas ($p < .001$).

Several prospective studies have linked hostility to risk of coronary heart disease (CHD) and premature mortality. Dembroski, MacDougall, Costa, and Grandits (1989) found that among men under age 47, greater hostility measured on entry into the Multiple Risk Factor Intervention Trial (Multiple Risk Factor Intervention Group, 1976) conferred an adjusted relative risk of 2.1 for subsequent MI or coronary heart disease (CHD) or both ($p = .001$) controlling for cigarette smoking, diastolic blood pressure, and serum cholesterol. In a 25-year follow-up of a sample of medical students, Barefoot, Dahlstrom, and Williams (1983) found CHD incidence density to be .9 per 1000 person-years of follow-up for those with hostility scores at or below the median versus 4.5 for those above the median. And in a 10-year follow-up of a male sample, Shekelle, Gale, Ostfeld, and Paul (1983) found the relative odds of an initial CHD event to be .68 for low- versus high-hostility groups after adjustment for age, systolic blood pressure, serum cholesterol, cigarette smoking, and alcohol intake ($p < .01$). In addition, cross-sectional studies have found associations between hostility and peripheral arterial disease (Joesoef, Wetterhal, DeStafano, Stroup, and Fronek, 1989), essential hypertension (reviewed in Diamond, 1982), and CHD (reviewed in Diamond, 1982; Barefoot et al., 1983).

Psychological Stress

Associations between SES and health may stem in part from differential exposure to and experience of greater stress. Stress has been characterized in two ways: (a) as exposure to life events that require adaptation, generally measured by a checklist of major events (e.g., divorce, death of a relative, job loss), or (b) as a state that occurs when persons perceive that demands exceed their abilities to cope, usually measured by self-reports of subjective experience. There is evidence for the role of both types of stress indicators in the SES-health link.

Life events presumably trigger perceptions of stress and negative emotion. These perceptions are known to alter neuroendocrine response and immune responses that may put persons at greater risk for a range of illnesses. Persons experiencing recent stressful life events have been found to be at greater risk for gastrointestinal disorders (Harris, 1991), menorrhagia and secondary amenorrhea (Harris, 1989), heart attacks (Theorell, 1974), and susceptibility to infectious agents (Cohen, Tyrell, and Smith, 1991, 1993; Stone et al., 1992). Perceptions of stress and negative affect have been similarly linked to heart disease (Byrne and Whyte, 1980; Tofler et al., 1990), stroke (Harmsen, Rosengren, Tsipogianni, and Wilhelmsen, 1990), and susceptibility to infectious agents (Cohen et al., 1991, 1993).

Higher placement in the SES hierarchy can reduce stress and its somatic correlates in two ways. First, higher SES diminishes the likelihood that individuals will encounter negative events. In a community survey, lower-income respondents were exposed to more stressful life events beyond their control than were higher-income respondents (Dohrenwend and Dohrenwend, 1970). Similarly, Dohrenwend (1973) found that families whose head of household had less than a high school education reported more stressful life events than did those headed by a high school graduate or some college. This relation held both for events whose occurrences were within respondent control and for those outside of their control. McLeod and Kessler (1990) found small but consistent associations between SES and exposure to negative life events. A second way in which higher SES placement can reduce stress results because as individuals descend the SES hierarchy, they may have fewer social and psychological resources to cope with stressful life events and thus will be more susceptible to the subjective experience of stress. Those lower in the hierarchy may have less opportunity to form, maintain, and access social networks that can buffer the effects of stressful life events (Cohen and Wills, 1985; House et al., 1991; McLeod and Kessler, 1990). In an analysis of 720 persons interviewed in a New Haven mental health catchment area, Kessler (1979) found that persons of lower SES were exposed to more stressful events than were upper-SES persons and that, given equal exposure, emotional functioning was more affected among lower- than among upper-SES individuals.

Evidence for a gradient relation between SES and appraisals of life as stressful was reported in an analysis of a national probability sample collected by the Harris Poll: Perceptions of stress decreased in a dose-response fashion in relation to both increased household income and education (Cohen and Williamson, 1988). In summary, higher socioeconomic status is associated with decreases in stressful events and stress perceptions, both of which may affect risk for illness.

Only one study has examined associations among education, stress, and mortality. Ruberman, Weinblatt, Goldberg, and Chaudhary (1984) examined mortality among 2,572 male survivors of MI who were assigned to the treatment condition in a clinical trial of a beta blocker for prevention of subsequent attacks. Educational level, social isolation, and life stress (as measured by questions involving occurrence and evaluation of events or circumstances such as experiencing major financial difficulties, not enjoying one's work, being in a low-status occupation, experiencing a divorce or violent event and reacting by being very upset, etc.) each showed an inverse gradient with mortality over a three-year period. Educational level itself was inversely related to life stress and to social isolation. Moreover, when both life stress and social isolation were high or low, education was no longer linked to differential mortality, suggesting that the zero-order association was due to the linkage of education with stress and social isolation. However, the measure of stress included measures of occupational status, which may have confounded the association with education, and replication of these findings with a better measure of stress is needed.

Effects of Social Ordering

Hierarchical position may have a direct effect on health as well as indirect effects through SES-related differences in the physical and social environment, health behaviors, or personality. In other words, one's relative position in the SES hierarchy, apart from the material implications of one's position, may affect risk of disease. Wilkinson (1992) has shown that among developed countries, per capita income is not as strongly related to life expectancy as is income distribution, with longer life expectancy associated with a greater proportion of income received by the least well-off 70 percent of the population. Effects of SES hierarchies are most strongly shown within countries rather than across countries, particularly in terms of life satisfaction, suggesting that relative status as opposed to absolute status may be most critical. Provocative research findings in both animals and humans provide evidence for this proposition.

Hierarchical social structures emerge in virtually all human social groups and serve to reduce intragroup aggression (LaFreniere and Charlesworth, 1983). These structures are stable over time and are present as early as the second year of life (Strayer, 1989; Strayer and Trudel, 1984; Vaughn and Waters, 1978). Dominance hierarchies in primate and subprimate groups have been inferred from observations of antagonistic, aggressive behaviors and were initially assumed to be driven primarily by survival-related competition for limited resources (e.g., food; Bernstein, 1976). More recently, evidence for stable, observable patterns of social dominance has appeared even within primate groups artificially constructed in laboratory settings with universal availability of food and other resources (Manuck, Kaplan, Adams, and Clarkson, 1988).

Hierarchical status in animal models in the laboratory and the natural environment relates to health endpoints and risk factors for disease. Sapolsky and Mott (1987), for example, found decreased levels of high-density lipoprotein cholesterol—a protective factor in CHD—among subordinate wild baboons. Other work in the same laboratory (Sapolsky, 1989) has revealed significant associations between social rank and serum cortisol levels, secretion of gonadal steroids, and immune function.

Conditions in the larger social environment will affect the direction and magnitude of status-related health effects. Manuck and colleagues (Kaplan, Manuck, Clarkson, Lusso, and Taub, 1982; Manuck et al., 1988) found decreased coronary atherosclerosis in socially dominant cynomolgus macaques, but only under stable social conditions. Under unstable conditions that presented recurrent threats to dominance status, dominant animals showed more atherosclerosis than did submissive animals. The atherogenic effects of dominance under unstable social conditions were reversed with a beta antagonist, propranolol, implying that autonomic arousal and cardiovascular reactivity may underlie the observed association. Similarly, Sapolsky (1989) showed that high social rank was protective in the context of a stable hierarchy but was a risk factor for disease under conditions of instability. This work has also produced limited evidence that profiles of protective versus pathogenic physiology change over time with changes in rank, suggesting that physiologic status is a function of hierarchical position rather than the reverse.

The possibility that dominance status can affect physiological and anatomic characteristics is further supported by research on the African cichlid fish, *Haplochromic burtoni*. Davis and Fernald (1990) showed that young, submissive male fish displayed slower phenotypic maturation, hypogonadism, and undersized neuronal cell bodies among the preoptic neurons responsible for secretion of gonadotropin-releasing hormone. Delayed phenotypic and anatomic maturation was found, however, only under rearing conditions in which older, territorial males were also present; in peer-rearing conditions, earlier maturation occurred as a result of more accelerated neuronal development in the preoptic area. These results suggest that the timing of central nervous system (CNS) maturational events are under social control and that dominance status within a given social context can exert profound influences on neurobiologic function.

Taken together, the studies on social order suggest the following general and preliminary observations regarding possible health effects of social dominance status per se: First, responses to hierarchical position may be encoded into the behavioral repertoire of individual organisms to protect the survival of the group and may be expressed at times even at the expense of individual well-being. Second, hierarchical position may have direct effects on physiological processes and neuroanatomic structures, which may in turn influence an individual's biologic vulnerability to agents of disease. Finally, the health effects of dominance status may be largely dependent on characteristics—particularly stability—of the larger social context in which position is assigned.

ISSUES OF METHODOLOGY AND ANALYSIS

Research on SES and health has been limited by several conceptual and methodological constraints. First as noted earlier, the vast majority of studies of SES and health have failed to examine the whole range of the SES hierarchy. Differentiations at upper as well as lower levels need to be examined.

Second, SES is typically measured by a single variable, such as income or education. Although various components of SES are intercorrelated, they are not identical. Socioeconomic status may function most powerfully in terms of combinations of variables. In studying psychiatric disorders, Rutter (1985) found that no single adverse condition affected risk but that "psychiatric risk went up sharply when several adversities co-existed" (p. 601). In many studies, moreover, race is used as a proxy for SES. Yet there is evidence that SES may operate differently within racial groups and may interact with race to affect health. For example, the association of race and health appears to be particularly strong among low-SES blacks, for whom the burden of discrimination may be more powerful (Klag, Whelton, Coresh, Grim, and Kuller, 1991).

Third, SES indicators have generally been measured at only one level. For example, income has generally been assessed either at the individual level (e.g., family income) or the aggregate level (e.g., mean income within a census tract). We know little about how these levels may function together to affect health outcomes. It may be that the health implications of low income are quite different for individuals living in relatively more affluent areas than in those residing in poorer areas. For example, Haan, Kaplan, and Camacho (1987) found that residing in a neighborhood that was federally designated as a poverty area (characterized by a high proportion of low-income families, substandard housing, many unskilled male laborers, etc.) was a risk factor for subsequent mortality above and beyond the characteristics of the individual. Using data from the Alameda County study, they found that residing in a poverty area predicted nine-year mortality rates, even controlling for the individual's own socioeconomic characteristics (e.g., income or education). Similarly, neighborhood residence continued to predict subsequent mortality when controls were entered for access to health care, for health behaviors, or for social isolation. Similarly, Krieger (1992) has shown that "contextual analyses" in which neighborhood (block group, a subdivision of a census tract, encompassing about 1,000 individuals) and census tract information is used in addition to individual data provide a better understanding of health behaviors and outcomes.

Fourth, almost all studies have used either simple correlation or regression analysis to examine the main effects of SES on a health outcome. Regression analysis is severely limited in its ability to disentangle the SES-health gradient. Only a small set of variables can be analyzed in a regression model, particularly if the goal is to evaluate the interactions as well as the separate effects of the variables. For example, Haan et al. (1987), cited above, examined individual and neighborhood data as independent predictors, assessing the contribution of the latter once a given individual-level variable was controlled for. However, this does not inform us about the joint and individual functioning of these factors. Because of the complexity of the expres-

sion of SES, we need more complete measures and use of statistical procedures to analyze complex, interrelated variables. One such approach is use
of tree-structured regression that examines combinations of conditions associated with poorer health outcomes (Segal and Bloch, 1989). This approach
partitions populations into subgroups and then identifies different paths to
given outcomes. It may be that individuals who have less than a high school
education *and* who smoke *and* who are depressed *and* who live in poor
neighborhoods show dramatically worse health outcomes. Taken individually these factors may have relatively weak associations with health
outcomes, but their combination may be strongly associated.

Alternatively, "grade of membership" (GOM) analysis provides a way to
deal with large numbers of variables. Clive, Woodbury, and Siegler (1983)
demonstrated that this technique, which uses "fuzzy sets," better portrayed
health status over time than did conventional models. GOM analyses
develop profiles or "ideal types" either theoretically or empirically. Individuals can then be classified in terms of how closely they match these profiles.
For example, Berkman, Singer, and Manton (1989) identified four profiles
based on multiple indicators of health and functioning in a community
sample of elderly individuals; then they compared how well Blacks and
Whites were characterized by these profiles. An advantage of GOM analysis is that it becomes more precise as more variables are added, rather than
becoming more unstable, as in regression.

A deeper understanding of the SES-health gradient may emerge if we
examine how variables across multiple dimensions and levels co-occur and
interact. Ideally, we would assess variables that characterize various aspects
of SES, including education, income, and occupational status; individual-
level variables, such as depression, hostility, sense of control, and health
behaviors; and social-level variables, such as characteristics of one's resi-
dential neighborhood (e.g., percentage of poverty, air quality), communities
(health access, community norms regarding health-relevant behaviors), and
work environments. Data-analysis strategies that can accommodate multiple correlated variables would allow us to determine which profiles or combinations of variables were associated with better health and lower morbidity
and mortality.

CONCLUSION

Individuals in lower social status groups have the highest rates of morbidity
and mortality within most human populations. Moreover, studies of the
entire SES hierarchy show that differences in social position relate to morbidity and mortality even at the upper levels of the hierarchy. This observation
calls into question traditional explanations for the relationship between SES
and health, which pertain primarily to the lower SES levels and the health
effects of poverty.

The review presented in this chapter suggests a series of analytic and
conceptual steps that should be taken in an effort to elucidate the impact of

SES on health. As a first step in increasing our understanding of the SES gradient, SES should be examined in terms of a set of variables beyond the standard SES indicators. On the basis of existing studies, we have suggested several domains of such factors, which include health behaviors, psychological factors, and perceptions of social ordering. Although not reviewed here, variables in the physical and social environments, such as crowding, pollution, and access to health care, should also be included (Stokols, 1992). The range of individual variables should be broad and should include those that may lower as well as increase risk of morbidity and mortality. It is very likely that some variables and domains will be more potent at lower levels, whereas others may be more relevant to the SES-health association at the upper levels. For example, Margolis et al. (1992) found that the prevalence of both acute and persistent respiratory symptoms in infants showed dose-response relationships with SES. When risk factors such as crowding and exposure to smoking in the household were adjusted for, relative risk associated with SES was reduced but still remained significant. The data further suggest that risk factors operate differently for different SES levels: being in day care was associated with somewhat reduced incidence in lower-SES families but with increased incidence among infants from high-SES families.

Many of the variables linking SES to health may be dynamically intertwined. Standard analytic methods such as linear regression cannot do justice to the complex relationships among these variables. Their impact on the SES-health gradient may therefore be best described by statistical methods such as regression trees and GOM that can disentangle the effects of variables that co-occur and interact. The application of these methods will enable us to build on the foundation provided by the analysis of individual factors and increase knowledge of the ways these factors directly and in interaction affect health outcomes at different points along the SES-health gradient.

We should not expect, however, that the results of these first stages of analysis will exhaustively explain the SES gradient. Alternatively, they may point to higher-order variables, which will account for aspects of the gradient not explained by the subordinate variables that interact and co-occur. The concept of individual control over existing life circumstances, for example, may be a higher-order variable that synthesizes or renders coherent a number of the factors reviewed here. There is evidence, largely from older populations, that the experience of control contributes to lower morbidity and mortality (Rodin, 1986a, 1986b). Individuals higher on the socioeconomic ladder may have more frequent or more significant opportunities to influence the events that affect their lives, compared with people at lower levels. This sense of control could affect education, occupation, housing, nutrition, health behaviors, medical care, and other aspects of social-class experience not previously discussed. New conceptualizations and measures of control will be needed to capture this type of cross-domain influence.

Social class is among the strongest known predictors of illness and health and yet is, paradoxically, a variable about which very little is known. Psychologists have an important role to play in unraveling the mystery of the SES-health gradient. Several plausible explanations for the puzzling and challenging gradient, including the role of stress, have been proposed, and it will be important to explore these possibilities in more depth in future research. Resolution of the conceptual and analytic dilemmas that have been the focus of this review will be key elements in the continuing, and we hope advancing, efforts to improve health and prevent disease.

NOTES AND ACKNOWLEDGMENTS

Preparation of this chapter was supported by the John D. and Catherine T. MacArthur Foundation Network on Determinants and Consequences of Health-Promoting and Disease-Preventing Behavior, chaired by Judith Rodin. We would like to thank Burton Singer and George Kaplan for consulting with us on this chapter, Kenneth Wallston for his helpful review and comments on an earlier draft, members of the MacArthur Network for their input, and Lynae Darbes for her assistance in the research.

1. In a few diseases such as malignant melanoma and breast cancer, a reverse gradient is found. In addition, the gradient may not emerge in every country or epoch. Although beyond the scope of this paper, study of the variation in the direction and degree of association of SES with specific diseases across time and countries would be valuable.

2. In the United States, research has tended to focus on health differences by race rather than by SES. Research has been hampered by limitations on national data. Although the census provides data on SES, this allows only for analyses of aggregate rather than individual data. Until last year, death certificates provided information only on race, they will now also include years of education. In contrast, Britain provides a ranking of occupational status, which provides a more uniform indicator of social standing (Smith and Egger, 1992).

3. It is interesting to note that a recent review of the contribution of psychosocial factors to disease etiology (Adler and Matthews, 1993) concluded that the evidence for the role of such factors in the etiology of cancer was much weaker than for other diseases, particularly cardiovascular disease.

REFERENCES

Adelstein, A. M. (1980). Life-style in occupational cancer. *Journal of Toxicology and Environmental Health, 6,* 953–962.

Adler, N. E., Boyce, T., Chesney, M., Folkman, S., and Syme, L. (1993). Socio-economic inequalities in health: No easy solution. *Journal of the American Medical Association, 269,* 3140–3145.

Adler, N. E., and Matthews, K. (1993). Health psychology: Why do some people get sick and some stay well? *Annual Review of Psychology, 45,* 229–259.

Antonovsky, A. (1967). Social class, life expectancy and overall mortality. *Milbank Memorial Fund Quarterly, XLV,* 31–73.

Barefoot, J. C., Dahlstrom, W. G., and Williams, R. B., Jr. (1983). Hostility, CHD incidence, and total mortality: A 25-year follow-up study of 255 physicians. *Psychosomatic Medicine, 45(1),* 59–63.

Barefoot, J. C., Dodge, K. A., Peterson, B. L., Dahlstrom, W. G., and Williams, R. B, Jr., (1989). The Cook-Medley Hostility Scale: Item content and ability to predict survival. *Psychosomatic Medicine, 51,* 46–57.

Barefoot, J. C., Peterson, B. L., Dahlstrom, W. G., Siegler, I. C., Anderson, N. B., and Williams, R. B. (1991). Hostility patterns and health implications: Correlates of Cook-Medley Hostility Scale scores in a national survey. *Health Psychology, 10,* 18–24.

Becker, M. H., Drachman, R. H., and Kirscht, J. P. (1974). A new approach to explaining sick-role behavior in low-income populations, *American Journal of Public Health, 64,* 205–216.

Berkman, L., Singer, B., and Manton, K. (1989). Black/White differences in health status and mortality among the elderly. *Demography, 26,* 661–678.

Bernstein, I. S. (1976). Dominance, aggression and reproduction in primate societies. *Journal of Theoretical Biology, 60,* 459–472.

Booth-Kewley, S., and Friedman, H. S. (1987). Psychological predictors of heart disease: A quantitative review. *Psychological Bulletin, 101,* 343–362.

Bouchard, C., Shepard, R. J., Stephens, T., Sutton, J. R, and McPherson, B. D. (eds.). (1990). *Exercise, fitness and health: A consensus of current knowledge.* Champaign, IL; Human Kinetics Books.

Byrne, D. G., and Whyte, H. M. (1980). Life events and myocardial infarction revisited: The role of measures of individual impact. *Psychosomatic Medicine, 42,* 1–10.

Carney, R. M., Rich, M. W., Freedlan, K. E., Sarni, J., TeVelde, A., Sineone, C., and Clark, K. (1988). Major depressive disorder predicts cardiac events in patients with coronary artery disease. *Psychosomatic Medicine, 50,* 627–633.

Cauley, J. A., Donfield. S. M., LaPorte, R. E. and Warhaftig, N. E. (1991). Physical activity by SES in two population-based cohorts. *Medicine and Science in Sports and Exercise, 23,* 343–352.

Centers for Disease Control. (1987). *Smoking, tobacco and health: A fact book.* Rockville, MD: U.S. Department of Health and Human Services, Public Health Service, Office on Smoking and Health.

Clive, J., Woodbury, M. A., and Siegler I. A. (1983). Fuzzy and crisp set-theoretic-based classification of health and disease: A qualitative and quantitative comparison. *Journal of Medical Systems, 7,* 317–332.

Cohen, S., Tyrell, D. A. J., and Smith, A. P. (1991). Psychological stress in humans and susceptibility to the common cold. *New England Journal of Medicine, 325,* 606–612.

Cohen, S., Tyrell. D. A. J., and Smith, A. P. (1993). Negative life events, perceived stress, negative affect, and susceptibility to the common cold. *Journal of Personality and Social Psychology, 64,* 131–140.

Cohen, S., and Williamson, G. M. (1988). Stress and infectious disease in humans. *Psychological Bulletin, 109,* 5–24.

Cohen, S., and Wills, T. A. (1985). Stress, social support and the buffering hypothesis. *Psychological Bulletin, 98,* 310–357.

Cunningham, L. S., and Kelsey, J. L. (1984). Epidemiology of musculoskeletal impairments and associated disability. *Journal of Public Health, 74,* 574–579.

Davis, M. R., and Fernald, R. D. (1990). Social control of neuronal soma size. *Journal of Neurobiology, 21,* 1180–1188.

Dembroski, T. M., MacDougall, J. M., Costa, P. T., Jr., and Grandits, G. A. (1989). Components of hostility as predictors of sudden death and myocardial infarction in the Multiple Risk Factor Intervention Trial. *Psychosomatic Medicine, 51,* 514–522.

Devesa, S. S., and Diamond, E. L. (1983). Socioeconomic and racial differences in lung cancer incidence. *American Journal of Epidemiology, 118,* 818–831.

Diamond, E. L. (1982). The role of anger and hostility in essential hypertension and coronary heart disease. *Psychological Bulletin, 92,* 410–433.

Dohrenwend, B. P. (1973). Social status and stressful life events. *Journal of Personality and Social Psychology, 28,* 225–235.

Dohrenwend, B. S., and Dohrenwend, B. P (1970). Class and race as status-related sources of stress. In S. Levine and N. A. Scotch (eds.), *Social stress* (pp. 111–140). Chicago: Aldine.

Dutton, D. B., and Levine, S. (1989). Overview, methodological critique, and reformulation. In J. P. Bunker, D. S. Gomby, and B. H. Kehrer (eds.), *Pathways to health* (pp. 29–69). Menlo Park, CA: Henry J. Kaiser Family Foundation.

Escobedo, L. G., Anda, R. F., Smith, P. F., Remington, P. L., and Mast, E. E. (1990). Sociodemographic characteristics of cigarette smoking initiation in the United States. *Journal of the American Medical Association, 264,* 1550–1555.

Feldman, J., Makuc, D., Kleinman, J., and Cornoni-Huntley, J. (1989). National trends in educational differentials in mortality. *American Journal of Epidemiology, 129,* 919–933.

Ford, E. S., Merrit, R. K., Heath, G. W., Powell, K. E., Washburn, R. A., Kriska, A., and Haile, G. (1991). Physical activity behaviors in lower and higher socioeconomic status populations. *American Journal of Epidemiology, 133,* 1246–1256.

Goldberg, E. M., and Morrison, S. L. (1963). Schizophrenia and social class. *British Journal of Psychiatry, 109,* 785–802.

Haan, M. N., Kaplan. G. A., and Camacho, T. (1987). Poverty and health: Prospective evidence from the Alameda County Study, *American Journal of Epidemiology, 125,* 989–998.

Haan, M. N., Kaplan, G. A., and Syme, S. L. (1989). Socioeconomic status and health: Old observations and new thoughts. In J. P. Bunker, D. S. Gomby, and B. H. Kehrer (eds.), *Pathways to health* (pp. 76–135). Menlo Park, CA: Henry J. Kaiser Family Foundation.

Harmsen, P., Rosengren, A., Tsipogianni, A., and Wilhelmsen, L. (1990). Risk factors for stroke in middle-aged men in Goteborg, Sweden. *Stroke, 21.* 23–29.

Harris, T. O. (1989). Physical illness: An introduction. In G. W. Brown and T. O. Harris (eds.), *Life events and illness* (pp. 199–212). New York: Guilford Press.

Harris, T. O. (1991). Life stress and illness: The question of specificity. *Annals of Behavioral Medicine, 13,* 211–219.

House, J. S., Kessler, R., Herzog, A. R., Mero, R., Kinney, A., and Breslow, M. (1991). Social stratification, age, and health. In K. W. Schaie, D. Blazer, and J. S. House (eds.), *Aging, health behaviors, and health outcomes* (pp. 1–32). Hillsdale, NJ: Erlbaum.

Illsley, R., and Baker, D. (1991). Contextual variations in the meaning of health inequality. *Social Science and Medicine, 32,* 359–365.

Joesoef, M. R., Wetterhal, S. F., DeStafano, F., Stroup, N. E., and Fronek, A. (1989). The association of peripheral arterial disease with hostility in a young, healthy veteran population. *Psychosomatic Medicine, 51,* 285–289.

Kahn, H. S., Williamson, D. F., and Stevens, J. A. (1991). Race and weight change in U.S. women: The roles of socioeconomic and marital status. *American Journal of Public Health, 81,* 319–323.

Kaplan, J. R., Manuck, S. B., Clarkson, T. B., Lusso, F. B., and Taub, D. M. (1982). Social status, environment and atherosclerosis in cynomolgus monkeys. *Arteriosclerosis, 2,* 359–368.

Kaplan, G. A., Roberts, R. E., Camacho, T. C., and Coyne, J. C. (1987). Psychosocial predictors of depression: Prospective evidence from the Human Population Laboratory studies. *American Journal of Epidemiology, 125,* 206–220.

Kaprio, J., and Koskenvuo, M. (1988). A prospective study of psychological and socioeconomic characteristics, health behavior and morbidity in cigarette smokers prior to quitting compared to persistent smokers and non-smokers. *Journal of Clinical Epidemiology, 41*, 139–150.

Kessler, R. C. (1979). Social status and psychological distress. *Journal of Health and Social Behavior, 20*, 259–272.

Kitagawa, E. M., and Hauser, P. M. (eds.). (1973). *Differential mortality in the United States: A study in socioeconomic epidemiology.* Cambridge, MA: Harvard University Press.

Klag, M., Whelton, P., Coresh, J., Grim, C., and Kuller, L. (1991). The association of skin color with blood pressure in U.S. Blacks with low socioeconomic status. *Journal of the American Medical Association, 265*, 599–602.

Kohn, M., and Schooler, C. (1978). The reciprocal effects of the substantive complexity of work and intellectual flexibility: A longitudinal assessment. *American Journal of Sociology, 84*, 24–52.

Kraus, J. F., Borhani, N. O., and Franti. C. E., (1980). Socioeconomic status, ethnicity, and risk of coronary heart disease. *American Journal of Epidemiology, 111*, 407–414.

Krieger, N. (1992). Overcoming the absence of socioeconomic data in medical records: Validation and application of a census-based methodology. *American Journal of Public Health, 82*, 703–710.

LaFreniere, P. J., and Charlesworth, W. R. (1983). Dominance, attention, and affiliation in a preschool group: A nine-month longitudinal study. *Ethology and Sociobiology, 4*, 55–67.

Manuck, S. B., Kaplan, J. R., Adams, M. R., and Clarkson, T. B. (1988). Studies of psychosocial influences on coronary artery atherogenesis in cynomolgus monkeys. *Health Psychology, 7*, 113–124.

Margolis, P. A., Greenberg, R. A., Keyes, L. L., Lavange, L. M., Chapman, R. S., Denny, F. W., Bauman, K. E., and Boat, B. W. (1992). Lower respiratory illness in infants and low socioeconomic status. *American Journal of Public Health, 82*, 1119–1126.

Marmot, M. G., Kogevinas, M., and Elston, M. A. (1987). Social/economic status and disease. *Annual Review of Public Health, 8*, 111–135.

Marmot, M. G., Shipley, M. J., and Rose, G. (1984). Inequalities in death: Specific explanations of a general pattern? *Lancet, 1*, 1003–1006.

Marmot, M. G., Smith, G. D., Stansfeld, S., Patel, C., North, F., Head, J., White, I., Brunner, E., and Feeney, A. (1991). Health inequalities among British civil servants: The Whitehall II study. *Lancet, 337*, 1387–1393.

Matthews, K., Kelsey, S., Meilahn, E., Kuller, L., and Wing, R. (1989). Educational attainment and behavioral and biologic risk factors for coronary heart disease in middle-aged women. *American Journal of Epidemiology, 129*, 1132–1144.

McLeod, J. D., and Kessler R. C. (1990). Socioeconomic status differences in vulnerability to undesirable life events. *Journal of Health and Social Behavior, 31*, 162–172.

Multiple Risk Factor Intervention Group. (1976). The Multiple Risk Factor Intervention Trial (MRFIT): A national study of primary prevention of coronary heart disease. *Journal of the American Medical Association, 235*, 825–827.

Murphy, J. M., Olivier, D. C., Monson, R. R., Sobol, A. M., Federman, E. B., and Leighton, A. H. (1991). Depression and anxiety in relation to social status. *Archives of General Psychiatry, 48*, 223–229.

Pappas, G., Queen, S., Hadden, W., and Fisher, G. (1993). The increasing disparity in mortality between socioeconomic groups in the United States, 1960 and 1986. *New England Journal of Medicine, 329*, 103–109.

Pincus, T., and Callahan, L. F. (1985). Formal education as a marker for increased mortality and morbidity in rheumatoid arthritis, *Journal of Chronic Diseases,* 38, 973–984.

Pincus, T., Callahan, L. F., and Burkhauser, R. V. (1987). Most chronic diseases are reported more frequently by individuals with fewer than 12 years of formal education in the age 18–64 U.S. population. *Journal of Chronic Diseases, 40,* 865–874.

Pugh, H., Power, C., Goldblatt, P., and Arber, S. (1991). Women's lung cancer mortality, socio-economic status and changing smoking patterns. *Social Science and Medicine, 32,* 1105–1110.

Remington, P. L., Forman, M. R., Gentry, E. M., Marks, J. S., Hogelin, G. C., and Trowbridge, F. L. (1985). Current smoking trends in the United States: The 1981–1983 behavioral risk factor surveys. *Journal of the American Medical Association, 253,* 2975–2978.

Rodin, J., (1986a). Aging and health: Effects of the sense of control. *Science, 233,* 1271–1276.

Rodin, J. (1986b). Health, control, and aging. In M. Baltes and P. Baltes (eds), *Aging and control* (pp. 139–165). Hillsdale, NJ: Erlbaum.

Ruberman, W., Weinblart, E., Goldberg, J., and Chaudhary, B. (1984). Psychosocial influences on mortality after myocardial infarction. *New England Journal of Medicine, 311,* 552–559.

Rutter, M. (1985). Resilience in the face of adversity: Protective factors and resistance to psychiatric disorder. *British Journal of Psychiatry, 147,* 598–611.

Sapolsky, R. M. (1989). Hypercortisolism among socially subordinate wild baboons originates at the CNS level. *Archives of General Psychiatry, 46,* 1047–1051.

Sapolsky, R. M., and Mott, G. E. (1987). Social subordination in wild baboons is associated with suppressed high density lipoprotein-cholesterol concentrations: The possible role of chronic social stress. *Endocrinology, 121,* 1605–1610.

Scherwitz, L., Perkins, L., Chesney, M., and Hughes, G. (1991). Cook-Medley Hostility Scale and subsets: Relationship to demographic and psychosocial characteristics in young adults in the CARDIA study. *Psychosomatic Medicine, 53,* 36–49.

Seccareccia, F., Menotti, A., and Prati, P. L. (1991). Coronary heart disease prevention: Relationship between socio-economic status and knowledge, motivation and behavior in a free-living male, adult population. *European Journal of Epidemiology, 7(6),* 166–170.

Segal, M. R., and Bloch D. A. (1989). A comparison of estimated proportional hazards models and regression trees. *Statistics in Medicine, 8,* 539–550.

Shekelle, R. B., Gale, M., Ostfeld, A., and Paul, O. (1983). Hostility, risk of coronary heart disease and mortality. *Psychosomatic Medicine, 45,* 109–114.

Smith, G. D., and Egger, M. (1992). Socioeconomic differences in mortality in Britain and the U.S. *American Journal of Public Health, 82,* 1079–1080.

Sobel, J., and Stunkard, A. J. (1989). Socioeconomic status and obesity: A review of the literature. *Psychological Bulletin, 105,* 260–271.

Stimson, G. V. (1974). Obeying doctor's orders: A view from the other side. *Social Science and Medicine, 8,* 97–104.

Stokols, D. (1992). Establishing and maintaining healthy environments: Toward a social ecology of health promotion. *American Psychologist, 47,* 6–22.

Stone, A.A.L., Bovbjerg, D. H., Neale, J. M., Napoli, A., Valdimarsdottir, H., Cox, D., Hayden, F. G., and Gwaltney, J. M., Jr. (1992). Development of the common cold symptoms following experimental rhinovirus infection is related to prior stressful life events. *Behavioral Medicine, 13,* 70–74.

Strayer, F. F. (1989). Co-adaptation within the early peer group: A psychobiological study of social competence. In B. H. Schneider (ed.), *Social competence in developmental perspective* (pp. 145–172). Norwell, MA: Kluwer Academic.

Strayer, F. F., and Trudel, M. (1984). Developmental changes in the nature and function of social dominance among young children. *Ethology and Sociobiology, 5,* 279–295.

Susser, M., Watson, W. and Hopper K. (1985). *Sociology in medicine* (3rd ed.). Oxford: Oxford University Press.

Theorell, T. (1974). Life events before and after the onset of a premature myocardial infarction. In B. S. Dohrenwend and B. P. Dohrenwend (eds.), *Stressful life events: Their nature and effects* (pp. 101–117). New York: Wiley.

Tofler, G. H., Stone, P. H., Maclure, M., Edelman, E., Davis, V. G., Robertson, T., Antman, E. M., Muller, J. E., and The MILIS Study Group. (1990). Analysis of possible triggers of acute myocardial infarction (The MILIS Study). *American Journal of Cardiology, 66,* 22–27.

Townsend, P. (1974). Inequality and the health service. *Lancet, 1,* 1179–1189.

U.S. Department of Health, Education and Welfare. (1979). *Smoking and health: A report of the Surgeon General 1979* (USDHEW Publication, No. 79–50066). Washington, DC: U.S. Government Printing Office, Public Health Service.

U.S. Department of Health and Human Services. (1989). *Promoting health/preventing disease: Year 2000 objectives for the nation.* Washington, DC: United States Department of Health and Human Services, Public Health Service.

Vaughn, B., and Waters, E. (1978). Social organization among preschooler peers: Dominance, attention and sociometric correlates. In D. R. Omark, F. F. Strayer, and D. Freedman (eds.), *Dominance relations: An ethological view of human conflict and social interaction* (pp. 359–380). New York: Garland STPM Press.

Wilkinson, R. G. (ed.). (1986). *Class and health: Research and longitudinal data.* London: Tavistock Publications.

Wilkinson, R. G. (1992). Income distribution and life expectancy. *British Medical Journal, 304,* 165–168.

Winkleby, M., Fortmann, S., and Barrett, D. (1990). Social class disparities in risk factors for disease: Eight-year prevalence patterns by level of education. *Preventive Medicine, 19,* 1–12.

14. Interrelationship Between Gender Relations and the HIV/AIDS Epidemic: Some Possible Considerations for Policies and Programs

Jacques du Guerny and Elisabeth Sjöberg

Today, more than 90 percent of adults newly infected with HIV have acquired the infection from heterosexual intercourse. As a result, developing countries now have as many newly infected women as men, and developed countries are slowly moving toward equal incidence in men and women.[1] Furthermore, the issue is becoming a matter of urgency as recent reports provide evidence of an increasing infection sex ratio to the disadvantage of women, and linkages to tuberculosis.[2]

The heterosexual spread of the epidemic is greatly facilitated by the inability of many women to protect themselves because of their lower cultural and socioeconomic status and their lack of influence on sexual relations. The objective of this chapter is to show how gender relations play a crucial role in the spread of HIV, and to demonstrate how a gender perspective could contribute to the design of policies and programs for combating the HIV/AIDS epidemic more effectively.

Our primary goal is to highlight the gender mechanisms through which women frequently end up with little control over their own lives and bodies, and so cannot protect themselves or their children from HIV/AIDS. Second, we discuss the danger of women's being pushed back into a traditional caring role, at the expense of self-empowerment and advancement toward equality with men. We argue that planners of programs to combat AIDS, implicitly or explicitly, expect women to take on the extra burden of caring for people with AIDS. However convenient this may appear, given the difficulty of finding other options in poor countries, we will try to show that this could trap women into weaker and more dependent positions, thus facilitating the spread of HIV/AIDS.

GENDER RELATIONS AND THE AIDS EPIDEMIC

We focus on the issue of "gender" rather than "women," because the problems of women in relation to AIDS are often seen in terms of their biological differences to men, and therefore focus only on medical issues. AIDS programs today continue to focus on health issues. While attention to health is necessary, the epidemic is also threatening to dramatically alter the economic and social fabric of many societies. In the absence of an effective and affordable vaccine, other measures must be taken urgently. In applying a gender-aware approach, we examine how the social relationships between men and women may reveal new cultural, social, and economic perspectives on the epidemic, and new responses to it. A related question is whether strategies that focus exclusively on women, or men, and which fail to address the system formed by male-female gender relations can be effective.

There are no easy solutions, but we believe that unless the complementary strategies outlined below are incorporated into HIV/AIDS programs, there can be no real progress. These strategies involve, first, raising the status of women, particularly through self-empowerment, since they may prove important for the prevention of AIDS and for the development of society in general, and, second, redesigning gender relations.[3]

Women and men are assigned different gender roles in different cultures. Women frequently take on most of the responsibility for household work and for caring for children, elderly and sick people (human reproduction or "reproductive work").[4] Men are often assigned the "productive work" (the income-generating work) and so frequently control the family income. While men's work is valued, either directly through paid remuneration or indirectly through status and political power, women's reproductive work often fails to be recognized as work.

In practice this means that women are likely to be in economically dependent positions, implying a lack of power, lower status, and limited influence on decisions concerning themselves and their families. At the same time, men often have a leadership role in the community and access to positions of direct authority.[5] Under such conditions, women often lack influence over sexual relations, and cannot generally demand the use of condoms, for example, even if they know that their husbands/partners may be HIV-infected. Thus the inequality between men and women fuels the spread of HIV/AIDS.

Women's lower status, especially in combination with poverty and culturally accepted gender roles, makes it possible for men to claim, buy, or enforce sexual favors from girls and women. The outcomes range from sexual violence against women to women trading sexual favors for material support, and prostitution. If young girls are educated to perform a mainly reproductive role, they often have to rely on older, established men as a strategy for survival. Classic examples are the "sugar daddy" or *"deuxième bureau"* phenomena in Africa, and the "minor" wife custom in parts of Southeast Asia. In such cases, the longer sexual history of the man means that he has had more opportunities for exposure to HIV infection than his young partner, so women are more likely to be infected at an earlier age than men.[6]

Prostitution, with its strong links to the feminization of poverty, is, with drug abuse, a major problem in controlling the spread of HIV/AIDS. Since prostitution is a direct outcome of women's gender subordination,[7] such links should be recognized by AIDS programs, and ways found to combat the traditions and sex tourism that preserve and fuel prostitution and the sex industry. Sex tourism is so profitable that tourist organizers in the West, and in the destination countries, repeatedly play down the risk of AIDS or suppress information for fear of losing customers.[8] Tradition also plays an important role in countries such as Thailand, where most men visit prostitutes more or less regularly.[9] Occasional commercial sex (for example, by women who have no other immediate means to pay a dept or bill) can lead to acceptance of risks which the woman might not accept otherwise. Strategies for raising the status of women, changing attitudes among men, and adding other means of income for women could have an important impact on reducing the spread of HIV/AIDS.

Societies have great difficulty in recognizing and accepting the sexuality of both men and women, but women in particular. Denial of sexuality and sexual behavior combined with double standards in the acceptance of certain behaviors, especially for women, make communication about sex between men and women extremely difficult. Meanwhile, the inability to discuss sexuality and sexual behavior, recognized for many years in family planning, is a central problem worldwide.[10] In combination with masculine cultures of machismo and stereotyped norms for female/male sexual behavior, this encourages risky behavior and perpetuates the spread of AIDS. A concrete example, representative for many regions, can be found in an account of an interview with an Ugandan man dying of AIDS:

> He knows it himself, but his two wives and his other relatives in the village do not. But even if they knew that Kamyambo is suffering from AIDS, this would not mean much. According to him, AIDS is still an unknown illness to them, even though it is plaguing almost all of Uganda.[11]

And so infection is passed on, and the epidemic spreads. Kamyambo's wives do not know about AIDS, so it is not known whether they or their children are HIV-positive. Cases from Zambia, and St. Lucia in the Caribbean, provide contrasting examples. Young schoolgirls may trade sexual favors for money from richer, older men looking for virgins, to enable them to buy shoes and books.

> When one asks them if they are not afraid of being infected, they answer in despair that it is a matter of surviving at present, rather than taking the risk of dying in 10 years' time.[12]

Another example from St. Lucia points to serious problem related to the lower status of women and their lack of bargaining powers. Schoolgirls are frequently picked up by bus or taxi drivers on their way to and from school and can be coerced into sexual activity or even assaulted. Male students and teachers demanding sex from female students either in the form of rape or by blackmail in schools and training centers is another problem, which causes girls to drop out early as they are forced to leave when they get pregnant.[13] Apart from the physiological and physical damage this causes the girls, it also jeopardizes future employment opportunities and might expose them to HIV infection at an early age.

Table 1 summarizes the many reasons why a woman may not be able to protect herself from HIV infection, all of which are direct outcomes of her lower status.

FACING THE CONSEQUENCES OF THE EPIDEMIC: THE NEED FOR CARE

Developing countries are increasingly bearing the brunt of the AIDS epidemic and, as the World Health Organization (WHO) points out, lack the health and social support infrastructure to cope with the clinical burden of HIV-related disease. An unknown number of children and elderly people are already being left without support,[14] and in some cities up to three-quarters of all hospital beds are already occupied by AIDS patients. Until a sufficiently cheap vaccine is found, the only form of support for AIDS patients is care. The provision of this care (in a broad sense) is therefore becoming a crucial component in the effect the epidemic has on women's lives.[15]

For women, the effects of HIV/AIDS go well beyond the suffering and death of the infected individual: the phrase *triple jeopardy* describes the dangers women face as individuals, mothers, and caregivers.[16] Women will likely have to care not only for their sick children and partners, possibly even while being infected themselves, but also for elderly people in need of care (whether infected or not) as well as infected dying relatives and friends, and their children. Women from all strata of society and of all ages are affected, but poor women have the heaviest burden.

Women and girls may feel under pressure to give up paid work or studies, which may result in economic dependence. Special attention should be paid to the fact that caring duties will, to a great extent, have to be taken over by elderly women and girls, as the young and middle-aged women fall ill. Equally, the strain on women who have to combine paid labor with reproductive work and caring for people with AIDS can be enormous.[17] As women start to break down under the burden of the caregiving role, and often themselves fall ill, the situation will become increasingly precarious.[18]

As men frequently fall ill before their wives or partners they leave the women to care for them, as well as for infected children. However, the situation is not symmetrical since ill women less commonly demand care from their husbands or partners. Overburdened women are forced to sacrifice

**Table 1. Illustration of Some Gender Factors Influencing
the Spread of the HIV/AIDS Epidemic**

Society assigns men and women gender roles and unequal status	
Women—lower status	Men—higher status
Lack of education/burden of household work and bringing up children, caring for elderly and sick AIDS epidemic increases burden of traditional roles	Better chances for education/little or no responsibility for children, household work, or caring for elderly and sick
Lack of personal freedom/limited freedom of movement/limited access to information Lack of information about the HIV/AIDS epidemic	Greater personal freedom/sexual freedom/freedom of movement/access to information, including information on AIDS
Low or no income/little control over family income and how it is spent Economic dependency Little bargaining power in personal relations Little influence over own and partner's sex life/inability to discuss sex with partner	Wage income, and control over it Power to make decisions Greater power to choose sexual partner/de facto right to have many sexual partners, right to visit prostitutes/right to control sexual relationship with wife/partner
Overall outcome	
Cannot demand safer sex	Can choose whether to practice safer sex
Areas to build upon	
Women's traditional roles make them good organizers Women have a tradition of organizing self-help groups which could be used to strengthen and empower women	Can choose to change lifestyle and practice safer sex Can choose to change attitude toward women and to actively fight the epidemic through leadership roles
Obstacles to overcome	
Dependency in various areas	Machismo, expected to live up to the male ideal, which includes taking personal risks and endangering lives of others

Effect on HIV/AIDS Epidemic

Power imbalance between gender roles facilitates the spread of the epidemic. By identifying the strong and the weak points of each gender role, focal points for intervention may be identified.

other activities defined by their gender role, such as food production, for which women are often largely responsible, particularly in Africa.[19]

STRENGTHENING POLICIES AND PROGRAMS

There is clearly a danger in relying on what is usually termed "community care" or "coping mechanisms" to care for AIDS patients in national and voluntary AIDS programs, which are presently emphasizing such strategies. When formulating strategies, planners should be careful not to conflict with the already identified need to raise the status of women in order to limit the spread of AIDS. To stress the traditional caring role of women, explicitly or implicitly, clearly diminishes the possibility of preventing and controlling the spread of HIV/AIDS by reinforcing and preserving inequality, and represents a "gender trap" for women.[20] There could be dangers, for example, in recommendations that seek to reinforce traditional health-promoting values and practices, such as home care, or in programs that seek cooperation primarily with women's organization,[21] especially when voluntary, unpaid work is expected. Behind these recommendations lies the general assumption that women's reproductive and care role can be transferred to the collective level, i.e. their community role in the form of women's associations. Instead, or parallel to such recommendations, ways to involve men (beyond their community leadership role) in both the public and private sector will have to be found.

The Importance of Gender Analysis for Information Programs

Focusing on sexual behavior to fight AIDS might also lead to another "gender trap" unless the status of women is raised, or men and women are addressed together. Such information often focuses on reducing the risk of HIV infection by avoiding penetrative sex, reducing the numbers of partners, or using condoms. Directing information and education to individuals whose sexual behavior is perceived to put them at increased risk of infection is not enough. Neither is it sufficient to provide information for spouses or partners (usually women) who might get infected because of their partners' sexual behavior. This information will have little impact on limiting the spread of the epidemic in the situations where a woman, because of her low status, is unable to protect herself, unless her partner himself chooses to do so. Unless both partners have equal influence over their sex lives, the heterosexual spread of AIDS is likely to continue to grow rapidly. For the same reason, programs which include the distribution of condoms are ineffective as long as one partner cannot demand their use. To influence or demand the use of condoms is practically impossible for many women worldwide. In cultures where women's primary task is to produce children, it is difficult to insist on the use of condoms. In some cultures women must prove their fertility by giving birth before marriage and female status is gained only through giving birth to many children.[22] A Sudanese physician states:

> We African women cannot protect ourselves or our children against this lethal disease. We have to gain the right not to be infected with HIV. Today we do not have this right because the men are totally ruling our sex life and because a women's only task is to be a sex partner and have children.[23]

Another example from Thailand, where studies show that 95 percent of all men over the age of twenty-one have visited a brothel at least once,[24] is given by the founder of the Prateep Foundation, a self-help organization working in the slums of Bangkok:

But it is difficult to get a Thai man to use a condom. It is not considered natural. But it is considered natural for a man to visit prostitutes. . . . People are tired of our information campaigns at present. Not until the victims crying from AIDS are visible will AIDS be part of people's lives.[25]

Programs for the distribution of condoms that target only men may be partly effective, but until women are empowered to make the same decisions as men regarding condom use, it will still be left to one sex to make this possible life-or-death decision. The same applies to the development of preventative measures that can be controlled by women, for example, the female condom or microbicides. Even if there is a need to develop immediate tools so women can protect themselves from HIV/AIDS, there is a danger of treating the prevention of HIV transmission to women as if it were simply a technical problem, i.e., the assumption is made that if the woman can use a condom herself, she does not have to rely on the man to do it, or on his consent. The core of the problem lies in whether men will allow the use of preventative measures, whether women can decide when to have sex, and whether it is culturally acceptable for women to purchase contraceptives. Female condoms are only likely to reach women who are already in a position to control their sexual relations and thus probably already in a position to insist on their partner's use of condoms. Therefore it is not clear whether the development of preventative measures that can be controlled by women will be able to reduce the spread of the AIDS epidemic, given the present situation in many countries. On the other hand, this is one way of offering greater freedom of choice to women.

The various microbicides (and virucides) that are being developed offer considerable potential for women's empowerment. When combined with contraceptive barrier methods, they may offer women a range of choices such as contraception alone, protection against HIV (and other sexually transmitted diseases) alone or a combination of both, and in theory women can make this choice without interference from their partners. However it is currently estimated that only 3 percent of those using family planning methods worldwide rely on spermicides as the primary method. This implies that an enormous effort would have to be made in developing countries if microbicides were to be promoted.[26] Besides the magnitude of the task, many problems will persist at a social level in developing countries, such as opportunities for purchase (confidentiality, availability, accessibility, affordability) and the possibility of keeping and using products at home. Unfortunately, even when microbicides are readily available, it may be difficult for women to use them without organizing social support, depending on the degree of inequality in gender relations at the collective and individual level. The most well-known example is that of sex workers, who can organize themselves to demand the use of condoms. For other women, different types of women's associations would have to be encouraged. This empowering of individual women through the organization of social support groups could perhaps make a more immediate contribution to saving women's lives than any technological solution. It is certainly an area that deserves much more research.

SUGGESTIONS FOR INTERRELATED AND COMPLEMENTARY STUDY

At least two complementary and interlinked strategies, with both short-term and long-term goals, are needed to combat AIDS more effectively by incorporating the gender dimension (Table 2).

Raising the Status of Women Through Self-Empowerment

Raising the status of women means changing lifelong patterns of gender role training. First and foremost it means channeling resources and investment to women, as well as a reevaluation of women's unpaid "reproductive" work.[27] For example, girls and women need equal access with men to education and vocational training, combined with both *de jure* and *de facto* equality regarding access to income, land, and credit.[28] The national machinery for the advancement of women, which is any organizational structure established with particular responsibility for the advancement of women at the central national level,[29] is an important key to the mobilization of governmental policies, programs, and resources. Since much national machinery is weak at present, it must be strengthened, which requires both political will

Table 2. Short-term and long-term goals

Short-term

Raising status of women
Focus on women's education and vocational training, in order to enhance women's economic independence
Stressing the importance of gender gender-sensitive AIDS information to men and women
Focus on community support to strengthen women's influence on, and control over, sexual relations
Re-distributing caring role
Actively seeking to re-distribute the caring role between the sexes and different actors: the public and private sector, and non-governmental organizations (not just women's groups)
Focus on involving men and boys and men's associations

Long-term

Programmes for changing attitudes to traditional gender roles, through tuition in schools, and other forms of public education
Attempts to change stereotyped images of women and men in school books and mass media
Reaching children and teenagers of both sexes early with information on AIDS and information on protection
Reducing women's economic dependence through legal, economic and social measures, such as access to land, credit and child-care and support to single mothers and female-headed households
Promote as a priority the development of contraceptive and barrier methods which are effective against sexually transmitted diseases and AIDS, which correspond better to women's and men's concerns and needs

and resources. It is of crucial importance that the national machinery become aware of the gender issues related to AIDS, and is prevented from considering AIDS as merely a health issue.

Redistribution of the Caring Role Between the Sexes and Different Actors

New networks for caring for the ill and for survivors without economic support need to be worked out using gender analysis. Focusing on coordination and the provision of frameworks, rather than merely funding, should be a priority when dealing with the role of the public and private sectors, since many developing countries lack the necessary resources. While it is important to recognize and support existing networks, such as women's organizations, that care for families and individuals with AIDS, it is also important to seek new ways of organizing caring networks involving, for example, youth associations and men's associations, in cooperation with the public and private sectors.

GENDER ANALYSIS AS AN AGENDA-SETTING STRATEGY FOR AIDS POLICIES AND PROGRAMS: A TENTATIVE CHECKLIST

It is not enough simply to add women or gender issues to already existing policies and programs, as if women were a "special group" treated on the margins rather than being considered at the core of such policies or programs. Neither has "mainstreaming" of women's issues been effective: so far the mainstreaming strategy most commonly used implies integrating gender issues within existing development strategies.[30] These seldom involve changing the development agenda. Paradoxically, while mainstreaming may lead to a material improvement for women, it does not necessarily improve their status, leaving women vulnerable to the AIDS epidemic. Instead, existing policies and programs need to be transformed, from a gender perspective, to combat the epidemic effectively. There is a growing realization that the consideration of gender issues will eventually lead to a resetting of the development agenda.[31]

This requires addressing women and men simultaneously in the gender system of society, with the aim of making this system more equal. In order to do this, a preliminary analysis of gender relations in different societies is needed. It is necessary to develop indicators, primarily statistical, and subsequent analysis based on data disaggregated by gender for a fuller understanding of gender inequality.[32] An important area for research would be the socioeconomic and cultural factors that contribute to the prevalence of HIV/AIDS among women. At present, data are generally available on women only as beneficiaries of programs, and very little attention has been paid to analyzing strategies that could be called transformative and empowering. So far, assistance policies and programs have not clearly targeted the achievement of gender equality in a measurable way. In order to transform the development agenda, such analysis and information should be given priority.[33] When applied to HIV/AIDS programs, gender analysis could start by asking some fundamental questions:

1. Given the present gender roles, what interventions will have most immediate effect on the epidemic in the short run?
2. Which gender roles need to be strengthened/modified for women and men in order to be able to combat the spread of the epidemic effectively in the long run?
3. How can gender roles linked to community caring be balanced for women and men, in order to solve the enormous problems of caring for those who fall ill, and the resulting consequences for the family? What other bodies or associations could be called upon?
4. What is the planned outcome of changing the roles (and what might happen if they are not changed) for men and women—in the gender system they form—for the epidemic and for society?

The next step is to identify how and where to intervene in gender roles, and to organize these interventions into a program. It is important to identify and design interlinked short-term and long-term programs, to identify priority areas and to establish quantitative targets.

Better methods of evaluating the gender impact of HIV/AIDS programs need to be identified. Such evaluation is of crucial importance to the outcome of AIDS programs, and we suggest that evaluation could be performed using the following basic questions: first, what impact has the program had on factors spreading the epidemic? Second, what impact has the program had on caring for AIDS patients? Third, what impact has the program had on the status of women and on gender relations (for example, the number of girls attending school, female employment and salaries, the sharing of household duties)?

Answers to such questions would provide important feedback and enable policies to be redesigned and improved. Two examples are given below to illustrate how different components of HIV/AIDS programs could be transformed into a more effective initiative using gender analysis: Information, Education and Communication (IEC) programs and the issue of caring for AIDS patients.

Illustration on Information, Education, and Communication (IEC) Programs

IEC programs today focus mainly on providing information, which is important but far from sufficient to combat the AIDS epidemic. Such programs generally fall short on education and communication because of insufficient resources. In addition, programs ought to consider (1) who the information is aimed at and why; how the information could be presented to men, women, boys, and girls, in order to alter the existing discriminating gender roles; how communication between the sexes on issues such as AIDS can be created or encouraged; (2) what impact the information is supposed to have, and for whom; (3) what *de facto* impact it has on the recipient, and on combating the AIDS epidemic.

Answers to basic questions such as these could result in concrete suggestions for action, and a call for a new and more complex interdisciplinary approach to IEC programs. It is particularly important that the information is coordinated for a coherent and collaborative approach, especially if it is to be formulated into a plan for the future by the women receiving the IEC. Messages, created on the basis of gender analysis, should target men and women in different age groups as well as, for example, teachers, youth leaders and different sorts of associations. In doing so, IEC programs should focus not only on attempting to change sexual behavior within existing gender roles, but rather on changing existing gender roles in order to change behavior.

Objectives and Contents

It is also important for IEC programs to focus on why people have unprotected sex instead of concentrating on how to practise safer sex. Rather than just informing on the necessity of using condoms, programs should attempt to work toward enabling and empowering both partners to do so on an equal basis. While women need to be empowered to influence their sex lives, men also need to be "freed" from attitudes and social pressures that dictate that it is "manly" not to use condoms, and to have unprotected sex with several partners—even if it puts their own and their families' lives at risk. This will require strengthening the "communication" component even though it is the most resource-consuming element of IEC.

Channels of Information

Gender analysis can identify the most effective channels for information campaigns. Simple questions may produce interesting answers: through what channels do people get their formal and informal information? Who gets what type of information, who is excluded and for what reasons? Who will be reached by using one channel, and how can this channel be utilized? Where can we reach women and men of different age groups? Integration of HIV/AIDS IEC into family planning programs is often recommended. However, this is a very complex and sensitive issue. Such integration needs to be worked out carefully and should be encouraged at a time when family planning programs are shifting emphasis toward a more client-centered approach and giving consideration to individual needs.[34] For example, one can start by introducing information on STD/AIDS and promoting measures, against reproductive tract infections (RTI). Meanwhile, other strategies such as the social marketing of condoms, can continue to be developed. Attempts could be made to combine health-related information (for example, posters in dispensaries and the like) with information that reaches people, particularly through peer-based education, at work or in cafés, bars, restaurants, at the football stadium, in the marketplace.

The long-term approach should focus on reaching children and teenagers through school and youth associations. Besides giving health information on AIDS, it requires removing teaching material with stereotyped pictures of men's and women's roles, and stressing the equal importance of girls and boys receiving education or vocational training leading to economic autonomy.

Illustration on Caring for AIDS Patients

We have argued that women's caring role is frequently taken for granted in HIV/AIDS policies and programs. In order to avoid this, policy-makers may be helped by the following initial checklist.

1. Is it assumed, implicity or explicity, that care for AIDS patients and orphans should be provided by female relatives, other women or women's groups? What is the role of men and boys in caring for AIDS patients? Why? Which gender is expected to carry the financial burden of caring?
2. What effects will the responsibility for caring have on women, their education, occupation, income possibilities, possibilities to rest, food production, and so on?
3. What consequences will it have for their families, particularly for the future of the daughters?
4. Would men who have to provide support for sick family members get support that women in the same situation would not receive (for example, from female relatives or public or private bodies)?
5. When a family member is found to be HIV positive, what could be done to plan for future sickness and loss of income, in order to limit the damage?
6. Why are men's organizations and unisex organizations not involved in community caring to the same extent, and to what extent do women participate in decision-making in organizing the provision of care?

Answering these questions will lead to a new set of important questions, such as, what organizational measures could be taken to distribute the caring role of women between the sexes, and what other bodies or associations could be found to participate? What type of community initatives and organizations could be strengthened in order to assist in the caring of patients? Who in the family, and which groups in the community, do health authorities, nongovernmental organizations (NGO), and private employers refer to in this matter?

The next step is to devise strategies to involve men, for example, by identifying men's organizations that could be approached, or by contacting schools, employers, trade unions, or religious associations. The organizations of the productive roles of men and how it could be changed (if necessary) to make it compatible with the assumption of caring roles by men could also be examined. This could be followed by an estimate of the type and amount of training needed, and how, when, and where it could be carried out. This will require, apart from a new way of thinking and approaching the problem, a lot of new ideas and creativity. Given the magnitude of the AIDS epidemic such considerations will be necessary in the long run, and time is running out.

CONCLUSION

The low cultural and socioeconomic status of women is facilitating and speeding up the heterosexual spread of AIDS in the world today. At the same time, the spread of HIV/AIDS is threatening to erase whatever progress has been made in raising the status of women over past decades by tying women to their caring roles, thus limiting their access to education and income-generating activities. For this reason, merely looking at women and AIDS from a health perspective is not enough—a gender analysis of the socio-economic and cultural causes and effects of the epidemic is necessary to achieve a more comprehensive picture of the magnitude of the problem and ideas on how to combat the epidemic effectively.

Using gender analysis to examine the spread of AIDS, we can develop a more effective approach to fight the epidemic. However, this requires new ways of thinking about HIV/AIDS. This chapter is intended to stimulate discussion, which we hope will generate further research and new ideas on how these issues could be addressed in AIDS policies and programs.

REFERENCES

1. National Commission on AIDS. *Report on HIV in Correctional Facilities*. Asian Population Studies Series No. 16 (E/CN.11/1212). Bangkok: National Commission on AIDS, 1975; World Health Organization: *Current and Future Dimensions of the HIV/AIDS Pandemic*. Geneva: WHO GPA; April 1991, p. 5; World Health Organization: *The Global Strategy for the Prevention and Control of AIDS, 1992 Update*. Geneva: WHO GPA, November 1991.
2. Barongo, L. R., Borgdorff, M. W., Mosha, F. F., et al. The epidemiology of HIV-1 infection in urban areas, roadside settlements and rural villages in Mwanza Region, Tanzania. *AIDS* 1992, 6: 1521–1528; Karim, Q. A., Karim, S.S.A., Singh, B., Short, R., Ngxongo, S. Seroprevalence of HIV infection in rural South Africa. *AIDS* 1992, 6: 1535–1539.
3. Economic and Social Council. *Development: Integration of Women in Development*. New York: United Nations, 1992, pp. 3–24.
4. Moser, C. Gender planning in the Third World: meeting practical and strategic gender needs. *World Development* 1989, 11: 1801.
5. Ibid.
6. Palloni, A., Lee, Y. T. *The Social Context of HIV and its Effects on Families, Women and Children*. Vienna: United Nations Office at Vienna; September 1990, pp. 5–21.
7. Smyke, P. *Women & Health. Women & World Development Series*. London: Zed Books, 1991, p. 55.
9. Maurer, M. Tourism-prostitution-AIDS. In *Report from Seminar on Action Against Traffic in Women and Forced Prostitution as Violations of Human*

Rights and Human Dignity. Strasbourg: Council of Europe. European Committee for Equality Between Women and Men, 1991, p. 1.

9. Soderberg, M. Interview with Prateep Ungsong Tham. *Världshorisont* 1992, 1: 8.

10. United Nations Economic and Social Commission for Asia and the Pacific: Husband-wife communication and practice in family planning. In *AIDS Reference Guide* 1991. Washington DC: Atlantic Information Service; March 1991.

11. Turan, F. Interview with Ugandan AIDS patient. *Världshorisont* 1992, 1: 8.

12. Dahlbom, A. Interview with Bawa Yamba, a Ghanaian cultural anthropologist. *Världshorisont* 1992, 1: 9.

13. Espling, M., Sjöberg, E., Waller, J. *An Evaluation of Moshi Vocational Centre, Tanzania*. Gothenburg: University of Gothenburg, 1988, pp. 11–14.

14. WHO, *The Global Strategy* (see note 1).

15. Schopper, D., Walley, J. Care for AIDS patients in developing countries: a review. *AIDS Care* 1992, 4: 1.

16. Muringo, Kiereini, E. Keynote. In *Report from Workshop on Women and AIDS*. Blantyre: Commonwealth Medical Association in cooperation with International Federation of Business and Professional Women, December 1992, 3.

17. Division for the Advancement of Women: *Women and AIDS. Women 2000*. Vienna: United Nations Office at Vienna 1989, 1: 10.

18. Dahlbom, A. Interview with Elizabeth Reid. *Världshorisont* 1992, 1: 6.

19. Armstrong, J. Socioeconomic implications of AIDS in developing countries. *Finance & Development*, December 1991: 17.

20. Division for the Advancement of Women: *A Gender Perspective on Population Issues*. Vienna: United Nations office at Vienna, 1992, p. 4.

21. WHO, *The Global Strategy* (see note 1).

22. United Nations Centre for Social Development And Humanitarian Affairs, Centre Français Sur La Population Et Le Développement/United National Population Fund, Université du Bénin: *Condition de la Femme et Population, Le Cas de l'Afrique Francophone*. Paris: CEPED, 1992: 17–32.

23. Atterstam, I. Interview with Dr Fathia Mahmoud. *Världshorisont* 1992, 1: 10.

24. Soderberg M. AIDS in the slums of Bangkok. *Världshorisont* 1992, 1: 4.

25. Soderbegr (see note 9).

26. Mati, J. Family planning, sexually transmitted diseases and AIDS. New York: Population Division, United Nations, October 1992.

27. Elson, D. *Male Bias in the Development Process*. Manchester: Manchester University Press, 1991, p. 186.

28. Economic and Social Council (see note 3).

29. Division for the Advancement of Women. *Directory of National Machinery for the Advancement of Women 1993*. Vienna: United Nations Office at Vienna, 1993.

30. Jahan, R. *Mainstreaming Women in Development in Different Settings*. Paris: Columbia University/Dhaka University/OECD DAC WID Expert Group, May 1992: 5–6.

31. Economic and Social Council (see note 3).

32. Ibid.

33. Division for the Advancement of Women (see note 29).

34. Division for the Advancement of Women. *Gender Perspective in Family Planning Programmes*. Vienna: United Nations Office at Vienna; 1992: 1–13.

15. Human Rights and AIDS: The Future of the Pandemic

Jonathan M. Mann

The central challenge facing HIV prevention efforts today is understanding and learning how to respond, both directly and concretely, to the societal determinants of vulnerability to HIV. Awareness of this need to address directly the societal dimensions of HIV/AIDS has experienced a gradual evolution. As with biomedical research, progress in understanding human behavior in the context of HIV prevention has involved a continuous and often frustrating, though occasionally exhilarating, process of discovery.

How society defines a problem determines the manner by which we confront it. Today, we can identify three periods in this history of conceptualization of behavior. During each period, available knowledge and experience produced somewhat different HIV prevention strategies. This chapter outlines the evolution of HIV prevention strategies as well as the various social factors identified as relevant to HIV/AIDS prevention. In addition, this chapter focuses on the inherent inadequacies of past and current prevention strategies, and offers an approach to HIV/AIDS prevention that focuses upon, and incorporates, the modern movement of human rights.

THE HISTORY AND CURRENT APPROACH TO HIV/AIDS PREVENTION STRATEGIES

The Three Periods of HIV Prevention Efforts

The first period began with the discovery of AIDS in 1981 and continued thorough 1984.[1] During this period, a series of epidemiological studies identified routes of spread and behaviors associated with increased risk of infection. Public health agencies acted primarily to alert people about the danger of the new disease and sought to translate epidemiological facts into comprehensible messages for the public. Public information campaigns of unprecedented vigor and boldness sought to inform and often, explicitly, frighten people into at least knowing that AIDS existed. Recall, for example, the central message of the informational program in the United Kingdom: "AIDS: Don't Die of Ignorance." Recall also the awkward and confusing use of the term "bodily fluids" as epidemiology met the mass media.

Uncertainty and urgency combined throughout the first period. In addition to little attention given to a guiding concept of behavior and behavioral change, messages were often disconnected and ad hoc. Though the alert was sounded, little behavioral change ensued.

During the second period, from approximately 1985 to 1988, public health focused on individual risk reduction. The emphasis shifted from alerting individuals about AIDS to the more complex tasks of informing, educating, and providing specific health and social services to help stimulate, support and sustain individual behavioral change. Programs were designed with a view, either explicitly or implicitly, of HIV-related behavior as fundamentally individualistic and rational. Therefore, whether based on the Health Belief Model,[2] the theory of Reasoned Action,[3] or Personal Self-efficacy,[4] preventive interventions focused on information and education, on counseling and other psychosocial support, and on teaching skills for sexual negotiation and condom use. In accordance with this understanding and approach to behavior, providing information, education, and health services to individuals at risk became the central mission of national AIDS programs, which the World Health Organization (WHO) fostered as part of its global AIDS strategy. This relatively traditional public health approach was the foundation of the unprecedented global mobilization of the mid to late 1980s.

The World Health Organization added a radically new element to this traditional formulation, namely, information/education plus linked health and social services. Based on field experience, WHO declared that coercion and discrimination toward HIV-infected people and people with AIDS undermined and reduced the effectiveness of HIV prevention programs. For example, wherever rumors spread that HIV testing facilities were providing lists of HIV-infected people to governments, participation in HIV testing declined precipitously. Conversely, where HIV testing facilities instituted anonymous testing, thus explicitly guaranteeing rather than merely promising confidentiality, participation in HIV testing and counseling activities by those at greatest risk of HIV increased. Thus, the World Health Organization developed a "public health rationale" for preventing discrimination toward those infected with HIV.

The public health rationale was a pragmatic step and did not reflect any ideological or philosophical commitment to human rights per se, but rather arose from an appreciation for the instrumental value of respecting the rights and dignity of HIV-infected and ill people. In this sense, discrimination was seen as a tragic and counterproductive side effect or result of the pandemic. In any event, for the first time in history, preventing discrimination toward those affected by an epidemic became an integral part of a global strategy to prevent and control an epidemic of infectious disease.

Finally, in the third period, beginning in the context of a steadily expanding and intensifying global epidemic in 1988, increasing efforts emerged to add and integrate a societal dimension with the previous individually centered, risk-reduction approach. The concept of vulnerability, or focusing on constraints and barriers to individual control over health, has been central to this effort. The vulnerability analysis considered the larger, societal contextual factors such as political, social, cultural, and economic considerations. These factors, of course, clearly influence individual behavior and decision-making. While this period witnessed a salutatory shift from a nearly exclusive focus on individual risk reduction toward an increasing concern with societal issues, public health has had great difficulty going beyond the stage of simply listing a broad range of contextual factors and influences.

The Future of the Pandemic: A Fourth Period

The difficulty in moving forward in understanding why, how, and in what ways a societal dimension can and must be added to HIV prevention reflects the combined and interconnected influences of the traditional public health paradigm and its core science, epidemiology. Epidemiology is a powerful tool, though it has important underlying assumptions and limits. Applying classical epidemiological methods to HIV/AIDS ensures, even predetermines, that "risk" will be defined in terms of individual determinants and individual behavior. Epidemiology has thus far failed to develop models and methods suited to discovering the societal dimensions that strongly influence and constrain individual behavior.

It was natural for public health to turn to epidemiology to describe the scope and distribution of infection and for discovery of routes of transmission. However, the direct translation of epidemiological data on risk behavior to public health, defined exclusively in individual terms, results inevitably in activities focusing on individuals in order to influence their risk taking behavior. This is accomplished through information, education, and services. Thus, we have the traditional public health approach: to consider diseases as dynamic events occurring within an essentially static social context. The reliance on classical epidemiology virtually ensures that this vision of disease and society will predominate.

The work of designing and implementing relatively traditional public health programs in order to assist individual risk reduction has been an enormous task. When focusing upon the positive, there is evidence from a range of settings worldwide that when implemented with care, sensitivity, and community involvement, the combination of information, education, and health services can substantially slow HIV spread. Indeed, such programs among injection-drug users, sex workers, gay men and heterosexual women and men have been as successful, if not more successful, than any other public health efforts relying on behavioral change. Focusing on the positive, however, does not represent the complete picture. Unfortunately, neither the scope, comprehensiveness, nor effectiveness of traditional HIV prevention programs has been optimal. Many people today still do not have access to these programs. Moreover, many programs do not provide the necessary services, nor provide them in a useful and appropriate manner.

Worldwide experience demonstrates that while the HIV risk-reduction approach is necessary and useful, it is not sufficient to control the pandemic. Though it has worked well for a few people, it has been somewhat helpful for many, and yet not very helpful for most. The focus on individual risk reduction was simply too narrow, for it was unable to deal concretely with the live social realities of women, men, and children around the world. For several years now, it has been clear to everyone working on AIDS that simply continuing to do what has thus far been done, albeit necessary, useful, and important, cannot bring the pandemic under control.

Faced with this painful situation of knowing that what we have been doing is necessary but clearly not sufficient, public health efforts in AIDS have reached a crossroads. One path leads us to those who have tacitly agreed to accept the inherently limited approach and its consequences. We see the subtle tendency to accept current limits appear in many ways. For example, in the United States, the predicition that forty thousand to eighty thousand people will become newly infected with HIV each year is deemed acceptable. As incidence figures plateau or even decline, there is increasing talk of "endemic" AIDS, thus taking advantage of the calming effect of leaving the word *epidemic* behind. Moreover, the slow slide into complacency takes an academic direction. For example, some debate endlessly whether this or that wording on a brochure or in a television spot would be best. In the end, we thereby focus on something we can deal with, rather than face the threatening reality of an expanding, intensifying, dynamic, and volatile epidemic.

Others, however, are taking a different path at the crossroads. Resisting the traditional public health tendency to learn to accept certain levels of preventable disease, disability, and premature death as the "normal background," they reject the idea that we can do no more. They refuse to accept the unacceptable. They are exploring ways forward, and asking, "What would need to be done to uproot the pandemic?"

This is precisely where we stand today. Can we find ways to deal concretely with the broader, societal factors that constrain, and influence to an enormous extent, individual behavior? Vulnerability to HIV reflects the extent to which people are, or are not, capable of making and effecting free and informed decisions about their health. Therefore, a person who is able to make and effect free and informed decisions is least vulnerable. Conversely, the person who is ill-informed, and with quite limited ability to make and/or carry out decisions freely arrived at, is most vulnerable. How, or more precisely, *through which conceptual prism* can we best identify and act positively upon the factors, beyond the individual, that constrain, limit, and interfere with the making and carrying out of free and informed choices about behavior? What are the societal preconditions for reducing vulnerability to HIV? The following analysis offers an overview and answers to some of these difficult questions.

THE INHERENT DIFFICULTIES OF HIV/AIDS PREVENTION PROGRAMS

Traditional Relevant Factors

In many places a variety of social factors have been identified as relevant to HIV/AIDS prevention. These can be grouped roughly into three categories: (1) political and governmental; (2) sociocultural; and (3) economic. Political factors include the inattention or lack of concern about HIV/AIDS, as well as governmental interference with the free flow of complete information about HIV/AIDS. Sociocultural factors involve social norms regarding gender roles and taboos about sexuality. Economic issues include poverty, income disparity, and the lack of resources for prevention programs.

Once identified, these contextual factors become potential objects of focused public health work and activism by nongovernmental organizations. Thus, specific governmental actions have been challenged, specific social norms have been highlighted and opposed, and many have pointed to economic constraints on successful HIV prevention work. Nevertheless, the efforts thus far to deal directly with these societal factors influencing HIV prevention have several important, limiting characteristics.

First, the prevention efforts are usually focused exclusively on HIV/AIDS. These efforts may involve challenges to proposed regulation requiring mandatory HIV testing, discrimination against gay men in the context of HIV and insurance, or the lack of resources to sustain successful HIV prevention programs. Second, this work lacks a coherent conceptual framework to describe and analyze the nature of the societal factors. The economist, political scientist, anthropologist, and social scientist all have their disciplinary perspectives. As a consequence, there is no consistent and accessible vocabulary to speak of and compare societal factors in situations arising in very different social, cultural, and political contexts.

What commonalities can be identified regarding the vulnerability of commercial sex workers in India, injection-drug users in the United States, street children in Brazil, and adolescents in sub-Saharan Africa? Without a coherent conceptual understanding and vocabulary, only the differences and local particularities can be seen. The current approach to the societal determinants of HIV vulnerability is essentially tactical, rather than strategic. There is no common understanding, let alone consensus, about the ways in which the societal factors should change to better promote and protect health.

Consequently, the societal-level work carried out thus far, while courageous and creative, remains inherently limited in its scope, applicability, and impact. It has become clear that a deeper understanding of the societal nature of the pandemic and the societal preconditions for HIV vulnerability is now required. To this end, insight can be derived from two lines of evidence: the evolution of the pandemic and the inherent limitations in the existing HIV prevention approach.

The Evolution of the Pandemic

A meta-analysis of the evolving HIV epidemics in countries around the world has revealed a feature of the pandemic that was previously unknown, unknowable, and hidden. The history of AIDS has shown that HIV can enter a community or country in many different ways. In each country, where HIV enters clearly defines the early history of the epidemic.

In the United States and France, white gay men were first noted to be affected. In Brazil, by contrast, the first cases occurred among members of the jet set in Rio de Janeiro and São Paolo. In Ethiopia, AIDS was initially noted among the social elite. With the passage of time, and as the epidemic matures, it evolves and moves along a clear and consistent pathway, which, although different in its details within each society, nevertheless has a single, vital, common feature. In each society, those people who before HIV/AIDS arrived were marginalized, stigmatized, and discriminated against became over time those at highest risk of HIV infection.

Regardless of where and among whom the epidemic may start, the brunt of it gradually and inexorably turns toward those who bear this societal burden. Thus in the United States, the epidemic has turned increasingly towards minority populations in inner cities, injection-drug users, and women. In Brazil, the HIV epidemic now rages through heterosexual transmission in the favelas around Rio and São Paolo. In Ethiopia, HIV is concentrated among the poor and dispossessed. The French have a simple term which says it all: HIV is now becoming a problem mainly for *les exclus,* the "excluded ones," living at the margin of society.

Inherent Limitations on Existing Prevention Efforts

The second source of insight about the societal dimensions of HIV prevention arises through a detailed analysis of limits and failures in existing prevention programs. To illustrate, married and monogamous women who receive the normal benefits of HIV prevention programs, including distribution of information, education, access to testing and counseling, and condom availability, may nevertheless be at risk of HIV infection. Indeed, in some countries, being married and monogamous is considered a "risk factor" for HIV infection. To understand this apparent paradox one must appreciate the real-life situations facing women.

Consider, for example, the recommendations given to both women and men to reduce the number of sexual partners, as part of risk-reduction approaches. Yet, as many have pointed out, this recommendation fails in the real world for several reasons. First, the risk to many women is related to the sexual behavior of their partner. Second, having multiple partners may be necessary for survival. Finally, women may often lack control over their sexual relationships. In marriage, the pervasive threat of physical violence or divorce, without legal recourse or legal rights to property, may totally disempower a woman. This can happen despite being educated about AIDS, even if condoms are available, and even if the woman knows her husband is HIV-infected. Clearly, therefore, the central issue is the inferior role and subordinate status of women. The disadvantages created by such a society cannot be addressed through individually focused information/education or HIV-specific health services.

This is one example among many. Consider gay and lesbian people, commercial sex workers, adolescents whose competence is rarely acknowledged and whose voice is rarely heard in any meaningful way, intravenous-drug users or people living in absolute or relative poverty within each society. This relationship between society, how people are treated within a society, risk for HIV infection, and inadequate HIV/AIDS care is something that has been "known" for a long time. It has been difficult to speak about, however, for at least three reasons.

First, as mentioned previously, a common conceptual approach and vocabulary was lacking for analysis and action. In the absence of an adequate conceptual framework, only the particular and unique features of each group and place could be seen. Second, members of vulnerable communities and AIDS workers feared that others would misuse these observations about society and AIDS to reinforce the false, yet persistent notion that AIDS is only a problem for the marginalized and thus is no longer a threat to the "general public." Third, many AIDS workers and organizations were reluctant to broaden the debate surrounding AIDS out of concern that limited resources would become too thinly spread.

A NEW APPROACH: FOCUSING UPON HUMAN RIGHTS

To move forward, there must be a mixture of the pragmatic and the theoretical, and a blend of insight and practical experience. Once we have determined that for HIV/AIDS, as for all other health problems, the major determinants are societal, it ought to be clear that since society is an essential part of the problem, a societal-level analysis and action will be required. In other words, the new public health considers that both disease and society are so interconnected that both must be considered dynamic. An attempt to deal with one, the disease, without the other, the society, would be inherently inadequate.

Fortunately, entirely outside the domain of public health or biomedical science, a series of concepts and a framework for identifying the societal preconditions for health had been developed. The modern movement of human rights, born in the aftermath of the Holocaust in Europe and born of the deep aspiration to prevent a recurrence of government sponsored violence, provides AIDS prevention with a coherent conceptual framework for identifying and analyzing the societal root causes of vulnerability to HIV. It also provides both a common vocabulary for describing the commonalities that underlie the specific situations of vulnerable people around the world, and a clarity about the necessary direction of health-promoting societal change.

Modern human rights involves the world's first efforts, necessarily incomplete and partial, to define the societal preconditions for human well-being. For this reason, promotion of human rights is one of the four principal purposes of the United Nations, founded in 1945. The Universal Declaration of Human Rights,[6] adopted by the UN General Assembly in 1948, provides a list of societal conditions considered essential for well-being, peace, and health.

The Universal Declaration can be thought of as the trunk of the human rights tree, with the UN Charter as its roots. The two major branches, the two major International Covenants on Civil and Political Rights, and on Economic, Social and Cultural Rights, emerge from and expand upon the trunk with further elaboration through many important treaties and declarations. Two such examples are the Convention on the Elimination of All Forms of Discrimination Against Women (CEDAW)[7] and the Convention on the Rights of the Child (CRC).[8]

These documents describe what governments and societies should not do to people—namely, torture them or imprison them arbitrarily or under inhuman conditions. In addition, the documents describe what governments and societies should ensure for all people in the society, namely shelter, food, medical care, and basic education. When and where human rights and dignity are respected, there will still be rich and poor, Mozarts and people who cannot carry a tune, but all will be ensured of a basic minimum in which their individual potential can be freely and fully developed.

We propose that, as respect for human rights and dignity is a *sine qua non* for promoting and protecting human well-being, the human rights framework offers public health a more coherent, comprehensive, and practical framework for analysis and action on the societal root causes of vulnerability to HIV/AIDS than any framework inherited from traditional public health or biomedical science. We propose that promoting and protecting human rights is therefore inextricably linked with our ability to promote and protect health. Clearly, human rights work will obviously not bring to a halt all preventable illnesses or premature deaths. However, the realization of rights and increasing respect for human dignity will reduce or even eliminate the societal contribution, which we know is the major contribution to this burden of disease, disability, and death.

What would it mean to incorporate a human rights dimension into HIV/AIDS prevention? It would mean that in addition to everything we already do, we would identify the specific rights whose violation contributes to HIV vulnerability in our particular community or country. It might involve the right to information, the equal status of women and men in marriage or its dissolution, the right to medical care, or even the basic proposition of nondiscrimination. Then we must work with those individuals and groups, whether official, nongovernmental, or private, who are already working to promote respect for human rights and dignity within the society.

We who are concerned about AIDS can add our voices, credibility, and knowledge to the work of others to promote rights by educating, seeking legal changes, catalyzing awareness, and by monitoring, identifying and drawing attention to human rights problems. It also suggests that helping to educate people about human rights may ultimately be as important, or even more important, for their health than any specific AIDS educational program. However, there is no need to choose one or the other. Both are needed. Human rights work for public health is not a substitute for traditional public health activities, though it is essential and necessary if we are to refuse the unacceptable about the HIV/AIDS pandemic.

Adding a human rights dimension to HIV prevention work will have major advantages, though it will also create some difficulties. Some major advantages will include acting at the deeper level of societal causes, so as to help *uproot* the pandemic. It will also be linking health issues with the mobilizing power of human rights and expanding the ability of people to see the connection between a "rights issue" and their health. In addition, it will enhance the capacity for cross-disciplinary work that occurs when people can identify a larger commonality of interest. Finally, the result will be revitalizing global thinking within the collective response to HIV/AIDS.

Some potential difficulties, however, will be the inevitable accusation that public health is "meddling" in societal issues that go far beyond its scope or competence. In addition, public health workers may be unfamiliar with rights concepts and language. Public health workers may desire to "own" the problem of HIV/AIDS, thereby keeping the discourse at a medical and public health level, thus assuring the preeminent role of health workers. Finally, critics may argue that issues of human rights inherently and inevitably put the person concerned with rights potentially at odds with governmental and other sources of power in the society.

Thus, as our capacity for understanding the pandemic deepens, so do the challenges of response become ever more difficult. It is clearly easier for public health agencies and organizations to alert the public about HIV/AIDS than to ensure comprehensive services to support individual risk reduction. Similarly, while quite difficult, attacking a single AIDS-related political issue is easier than developing and undertaking a human-rights-based analysis of and response to the pandemic.

The history of the response to HIV has demonstrated that we can bring the best of traditional public health together with new societal insights and understanding. This brings us to the threshold of *empowerment,* which is a critical concept not only for others, but also for ourselves. This empowerment rests on two pillars. One is knowledge: an understanding of the importance of societal determinants of health, of the ways in which human rights helps us to analyze and respond to societal deficiencies that underlie vulnerability to preventable disease, disability, and premature death. The second pillar is equally critical: the belief, faith, and confidence that the world can change. This belief, while it may be inspired by historical examples, or fostered by peers and participation in community organization and social movements, is ultimately quite personal. It is not clear exactly how people who have considered themselves powerless may begin to believe in the *possibility of change,* but this step is at the heart of personal and, ultimately, societal transformation. That next step, that possibility for change toward a more human world, will require a leap of confidence based on analysis, reflection, and hard work. Only we can empower ourselves.

CONCLUSION

Once we acknowledge that the goal of public health, beyond HIV/AIDS, is to "ensure the conditions in which people can be healthy,"[9] and recognize the enormous burden of evidence which tells us that societal factors are the dominant determinants of health status, we realize that, ultimately, to work for public health is to work for societal transformation. Linking human rights with health offers us a coherent vision of how to add the critical societal dimension to our public health work, which all too often has stopped at the threshold of real societal issues.

For this reason, since 1990 all graduates of the Harvard School of Public Health receive two scrolls at commencement. The first is the degree they have earned. The second is a copy of the Universal Declaration of Human Rights, their common birthright. The dean reminds graduates that the Universal Declaration of Human Rights is as vital to their future in public health as the Hippocratic Oath or similar document would be to a medical doctor. In this way, we symbolize the inherent, rich, complex, difficult, and ultimately indispensable linkage between society and health, for which we in public health have a special role and responsibility.

I believe it is for this reason that after fifteen years of struggle against a global pandemic, despite the burden of death and illness, those working on HIV/AIDS can carry forward a message of hope and confidence—not only a confidence in our ability to continue learning and understanding, but a confidence in our belief about the value of human rights and human dignity. This gives us hope and confidence in each other, in ourselves, and ultimately in our world and its future.

NOTES AND REFERENCES

1. Centers for Disease Control, "Pneumocystis Pneumonia—Los Angeles," 30 *Morbidity and Mortality Weekly Report* 30, 21 (1981): 250–252.
2. For a discussion of the Health Belief Model, see Irwin M. Rosenstock, "Historical Origins of the Health Belief Model," *Health Education Monographs* 2, 329 (1974); see also, Irwin M. Rosenstock, "The Health Belief Model and Prevention Health Behavior," *Health Education Monographs* 2, 354 (1974).
3. For a discussion of the Theory of Reasoned Action, see Martin Fishbein and Susan E. Middlestadt, "Using the Theory of Reasoned Action as a Framework for Understanding and Changing AIDS-Related Behaviors," in Vickie M. Mays et al. (eds.), *Primary Prevention of AIDS: Psychological Approaches* (1989), pp. 93–110.

4. For a discussion of the Personal Self-Efficacy Theory, see Albert Bandura, "Self-Efficacy: Toward a Unifying Theory of Behavioral Change," *Psycholological Review* 84, 191 (1977).

5. Epidemiology is the branch of medicine that focuses upon detecting the sources and underlying causes of epidemics in a society.

6. Universal Declaration of Human Rights, G.A. Res. 71, U.N. GAOR, 3d Sess., art. 17, 2, U.N. Doc A/810 (1948).

7. Convention on the Elimination of All Forms of Discrimination Against Women, *opened for signature* Mar. 1, 1980, 19 I.L.M. 33 (entered into force Sept. 3, 1981).

8. Convention on the Rights of the Child, G.A. Res. 44/25, U.N. GAOR, 44th Sess., Supp. No. 49, at 166, U.N. Doc A/44/736 (1989).

9. Institute of Medicine, *Future of Public Health* (1988).

Reflections on 16.
Emerging Frameworks
of Health and Human Rights

Lynn P. Freedman

Public health and human rights are "powerful, modern approaches to defining and advancing human well-being" and so are potentially powerful tools for generating change.[1] Yet public health and human rights have also, at times, been powerful tools for maintaining the status quo, reinforcing hierarchies of power and domination based on race, gender, and class. Thus, just because a concern or policy or program adopts the label "health" or "human rights" does not give it unqualified value. To create a workable framework for health and human rights collaboration, we need first to define human well-being; only then will it be possible to clarify how the tools of public health and human rights can be used to advance that vision of it.

Of course, defining human well-being is a rather tall order, which I don't pretend to fill in this chapter. My aim is much more modest: in these reflections I try to expose some of the assumptions about human well-being that underlie traditional views of public health, human rights, and the connections between them, and to suggest some possible alternative directions for future discussion, elaboration, and action. In doing so, I write primarily from my perspective as a women's health advocate with a focus on reproductive health and reproductive rights. My approach is shaped not only by my academic training (in law and public health), but also by my engagement with fields traditionally described as population, family planning, maternal/child health, women's rights, and human rights, and by my understanding of the forces that have historically driven programs, policies, and scholarship in those fields.

Perhaps because of this background and orientation, I view health and human rights advocacy as an essentially subversive activity, in the sense that my vision of "defining and advancing human well-being" ultimately requires overturning deeply rooted social and political structures that produce ill health and that prevent all people—women and men—from fulfilling their highest potential as human beings. But the goal is not to destroy: it is to transform and create. The structures that now obstruct human well-being must be changed into modes of social organization and interaction that will promote and support it. The disciplines of public health and human rights offer ways of thinking, of working, and of organizing that can ultimately give expression and concrete direction to that endeavor.

THE TOOLS OF PUBLIC HEALTH

Public health is a quintessentially social enterprise. Whereas medicine looks at the biological mechanisms of disease in individual people, public health looks at patterns of health and disease in populations. Most critical for present purposes, public health focuses on the links between an individual and the environment (physical, social, cultural, political, and/or economic) in which she lives, seeking in that linkage both an explanation for her health status and a potential entry point for policies and programs to address it.

The primary research and analytical tool of public health is epidemiology. Using statistics and probability theory, epidemiologists document a particular health phenomenon (e.g., maternal death) and measure the strength of its association with particular "risk factors" (e.g., maternal age or parity). Through this measurement, epidemiologists quantify risk; they measure the probability that a particular health phenomenon will occur if a particular risk factor is present. When a sufficient likelihood of an association is repeatedly found, the epidemiologist can state with reasonable confidence that the association is "real," i.e., it is not due to chance, bias, or poor study design. From such an association between a phenomenon and a risk factor, as well as additional information, the epidemiologist can *infer*—not prove—causality. That understanding of possible causal relationships can then form the basis for making effective public health policies and programs.

To many activists this may sound like a dry and tedious exercise, but in fact it has truly revolutionary potential. Nancy Krieger, in an insightful article about the politics of public health data, tells the story of how Louis René Villermé (1782–1863), one of the founders of epidemiology, used his classic study of mortality in early-nineteenth-century Paris to challenge theories of disease causation that had prevailed in European medical thought for nearly two thousand years.[2] In this study, Villermé first documented and ranked variations in mortality rates across different neighborhoods in Paris. He then attempted to correlate the variation in mortality with variations in environmental factors such as altitude, seasonal temperature, humidity, and quality of air, water, and soil, all of which were thought to cause disease. In this first-ever systematic test of long-accepted environmental theories of disease causation, it turned out that none of these factors could account for the differences in mortality rates.

Looking for an alternative explanation, Villermé turned to the field of sociology, just then emerging in Europe, to develop hypotheses about the effects of social factors such as poverty and wealth on health. This time he calculated the proportion of households in each neighborhood that were exempt from rent tax, which was levied only on the wealthy, in order to arrive at a proxy measurement for poverty. He then correlated those proportions with the mortality data. The result was an "almost perfect fit": the neighborhoods with the lowest mortality also had the lowest proportion of tax-exempt households (i.e., were the wealthiest), while the neighborhoods with the highest mortality rates had the highest portion of tax-exempt households (i.e., were the poorest).[3] Villermé thus concluded that social factors such as wealth and poverty (factors amenable to manipulation through public policy) were the principal causes of wide variations in mortality—a conclusion that, as Krieger pointedly notes, was not unrelated to the politics of his own time and place:

> Villermé's ability to reach this conclusion in turn was shaped by the rapidly changing political realities and debates of his times: living in an era that saw the rise of industrial capitalism and the defeat of monarchies and mercantilism, Villermé, a firm supporter of the free market, could conceive of and receive public funds for investigating relationships between societally-produced—as opposed to divinely ordained—wealth, poverty, and disease.[4]

Villermé's study is a classic example of the basic methodology employed by epidemiologists; it also helps demonstrate several points that are key to this discussion about the potential for health and human rights collaboration. As Krieger points out, Villermé's important findings about the nature of disease "did not depend on technological or biomedical breakthroughs, but upon broadening the 'natural' discourse of science with explicitly political concepts."[5] Moreover, I would add, what was (and is) uncritically accepted in science as "natural" and therefore immutable has often served as effective camouflage for those in power to promote their own social and political goals—a phenomenon repeatedly uncovered in the histories of medical and "scientific" approaches to women's reproduction,[6] to racial differences,[7] and to colonial health policy.[8]

The influence of political ideology on health research and policy-making is fairly easy to see and accept in historical studies, especially with the benefit of nearly two centuries of hindsight, as in the example of Villermé. It is far more difficult to recognize and expose such assumptions when they are embedded in the daily discourse and routine work of public health today. To illustrate how politically or culturally conditioned assumptions about women's roles and lives influence current public health research and practice, I examine one article from the growing literature on the health effects of structural adjustment programs.

In an essay entitled "A Public Health Approach to the 'Food-Malnutrition-Economic Recession Complex,'" Leonardo Mata challenges the contention that shrinking food availability caused by economic crisis has led to declining child health.[9] He questions whether economic conditions have significantly changed the "nutritional state and survival of children in less developed countries" because, in fact, the unavailability of food is not the usual cause of malnutrition and infant/child death. He demonstrates that infant and child mortality in developing countries is more often a complex interaction between malnutrition and infection conditioned by a multitude of factors other than the mere lack of food.

Mata then points to the fact that, given precisely the same financial resources and physical environment, certain children thrive while others are swept into the spiral of malnutrition and infection that ultimately ends in death or permanent disability. From this observation, Mata concludes that the true cause of poor child health is not lack of food; it is what Mata calls "deficient maternal technology." He defines "good" maternal technology as consisting of the following:

> (a) adequate knowledge and technique for preparation and administration of weaning foods; (b) appropriate handling of human and animal feces; (c) knowledge about signs and symptoms of dehydration and other life-threatening conditions; (d) acceptance of immunizations and other elements of modern medicine; (e) basic nutrition and health education; and (f) proclivity towards family planning.

Perhaps "technology" is the key word here, for Mata perceives a woman's inability to promote her children's health as primarily a failure to learn the technical lessons of primary health care. Nodding slightly to some vague social factors that may influence a woman's ability to protect her children, Mata tries to be careful not to lodge moral blame against mothers who fail. On the other hand, Mata stresses, faced with similar circumstances, some women seem to do just fine:

> Mothers are not entirely responsible for inadequacies in maternal technology, inasmuch as they are trapped in ecosystems and societies that have not permitted them to acquire an understanding and knowledge of the ubiquitous fecal contamination of food and environment and other threats to child nutrition and survival. On the other hand, many women in villages and slums possess effective maternal technologies, and their children thrive well despite the odds and hardships.

For Mata, the implications of his insight are clear: food programs to buffer the effects of economic crisis and structural adjustment are not the solution, because lack of food is not the problem. Rather, poor mothers are the problem; thus improving maternal technology—creating better mothers—must be central to the solution.

Of course, Mata is not wrong when he states that a mother who makes sure the family's food is free from fecal contamination is more likely to have a healthy child than a mother who ignores the risks of contamination. Indeed, Mata and others who support his view probably would concede quite readily that in many cultures, the subordination of women does much to prevent them from learning or implementing the lessons of sanitation. The problem with the view exemplified by the Mata article is that it fails to invest that subordination of women with any importance, programmatically or theoretically.

By failing to pay attention to the elements of women's lives that lie outside the mother-child relationship—by failing to ask the right questions in his comparison of the children who thrive and those who die—he fails to see the multiple, fundamental ways in which economic crisis jolts women's lives and intensifies unequal gender and power dynamics within their households. These are dynamics that all too often lead to violence, marital breakdown, mental illness, and abject despair, and so to an inability to cope with the effects of economic crisis.[10] At the same time, the intense focus on the mother-child relationship, and the tendency to view women as isolated actors whose sole role in life is the birth and rearing of children, obscures the incredible strength, assertiveness, and resourcefulness that many women have shown in the face of crisis, developing and carrying out strategies that require them to go well beyond conventional gender roles of wife and mother in order to ensure their own and their families' survival.[11]

Thus, where Mata points to "maternal technology" as the solution to children dying from malnutrition-infection complex, other defensible solutions could be to change (or abandon) structural adjustment programs so that even children in families least able to cope with crisis can survive, and/or to facilitate women's ability to cope by taking measures to increase their autonomy, power, and rights within the families and communities devastated by adjustment programs. The public health practitioner trained only in the techniques of primary health care, and conditioned to think of them as "magic bullets" of unquestioned benefit, all too often will accept uncritically a conclusion such as Mata's. But the feminist or human rights activist attuned to the political implications of medical practice and health policy will likely ask a different set of questions to understand the dynamics of the household and communities in which children die during economic crisis. Such questions yield a different range of policy conclusions, possibly with primary health care (albeit wrapped in a different implementation package) among them.

Finally, there is another, more general observation to make about the approach exemplified in the Mata article. Even when the potential influence of social factors such as macroeconomic crisis and structural adjustment programs is acknowledged, public health policy-makers and practitioners often resort, almost reflexively, to the same kind of solution: individuals must modify their own behavior. In the case of women, this often means they must become "better" wives, mothers, or homemakers. This is a theme that has been repeated over and over again in current public health discourse and practice, particularly when it comes to health problems prevalent in marginalized populations.

For example, individual behavior change has long been the central theme in HIV/AIDS prevention policy, exhorting all people to "just say no" or to engage only in safer sex practices. Yet, for women who are powerless and vulnerable, caught in marital and sexual relationships over which they have little control, such advice may be worse than useless. Programs that address, or at least recognize, the power imbalances that shape women's lives are now beginning to receive increased attention as the HIV/AIDS pandemic continues to ravage vast parts of the world.[12] But in the United States, at least, this focus on individual behavior as the source of and solution to all social ills is now reaching new rhetorical heights with the Republicans' Contract with America and its cynically titled centerpiece, "The Personal Responsibility Act," which purports to address the public health issues of "teenage pregnancy and illegitimacy," as well as the budget deficit, by penalizing indigent women who have children.[13]

I certainly do not mean by this discussion to imply that individual behavior change is irrelevant to improving health and preventing disease. Indeed, I would argue that, *as a matter of human rights,* individuals must be empowered to make the kinds of decisions about their lives that will enable them to protect their health. But it is also critical to recognize that the decision to focus on individual behavior to the exclusion of other social determinants of ill health is a *political choice;* it is not an inescapable answer compelled by an indisputable, "scientifically correct" understanding of disease causation. Moreover, the model of behavior modification that typically underlies public health campaigns incorporates a kind of individualism, associated with biomedical approaches to health, that actually does little to empower people to make such changes. As Elizabeth Fee and Nancy Krieger explained it in their article on the history of HIV/AIDS paradigms:

> The biomedical model is also premised on the ideology of individualism. Adopting the notion of the abstract individual from liberal political and economic theory, it considers individuals "free" to "choose" health behaviors. It treats people as consumers who make free choices in the marketplace of products and behaviors, and it generally ignores the role of industry, agribusiness and government in structuring the array of risk factors that individuals are supposed to avoid. There is little place for understanding how behaviors are related to social conditions and constraints or how communities shape individuals' lives.[14]

This kind of abstract individualism will surface again in subsequent sections that consider the prevailing conceptions of rights which, like biomedicine, are influenced by liberal theory. But to summarize here: public health tools, and epidemiology in particular, expand our ability to see, to understand, indeed to measure, important aspects of the individual's relationship with the world. The fact that epidemiology is grounded in specific contexts, that it is based on statistical measurements that are testable and repeatable, is critically important to practice and effective advocacy. But we must beware of the "false conflation between scientific objectivity and value-free science."[15] Epidemiology—whether the question is which data to gather, how to interpret data we have or how to craft policies and programs based on the data—will never be value-free, nor do I argue that it should be. But epidemiology and the tools of public health are just that—tools and methodology. The values that drive their theory and practice cannot be found internally within epidemiology; they must come from outside of it.[16]

Can health, then, be a value, a "good," in and of itself? My answer is emphatically *yes*. Only a person blessed with perfect health and blind to the suffering of others could have the arrogance to seriously propose otherwise. Hence, my point here is not to deny that health has biological dimensions or to belittle the importance of physical health as a worthwhile policy goal; rather, my point is to show that even an individual's physical health—not to mention her mental and emotional health—is inextricably tied to the wider conditions of her life. Thus physical health cannot be detached from political and social concerns, posited as an objective state of biological being, and then treated as though the choices we make in pursuit of it are apolitical and compelled by some internal logic that derives solely from health itself.

Yet the influence of this detached and narrowly bounded view of health is so deep and pervasive in Western biomedical models and the social policies that derive from them that its impact and operation can be extremely difficult to recognize and even harder to contest.[17] Of course, the inability to perceive the influence of narrow health models or to gasp the fundamental truth that health is socially produced is a malady that primarily afflicts those of us who are academics, theorists, policy analysts, or health professionals and have been born, bred, and/or trained in the ideology of science and Western biomedicine.[18] By contrast, for the people in every part of the world, North and South, who live the reality of deprivation and discrimination in its harshest forms, the truth of the social production of health and disease is painfully obvious—even if its solutions are not.

Human rights is fundamentally about the struggle to make *their* voices heard and heeded. In a sense, then, the collaboration between health and human rights begins here, with the struggle to decide whose view of health will control the policies and programs that address it. Perhaps nowhere is this struggle more contentious, or the collaboration between health and human rights more urgent, than in the area of women's reproductive health and reproductive rights.

ALTERNATIVE VISIONS OF HEALTH AND RIGHTS

The reproductive health and reproductive rights movements grow from the conviction that at the core of human dignity lies the ability to be an effective agent in guiding the course of one's own life. Much of the work by activists and theorists in this field is devoted to understanding what exactly this means across different cultures and political systems, and to finding the social structures and cultural configurations that will promote and support it. That work is under way but far from complete. The evolving understanding of reproductive health advocated by women's movements and many others in the public health field incorporates a broad, holistic, multifaceted approach to women's health and health care; as theoretical understandings of reproductive health continue to develop, important initiatives on the ground can and do address specific health concerns in effective ways.[19] There is certainly much to be said from a clinical or programmatic perspective about how such reproductive health initiatives are being designed and implemented (and, indeed, about how they contribute to the advancement of human rights, even if they are not ever perceived as human rights initiatives). But, for explanatory purposes here, it is perhaps easier to describe what reproductive health and reproductive rights are by showing what they are not, or rather, by showing what these movements have reacted against.

In the health field, they have reacted against population control efforts that treat women as "targets" of contraceptive programs, blatantly manipulating their reproductive capacity in order to achieve demographic goals— goals set by dominant elites in pursuit of any number of different political agendas. They have reacted against maternal/child health policies that view the health of women as an instrument to ensure the health of children, and not as an important or valuable matter in its own right. They have reacted against medical institutions that focus on different pieces of women's bodies as discrete biological systems to be prodded, probed, and fixed, rather than seeing women's health as *women live it,* as part of complex interactive systems tied inextricably to the broader conditions of their lives. And they have reacted against domination by health professionals who present "risk" as if the only thing at stake in deciding whether or not to conceive or give birth is the possibility of physical injury; who obsess about reproduction but ignore sexuality; who preach about "personal responsibility" but fold on questions of power and resources, of vulnerability and discrimination.

This struggle around reproduction goes far beyond the health field, for women's reproduction is viewed as the primary tool for many other political projects as well. Thus, in many societies, a woman's sexuality and reproduction are symbols of her family's honor, to be guarded, watched, and controlled. They are the weapons with which the wars of identity politics are waged; most brutally, they are the scene of "ethnic cleansing." It is these political projects, and many others like them, against which the reproductive health and reproductive rights movements have been forced to define themselves.

Thus, stated in the negative, reproductive health and reproductive rights—indeed, human dignity—are about the right not to be alienated from one's own reproductive and sexual capacity; the right not to have that capacity used as an instrument to serve the interests of other individuals, collectivities or states without one's consent and without the opportunity to participate in the political processes by which such interests are defined. Stated in the affirmative, the reproductive health and reproductive rights movements are about shifting perspectives, about changing whose point of view, whose values, whose experience, whose choices will control women's reproduction.

Such a shift in perspective will not happen automatically by force of logic, nor will it grow out of a movement that focuses on health alone, or on health as a biological problem to be addressed solely through improved medical techniques. It can happen only when health is understood as a function of the same forces that structure a woman's relationship to the physical and social world around her, and is addressed in policies, programs, and activist movements as such.

Once health is understood in this way, then improving health necessarily means dismantling the systems that have wrested away from women the ability and entitlement to decide the meanings and uses of their bodies and their lives. But it also means building social systems that promote and support women as effective actors who are vested, committed, inseparable, and indispensable parts of the families, communities, and states within which they live. This second task, the task of renovating or rebuilding, is not an optional after-thought. It is the essence of the search for human dignity and social justice that is the basic motivation for human rights advocacy. But for that search to be successful, human rights will need to be reclaimed and reshaped to fit a movement that seeks to reflect the experiences and serve the visions of women in diverse cultural and political settings.

RECLAIMING HUMAN RIGHTS

If "health" as a political category has a problematic history for women's advocates, so too do "rights." Indeed, feminist theorists have been among the most articulate critics of rights-based legal régimes. While it is surely important for women's advocates and activists to consider these arguments, it is also essential to look beyond the academic debate surrounding rights; to acknowledge the different historically grounded meanings that "rights" can have to the people who assert them; to assess the ways that rights language has been used and manipulated in international discourse; and then to make a strategic decision about the potential utility of health and human rights collaboration in advancing the ultimate goals of their work.[20] This is an ongoing, dynamic process that will not yield one "correct" strategic answer, but rather, different answers at different times and places, all of which can effectively contribute to the same, shared political goals. Moreover, it is an exceptionally complex inquiry because it involves not only sensitivity to political dynamics at the international level (e.g., in UN conferences, in bilateral or multilateral governmental relationships, and in the increasingly influential world of international nongovernmental organizations) but also a sensitivity to the multitude of ways in which international developments interact with very diverse and specific local realities in every part of the world.

Of course, a full treatment of all these issues is well beyond the scope of these preliminary reflections about health and human rights. In the section that follows, therefore, I attempt only to give a very broad-brush, almost impressionistic sense of conventional approaches to human rights, women's responses to them and the political use that various forces have found for both. In doing so, I focus most heavily—even if still only superficially—on a few key aspects of a much bigger set of problems and on one key area of concern (reproductive health and rights) in the hope of stimulating more critical attention to the broader challenges we face as the field of health and human rights develops.

Conventional Approaches and Feminist Critiques

Human rights is conventionally approached as a formal body of law codified in treaties, conventions, and covenants. This law was first articulated in its contemporary form in the Universal Declaration of Human Rights (1948) and then further elaborated in legally binding instruments in the International Covenant on Civil and Political Rights (ICCPR) and the International Covenant on Economic, Social and Cultural Rights (ICESCR) (1966), all of which together form what has sometimes been called the "International Bill of Rights." As an expression of basic values of human dignity and social justice, human rights draws inspiration from and resonates with historical and contemporary legal traditions of many different societies and cultures around the world.[21] However, as a body of formal law dealing primarily with the relationship between individual citizens and their governments, human rights took its initial doctrinal inspiration from concepts of civil liberties found in Western legal systems, which, in turn, derive largely from liberal political and economic theory.

That theory, in its classical formulations, embraces an ideology of individualism that has been the lightning rod for much of the criticism of rights. Closely associated with the theory and operation of a capitalist free market economic system, liberal individualism views people abstractly, as self-made, self-contained, separate individuals, isolated from others, pitted against the collective, pursuing their economic self-interest without reliance on the state. In a world so conceived, the purpose of rights is to stake out and protect a sphere of personal freedom; but that freedom is imagined as one built on boundaries: its essence is the right to keep others out, the right to be left alone.

In a legal system premised on such a worldview, freedom from others also depends on enforcing the separation between the public and the private: rights are theoretically meant to keep the state out of the private sphere altogether, and to operate most meaningfully in the public sphere, where they regulate the individual's participation in public life and civil society and his or her interaction with the law enforcement mechanisms of the state (police and court systems). Thus civil and political rights include such areas as freedom of speech and association, freedom from torture and from cruel, inhuman or degrading treatment and punishment, and the rights to a fair trial and to life, liberty and security of person (traditionally interpreted to refer to matters such as genocide, arbitrary arrest and detention, and execution). These civil and political rights, codified in the ICCPR, are often called "negative" rights because they are aimed at limiting the state's ability to encroach on individual freedom, at stopping the state from arbitrary or coercive actions.

By contrast, economic, social, and cultural rights, often called "positive" rights, deal with the state's obligation to create the affirmative conditions that help ensure human well-being. They include such matters as rights to health, education, employment, and housing. By ratifying the ICESCR, a state party "undertakes to take steps . . . to the maximum of its available resources, with a view to achieving progressively the full realization of the rights recognized in the present Covenant by all appropriate means, including particularly the adoption of legislative measures."[22] Although these positive rights were certainly central to the initial expansive conception of human rights embodied in the 1948 Universal Declaration, for a variety of reasons—some practical and some political—work in the human rights field has centered almost exclusively on the protection of civil and political rights. Most human rights NGOs have chosen not to address economic, social, and cultural rights, in part because of the near total absence of any methodology to monitor enforcement or define violations of them. Not surprisingly, governments have been equally reluctant to tread on this uncharted territory, where implementation implies not just refraining from wrongful action but also affirmative steps to alter the distribution and spending of public and private resources.

Failure to maintain the interconnection between positive and negative rights is among the primary criticisms that have been leveled against liberal theory and the rights-based legal systems it spawned. At the heart of these criticisms is a fundamental challenge to the notion that people exist as atomistic, disconnected, self-enclosed individuals. A legal system premised on a strict dichotomy between individuals and the collective ignores the extent to which individuals define themselves through, and take meaning from, their relationships with others; it fails to recognize the extent to which "we come into being in a social context that is literally constitutive of us."[23]

Seeing the individual primarily in opposition to the collective, liberalism supports the prevailing "negative" view of rights that is designed essentially to keep the state in check and as far out of social and economic life as possible. Within the international human rights scheme, this means emphasizing civil and political rights rather than economic, social, and cultural rights and maintaining a strict distinction between them. As women's human rights advocates have repeatedly pointed out, this distinction results in a formalistic and ultimately hollow view of rights. For example, the right to decide on the number and spacing of children, however important to a women's health in theory, actually means little in a woman's life if there are no health services in place and no contraceptives available.[24]

More specifically, feminist critics of liberal, rights-based legal systems have demonstrated how conventional interpretations of such laws—including international human rights law—reflect the experience and interests of male elites and fail to accommodate or acknowledge the realities of women's lives.[25] Their analyses elucidate the myriad ways in which the separation of the public and the private deflects the reach of rights from the site of women's most pervasive exploitation and deepest vulnerability—the domestic sphere—and obscures the crucial role that women play in the public sphere as well.[26] Though liberal legal systems purport to eschew all interference in the private sphere, particularly the family, feminist critics have shown that it is precisely the operation of such systems of law that structures the most intimate matters of private and family life, rendering the stated ideal of non-interference an incoherent principle and the purported neutrality of law an illusion.[27]

The Political Context of Debates Over Human Rights

At the international level, the debate over human rights has other, highly explosive dimensions that take the discussion well beyond theory, into the harsh political reality within which women's movements operate internationally. Thus, any attempt to find a workable collaboration between health and human rights must also consider the ways that rights language has been manipulated for political ends that may have little to do with the defense or denial of the idea of rights per se.

In international discourse, the problem of rights is often posed as a series of oppositional dichotomies: universalism vs. cultural relativism; the individual vs. the collective; civil and political rights vs. economic, social, and cultural rights; North vs. South or East vs. West. The tensions that lie behind these dichotomies are real ones that need to be addressed carefully by the human rights community. I do not purport to do that here, nor do I mean to dismiss such tensions lightly; rather, I wish to make a different point: while the tensions are real, the choice to pose the issues as either/or dichotomies presumes that the two poles exist only in opposition to each other, that the resolution can be only to choose one pole or the other. That is a presumption that serves particular political interests, as becomes clearer when we examine who is using these dichotomies and how they benefit from doing so, and when we see how structuring the problem this way becomes a tactic to be used against women internationally, in an effort to divide and silence us.

Perhaps a start in the bigger task of unpacking and analyzing these dichotomies is to recognize that lying at the crux of the problem is this: foes of women's rights typically characterize any expression by women of their entitlement to guide the course of their own lives as a rejection and denial of any and all ties or responsibility to others or to the collective. In their scenario, there is no such thing as a woman who seeks and gains control over the conditions of her existence yet chooses to live a life built around commitments and connections to others; given the chance allowed to escape from the domination of patriarchal families and communities, it is presumed that women will abandon those families and communities altogether, in a ghastly display of selfish and hedonistic individualism. This basic conception of the "uncontrolled" woman as a dangerous and destructive force explains, in part, why human rights, with its apparent defense of the individual *as against* the collective, has become so explosive, particularly when applied to women's reproduction and sexuality, the area in which control over women is guarded most jealously.[28]

Lest this seem like a melodramatic overstatement of the position of those who oppose women's rights, consider some of the recent pronouncements of leaders of that opposition. For example, in 1992, urging voters to reject the proposed Equal Rights Amendment that would have explicitly prohibited discrimination on the basis of gender, Pat Robertson, leader of the increasingly powerful Christian Coalition in the United States, made this now infamous statement:

> The feminist agenda is not about equal rights for women. It is a socialist, anti-family political movement that encourages women to leave their husbands, kill their children, practice witchcraft and become lesbians.[29]

His statements were echoed in more apocalyptic, even if somewhat less picturesque, terms by representatives of the Holy See who, in 1994, led a determined effort to derail the International Conference on Population and Development (ICPD) and to undermine its Programme of Action, a document that explicitly endorsed concepts of reproductive health and reproductive rights and acknowledged their link to human rights. Portraying the Cairo conference as "basically about a type of libertine, individualistic life style" being imposed by the United States under the sway of "a pervasive feminist influence" that amounted to "cultural imperialism,"[30] the Vatican made no bones about how serious it deemed the threat to be: "Civilization is at stake. We should be foolish to see in the Cairo conference anything else."[31]

The Vatican found willing allies for its position in parts on the Muslim world. In statements condemning the conference, officials at Cairo's Al Azhar University, perhaps the most prestigious institution for Islamic scholarship in the world, challenged the Programme of Action reportedly because it "aims to defend sexual relations outside legal marriage," "undermines parental authority," and "might encourage prostitution."[32] Such statements helped touch off a wave of threats from Muslim extremists opposed both to the conference and perhaps, more significantly, to the Egyptian government. Such opposition was broadcast over loudspeakers during sermons in neighborhood mosques: "We reject this conference. . . . It is a Zionist and imperialist assault against Islam. This is a policy imposed on Egypt by the United States."[33]

Others, speaking to the international press, took their campaign to a more chilling level. As one leader of a militant group based in Cairo is reported to have commented:

> Some brothers are preaching against this corrupt, immoral conference in the mosques. But others may decide to defend Islam by killing, and they would be willing to die in the process. If the West is afraid of blood, it should stay away from us.[34]

It is thus a slippery slide between and among women's assertion of the right to control their reproductive lives; charges of destructive individualism; the specter of cultural imperialism; and the evocation of North and South, East against West. Of course, as implied by the discussion of liberalism above, this is not a wholly frivolous position: human rights as classically formulated *are* Western in origin; and the kind of oppositional relationship between individual and collective that was projected by human rights theory, at least in its conventional formulations, *does* differ from that lived in most social and cultural arrangements, North and South. Moreover, governments clearly have been selective in the accusations of human rights violations made against one another, often having economic or other ideological interests as the primary consideration. And interactions involving human rights NGOs do sometimes suffer from the same arrogance and myopia that plague all kinds of cross-cultural exchanges. These are issues in the human rights field that must be taken seriously and handled with honestly and circumspection.

Nevertheless, the structuring of the discussion as a set of oppositional dichotomies and, worse, the conflation of each dichotomous relationship with the others are disastrous for women in both North and South. When any assertion of individual entitlement by women is automatically characterized as betrayal of the collective, when women are forced to choose between an assertion of themselves and assertion of their national, ethnic, or religious identity, then they have lost the first battle: the battle to set the terms of the debate. When this battle is lost then the result is silence: silence from those in the South who fear the accusation that they are "feminist" or "Western"; silence from those in the North who fear the accusation that they are "cultural imperialists."

The characterization of feminism or women's rebellion against patriarchal structures as simply an alien, Western import denies and attempts to suppress the leading role that women from Asia, Africa, and Latin America have played in defining the terms and setting the direction of women's human rights movements and reproductive health and rights movements in their own countries and on the international stage.[35] Moreover, it makes invisible the long and rich histories of women's resistance as individuals or as organized movements in those countries and in relation to the diverse cultures within them.[36] Finally, this conflation of dichotomies takes the genuine and appropriate circumspection of women in the North, who are seriously concerned that their own voices and perspective have dominated some parts of the women's movement, and converts that self-reflection and self-criticism into a paralyzing prescription for political correctness that prevents these women in the North from hearing and supporting those women in the South who are taking courageous stands to assert their own visions of human rights. At the same time, it prevents women in the South from building alliances with or supporting the struggles of women in the North by characterizing any attempt to make such alliances or connections, even on an *ad hoc* basis for special purposes, as a breach of a different prescription of political correctness, one that views everyone located in the North as undifferentiated agents of imperialism and Western hegemony.

There is obviously much more work to be done to understand the historical and contemporary connections among all these phenomena and to understand their political use in international discourse about human rights generally and women's human rights and reproductive rights in particular, and the strategic options for resisting them. That work is now urgent, as the politico-religious right will clearly remain a powerful force in international politics for a long time. But it is also important for women's health and rights advocates to remember that these are not the only forces threatened by the idea of women's control over their own reproductive and sexual lives. For many years, resistance to women-centered reproductive health and reproductive rights has also come from much quieter, even if more powerful, quarters. Perhaps the most influential of these are certain of the most conservative segments of the population "establishment" that has set the direction for many of the population policies that national governments have implemented over the last four decades often with the help of, under pressure from, bilateral and multilateral aid agencies.[37]

This part of the population establishment certainly operates from a political agenda very different from that of the politico-religious right. It is therefore instructive to see the extent to which both camps have been driven by similar assumptions, particularly the belief that if women are allowed to escape the control of patriarchal families, communities, and states, they will abandon responsibility for and commitment to the collective. Although this belief rarely surfaces in a strident or even explicit way in the writing or work of population and family planning specialists, its influence can be teased out nevertheless. For example, Susan Cotts Watkins, in an article entitled "If All We Knew About Women Was What We Read in *Demography,* What Would We Know?" examines twenty-five years of this leading academic journal to try to understand the views of women that have driven demographers, work. She knows that demography as a field tends to share the basic view of liberal theory in which women are conceptualized as "separate selves," as "autonomous and impervious to social influence," and ultimately concludes that

> if all we knew about women was what we read in the articles on fertility, marriage, and the family, we would conclude that women are primarily producers of children and of child services, that they produce with little assistance from men, that they are socially isolated from relatives and friends; *and that their commitment to the production of children and child services is expected to be rather fragile* [emphasis added].[38]

This description of demographers' views of women is startlingly contrary to many women's own views of themselves, their feelings of commitment, their experience of connectedness, and their valuing of relationships (including relationships with their own and others' children, relatives, and friends) as expressed in narratives, demonstrated in everyday life, and even proven in social science research.[39] Yet in many parts of the world, population and health policies have been routinely built *not* around women's own experience of the world (as advocated by the reproductive health and reproductive rights movements), but around the assumptions and worldview exposed by Watkins. The result is precisely the kinds of programs that evidence a deep distrust of women and of what decisions they might make if given the chance. Thus, population policies and family planning and decision-making processes, and instead impose on them, through methods involving varying degrees of persuasion or coercion, the so-called professional's view of what is good for society, for families, for health and for women and have the power of the state to back them up.[40]

Given this orientation of the population establishment, it is important to recognize and question why they have historically been among the strongest advocates of recognizing "the right to decide freely and responsibly on the number and spacing of children" as a human right. Elsewhere, I have shown that when this was first articulated as a human right, at the 1968 Teheran Conference on Human Rights, a primary motivation was to find a wedge to get contraceptives into the many countries (especially in the South) where they were then illegal or otherwise blocked, in order to control population growth.[41] Although those within the population movement who advocated this human right no doubt genuinely believed that individuals have the right to use contraceptives and to control their fertility, they perceived the limits on an individual's right to decide whether to have children very different from the way women's movements understood the same right when they promoted it.[42] In short, the primary goal of the population movement was to lower population growth, not to ensure that women themselves had both the right and the ability to control their bodies and lives; thus the "freedom" of the individual to decide was, in the view of the population movement, readily limited by the "responsibility" to make the fertility-limited decision imposed by government population policies purportedly in furtherance of the greater good. As Susan Watkins put in, commenting on the special issue of *Demography* on family planning that was published in 1968, the year of the Teheran Conference, "even when the language seems to empower to choose to control their fertility, they are expected to use this power to control world population growth."[43]

Apparently, then, the population control movement believed that in the human rights framework as conventionally understood, it had found a useful tool for advancing towards its own view of human well-being. Thus, one lesson is clear: human rights, like public health, can be wielded as a tool to promote quite particular political goals that might be substantially different from or even contrary to the goals of women's advocates. This takes us back to the point made at the very start: while public health and human rights can be powerful tools for generating change, they can also be powerful tools for maintaining hierarchies of power and domination based on gender, race, and class.

THEN WHY BOTHER WITH HUMAN RIGHTS?

If rights, in their conventional interpretations, have failed to recognize or redress women's experience of violation, and if the human rights paradigm, when manipulated either by those who purport to accept it or by those who vehemently reject it, provides fodder to precisely the forces that seek to oppress women, then one might legitimately ask, why bother to use human rights at all? Aren't they more trouble than they are worth, particularly given the notoriously weak enforcement mechanisms in the international system?

My answer begins with the refusal to accept the dichotomies routinely imposed on the discussion. Human rights are strategically valuable because they express, in the broadest terms, basic values of human dignity and social justice that have historical contemporary roots in cultures throughout the world. But those values do *not* dictate a particular lifestyle, or identity, or way of being in the world. Rather, they affirm the fundamental value of human agency: the nature of human beings as effective social actors.

When read carefully and interpreted in its fullest dimensions, the human rights paradigm enables us to reject as inaccurate and destructive the abstract individualism of liberal theory, the notion of individuals operating in isolation and crude self-interest, seeking to keep others at bay, even while imposing their will on everything, animate and inanimate, around them. At the same time, the human rights paradigm rejects treatment of any person as property, chained to another's or a group's will, to be dominated, controlled, and used. Rather, it seeks to create a world in which human dignity adheres in the still distant ideal of choice: the notion that human beings, constituted through relations with others, can still make choices about their lives, can still have something to say about how to structure and maintain relations with others, be they family, community, or state.

Such an ideal has particular power and importance in our time. In a world increasingly consumed by the most brutal struggles of "identity politics," a politics in which access to power and resources is sought to be determined by group identification, and group identification is prescribed by allegedly immutable characteristics of birth (e.g., race, ethnicity, even religion), then women—whose appearance, behavior, and, particularly, sexual conduct are made to be the symbols of "purity," the quality that is believe to ensure group strength and continuity—are most vulnerable to control and domination.[44] At the same time, our world is increasingly, and irrevocably, international: in economies, politics, and communications, we are all now bound to each other through complicated webs of dependence, infiltration, and, most painfully, inequality and domination. In such a world, human rights affirms the basic entitlement of *all* people to resources and to the resources and to the respect and dignity that comes from the ability to consciously, willfully participate in setting the terms of their interactions with the world around them.

No one fools herself into believing that we are close to such an ideal. No one fools herself into thinking that its attainment will be easy or that it will come without massive social change, in which some will be required to relinquish power over others. But in the area of health, in which we can see in the most obvious physical terms the results of structures of inequality large and small, we have perhaps the best chance to make a difference, to determine and implement social configurations that can support and promote human well-being. In short, when human rights principles are applied to health, we begin to have the strategic political basis upon which to mobilize across the divides of nation, culture, class, race, and religion in support of each other and in pursuit of change.

RETHINKING THE CONNECTIONS BETWEEN HEALTH AND HUMAN RIGHTS

To use health and human rights collaboration in this way means rebuilding our understandings of both health and human rights, as well as the vision of human well-being they define and advance, from the ground up. It means taking full account of the very real differences that shape our lives, while giving full respect to our common humanity. It means approaching health and human rights collaboration not as a theoretical puzzle that is worked through in a political vacuum, but rather as a very concrete, contextualized inquiry that begins from the experience of those whose health and human rights are most at stake.

Such work will require the combination of many different approaches at the same time. For example, the women's human rights movement has effectively used the analytically simple, but emotionally and rhetorically powerful, method of personal testimony to force recognition of women's violation, entitlement and need. This has happened most notably in the area of violence against women, where substantial progress has been made in changing perceptions in both the human rights field[45] and the international health field.[46] To a significant extent, such progress has come as a result of women's demand, quite simply, to be heard. In "tribunals" held in all parts of the world and also in international fora, women's often courageous testimonies of violence inflicted with impunity in both the private and public spheres demonstrated more powerfully than any amount of academic analysis ever could that both fields, locked into formalistic, narrow ways of understanding both rights and health, had failed to listen to or acknowledge the impact or importance of such experiences and so had effectively excluded this aspect of women's lives from their purview.

In the area of reproduction and sexuality, enormously valuable work that will ultimately contribute to new understandings of health and human rights is being done in multidisciplinary, action-oriented field research. This includes, for example, the project being conducted by the International Reproductive Rights Research Action Group (IRRRAG) in seven countries in Africa, Asia, Latin America, and North America to uncover and document the ways that women themselves understand and express their entitlement in matters of reproduction and sexuality.[47] Another project, conducted jointly by Health Action Information Network in the Philippines and the Institute for Development Research in the Netherlands, through participatory action-research in multiple countries focuses more specifically on women's experiences of fertility-regulating methods and reproductive health care.[48]

Such reconceptualizing of health and rights, beginning with the experiences of women, will also require working at a more theoretical level to transform the way the very words we use in health and human rights work are interpreted and understood. For example, Rosalind Petchesky, in an essay entitled "Body as Property: A Feminist Re-Vision," attempts to "recuperate the notion of self-propriety"—the idea of "owning" or controlling one's body—by looking "at the variety of local meanings that women in noncapitalist societies, radical democrats, and slaves have given to the idea of owning their bodies, as well as the value that contemporary feminists of color are placing on re-owning their bodies as an aspect of self-definition."[49] As she puts it, "The 'objects of property' may have more to tell us from their vantage point than we can learn from positioning ourselves within the debates of the treatises, the lawbooks, and the political-theory canon."

As with women's approach to human rights more generally, Petchesky's point is not to make women's lives and claims fit within the four corners of the law as it currently is interpreted; rather, her point is to see how the powerful language so basic to that law in this case, the concept of "property," can be reshaped to serve the political goals defined by women. The aim is to understand "the language of self/body ownership as a rhetorical strategy for political mobilization and defining identities, not a description of the world." From this perspective, the very notion of "property" is given new meaning:

> Rhetorical claims on behalf of women's ownership of their bodies invoke meanings of ownership as a relationship of right, use, and caretaking meanings that have different cultural moorings from the commercial idea of property that the regime of triumphal international capitalism conventionally takes for granted.[50]

The project she envisions has distinctly political importance:

> Perhaps there are good reasons to defend this language particularly as it pertains to people's relationship to their bodies. Perhaps owning one's body is a necessary element of citizenship in an affirmative but noninterventionist state.[51]

All of these projects that focus intensely on the meanings that women in a wide range of different political, social, and cultural settings express for themselves are vitally important for the ultimate collaboration between health and human rights. But if we are really to escape the abstract individualism of liberal theory and the biases it has imposed onto biomedicine and conventional rights interpretations—that is, if we are to demand that rights be understood not primarily as a right to build boundaries or to be left alone, but rather as a right to live with dignity in the context of social commitments and relationships; and if we are to demand that health and disease be understood not simply as a function of "free" individual behavioral choices, but rather as a result of lives constrained by social forces such as poverty and discrimination—then we will also need to develop a much more structural critique than can be gleaned from case studies or narratives or anecdotal evidence alone.

This is where public health and its tools hold great potential in strategic collaboration with human rights. As discussed much earlier, public health seeks to understand health and disease not simply as a function of self-contained biological systems of the human body, but also as a function of the wider conditions of a person's life. By looking not just at the health of the individual but at patterns of health in populations, public health allows us to go beyond isolated anecdotes or incidents and to see social patterns and configurations associated with what is experienced as individual phenomena of death, disability, or disease.

An excellent example of this is an article by Susan Greenhalgh and Jiali Li that explicitly attempts to demonstrate how feminists can use the discipline and methodology of demography to reveal patterns and practices not observable through qualitative research.[52] Working with data from a rural area of China, they show how the one-child policy has in practice been shaped over time through "politics of resistance," then "negotiation," then "submission." By projecting to the population level and documenting the shocking shifts in sex ratios in different age and birth-order cohorts, they enable us to see more than simply a rash of cases of selective abortion or infanticide; rather, they can demonstrate how a policy that began as gender-neutral ultimately has come to involve massive violence and discrimination against the youngest girls in China and, in the most profound ways, has inflicted terrible damage on the wider society as well. Arguing for the importance of developing a feminist demography, they point out:

> [I]t may be that the more politicized the arena of reproduction, the more crucial demographic evidence becomes, for where reproduction is heavily contested, people work hard to hide their secrets, not only from other members of their society but from social scientists as well. In China the discrimination and violence directed against little girls were thickly cloaked until large-scale demographic evidence brought them to light.[53]

Not only do public health tools (including epidemiology and demography) help us identify and describe health issues as socially constructed human rights issues, they also begin to tell us what to do about them. This is critical in the area of positive rights, where the objective is not just to get the state to stop committing a violation, but rather to get the state to do the right thing to improve the social condition in question. Thus, not only can epidemiological evidence show us the extent of a health problem and its general association with social conditions, it can also show us in far more refined ways how particular social conditions interact with biological factors to yield patterns of ill health.[54] It thus can help us determine where to begin to address state responsibility for dealing with a particular health issue.

But, as the earlier discussion of "deficient maternal technology" in the context of structural adjustment programs demonstrated, this is not a value-free exercise. When health data are analyzed from a feminist perspective (such as demonstrated in the Greenhalgh and Li article), essentially bringing a politicized view of human well-being to the endeavor, then the understandings developed from health research can begin to acquire the dimensions necessary to organize and advocate effectively within the framework of human rights law. Rather than simply shouting that something must be done to meet, for example, obligations to ensure a right to health under the ICESCR, we can begin to show that "progressive achievement of rights" requires very specific steps, and then demand that such steps be taken.[55]

Finally, it is important to see that health research can also be used the other way around. Not only can we study particular health phenomena to understand how they are socially produced and can be socially ameliorated; we can also study particular human rights phenomena to understand their implications for health. Mann and colleagues point out that a "coherent vocabulary and framework to characterize dignity and different forms of dignity violations are lacking" and suggest that "a taxonomy and epidemiology of violations of dignity may uncover an enormous field of previously suspected, yet thus far unnamed and therefore undocumented, damage to physical, mental, and social well-being."[56] While this is certainly true, from the perspective of the affirmative building of health and human rights collaboration, we also need to study advancements in human rights. For example, while some feminist theorists are working from within legal and social science frameworks to "reconceive" the concept of autonomy (in somewhat the same way that Petchesky is doing with "property"),[57] demographers and public health researchers are attempting to understand how changes in women's status/power/autonomy (variously defined) in many different social and cultural settings affect the health and well-being of women, their children and families, and their wider communities.[58]

It is perhaps this research, as much as anything else, that actually built the momentum for the major shifts in perspective within the population and family planning community that were ultimately incorporated in the Cairo Programme of Action. Many years of careful public health research and writing provided the fuel for advocates of reproductive health and reproductive rights to elaborate and assert a women-centered approach. In the end, the proof that the well-being of all people—men, women and children—depends on dramatic changes in the ability of women to set the course of their lives became undeniable. To a significant extent, that understanding is now incorporated in the theoretical literature and rhetorical statements that shape the population/family planning/maternal-child health fields, and thus the evolving reproductive health field is beginning, slowly, to convert them, in substantial part, in the reproductive health field. But it will take a human rights movement, one that insists on our common humanity yet respects our diversity, to give those statements real meaning in transforming the relationships of power that shape the health and lives of us all.

NOTES AND REFERENCES

1. J. Mann et al., "Health and Human Rights," *Health and Human Rights* 1(1994): 8.
2. N. Krieger, "The Making of Public Health Data: Paradigms, Politics, and Policy," *Journal of Public Health Policy* (Winter 1992): 412–427.
3. Ibid., p. 416.
4. Ibid.
5. Ibid.
6. E. Martin, *The Woman in the Body: A Cultural Analysis of Reproduction* (Boston: Beacon Press, 1987).
7. See Krieger's description of the early work of Dr. James McCune Smith, and her own work on racial differences in infant mortality in the United States (note 2).
8. E.g., D. Arnold, *Colonizing the Body: State Medicine and Epidemic Disease in Nineteenth-Century India* (Delhi: Oxford University Press, 1993). Arnold shows that colonial medicine was not simply a process of importing European ideas and practices wholesale and then imposing them on colonial populations. Rather, the entrenchment of Western medicine in colonies such as India was very much a process shaped by interaction between the colonizers and the colonized, a process that continues to have important ramifications for work by epidemiologists in South Asia, at least. K. S. Khan, "Epidemiology and Ethics: The Perspective of the Third World," *Journal of Public Health Policy* (Spring 1994): 218–225.
9. L. Mata, "A Public Health Approach to the Food-Malnutrition-Economic Recession Complex, in D. Bell and M. Reich (eds.), *Health, Nutrition and Economic Crisis: Approaches to Policy in the Third World* (Dover, Mass.: The Auburn Publishing House, 1988).
10. See, e.g., C. Moser, "The Impact of Recession and Adjustment Policies at the Micro-level: Low Income Women and Their Households in Guayaquil, Ecuador," in UNICEF, *The Invisible Adjustment: Poor Women and the Economic Crisis* (Santiago, Chile: UNICEF,1989); L. Beneria and M. Roldan, *The Crossroads of Class and Gender: Industrial Homework, Subcontracting and Household Dynamics in Mexico City* (Chicago: University of Chicago Press, 1987).
11. UNICEF, *The Invisible Adjustment: Poor Women and the Economic Crisis* (Santiago, Chile: UNICEF, 1989); Commonwealth Secretariat, *Engendering Adjustment for the 1990s*, in Report of a Commonwealth Expert Group on Women and Structural Adjustment (London: Commonwealth Secretariat, 1989).
12. L. Heise and C. Elias, "Transforming AIDS Prevention to Meet Women's Needs: A Focus on Developing Countries," *Social Science and Medicine* 40, 7 (1995): 931–943, E. Fee and N. Krieger, "Understanding AIDS: Historical Interpretations and the Limits of Biomedical Individualism," *American Journal of Public Health* 83, 10 (1993): 1477–1486.
13. The Personal Responsibility Act of 1995, H.R. 4 (104th Congress, 1st session).
14. Fee and Krieger (see note 12), p. 1481.
15. Krieger (see note 2), p. 421.
16. K. S. Khan (see note 8).
17. See, e.g., J. Walsh and K. Warren, "Selective Primary Health Care," *New*

England Journal of Medicine 30 (1979): 967–974, an extremely influential article in the development of primary health care strategies, for an example of how this kind of thinking has driven health policies in a way that is, on its face, objective and scientific, but in fact incorporates unarticulated values about whose health is more socially valuable. For a discussion of how this notion affects our understanding of risk in reproductive decision-making, see D. Maine, L. P. Freedman, F. Shaheed, and S. Frautschi, "Risk, Reproduction, and Rights: The Uses of Reproductive Health Data," in *Population and Development: Old Debates, New Conclusions,* ed. R. Cassen (Washington, D.C.: Overseas Development Council, 1994).

18. Although this view of health originates most strongly in Western medicine, it is not only people in the North who are trained and conditioned into understanding health and health policy this way. See Kausar Khan's discussion of the ethical dilemmas faced by epidemiologists and other health professionals in Pakistan and, presumably, other Southern countries who, feeling an intellectual and professional affinity with their colleagues in the North, find themselves to be what she calls "First World 'Islanders'" who "inadvertently violate local beliefs and practices, and thereby also their (local populations among whom they conduct research) value systems" (see note 8), p. 219.

19. The most commonly used definition of reproductive health is Mahmoud Fathalla's: a condition in which the reproductive process is accomplished in a state of complete physical, mental, and social well-being and is not merely the absence of disease or disorders of the reproductive process. Reproductive health, therefore, implies that people have the ability to reproduce, to regulate their fertility and to practice and enjoy sexual relationships. It further implies that reproduction is carried to a successful outcome through infant and child survival, growth and healthy development. It finally implies that women can go through pregnancy and childbirth, that fertility regulation can be achieved without health hazards, and that people are safe in having sex. M. F. Fathalla, "Reproductive Health: A Global Overview," *Annals of the New York Academy of Sciences* 626 (1991): 1–10.

20. See P. J. Williams, *The Alchemy of Race and Rights* (Cambridge, Mass.: Harvard University Press, 1991), particularly the essay entitled "The Pain of Word Bondage," for a powerful statement of the need to assess the value of rights not only from the privileged position of those who have always had them, but also from the position of those to whom they have been denied: "For the historically disempowered, the conferring of rights is symbolic of all the denied aspects of their humanity: rights imply a respect that places one in the referential range of self and others, that elevates one's status from human body to social being. For blacks, then, the attainment of rights signifies the respectful behavior, the collective responsibility, properly owed by a society to one of its own," p. 153.

21. See, e.g., A. An-Na'im, *Toward an Islamic Reformation: Civil Liberties, Human Rights, and International Law* (New York: Syracuse University Press, 1990), R. T. Nhalapo, "International Protection of Human Rights and the Family; African Variations on a Common Theme," *International Journal of Law and the Family* 3 (1989): 1–20.

22. International Covenant on Economic, Social and Cultural Rights, GA Res.2200 (XXI), UN GAOR, 21st Sess., supp. No. 16, at 49, UN Doc. A/6316 (1966).

23. J. Nedelsky, "Reconceiving Autonomy: Sources, Thoughts and Possibilities," *Yale Journal of Law and Feminism* 1 (1989): 7–36.

24. See, e.g., S. Corrêa and R. Petchesky, "Reproductive and Sexual Rights: A Feminist Perspective" in G. Sen, A. Germain, and L. Chen (eds.), *Population Policies Reconsidered* (Cambridge, Mass: Harvard University Press, 1994).

25. H. Charlesworth, C. Chinkin, and S. Wright, "Feminist Approaches to International Law," *American Journal of International Law* 85 (1991): 613; C. Bunch, "Women's Rights as Human Rights: Toward a Re-Vision of Human Rights," *Human Rights Quarterly* 12 (1990): 486.

26. H. Charlesworth, "The Public/Private Distinction and the Right to Development in International Law," *Australian Year Book of International Law* 12 (1992): 190–204.

27. F. E. Olsen, "The Myth of State Intervention in the Family," *Journal of Law Reform* 18 (1985): 835.

28. See, for example, an article by Fatima Mernissi that examines the *Qur'anic* concept of *nushüz* (women's rebellion), its relation to *bid'a* (innovation), and the fear of individualism, which she believes explains much about the rise of religious extremism and its focus on the behavior of women in some parts of the Muslim world today. F. Mernissi, "Femininity as Subversion: Reflections on the Muslim Concept of *Nushüz*," in D. Eck and D. Jain (eds.), *Speaking of Faith* (Philadelphia: New Society Publishers, 1993).

29. *Washington Post,* August 23, 1992.

30. "Vatican Fights U.N. Draft on Women's Rights," *New York Times,* June 14, 1994.

31. J. Navarro-Valls, "The Courage to Speak Bluntly," *Wall Street Journal,* September 1, 1994.

32. "Muslims Protest U.N. Draft on Population," *New York Times,* August 12, 1994.

33. "Muslim Preachers in Egypt Condemn Population Conference," *New York Times,* August 23, 1994.

34. Ibid.

35. See, e.g., S. Corrêa in collaboration with R. Reichman, *Population and Reproductive Rights: Feminist Perspectives from the South* (London and New Jersey: Zed Books Ltd., and New Dehli: Kali for Women, 1994).

36. See K. Jayawardena, *Feminism and Nationalism in the Third World* (New Jersey: Zed Books Ltd. 1986); L. Ahmed, *Women and Gender in Islam: Historical Roots of a Modern Debate* (New Haven: Yale University Press, 1992).

37. Although the population field includes a fairly diverse range of organizations and individuals in the North and South, who actually lie along a fairly broad spectrum of political positions, it is possible to generalize about the theories and forces that have motivated decision makers in this field. See L. P. Freedman, "Censorship and Manipulation of Reproductive Health Information: An Issue of Human Rights and Women's Health," in *The Right to Know: Human Rights and Access to Reproductive Health Information* (London: Article 19, U. Pennsylvania Press, 1995).

38. S. C. Watkins, "If All We Knew About Women Was What We Read in *Demography,* What Would We Know?" *Demography* 30, 4 (1993): 553.

39. See C. Gilligan, *In A Different Voice: Psychological Theory and Women's Development* (Cambridge, Mass.: Harvard University Press, 1982), and also numerous studies demonstrating that, even in times of severe economic crisis, women tend to use their time and such income as they control to promote the well-being of the family over their own personal needs, whereas men often spend such resources on themselves; Commonwealth Secretariat, *Engendering Adjustment for the 1990s* in *Report of a Commonwealth Expert Group on Women and Structural Adjustment* (London: Commonwealth Secretariat, 1989); J. Leslie, M. Lycette and M. Buvinic, "Weathering Economic Crisis: The Crucial Role of Women in Health," in D. E. Bell and M. R. Reich (eds.), *Health, Nutrition and Economic Crisis: Approaches to Policy in the Third World* (Dover, Mass.: The Auburn Publishing House, 1988).

40. D. Maine, L. P. Freedman, F. Shaheed, and S. Frautschi, "Risk, Reproduction, and Rights: The Uses of Reproductive Health Data," in R. Cassen (ed.), *Population and Development: Old Debates, New Conclusions* (Washington, D.C.: Overseas Development Council, 1994); and L. P. Freedman (see note 37).

41. L. P. Freedman and S. L. Isaacs, "Human Rights and Reproductive Choice," *Studies in Family Planning* 24 (1993): 18–30.

42. Ibid.

43. Watkins (see note 38), p. 557.

44. See H. Papanek, "The Ideal Woman and the Ideal Society: Control and Autonomy in the Construction of Identity," in V. M. Moghadam (ed.), *Identity Politics and Women: Cultural Reassertions and Feminisms in International Perspective* (Boulder, CO: Westview Press, 1994).

45. For example, General Recommendation 19, issued by the committee that oversees the Convention on the Elimination of All Forms of Discrimination Against Women. See also Vienna Declaration and Programme of Action, World Conference on Human Rights, UN Doc. A/CONF.157/24 (1993).

46. For example, L. Heise, J. Pitanguy, and A. Germain, "Violence Against Women: The Hidden Health Burden," World Bank Discussion Paper no. 255 (Washington, D.C.: The World Bank, 1994).

47. "Reproductive and Sexual Health as Women's Human Rights," a workshop held by IRRRAG during the 1994 ICPD as part of the series "Human Rights Dimensions of Reproductive Health." Transcripts available from the author.

48. *Gender, Reproductive Health and Population Policies,* Reports from the Manila Workshop, 7–10 April 1994 (Quezon City, Philippines: HAIN and InDRA, 1995).

49. R. Petchesky, "The Body as Property: A Feminist Re-Vision," in F. Ginsburg and R. Rapp, *Conceiving the New World Order: The Global Politics of Reproduction* (Berkeley: University of California Press, 1995).

50. Ibid.

51. Ibid.

52. S. Greenhalgh and J. Li, "Engendering Reproductive Policy and Practice in Peasant China: For a Feminist Demography of Reproduction," *Signs* 20 (1995): 601–641.

53. Ibid., p. 636.

54. Compare, for example, the framework of biological and social determinants that has been used effectively to address infant mortality with that which should be used to address maternal mortality. W. H. Mosley and L. Chen, "An Analytical Framework for the Study of Child Survival in Developing Countries," *Population and Development Review,* supp. to vol. 10 (1984): 25–45; J. McCarthy and D. Maine, "A Framework for Analyzing the Determinants of Maternal Mortality," *Studies in Family Planning* 23(1992): 22–33.

55. L. Freedman and D. Maine, "Facing Facts: The Role of Epidemiology in Reproductive Rights Advocacy," *American University Law Review* 44 (1995): 1085–1092.

56. Mann et al. (see note 1).

57. Dutch anthropologist J. Schrijvers traces the first use of "autonomy" as a feminist concept to a 1979 seminar in Bangkok, involving mostly women from Asia and other countries of the South, where the term was put forward to describe an element of the long-term goals of feminism. Schrijvers herself later used very specific case studies in Sri Lanka to try to understand and describe the personal qualities and social configurations that allowed certain women to resist violence in domestic relationships, working from those observations to define the

elements of autonomy. J. Schrijvers, "Feminist Science and Research Philosophy: History and General Principles," in *Gender, Reproductive Health and Population Policies* (see note 48). Theoretical work in this area is also being done from a legal perspective. See, e.g., Nedelsky (see note 23).

58. See generally, S. Mahmud and A. M. Johnston, "Women's Status, Empowerment, and Reproductive Outcomes," in G. Sen, A. Germain, L. Chen (eds.), *Population Policies Reconsidered: Health Empowerment and Rights* (Cambridge, Mass.: Harvard University Press, 1994); R. Dixon-Mueller, *Population Policy and Reproductive Rights: Transforming Reproductive Choice* (Westport, CT: Praeger Publishers 1993); N. Sadik, *Investing in Women: The Focus of the 90s* (New York: United Nations Population Fund, 1991); K.O. Mason, "The Status of Women: Conceptual and Methodological Issues in Demographic Studies," *Sociological Forum* 1 (1986): 284–300; J. Caldwell and P. Caldwell, "Women's Position and Child Mortality and Morbidity in LDCs," paper presented at the Conference on Women's Position and Demographic Change in the Course of Development, Oslo, Norway, June 15–18, 1988; J. Caldwell, "Routes to Low Mortality in Poor Countries," *Population and Development Review* 12 (1986): 171–200.

Gender, Health, and Human Rights 17.

Rebecca Cook

Motherhood can take a woman to the heights of ecstasy and the depths of despair; it can offer her protection and reverence. But it can also deny a woman consideration as anything more than a vehicle for human reproduction. Women's reproductive function fits within a social framework of gender that affects women's capacities and health. While traditional cultures established laws to protect women's reproductive functions, these laws have confined women to the extent that they have been denied almost all additional and alternative opportunities to flourish as individuals and to achieve complete health in their communities and wider societies. Emphasizing that health is more than a matter of an individual's medical condition, the World Health Organization (WHO) asserts that "health is a state of complete physical, mental and social well-being and not merely the absence of disease or infirmity."[1]

It has been only recently recognized that states must address the protection and advancement of women's health interests through gender planning, to achieve not simply the abstract value of justice, but to conform to legally binding international human rights obligations as well. Gender planning concerns both practical and strategic needs of women in developing and industrialized countries.[2] Their practical needs are addressed through programs such as the Safe Motherhood Initiative, co-sponsored by several UN agencies and international nongovernmental organizations.[3] This program focuses on reducing the rates of maternal mortality, unwanted pregnancy, and sexually transmitted diseases, including HIV infection. Comparable programs address women's health and nutritional needs throughout the life cycle.[4]

Women's strategic needs transcend such practical needs, however, because they address the value of women to society—a value extending beyond motherhood and service in the home. Focusing on strategic needs promotes women's roles in such areas as the economic, political, spiritual, professional, and cultural life of communities. Most important, it opens the way to women's achievement of complete health as defined by WHO.

There is a paradox in addressing women's practical and strategic needs: those concerned with practical needs may develop concepts whose effects, and perhaps whose purpose, confine women to maternal, domestic, and subordinate social roles. This denies women's legitimate strategic needs and prevents them from flourishing to their full capacity within the family, community, and society.

This chapter addresses how the gender role in society occupied primarily by women has constrained women's growth to the detriment of their complete health. It also outlines how international human rights law obliges states to liberate women from this constraint to permit women's pursuit of health and achievement in areas of their own choice.

SEX AND GENDER

Medicine has historically used male physiology as the model for medical care, based on research studies involving exclusively men.[5] Accordingly, women have been considered only to the extent that they are different from men, focusing medical attention on reproductive characteristics.

Further, medicine progressed from being an art of human interaction to a science dominated by biological revelations achieved in laboratories. More and more, it is driven by the institutional demands of hospital-based medicine, where results of laboratory science and, more recently, medical engineering and technology can be applied. In moving the locus of their functions from the community to the laboratory and hospital, doctors have become isolated from those social realities that condition the lives and health status of their patients.

In many regions of the world, health agencies are increasingly recognizing how functions performed by community members can protect and enhance people's health, and how important it is to reassess how an individual woman's self-esteem and health status are affected by the value placed on women by her community.[6] Health professionals themselves are becoming more sensitive to the health impact of patients' social experiences. For example, the 1994 World Report on Women's Health, issued by the International Federation of Gynecology and Obstetrics, concluded that future improvements in women's health require not only improved science and health care, but also social justice for women and removal of socially and culturally conditioned barriers to women's equal opportunity.[7]

The experiences of women in their families and communities are different from those of men. The difference transcends reproductive functions, although the reproductive role of women in the creation and maintenance of families has commonly been used to justify women's subordination and denial of equal opportunity. The dominant view that women are distinguishable from men only as regards their biological constitution and reproductive role hides the profound psychological and social differences based on gender that societies have created, and that compromise women's complete health.[8]

The terms *sex* and *gender* are frequently used interchangeably. The latter is often preferred over the crude and salacious connotations of the former; but strictly speaking, the terms are different. Sex is a matter of biological differentiation, whereas gender is a social construct by which various activities and characteristics are associated with one or the other sex. For instance, leadership through success in battle is male-gendered, whereas caring for the dependent young, sick, and elderly is female-gendered. Popular imagery of leadership in, for example, politics, commerce, industry, the military, and religion is male-gendered, whereas nursing and domestic service are female-gendered. It is obvious that women can be political and industrial leaders, and that men can be caregivers, but it has been considered exceptional for people to assume a gender role at variance with their sex. Activities and characteristics are preconceived via gender stereotypes, which determine the parameters of the normal. "Masculine" behavior in women and "feminine" behavior in men have long been considered deviant. That which is normal or self-evident escapes special attention, because it is taken as the norm from which only departures are of interest. Behavior that is in accordance with conventional expectations and presuppositions of gender roles is generally unremarkable.

WOMEN'S SUBORDINATION AND EXCLUSION

In societies around the world, female-gendered status is inferior and subordinate to male-gendered status. The male protects the female through the attributes of gallantry and chivalry; he is bold in courtship, aggressive in initiative and forthcoming among peers. The female is passive, renders service in modest fulfillment of duty and offers comfort in responsive obedience. Societies have modeled their role expectations on these assumptions of the natural order of humankind. Historic social structures, including the organization and conduct of warfare, the hierarchical ordering of influential religious institutions, the attribution of political power, the authority of the judiciary, and the influences that shape the content of the law, reflect this gender difference of male dominance and female subordination.

Because women naturally tend to behave in female-gendered ways, they have been vulnerable to confinement to female status by social, political, religious and other institutions, populated exclusively by men, that act in male-gendered ways. Women have accordingly been subordinated to assume only inferior, servile social roles, and have traditionally been excluded from centers of male-gendered power by legal and other instruments. These include legislatures, military institutions, religious orders, universities, and the learned professions, including medicine. This is still the age of "first women," such as the first woman medical school dean, the first woman Supreme Court justice, and the first woman head of a medical association.

The historic subordination, silencing, and imposed inferiority of women (beginning at birth as an expendable and often unwanted girl child) has been invisible because it has been considered not simply a natural feature of society, but the very condition by which society can exist. Traditional forces emphasizing that women's "natural place" is in the home and that their natural functions in the rearing of children must always be protected cannot envisage that women can aspire to and achieve the same advances in areas of male-gendered activities as men; nor do they acknowledge that it is oppressive of women's human rights to confine them to servile functions traditionally considered natural to their sex.

It is becoming increasingly recognized that an individual's health status is determined not only by chance genetic inheritance and the geographical availability of nutritional resources, but also by socioeconomic factors.[9] Relatively affluent people, and those content with their lives, enjoy better health status than impoverished, frustrated, and oppressed people who suffer disrespect in their communities and poor self-image. The determinants of earned income, including education, literacy, employment opportunities and, for instance, financial credit for launching income initiatives, all show how women have been disadvantaged by their inferior gender role. Even within affluent families, women have often suffered frustrations—through male preference in inheritance, education preceding marriage, and training to occupy positions of influence and power within their communities. Women have been denied a commitment of family resources for these opportunities in the belief that upon marriage they will attenuate association with their own families (reflected, for example, in their shedding family names) and will assume a role of service within their husbands' families.

Complex social dynamics have produced a modern reality, common to communities across the full spectrum of economic and industrial development, of women being primary or sole economic supports of their families, and also being unmarried, widowed, or abandoned mothers of their children. Women's unequal opportunities to participate in the resources and well-being of their communities and to contribute to political, economic, spiritual, and related leadership has a serious impact. It deprives those families that financially depend on women of equal opportunities for well-being, and it robs women themselves of the economic, psychological, and social determinants of health. Women's vulnerability to sexual subordination through the greater physical, military, and social force of men produces harmful health consequences in women extending beyond pain, indignity, unwanted pregnancy, and venereal infection.

HOW HEALTH PROFESSIONS HAVE CONSTRUCTED WOMEN

Members of the health professions have done much to mitigate the health consequences of women's gendered disadvantage. They have cared for the distressed and violated, relieved physical pain, and eased women through unwanted and, at times, violently imposed pregnancy. As participants in traditional communities, however, undertaking the male-gendered functions of decision-making and leadership, doctors have tended to share prevailing perceptions of women's natural role and exhibit blindness toward women's gender-specific health risks. Indeed, in the past, doctors have considered women constitutionally unsuited to political, commercial, and professional life, prone to swoon under stress and to require nine months of bed rest while pregnant.

When society blamed women for resorting to prostitution as a means of economic maintenance while denying them alternative opportunities to support themselves and their families, doctors, among others, promoted the image of women as vectors of disease. Accordingly, when, for instance, victorious soldiers returned to the United States between 1918 and 1920, eighteen thousand women—alleged to be prostitutes—were detained in a medically supported governmental initiative, for fear that they would spread venereal infection.[10] Women's image as vectors of disease to sexual partners and to children they conceive has been recycled in the modern pandemic of AIDS.[11]

In many parts of the world, medicine retains marks of its gendered practice, for instance in placing women under the patriarchal control of men and others who exercise male-gendered authority. For example, in some countries, a woman's request for health care is accepted only with the express authorization of her husband.[12] Women's requests for control over their reproduction have so threatened male dominance of women's fertility that birth control and voluntary sterilization were condemned until recently as crimes against morality.[13] Voluntary abortion remains a major point of contention almost universally within institutions of traditional power, which are male-gendered. Whether it is discriminatory and socially unconscionable to criminalize a medical procedure that only women need is a question that usually goes not simply unanswered but unasked.

MEDICINE SERVING THE STATUS QUO

By focusing its attention on the distress of individual women in clinical settings, medicine in general and psychiatry in particular have inadvertently served as agents of the continued subordination and oppression of women.[14] Women have suffered feelings of ill health and emotional dissonance with family and community as a reaction to denial of equal opportunities to seek their own achievements and their confinement to seeking satisfaction in the care of children, the sick, and the dependent. Health professionals have conscientiously looked for physiological and psychiatric causes of maladjustment in patients' lives, and for other medical reasons for unhappiness and discontent.[15] Illness alone was used to explain women's unhappiness in the midst of affluence and caring family members, a situation that by conventional standards should produce contentedness.

One effect of modern feminist sensitivity has been to expose feelings of frustration and anger as being not unnatural reactions to natural conditions but natural, healthy reactions to social injustice. By diagnosing women's discontent and "disorders" as medical problems, physicians have reinforced and perpetuated the injustice of the prevailing social order, which prejudices women's health, rather than acting as instruments of remedy.

Medicine has a history of paternalism. Patients have been infantilized and denied social status, for example, by being called by their first names and presumed incapable of exercising informed choice among treatment options. A legal recognition of only recent evolution is that treatment choices are not to be medically dictated, but are to be medically informed personal choices made by patients as acts of self-determination. Physicians are increasingly required by law to afford patients respect as equals—capable of and responsible for making critical life decisions—by providing them the medical information they need to fully exercise choice.

However, while meeting this objective standard of medical disclosure, doctors must recognize how women's experiences in female-gendered roles have affected their medical histories and health prospects. The critical transition is from doctors treating women as inferior to men, physiologically different only in reproductive functions, to recognizing women as equal to men, different only because of the gendered experiences that affect their health.

As the health care system moves from a biomedical model of practice to a health promotion model, health professionals must meet the challenge and opportunity of reshaping their understanding of how women's experiences affect health. Restoration of health in reaction to illness and dysfunction can no longer concentrate only on the sciences, including physiology, biology, chemistry, and pharmacology. At the clinical level, these disciplines are essentially impersonal and neutral to the social, political, and environmental conditions that influence health. When health professionals concentrate on promoting health rather than just treating disease and dysfunction, they are compelled to consider the social, economic, and, for instance, environmental determinants of health. They must confront, among other influences, gender-based discrimination that denies women opportunities for achieving physical and mental health.[16]

Clinically trained health professionals enhance their diagnostic and therapeutic capacities via recognition of the links between women's health status and the social environments they inhabit. Their knowledge about gender-based vulnerabilities to, for example, domestic violence and unwanted pregnancy, and their awareness of gender-based social constraints on career ambitions, will educate health professionals about the many factors beyond clinical services that contribute to women's health. As health professionals come to realize the extent to which health is compromised as a result of gender discrimination, they may turn to human rights principles and instruments in order to find ways in which discrimination may be remedied or even prevented.

THE DEVELOPMENT OF HUMAN RIGHTS

The function of modern human rights is to redress the imbalance between society's privileged and unempowered members.[17] Countries may now be held to international account for internal policies, practices, and failures of public intervention by which an individual's human dignity is violated. It usually falls to the weak and vulnerable of a society, and to those who advocate on their behalf, to invoke inherent human rights for the protection and promotion of their interests. Similarly, those who enjoy the privilege of power and protection resist challenges to their conventional authority. While at times sympathetic to rights rhetoric that may advance their own claims to entitlement, the privileged often resist service to rights that requires them to yield or share their privilege, observe duties related to rights, or support action that would reduce their privilege to no more than the rights that are shared by all others.

The United Nations was founded in 1945 on principles of respect for individual human rights, and it paid tribute to its inspiration in its 1948 Universal Declaration of Human Rights. Postwar reconstruction and the Cold War preoccupied much of the early UN work to advance human rights. Rights of sexual equality were submerged in efforts against colonialism, of relieving the plight of refugees and of resisting apartheid. General international human rights conventions that gave legal substance to the Universal Declaration, namely, the International Covenant on Civil and Political Rights, and the International Covenant on Economic, Social and Cultural Rights, condemned sexual discrimination in only nominal terms. The several related regional human rights conventions were no more vigorously applied in this area.

It was not until 1966 that the UN adopted the International Convention on the Elimination of Racial Discrimination. The move to advance women's equality was more prolonged, because violations of women's rights were not as visible to male authorities as those suffered on racial grounds. However, one of the most dynamic perceptions of the late twentieth century has been growing recognition of the unjust exclusion, oppression, and subordination of women through gender stereotyping practiced by such reputable institutions as, for instance, democratic governments, organized religions, and higher education, as well as such professions as medicine and law.

In 1979, the UN adopted the Convention on the Elimination of All Forms of Discrimination Against Women (the Women's Convention), and ratifications brought the convention into legal effect with unusual speed. The convention is currently ratified by at least 140 countries, although it remains subject to such extensive exceptions of applicability by some ratifying states that it is legitimate to ask whether, by tests of international treaty law, these states are truly parties.[18] Nevertheless, the Women's Convention reinforces previous general and regional human rights conventions and provides language to express those specific and binding entitlements to respect for individual dignity that constitute the human rights of women.

The points at which women's social inequality and negative stereotyping can be demonstrated are recognized more and more. Modern analysis has shown systemic denial and suppression of information concerning women's victimization by violence and rape in their homes.[19] In fact, rape has been recharacterized by feminist scholarship not as a sexual act perpetrated by force, but as a violent act perpetrated through sex.[20] Certain countries, including Canada, now grant refugee status to women fleeing their countries due to a well-founded fear that they or their daughters will be circumcised.[21] Sexual abuse in military conflict has been exposed as an act of dominance against women that amounts to torture. Additionally, it is often intended as a means of aggression towards men, who consider the chastity and sexual availability of women in their communities to be their exclusive possession. Recently the Inter-American Commission on Human Rights, in a report on the situation of human rights under the administration of Raoul Cedras, determined that the rape and abuse of Haitian women constituted violations of their rights to be free from torture and inhuman and degrading treatment, and their right to liberty and security of the person.[22]

HUMAN RIGHTS RELATING TO WOMEN'S HEALTH

The International Covenant on Economic, Social and Cultural Rights explicitly names the right to the highest attainable standard of health and to enjoyment of the benefits of scientific progress. But because the determinants of health, including socioeconomic status and the capacity to realize reasonable life ambitions, are multifaceted, most if not all named human rights contribute in differing degrees to the protection and promotion of health.[23] In its preamble, the Women's Convention observes that the need for this separate legal instrument to reinforce the sexual nondiscrimination provisions of previous international conventions arises from the concern that "despite these various instruments, extensive discrimination against women continues to exist." It goes on to state that "in situations of poverty, women have the least access to food, health, education, training and opportunities for employment and other needs." By Article 12(1) of the Women's Convention, states parties agree that they will "take all appropriate measures to eliminate discrimination against women in the field of health care in order to ensure, on a basis of equality of men and women, access to health care services, including those related to family planning."

Promotion of women's health depends upon the interaction of most if not all human rights. Rights relevant to health include those to protect women's employment and grant equal pay for work of equal value; to education; to information; and to political participation, influence, and democratic power within legislatures. These last rights permit women's rights to be respected in the general conduct of states.

In international and regional human rights conventions, the common prohibition of discrimination on grounds of sex has not been applied to condemn discrimination on grounds of gender. Elimination of sexual discrimination alone would bring women's status closer to that of men and afford women the means that men enjoy to protect and advance their health. However, the wider health disadvantage that women suffer on grounds of gender must be tackled. Further, it must be based not only on the biological difference between the sexes, but on socially structured gender differences that compromise women's achievement of "the highest attainable standard of health." By Article 5(1) of the Women's Convention, states parties agree to deconstruct gender discrimination by taking appropriate measures to modify the social and cultural patterns of conduct of men and women. This is agreed upon with a view toward eliminating prejudices and customary and all other practices based on the inferiority or superiority of either sex or on stereotyped roles for men and women.

Women's poor physical and psychological health may represent a metaphor for the poor health of women's rights in the body politic and in influential community institutions, whether political, economic, religious, or health care. Application of human rights law may provide a remedy that results in improvements in women's health status. While this legal application faces formidable challenges, these challenges are increasingly being addressed by developments in legal doctrine.

LEGAL APPROACHES TO APPLY HUMAN RIGHTS TO HEALTH

Human rights law makes an important distinction between *negative* and *positive* rights. Of the two, negative rights are more easily applied, as they require states to do nothing but permit individuals to pursue their own preferences. In fact, states have not trusted women to make decisions affecting their own lives; rather, they have encumbered those women pursuing reproductive and other health interests with burdens, conditions, and, at times, ferocious penalties.

Male-gendered institutions of government, religion, and the health professions have justified intervention in women's reproductive self-determination by invoking their own principles of public order, morality, and public health. Laws have been developed in many countries that punish women, and those who assist them, for resorting to contraception or abortion, and women's access to health examinations and services have been made dependent upon authorization by husbands and fathers. Women's negative human rights require that states remove all such barriers to women's pursuit of their health interests, except for those governing safety and efficacy of health services in general.

Positive rights require more of states—even amounting in some cases to social reconstruction. For example, the Colombian Ministry of Health's interpretation of the Women's Convention led it to introduce a gender perspective into national health policies. These policies consider "the social discrimination of women as an element which contributes to the ill-health of women."[24] One ministerial resolution orders health institutions to respect women's decisions on all issues that affect their health, lives, and sexuality, and to respect rights "to information and orientation to allow the exercise of free, gratifying, responsible sexuality which cannot be tied to maternity."[25]

Human rights regarding health require that the state provide health care that individuals are not able to obtain or provide on their own. This includes clinic and hospital-based services dependent on specialized skills of health care professionals, surgical interventions, and medical technologies. It also includes less sophisticated means, such as the supply of routine antibiotics and contraceptives that require little more than minimum counseling, nursing, and pharmaceutical services.

Positive rights may be difficult to observe in states with strained resources. However, it is a notorious fact that states invoking poverty to justify nonobservance of duties to defend women's health often provide disproportionately large military budgets. This is consistent with male-gendered perceptions of a population's needs.

Epidemiological data can be used to show how human rights can be made relevant to women's health. For example, international law has not yet developed the right to life beyond the duty to apply due process of law in cases of capital punishment. The right to life has not been invoked on behalf of the estimated half-million women annually who die of pregnancy-related causes because of lack of appropriate care.[26] Supplying appropriate care for women may be characterized as a duty of positive human rights to which states must allocate resources. An estimated two hundred thousand of these deaths are due to unsafe abortion alone.[27] Health indications for abortion include pregnancies that come too early, too late, too frequently, and too closely spaced. Permitting women access to qualified health personnel willing to perform the procedure is a negative human right that states are increasingly recognizing. The challenge remains of requiring states to satisfy the positive duty of providing qualified services when women have no access to them on their own.

Feminist legal analysis exposes further areas of human rights observance to which states can be held. A distinction is commonly drawn between public and private law. Typically, the state engages its machinery for public law concerns such as governmental administration and maintenance of public order but excludes itself from such private law matters as family relationships and functioning. Feminists identify domestic violence, discrimination against female children, women's exclusion from family inheritance, and demands for husbands' authorization of wives' medical care as oppression and subordination. They point out that these impair women's health but are not observed and remedied by the state.[28] In many countries, laws excluded husbands from liability for rape of their wives until recently, while these laws are still maintained in others. Feminist theories show how such male-gendered laws are structured and enforced at a cost to women's health. Similarly, laws permitting younger marriage of girls than boys promote the stereotyping of women in childbearing and service roles, and exclude them from the education and training that boys receive to fulfill their masculine destiny as family and social leaders.

CONCLUSION

Recognition of gender stereotyping exposes the underlying social conditions that compromise women's health. International human rights law requires state action to remove stereotyping that negatively affects women's status and health. Further, it justifies individual and nongovernmental organization initiatives both to assist states in conforming to the law and to hold states accountable for their failures.

Achieving respect for each person's right to the highest attainable standard of health is in itself an important goal of international law, but that right is interdependent with many other human rights. Good health is the precondition to individuals' exercise of rights to equal participation in communal and social life. At the same time, an individual's capacity for participation in activities of their choice enhances their health status.

REFERENCES

1. Constitution of the World Health Organization, signed July 22, 1946, and entered into force on April 7, 1948, in *Basic Documents*, 39th ed. (Geneva: World Health Organization, 1993).
2. C. O. N. Moser, "Gender Planning in the Third World: Meeting Practical and Strategic Needs," *World Development* 17 (1989): 1799–1825.
3. See, generally, T. Turman, C. AbouZahr, and M. Koblinsky (eds.), "Reproductive Health: The MotherCare Experience," *International Journal of Gynecology and Obstetrics* 48, supp. (1995).
4. See, generally, World Bank, *A New Agenda for Women's Health and Nutrition* (Washington, D.C.: World Bank, 1994).
5. A. C. Mastroianni, R. Faden, and D. Federman, *Women and Health Research*, 2 vols. (Washington, D.C.: National Academy Press, 1994).
6. R. de los Rios, "Gender, Health, and Development: An Approach in the Making," in *Gender, Women, and Health in the Americas* (Washington, D.C.: Pan American Health Organization, 1993), pp. 3–17.
7. M. F. Fathalla, "Women's Health: An Overview," *International Journal of Gynecological Obstetrics* 46 (1994): 105–118.
8. C. Gilligan, *In a Different Voice: Psychological Theory and Women's Development* (Cambridge, Mass.: Harvard University Press, 1982).
9. J. S. Stein, *Empowerment and Women's Health: A New Framework* (London: Zed Press, 1996).
10. A. M. Brandt, *No Magic Bullet: A Social History of Venereal Disease* (New York: Oxford University Press, 1985).
11. G. Seidel, "The Competing Discourses of HIV/AIDS in Sub-Saharan Africa: Discourses of Rights and Empowerment v. Discourses of Control and Exclusion," *Social Science and Medicine* 36 (1993): 175–194.
12. R. J. Cook and D. Maine, "Spousal Veto Over Family Planning Services," *American Journal of Public Health* 77 (1987): 339–344.
13. On Canada, see B. M. Dickens, *Medico-Legal Aspects of Family Law* (Toronto: Butterworths, 1979), p. 28.
14. V. Franks and E. D. Rothblum (eds.), *The Stereotyping of Women: Its Effects on Mental Health* (New York: Springer Publishing Co., 1983).
15. E. D. Rothblum, "Sex-Role Stereotypes and Depression in Women," in V. Franks and E. D. Rothblum, *The Stereotyping of Women: Its Effects on Mental Health* (New York: Springer Publishing Co., 1983), pp. 83–111.

16. N. Lewis, S. Huyer, B. Hettel, and L. Marsden, *Safe Womanhood: A Discussion Paper* (Toronto: Gender, Science and Development Programme, The International Federation of Institutes for Advanced Study, 1994).

17. R. Dworkin, *Taking Rights Seriously* (Cambridge, Mass.: Harvard University Press, 1977).

18. R. J. Cook, "Reservations to the Convention on the Elimination of All Forms of Discrimination Against Women," *Virginia Journal of International Law* 30 (1990): 645–716.

19. Human Rights Watch, *Criminal Injustice: Violence Against Women in Brazil* (New York: Human Rights Watch, 1991).

20. S. Brownmiller, *Against Our Will: Men, Women and Rape* (New York: Simon and Schuster, 1975).

21. C. Farnsworth, "Canada Gives a Somali Refuge from Genital Rite," *New York Times*, July 21, 1994.

22. OEA/Ser.L/V/II.88, February 9, 1995: 12–13, 39–47, 93–97.

23. R. J. Cook, *Women's Health and Human Rights* (Geneva: World Health Organization, 1994).

24. M. I. Plata, "Reproductive Rights as Human Rights: The Colombian Case," in R. J. Cook (ed.), *Human Rights of Women: National and International Perspectives* (Philadelphia: University of Pennsylvania Press, 1994), pp. 515–531.

25. Ibid.

26. C. AbouZahr and E. Royston, *Maternal Mortality: A Global Factbook* (Geneva: World Health Organization, 1991), p. 1.

27. World Health Organization, *Coverage of Maternity Care: A Tabulation of Available Information*, 3rd ed. (Geneva: World Health Organization, WHO/FHE/MSM/93.7, 1993), p. 12.

28. S. Goonesekere, *Women's Rights and Children's Rights: The United Nations Conventions as Compatible and Complementary International Treaties* (Florence: UNICEF, 1992).

Health, Human Rights, and Lesbian Existence

18.

Alice M. Miller, AnnJanette Rosga,
and Meg Satterthwaite

When [my parents] found out that I was a lesbian, they tried to force me to find a boyfriend, but I could not fit in with what they wanted. . . . My parents decided to look for a husband on my behalf so they brought several boys home to meet me but I was not interested so in the end they forced an old man on me. They locked me in a room and brought him every day to rape me so I would fall pregnant and be forced to marry him. They did this to me until I was pregnant, after which they told me I was free to do whatever I wanted but that I must go and stay with this man or else they would throw me out of the house. They did throw me out eventually. . . . I did not contact them for six months. The police were looking for me so I used to move during the night only. In the end, the police found me and took me home where I was locked up and beaten until I could not even lift my arms or get up.[1]

The treatment began with three weeks of sleep therapy. Then I had three sessions of analysis. . . . They carried me on a stretcher, in a wheelchair, and finally kicking and screaming, because the psychiatrist decided they would have to give me shock treatment. . . . Meanwhile, there were drug treatments . . . hot and cold baths, etc. . . . The psychiatrist, always very aggressively . . . taught me what it meant to be a homosexual: to suffer a lot, to be wretched. . . . His treatment consisted [in part] of . . . injections to induce nausea. . . . I spent long hours in an armchair with him projecting slides. They were women undressed. . . . I came to see it with hatred instead of naturally. I started saying exactly what he wanted to hear.[2]

As can be seen from the examples above, the "health" issues faced by lesbians are often inextricable from their most basic human rights. Yet, having been invited to contribute this commentary on lesbian health and human rights, we find ourselves faced with a rather extraordinary challenge. In the

United States and in a few other countries such as Canada and the United Kingdom, lesbian *health* movements have begun to appear. Simultaneously, there have emerged several successful international demands for gay (and lesbian) *human rights* in the past decade. We have not, however, been successful in our search for scholarly literatures, grassroots movements, or legal argumentation that specifically combine the concept of lesbian health with the call for lesbian human rights, or that identify health *as* a human right for lesbians.

This chapter represents our attempt to initiate such a conversation. In the following pages we will briefly sketch out some of the obstacles to, and potential locations for, a lesbian right to health. We will focus primarily on the issue (and absence) of lesbian health within current human rights norms, rather than, for instance, on how human rights standards might be brought to bear upon lesbian health movements in particular countries or contexts.[3]

To begin our discussion, it must be noted that health itself is a fraught location for lesbians. Indeed, for lesbians, "'health' has often been a site of oppression."[4] In the United States and Europe, "lesbians were said to harbor the same sickness and evil found in gay men; however, several medical theories warned of even greater danger associated with female homosexuality."[5] Given a history in which lesbianism has been defined as an illness in need of treatment, it might be said that "lesbian health" is something of an oxymoron. Moreover, some of these "treatments" could themselves be described as direct attacks on lesbian health and human rights. For instance, in the United States, as in other countries, treatments for lesbianism have included "psychiatric confinement, electroshock treatment, genital mutilation, aversive therapy, psychosurgery, hormonal injection, psychoanalysis, and psychotropic chemotherapy."[6]

It is crucial that we challenge the medicalization of lesbians; however, it is also clear that lesbian well-being depends upon the articulation and recognition of a whole-person analysis that takes into account the dynamics of individual and social relations, as well as basic human needs for "peace, shelter, education, food, income, a stable eco-system, sustainable resources, social justice, and equity."[7] Indeed, the Institute of Medicine's definition of public health suggests the elements, both material and political, to be included in any dynamic construction of lesbian well-being: "Public health is what we as a society do collectively to ensure conditions in which people can be healthy."[8] By allowing a whole-person analysis, the health and human rights paradigm may offer lesbians a way to articulate rights claims while avoiding some of the pitfalls that have plagued lesbians' appearance in the few human rights frameworks in which they have been marginally included thus far. It is our contention that the field of health and human rights could become a particularly useful one for lesbians.

However, although strategies for achieving a human right to health may indeed hold special promise for lesbians, recent efforts within this new field—for complex historical and political reasons—have tended to focus on issues not central to lesbians' lives. This chapter examines the intersection of emerging paradigms of health and human rights with two other critical human rights movements: women's human rights and the human rights of homosexuals. We conclude that within international frameworks defining a woman's right to health, reproductive health has played a predominant role, and when discussions of health and human rights have addressed homosexuality, they have tended to focus on the explosive conjunction of AIDS and discrimination in the lives of gay men. While neither reproductive health nor HIV is irrelevant for lesbians around the world, an explicit focus on lesbians requires us to interrogate the ways in which existing frameworks may preclude our ability to name strategies more conducive to a full range of protections for lesbian health.

A discussion of lesbian health and human rights should not proceed without mentioning two crucial obstacles within international human rights frameworks that have been particularly cumbersome for lesbians attempting to articulate their human rights. The first analytical difficulty has been described in feminist critiques of international human rights law. This critique has called attention to the fact that human rights norms focus on the public sphere as the locus of protected rights, yet women also traditionally face great obstacles and violations in the private spheres of family and home.[9] This problem is linked to the absence of developed systems of international state accountability for violations of human rights by domestic non-state actors as well as for violations resulting from the policies and practices of international financial institutions and transnational corporations. "By focusing almost exclusively on the behavior of government actors rather than private parties, human rights advocates have tended to exclude numerous aspects of women's lives—and lesbians' lives in particular—from international scrutiny."[10]

Secondly, as the universal nature of human rights is one of the most powerful aspects of their claim to legitimacy and respect, any articulation of lesbian claims to these rights must answer to what may appear to be contradictory claims to particularity and cross-cultural relevance. "Not only do individuals who engage in same-sex practices have differing perceptions of their homosexual identity which are linked to their culture, but lesbians have needs and objectives for human rights law that are often distinct from those of gay men."[11] In an international context, especially, the meaning of *lesbian* is far from transparent. Further, converging with the first difficulty, existing models for understanding identities such as lesbian have largely relied upon the expression of those identities through actions in the public sphere. Since women in many areas have had limited access to a public sphere, models of identity that rely upon public expression may preclude the "appearance" of lesbians in international human rights discourse.

With our use of the term *lesbian* in this chapter, we do not want to assume that a lesbian identity or orientation—that is, a sustained affectional and sexual identification with other women—is uniformly present across cultures.[12] Nonetheless, women who are identified by state or private actors as "deviant" because of their same-sex relationships may be stoned to death, raped, forced into marriage, or denied housing, jobs, or education despite their apparent lack of a public lesbian identity.[13] We wish to extend our analysis to include such women regardless of whether they are explicitly understood to be lesbians.[14]

ENGENDERING HUMAN RIGHTS: LESBIANS AS WOMEN

The goal of putting women on the human rights agenda has entailed painstaking review of existing human rights norms and standards in all areas—civil, political, social, cultural, and economic. Some of these strategies have focused on the application of sex-based antidiscrimination norms to rights within existing human rights treaties; others attempt to reconceptualize human rights norms or to integrate gender perspectives into existing institutions.[15]

One of the most critical aspects of the international women's rights movement has been its development of a gender-specific notion of discrimination within international human rights standards. "Discrimination" is defined by the Women's Convention and elaborated by the Committee on the Elimination of Discrimination Against Women (CEDAW) to address issues of great concern to women such as violence and the right to equality within the family.[16] However, CEDAW has as yet addressed only a few particular aspects of women's right to health, for example, discrimination against women in the context of HIV/AIDS, education concerning the health effects of "female circumcision," and issues involving family planning and reproductive choice.[17] The value of the Women's Convention's construction of nondiscrimination for lesbians has yet to be explored, although theoretically it might allow for review of laws and practices that discriminate against lesbians *as women* in public life and private spheres such as employment, family, and health care.

From the Women's Convention definition of discrimination comes, in part, the recognition of violence against women—including its adverse health effects—as a human rights concern. Indeed, the recognition that violence is a public health issue has been internationally accepted in the context of women's rights, and represents perhaps the most useful arena in which to seek protections for lesbian health.[18] The Declaration on the Elimination of Violence Against Women, adopted in December of 1993 by the UN General Assembly, defines violence occurring in the family, in the community, or "perpetrated or condoned by the State" as a violation of human rights.[19] By recognizing that violence against women violates, impairs, or nullifies the enjoyment of their human rights and fundamental freedoms, the declaration uniquely addresses "physical, sexual, and psychological violence" in public *and* private life.

The declaration would appear to be an especially promising site for the protection of lesbians, who often face violence in their families and communities, and for whom legal systems for protection or redress are inaccessible or nonresponsive. As yet, violence that targets women because of their homosexual practices, or something that might be called their "sexual identity" or "orientation" (whether committed in the name of "medical treatment" or in the course of other forms of torture), has not been addressed by international human rights mechanisms or bodies. However, recent attention to *sexual* violence begins to indirectly suggest the possibility of an articulation of bodily integrity that includes the protection of sexual identity and/or expression.[20]

Finally, the preparatory processes leading up to the Fourth World Conference on Women in Beijing have provided a setting for some of the first sustained lobbying campaigns for recognition of sexuality as an axis of women's personhood. An international network of lesbian activists and supportive organizations has contributed to official delegation submissions to the draft of the Platform for Action stating the need to end "discrimination on the grounds of sexual orientation."[21] Also included in the draft is recognition of sexual orientation as a factor akin to "race, language, ethnicity, culture, religion ... disability, socio-economic class" or status as migrant or refugee women.[22] However, there are only three references to sexual orientation, all "bracketed," throughout a document that addresses such varied areas of concern as the burden of poverty on women, unequal access to education, inequalities in health care and services, violence against women, armed conflict, inequality between women and men in decision-making, access to economic structures, and women and the environment.[24]

WOMEN'S HUMAN RIGHTS, WOMEN'S HEALTH: (HETERO)SEXUALITY AND REPRODUCTION

The women's international health movement has emerged from a creative and dynamic collaboration among health professionals and activists, human rights activists, and legal scholars. It is broadly international in rhetoric, if not yet fully international in reality, and it is committed to elucidating the connections between women's right to health and the construction of gender in family and society.[24] It has also devoted itself to the critical examination of institutionalized distinctions between public and private life and the nature of state obligations in relation to nonstate actors.

The field of women's human right to health has included attention to three aspects of the interrelation of human rights and health.[25] First, there has been a particularly sustained focus on family planning programs and public health policies governing reproduction and their assumptions about, and effects on, women's roles in various societies. Second, there has been a reexamination of human rights violations as direct hazards to women's *health*, as well as an effort to broaden the interpretation of existing human rights law to include gender-specific violations. There has been increasing recognition that violence, sexual violence in particular, violates human rights to bodily integrity and privacy, and that these abuses have disastrous effects on women's ability to enjoy their human right to health. Third, international women's rights advocates recognized early that a woman's social, economic, and political status is inextricably linked to her health.[26]

Despite this rich and varied set of interventions, however, the call for women's human right to health has achieved most attention and controversy at the international level in relation to reproductive health. As a result, the gendered impacts of health concerns such as anemia, tuberculosis, and occupational health have been overshadowed by debates about sexual and reproductive health and, in turn, concepts of sexual health have been defined to a large degree in relationship to reproductive health.

The link between sexual and reproductive health has derived in part from the success of women's rights advocates in forcing the dual recognition that women's human rights must take into account not only civil and political rights, but also social and economic rights, and that women's equality with men in all spheres is intimately related to their sexual and reproductive freedom. This success has combined synergistically with global concern over population growth and recently led to an important consensus at the Cairo International Conference on Population and Development. The Cairo Conference's Programme for Action notes a significant connection between sexuality and equality in gender relations: "Human sexuality and gender relations are closely interrelated and together affect the ability of men and women to achieve and maintain sexual health and manage their reproductive lives."[27]

While recognition that women's reproductive rights are dependent upon equality with men is certainly useful, it has also, unfortunately, continued the conflation between reproductive and sexual rights.[28] A similar conflation can be seen even in the more promising articulation of sexual rights that appeared in a preparatory draft of the Beijing Platform for Action. In "bracketed" language, the draft's section on health defines sexual rights as "includ[ing] the individual's right to have control over and decide freely in matters relating to her or his sexuality, free of coercion, discrimination and violence."[29] While this language is encouraging for lesbians, the right is contained by the context of heterosexual relations. The next and final sentence of the paragraph again links sexual rights with reproduction: "Equal relationships between women and men in matters of sexual relations and reproduction . . . require mutual consent and willingness to accept responsibility for the consequences of sexual behavior."[30]

By linking sexual rights to heterosexual couples' reproductive rights, lesbians are effectively excluded. For lesbians, sexual rights and reproductive rights, while both important, require conceptual frameworks that do not conflate the two. While lesbians have reproductive health concerns, and certainly face problems stemming from gender inequality, connecting one to the other will not address the most significant health or human rights concerns faced by lesbians.

Some of these health concerns have begun to be named at national levels; reviews of the English-language literature reveal that there is a small but growing body of medical and public health work addressing lesbian health.

These studies tend to discuss two factors negatively affecting lesbians' right to health in the countries they address: systemic barriers to effective health care services such as heterosexism, homophobia, or inadequate research on issues such as breast and cervical cancers in the context of lesbian health; and specific health problems manifested by lesbians, such as alcoholism, suicide, or mental and physical effects of homophobia, externally manifested and/or internalized.[31] Such studies are obviously limited in their international applicability, as they rely both upon Western constructions of identity and personhood and upon particular assumptions about the available systems of medical care. Both cross-cultural and cross-disciplinary research integrating human rights analyses with discussion of the conditions necessary for lesbian health—at home, in the workplace, in communities—have yet to be done.

BREAKING THE SILENCE: LESBIANS AS HOMOSEXUALS

Over the last fifteen years, important strides have been taken toward fulfilling the promise that all human rights should apply to all people. The movement for the human rights of homosexuals has rested on the understanding that gay rights are not "special rights" separate from "general" human rights; instead they require the application of general human rights norms without heterosexual bias.[32] Through a range of strategies, especially via legal challenges to sodomy statutes, this understanding has been upheld; a few key regional and international legal decisions and some first steps by mainstream human rights nongovernmental organizations demonstrate that the human rights of homosexuals have found an early voice in some fora.

The idea that lesbian and gay rights are an integral part of international human rights has been most widely accepted in Europe. The two most successful strategies have built upon protection of the rights to privacy and nondiscrimination.[33] While it may seem that protecting the human right to privacy would be a progressive step for lesbians who, as we have noted, may not have a strong "public" identity, the principle has not yet been explicitly extended to cover the right to privacy for lesbians.[34] Thus far, the three successful cases have dealt only with laws prohibiting male homosexual conduct.[35]

The seemingly more promising strategy for gay rights—the right to nondiscrimination on the basis of "other status" or sex—has been less widely accepted. The proscription of discrimination against minorities has achieved special prominence in Europe; it is a well-developed strategy for other statuses and identities in the international arena (e.g., race, ethnicity, religion, sex, or status as a refugee, a child, an indigenous person, or a member of a linguistic minority).[36] On the other hand, it has raised particular obstacles to the assertion of a whole-person analysis, one that does not parse the individual into isolated and independently affected identity fragments. If homosexuals wish to assert their right to live free from antigay discrimination, will they need a new convention definitively articulating homosexuality as a transnational identity (akin to the Convention on the Elimination of

All Forms of Racial Discrimination, the Convention on the Rights of the Child, the Convention Concerning Indigenous and Tribal Peoples, or the Women's Convention)? Problems with such an approach are manifold (not least, the reduction of an individual to his or her sexual behavior) and are quickly glimpsed when one considers how this strategy might affect lesbians. In the brief history of international attempts to protect homosexual rights, sexual orientation has been discussed apart from gender. Without specific attention to gender as an axis both of identity and oppression, the "lesbian" in lesbian and gay rights has tended to disappear.[37]

Recently, the right to nondiscrimination has gained a unique international hearing in a case combining this principle with the right to privacy for homosexuals. In *Toonen* v. *Australia*, a petition reviewed in the spring of 1994 before the United Nations Human Rights Committee, Tasmanian statutes that criminalized homosexual sodomy were found to violate both the right to privacy and the right to nondiscrimination protected by the International Covenant on Civil and Political Rights (ICCPR).[38] But the *Toonen* decision foregrounds the critical paradox confronting advocates for gay and lesbian human rights. Its strength lies in the fact that it interprets an existing international human rights covenant to *include* prohibition of discrimination based on sexual orientation, thus implicitly assuming that sexual orientation is an aspect of the totality of an individual's makeup. This would seem to suggest that the additional and problematic step of explicitly drafting, for instance, a nondiscrimination convention to protect homosexuals is unnecessary. Without an explicit statement from an authoritative body guaranteeing nondiscrimination based on sexual orientation, however, the future of homosexual antidiscrimination claims is tenuous at best.[39]

A third strategy, one that aims to protect homosexuals from state-sponsored violence such as torture, ill-treatment, and extrajudicial execution has perhaps been the most prominent in international arenas.[40] It has proceeded most smoothly because it addresses harms traditionally recognized by international human rights instruments: violations of civil and political rights by state actors. For the same reason, it leaves lesbians unprotected against many types of abuse. While lesbians do sometimes face traditional human rights violations, the limited information we possess about lesbians in different countries would seem to indicate that they are especially vulnerable to abuses in the private sphere by nonstate actors.[41]

HOMOSEXUALITY AND THE RIGHT TO HEALTH

Although the AIDS pandemic has proven to be a crucial arena for the developing field of health and human rights, especially in the context of gay men struggling against discriminatory practices and violence targeted at them, it has obscured more than it has clarified in regard to lesbian health needs.[42] Lesbians have a special status in demands for human rights in the face of HIV/AIDS: one that marginally includes lesbians in legal victories but also obfuscates the realities of lesbians' lives as distinct from those of gay men.

Discrimination against groups perceived to be "carriers" of HIV has been a constant in the pandemic. In many parts of the world, the spread of HIV has been associated primarily with gay men. This has led to discrimination and human rights violations against men who are, or who are perceived to be, homosexual. "Gay men are often considered to be 'AIDS carriers,' and as a result, may be subjected to ill-treatment at the hands of government authorities. In addition, activists who are working to prevent the spread of the AIDS virus in gay communities may be targeted for human rights abuses."[43] Although attention has focused principally on gay men, in some instances lesbians, because of their homosexuality, have been similarly labeled as "carriers" of HIV.[44]

Ironically, human rights abuses such as these have indirectly led to some of the first legal victories for the protection of homosexuals from discrimination. In the *Toonen* decision discussed above, the Tasmanian state government had defended the Tasmanian statute proscribing male same-sex sexual activity by arguing that it served as a public health measure against AIDS. The Human Rights Committee "openly acknowledge[d] the anomaly of using criminal sanctions to prevent the spread of HIV infection," and called on the Australian government to repeal the law.[45] This victory and others like it have the potential to protect lesbians as well as gay men, but, as we have tried to show, such protection will be far from automatic.

A second consequence of the association of HIV/AIDS with gay men has been reinforcement of the general lack of attention paid to women's health needs. Effects of this discrimination are particularly dangerous, since women are at high risk for infection in many areas of the world. When AIDS prevention policies have not been limited to gay men, they have tended to figure women similarly, as "carriers." They have often focused exclusively on women in their roles as sex partners of men, or as childbearers—that is, as threats of contagion to men and infants. This obscures the fact that in many cases women are placed at risk because of their exclusion from information, or as a result of their lesser power to negotiate safe sex in heterosexual relations, whether within a couple or family or in commercial sex situations.[46]

Unfortunately, a more accurate inclusion of women within the international HIV/AIDS picture, however crucial, is still at several steps' remove from drawing lesbians into the realm of health and human rights. To the extent that lesbians suffer from the effects of HIV/AIDS and the medical neglect and human rights abuses that often accompany it, it is to be hoped that health and human rights policies developed in relation to HIV/AIDS will benefit lesbians as well as gay men and nonlesbian women. However, as a result of the international emphasis on risk *groups* rather than risk *behaviors* in the transmission of HIV, the field of health and human rights has been caught up in efforts to protect perceived at-risk groups: predominantly gay men, and more recently, men and women involved in heterosexual sexual activity. Thus, the alchemy of history, discrimination, activism and policymaking has created a situation in which lesbians (as a putative group) have effectively been constituted out of the most vital arena of health and human rights to develop so far.

CONCLUSION

This article emerged out of our recognition that a literature on lesbian health *and* human rights simply does not exist. As some have observed, professional concepts of "health" in lesbian lives have been either absent or malevolent. Where efforts have been made to directly address lesbian health, they have primarily been directed at undoing the harms experienced by lesbians at the hands of health care practitioners and funding institutions. Attempts to articulate international human rights for lesbians are even less well developed. To speak of lesbians in the field of health and human rights, then, is to strain even the reach of a *transitive* property: if lesbians are both homosexual and female, and, if it can be argued that women and homosexuals appear within the emerging health and human rights movement, then perhaps lesbians may find a space there as well.[47]

As we have tried to show, there are two emerging arenas within international human rights in which the coalescence of health and human rights could have been usefully extended to include lesbians: women's sexual and reproductive health, and homosexual rights in the context of HIV/AIDS. The convergence of health and human rights that is occurring in these realms is important and productive. Yet as the health and human rights conversation has veered in one direction within the international movement for women's right to health and in others within the mutual constitution of gay rights and AIDS policies, it is clear that lesbians have fallen through the cracks. If lasting policies for health and human rights—those that include attention to human sexuality—are developed principally within the arenas of heterosexual couple-based reproduction and AIDS, the danger exists that their very structure will continue to preclude articulation of a lesbian human right to health.

Our consideration of these potential locations for a lesbian human right to health has foregrounded the absence of protection for sexual autonomy and the multiple processes of sexual definition. Mindful of the warnings with which we began, we cannot comfortably end our discussion with any simple call for global recognition of "lesbian identity" or the need for "lesbian health care." Instead, we would like to advocate development of more mobile and dynamic models of sexual selves—or rather, selves that may choose to express themselves sexually. Ideally, such selves should be protected not so much by guarantees of the expression of particular named identities as by the conditions necessary for multifaceted human development. The sexual self we envision is one that can be expressed publicly, yet is not solely defined by public expression—one that can also be freely developed privately, within conditions of both public and private safety. We recognize, however, that under current conditions, the full enjoyment of a complete range of human rights by lesbians may remain elusive without an explicit articulation of a right to a "sexual self" in international law.

Nevertheless, we are encouraged by the promises of the developing field of health and human rights. Paradoxically, consideration of health and human rights as a conjunction may offer lesbians the potential to counteract the harms and erasures that have evolved within each arena independently. As their interrelationship has been posed by Mann and colleagues and others, the confluence of these two arenas provides unique opportunities for the formulation of whole-person analyses within international human rights laws and guidelines. Not only can lesbians benefit from such analyses, but inclusion of lesbian health concerns may also help advance the work of health and human rights activists by forcing sustained attention to the difficulties of constructing common principles that will allow people to be both different and healthy across a wide range of cultural contexts.

ACKNOWLEDGMENTS

The authors express their gratitude for the work of Laurence Helfer and the assistance of Julian Schreibman.

NOTES AND REFERENCES

1. T. M., anonymous lesbian in *GALZ (Gays and Lesbians of Zimbabwe)* newsletter, 14 (1994): 16–17.
2. S. Likosky, *Coming Out: An Anthology of International Gay and Lesbian Writings* (Brazil)(New York: Pantheon Books, 1992), pp. 20–21.
3. Our analysis will not follow the standard progression through the accepted hierarchy of international instruments. However, our goal in this commentary is to suggest directions and identify key concepts that might promote, or prove to be barriers within, current trends in health and human rights analyses. Lesbians have not been explicitly addressed as a sector of society deserving protection in any international treaty or decision interpreting such a treaty. This international silence (albeit somewhat broken in the European region) necessarily leads us to conduct a multilevel search for the locations in which lesbians have emerged. These sites, scattered and irresolute, allow for only a fragmentary analysis of their rights.
4. W. Rubenstein, "Health *and* Human Rights?: The Experience of Lesbians, Gay Men and Bisexuals in the U.S.," presented at the Harvard School of Public Health, March 7, 1995.
5. P. Stevens and J. Hall, "A Critical Historical Analysis of the Medical Construction of Lesbianism," in E. Fee and N. Krieger (eds.), *Women's Health, Politics, and Power* (Amityville, NY: Baywood, 1994), pp. 233, 239.
6. P. Stevens, "Lesbian Health Care Research: A Review of the Literature from 1970 to 1990," in P. Noerager Stern (ed.), *Lesbian Health: What Are the Issues?* (Washington, D.C.: Taylor and Francis, 1992), pp. 1–30.
7. Ottawa Charter for Health Promotion, presented at the First International Conference on Health Promotion (Ottawa, November 21, 1986).
8. Quoted in *Economic, Social and Cultural Rights and Health* (Cambridge, Mass.: Harvard Law School Human Rights Program, 1995), p. 17.
9. See, generally, Celina Romany, "State Responsibility Goes Private: A Feminist Critique of the Public/Private Distinction in International Human Rights Law," in R. Cook (ed.), *Human Rights of Women: National and International Perspectives* (Philadelphia: University of Pennsylvania Press, 1994), p. 85; D. Sul-

livan, "The Public/Private Distinction in International Human Rights Law," in J. Peters and A. Wolper (eds.), *Women's Rights, Human Rights* (New York: Routledge, 1995), p. 126.

10. L. Helfer and A. Miller, "Human Rights and Sexual Orientation: Developments in the United Nations, the United States and Around the World," unpublished ms. (1994), pp. 27–28.

11. Helfer and Miller (see note 10), p. 5.

12. Stevens and Hall (see note 5), p. 234.

13. Amnesty International USA, *Breaking the Silence: Human Rights Violations Based on Sexual Orientation* (1994) and *Human Rights Are Women's Rights* (1995); R. Rosenbloom (ed.), *Unspoken Rules: Sexual Orientation and Women's Human Rights* (San Francisco: International Gay and Lesbian Human Rights Commission, 1995).

14. It is important to note that self-identified lesbian groups do exist in many countries and on every continent. See *Breaking the Silence* (see note 13) and J. Dorf and G. Careaga Perez, "Discrimination and the Tolerance of Difference: International Lesbian Human Rights," in J. Peters and A. Wolper (eds.) *Women's Rights, Human Rights* (New York: Routledge, 1995), p. 324. Additionally, as noted below in the context of discussions on women and HIV/AIDS, exclusive focus on one aspect of lesbian identity—such as definitions that limit the application of the term *lesbian* to women who have not had sex with a man in a particular number of years—may contribute to inadequate or inappropriate health care. Similarly, women who self-identify as lesbians but in fact have heterosexual relations—for example, in the context of commercial sex—may have health concerns overlooked for the opposite but equally problematic definitional reason.

15. See, generally, A. Bayefsky, "The Principle of Equality or Non-Discrimination in International Law," *Human Rights Law Journal* 11 (1990): 1–34; R. Cook, "International Human Rights Law Concerning Women: Case Notes and Comments," *Vand. J. Transnat'l L.* 23 (1990): 779–818. Additionally, much of the progressive work in applying the UN Convention on Refugees and its Protocol should be considered in this context. See N. Kelly et al., *Guidelines For Women's Asylum Claims* (Cambridge: Women Refugees Project, 1994); Immigration and Refugee Board, *Women Refugee Claimants Fearing Gender-Related Persecution* (Ottawa: Immigration and Refugee Board, 1993). It is also important to note the strategies for addressing homosexuals as a social group for purposes of refugee protection; see note 38. For an introduction to the work applying feminist theory to international law see, generally, C. Bunch, "Women's Rights as Human Rights: Toward a Re-Vision of Human Rights," *Human Rights Quarterly* 12 (1990): 486–498; A. Byrnes, "Women, Feminism, and International Human Rights Law—Methodological Myopia, Fundamental Flaws or Meaningful Marginalisation? Some Current Issues," *Australian Year Book of International Law* 12 (1992): 205–241; H. Charlesworth, C. Chinkin, and S. Wright, "Feminist Approaches to International Law," *American Journal of International Law* 85 (1991): 613–645; K. Knop, "Why Rethinking the Sovereign State Is Important for Women's International Human Rights Law," in R. Cook (ed.), *Human Rights of Women: National and International Perspectives* (Philadelphia: University of Pennsylvania Press, 1994), pp. 153–164.

16. The Convention on the Elimination of All Forms of Discrimination Against Women (hereinafter Women's Convention) defines discrimination as "any distinction, exclusion or restriction made on the basis of sex which has the effect or purpose of impairing or nullifying the recognition, enjoyment, or exercise by women, irrespective of their marital status, on a basis of equality of men and women, of human rights and fundamental freedoms in the political, economic,

social and cultural, civil or any other field." Article 1, Convention on the Elimination of Discrimination Against Women, adopted by GA Res. 34/180, UN GAOR, 34th Sess., Supp. No. 46, UN Doc. A/34/46 (1980), entered into force September 3, 1981.

17. See General Recommendations nos. 12, 19 (violence against women); no. 14 (female circumcision); no. 15 (avoidance of discrimination against women in national strategies for the prevention of acquired immunodeficiency syndrome [AIDS]); no. 21 (equality in marriage and family relations). General Recommendations adopted by the Committee on the Elimination of Discrimination Against Women as included in *Compilation of General Comments and General Recommendations Adopted by Human Treaty Bodies,* UN Doc. HRI/GEN/1/ Rev.1 (1994).

18. See, generally, L. Heise, "Violence Against Women: Translating International Advocacy Into Concrete Change," *American University Law Review* 44, 4 (1995): 1206, and specifically her discussion of attention to violence against women by both WHO and PAHO, pp. 1210–1211.

19. Declaration on the Elimination of Violence Against Women, UN Doc. A/RES/48/104 (February 23, 1994).

20. For examples in the mainstream of human rights reporting, see Human Rights Watch/Women's Rights Project, *A Matter of Power: State Control of Women's Virginity in Turkey* (Washington, D.C.: Human Rights Watch, 1994); A. Tierney Goldstein, *Recognizing Forced Impregnation as a War Crime Under International Law* (New York: The Center for Reproductive Law and Policy, 1993); International Human Rights Law Group, *Token Gestures, Women's Human Rights and UN Reporting: The UN Special Rapporteur on Torture* (Washington, D.C.: International Human Rights Law Group, 1993); and R. Copelon, "Gendered War Crimes: Reconceptualizing Rape in Time of War," in J. Peters and A. Wolper (eds.), *Women's Rights, Human Rights* (New York: Routledge, 1995), pp. 197–214.

21. Proposals for Consideration in the Preparation of a Draft Declaration and the Draft Platform for Action (hereinafter Platform for Action), paragraph 232 (h), UN Doc. future A/CONF.177/L.1 (May 15, 1995) (advance unedited version).

22. Platform for Action (see note 21), paragraphs 46, 226. The further contentiousness surrounding sexual orientation within the Beijing process is demonstrated by response to the use of the term *gender* throughout the Platform for Action. This debate explicitly surfaced some delegates' fears that *gender* was a concept disguised to introduce the social toleration of multiple forms of sexuality—specifically homosexuality, transsexuality, and bisexuality.

23. Language in the Platform for Action about which participating governments could not come to agreement at the final prepatory meeting has been placed in brackets. It will be the subject of further negotiations prior to and during the Beijing Conference.

24. D. Sullivan, "Introduction to the Conference on the International Protection of Reproductive Rights," *American University Law Review* 44, 4 (1995): 969–973.

25. See the articulation of a provisional framework for health and human rights in J. Mann, L. Gostin, S. Gruskin et al., "Health and Human Rights," *Health and Human Rights* 1 (1994): 7–23.

26. See, generally, L. Freedman and S. Isaacs, "Human Rights and Reproductive Choices," *Studies in Family Planning* 24, 2 (1993): 18–30; and R. Cook, "International Human Rights and Women's Reproductive Health," *Studies in Family Planning* 24, 2 (1993): 73–86. For a discussion on violence as a health problem, see L. Heise (see note 18).

27. Programme for Action of the International Conference on Population and Development (hereinafter ICPD), Ch. VII, sec. D, Report of the International Conference on Population and Development, 5–13 September 1994, UN Doc. A/CONF.171/13.

28. ICPD (see note 28).

29. Platform for Action (see note 21), paragraph 97.

30. Ibid. Further, the equation between sexuality and reproduction has recontained both within the heterosexual family structure. This raises the intriguing question of whether there may be room within current international human rights standards to articulate the right to found an alternative family. The intensity of the debates over families and alternative families within the ICPD and the final Programme for Action of the World Summit for Social Development suggest that this nexus has been recognized. A resolution to this question will be crucial, since such authoritative documents as the Universal Declaration of Human Rights and the International Covenant on Economic, Social and Cultural Rights recognize the family as "the natural and fundamental group unit of society." However, these discussions have not by their terms included alternative lesbian families.

31. R. Friedman and J. Downey, "Homosexuality," *New England Journal of Medicine* 331 (1994): 923–929; Janice Hitchcock, "Bibliography: Lesbian Health," *Women's Studies* 17 (1989): 139–144; P. Noerager Stern (see note 6).

32. See A. Clapham and J. Weiler, "Lesbians and Gay Men in the European Community Legal Order," in K. Waaldjik and A. Clapham (eds.), *Homosexuality: A European Community Issue: Essays on Lesbian and Gay Rights in European Law and Policy* (Boston: Martinus Nijhoff, 1993), pp. 7–69. See also J. Wilets, "International Human Rights Law and Sexual Orientation," *Hastings International and Comparative Law Review* 18, 1 (1994): 1–120.

33. Helfer and Miller (see note 10), p. 3. See also Wilets, Clapham, note 32.

34. Even the right to privacy, as it is linked to protections guaranteed against interference with family life, was refused to lesbians by the European Commission, in a case upholding denial of a permanent residence permit to the foreign partner in a lesbian couple and their daughter. *X. and Y. v. United Kingdom*, App. No. 9369/81, 32 Eur. Comm'n H.R. Dec. and Rep. 220 (1983).

35. Specifically, this refers to the right to respect for private life enshrined in the European Convention on Human Rights, as interpreted in *Modinos v. Cyprus*, 259 Eur. Ct. H.R. (ser. A) (1993), *Norris v. Ireland*, 142 Eur. Ct. H.R. (ser. A) (1988), and *Dudgeon v. United Kingdom*, 45 Eur. Ct. H.R. (ser. A) (1981).

36. "Homosexuals in Europe are perceived less as a criminal class and more as a nonethnic minority" Clapham and Weiler (see note 32), p. 14. See, for example, the 1984 European Parliament Resolution on Sexual Discrimination in the Workplace, which called for an end to discrimination in laws and practices at the national and EC/EU level; Peter Ashman, "Introduction," in K. Waaldjik and A. Clapham (eds.), *Homosexuality: A European Community Issue* (Boston: Martinus Nijhoff, 1993), p. 4. Also, the European Parliament, in its 17 May 1995 Intergovernmental Conference Resolution, stated that prohibitions on discrimination based on sexual orientation should be included in the revision of the Treaty of the European Union; Rex Wockner, "Euro Parliament Endorses Gay Protections," *International News* 58 (June 8, 1995).

37. See for example, A. M. Smith, "Resisting the Erasure of Lesbian Sexuality: A Challenge for Queer Activism," in K. Plummer (ed.), *Modern Homosexualities* (London: Routledge, 1992): 201–212.

38. *Nicholas Toonen v. Australia*, UN GAOR, Hum. Rts. Cte., 15th Sess., Case 488/1992, UN Doc. CCPR/c/50/D/488/1992 (April 1994).

39. The committee located its protection of sexual orientation in the prohibition against discrimination on the basis of "sex" rather than "other status." For a discussion of the potential implications of this aspect of the decision, see, for example, Helfer and Miller (see note 10). Also see Robert Wintemute, "Sexual Orientation Discrimination as Sex Discrimination: Same Sex Couples and the Charter in Mossop, Egan and Layland," *McGill Law Journal* 39 (1994): 429–478; Andrew Koppelman, "Why Discrimination Against Gays and Lesbians Is Sex Discrimination," *New York University Law Review* 69 (1994): 197–286. Additionally, *Toonen* again concerned a law that criminalized only male homosexual sex. As we have noted, abuses suffered by lesbians do not appear to stem as frequently from the specific criminalization of their sexual activity, as is the case for gay men. However, the committee's broad language in *Toonen* offers the prospect that prohibitions against lesbian same-sex activity may be similarly construed to violate protections guaranteed in the ICCPR, though as yet this has not been tested.

40. *Breaking the Silence* (see note 13) and Wilets (see note 32). Additionally, the successful strategies for obtaining political asylum for persecuted homosexuals directly manifest this traditional recognition of harms. See S. Goldberg, "Give Me Liberty or Give Me Death: Political Asylum and the Global Persecution of Lesbians and Gay Men," *Cornell International Law Journal* 26, 3 (1994): 605–623.

41. *Breaking the Silence* (see note 13); J. Dorf and G. Careaga Perez, "Discrimination and the Tolerance of Difference: International Lesbian Human Rights," in J. Peters and A. Wolper (eds.), *Women's Rights, Human Rights* (New York: Routledge, 1995), pp. 324–334.

42. "AIDS is the first worldwide epidemic to occur in the modern era of human rights. For the first time, public health practitioners [were] being held to a dual standard in the design and implementation of public health programs, in this case to prevent HIV transmission. . . . As understanding of the pandemic evolved, the relationship between societal discrimination or marginalization and the risk of becoming HIV-infected became more evident." K. Tomasevski, S. Gruskin, Z. Lazzarini, and A. Hendriks, "AIDS and Human Rights," in J. Mann, D. Tarantola, and T. Netter (eds.), *AIDS in the World: A Global Report*, (Cambridge: Harvard University Press, 1992), p. 538.

43. *Breaking the Silence* (see note 13), p. 34. Two HIV educators working in the gay community in Mexico were sentenced to imprisonment following an unfair trial, and in Turkey twenty-eight gay rights advocates from outside the country were asked to submit to HIV tests during detention for their activism (p. 35).

44. Rubenstein (see note 4).

45. Helfer and Miller (see note 10), p. 11. The *Toonen* opinion builds upon a recognition in international and national fora of the need to apply the norm of nondiscrimination to homosexuality in the context of HIV/AIDS. See, for example, the Resolution of the European Parliament of 30 March 1989 on the fight against AIDS, *Official Journal of the European Community* 158 (June 26, 1989): 477.

46. Women (whatever their sexual orientation) involved in commercial sex face a variety of working conditions variously affecting their vulnerability to HIV infection. Forced prostitution poses particular risks, as H. H. Pyne notes when discussing Burmese women forced into prostitution in Thailand: "The HIV/AIDS pandemic has given a new urgency to the problem of trafficking women and girls into prostitution. The women lack access to health care, information, and

support networks. They possess no bargaining power with either brothel owners or clients, and live in constant fear of torture and psychological abuse. All
these factors place [them] in a position of extreme vulnerability to the AIDS
virus." H. H. Pyne, "AIDS and Gender Violence: The Enslavement of Burmese
Women in the Thai Sex Industry," in J. Peters and A. Wolper (eds.), *Women's
Rights, Human Rights* (New York: Routledge, 1995), p. 223.

47. This is an extension of Meg Satterthwaite's remark that lesbians might be said to
derive human rights by "the transitive property: if lesbians are women, and
women have human rights, then lesbians have human rights." Keynote address,
Amnesty International USA, Southern Regional Conference, Atlanta, Georgia,
February 25, 1995.

PART V

Medicine and Human Rights

Since Hippocrates, physicians have shared an ethic that puts the best interests of their patients at the core of their professional responsibilities. Since World War II, this ethic has come under increasing criticism for being overly paternalistic and for ignoring the autonomy and equality of patients. A human rights perspective, which takes individual rights to information, privacy, and bodily integrity seriously and treats all people as equals, has already transformed approaches to the physician-patient relationship in many countries. Although this transformation is most apparent in democratic countries, it seems likely that the development of an international patient bill of rights could help bring universal recognition of the rights of patients.

The first major document incorporating human rights principles that centered on the professional responsibilities of physicians was the Nuremberg Code. This code was formulated by U.S. judges sitting in judgment of the Nazi doctors at Nuremberg in 1946 and 1947. The Nazi doctors were being tried for crimes against humanity and war crimes involving the murder and torture of concentration camp prisoners in a variety of barbaric human "experiments." The first chapter in this section begins with an edited version of the opening statement by General Telford Taylor, the chief prosecutor. The Doctors' Trial was the first of the twelve so-called subsequent proceedings at Nuremberg, all of which were held under the jurisdiction of the United States as the occupying power of the section of Germany surrounding Nuremberg. Prior to these proceedings, the International Military Tribunal (IMT), an international tribunal made up of judges from the United States, the United Kingdom, France, and the USSR sat in judgment of the major Nazi war criminals. It was this tribunal that determined the existence of war crimes and crimes against humanity, that individuals could be found personally accountable for committing these atrocities, and that the excuse of obeying orders was no defense. As Taylor outlines in his opening statement, he expected the U.S. judges to apply the law of the IMT to the Nazi doctors. The judges did, and the result is their articulation of a ten-point code of conduct for human experimentation: the Nuremberg Code (p. 298). This code stands to this day as the most authoritative and definitive statement of rules for the proper conduct of research on human subjects. Its first provision, the requirement of voluntary, competent, informed and understanding consent, now generally applies not just to experimentation but to therapy as well.

The second chapter, from George J. Annas and Michael Grodin, is a reflection on the importance of the Doctors' Trial and the Nuremberg Code, and how its critical human rights perspective can be more generally incorporated into medical practice. The authors give the history of the code, noting not only its successes but also continuing resistance to its teachings and consistent attempts to subvert and marginalize it with, for example, the more physician-oriented Helsinki Declaration. This chapter is followed by a comprehensive discussion of contemporary human experimentation by Annas that concentrates on the many and varied motives involved in the conduct of research on human subjects. Annas suggests that we often use language to obscure rather than clarify the human rights issues involved in human experimentation, and that both researchers and their subjects have an interest in trying to transform human experimentation (in which a hypothesis is tested to gain generalizable knowledge) into a therapeutic activity (in which physicians treat patients for their own good), especially in the context of research on dying patients. The chapter concludes with specific recommendations designed to better safeguard the human rights of research subjects.

Research in industrialized countries is challenging, but research in developing countries is many times more complex, pointing as it does to problems of resource allocation, poverty and cultural relativism arguments, all of which are often enmeshed with the worldwide problems of racism and sexism. This group of chapters begins with a discussion of the controversial practice of female genital cutting by Catherine Annas. She graphically describes the various practices, refutes their status as religious requirements and explores how these practices (which combine human rights issues relating to torture and experimentation) affect both women and their daughters. The core of this chapter details the human rights of women and girls (especially the differences in the status and rights of adults and children), and the role of international human rights and the medical profession in attacking this practice. The chapter concludes with concrete suggestions for action.

The next two chapters deal with the continuing controversy over how AIDS-related research should be conducted in countries on the African continent. In the first, Carel Ijsselmuiden and Ruth Faden discuss the question of whether informed consent is universal, and if its application is possible in the

African context. They conclude that informed consent is both necessary to protect individual rights and that its application in developing countries may be challenging, but is appropriate and can be reasonably accomplished.

George J. Annas and Michael A. Grodin briefly discuss the specific issue of the role of economic resources in research ethics. They argue that it is insufficient to justify research because it focuses on a drug or other intervention that is "affordable" in the host country. Instead, they insist that for research to be ethical and nonexploitative, a concrete and practical plan to make the research drug or intervention available to the community in which the research is being carried out must be in place *before* the research is commenced. This requirement has almost never been met.

The final chapter in this section continues the discussion of economic exploitation of poorer countries and communities by richer ones, and combines it with the issues of informed consent and research on human subjects. The chapter is from a 1997 report of a U.S. National Academy of Sciences committee whose charge was to evaluate the human genome diversity project, a vague plan to collect and analyze DNA from various ethnic groups around the world. In concluding that no such international project was in existence (but rather a variety of not-too-well-coordinated research projects), the committee decided to summarize the human rights issues (and ways to deal with them) involved in collecting and analyzing these samples (usually taken from blood and saliva) from members of isolated populations, sometimes mistakenly termed "vanishing tribes." The chapter contains the committee's deliberations and conclusions on the applicability of the human rights framework, and concludes that human rights protections must be made an integral part of any proposal to study human genetic variation.

These chapters underline the interconnectedness of human rights and medicine, and the increasingly shared belief of the international community that taking human rights in medicine seriously is as important as curing and research themselves.

19. The Nuremberg Doctors' Trial

(a) Opening Statement of the Prosecution, Dec. 9, 1946

Telford Taylor

The defendants in this case are charged with murders, tortures, and other atrocities committed in the name of medical science. The victims of these crimes are numbered in the hundreds of thousands. A handful only are still alive; a few of the survivors will appear in this courtroom. But most of these miscrable victims were slaughtered outright or died in the course of the tortures to which they were subjected.

For the most part they are nameless dead. To their murderers, these wretched people were not individuals at all. They came in wholesale lots and were treated worse than animals. They were 200 Jews in good physical condition, 50 Gypsies, 500 tubercular Poles, or 1,000 Russians. The victims of these crimes are numbered among the anonymous millions who met death at the hands of the Nazis and whose fate is a hideous blot on the page of modern history.

The charges against these defendants are brought in the name of the United States of America. They are being tried by a court of American judges. The responsibilities thus imposed upon the representatives of the United States, prosecutors and judges alike, are grave and unusual. It is owed, not only to the victims and to the parents and children of the victims, that just punishment be imposed on the guilty, but also to the defendants that they be accorded a fair hearing and decision. Such responsibilities are the ordinary burden of any tribunal. Far wider are the duties which we must fulfill here.

These larger obligations run to the people and races on whom the scourge of these crimes was laid. The mere punishment of the defendants, or even of thousands of others equally guilty, can never redress the terrible injuries which the Nazis visited on these unfortunate peoples. For them it is far more important that these incredible events be established by clear and public proof, so that no one can ever doubt that they were fact and not fable; and that this court, as the agent of the United States and as the voice of humanity, stamp these acts, and the ideas which engendered them, as barbarous and criminal.

We have still other responsibilities here. The defendants in the dock are charged with murder, but this is no mere murder trial. We cannot rest content when we have shown that crimes were committed and that certain persons committed them. To kill, to maim, and to torture is criminal under all modern systems of law. These defendants did not kill in hot blood, nor for personal enrichment. Some of them may be sadists who killed and tortured for sport, but they are not all perverts. They are not ignorant men. Most of them are trained physicians and some of them are distinguished scientists. Yet these defendants, all of whom were fully able to comprehend the nature of their acts, and most of whom were exceptionally qualified to form a moral and professional judgment in this respect, are responsible for wholesale murder and unspeakably cruel tortures.

It is our deep obligation to all people of the world to show why and how these things happened. It is incumbent upon us to set forth with conspicuous clarity the ideas and motives which moved these defendants to treat their fellow men as less than beasts. The perverse thoughts and distorted concepts which brought about these savageries are not dead. They cannot be killed by force of arms. They must not become a spreading cancer in the breast of humanity. They must be cut out and exposed, for the reason so well stated by Mr. Justice Jackson in this courtroom a year ago. "The wrongs which we seek to condemn and punish have been so calculated, so malignant, and so devastating, that civilization cannot tolerate their being ignored because it cannot survive their being repeated."

To the German people we owe a special responsibility in these proceedings. Under the leadership of the Nazis and their war-lords, the German nation spread death and devastation throughout Europe. This the Germans now know. So, too, do they know the consequences to Germany: defeat, ruin, prostration, and utter demoralization. Most German children will never, as long as they live, see an undamaged German city.

To what cause will these children ascribe the defeat of the German nation and the devastation that surrounds them? Will they attribute it to the overwhelming weight of numbers and resources that was eventually leagued against them? Will they point to the ingenuity of enemy scientists? Will they perhaps blame their plight on strategic and military blunders by their generals?

If the Germans embrace those reasons as the true cause of their disaster, it will be a sad and fatal thing for Germany and for the world. Men who have never seen a German city intact will be callous about flattening English or American or Russian cities. They may not even realize that they are destroying anything worthwhile, for lack of a normal sense of values. To reestablish the greatness of Germany they are likely to pin their faith on improved military techniques. Such views will lead the Germans straight into the arms of the Prussian militarists to whom defeat is only a glorious opportunity to start a new war game. "Next time it will be different." We know all too well what that will mean.

This case, and others which will be tried in this building, offer a signal opportunity to lay before the German people the true cause of their present misery. The walls and towers and churches of Nuernberg were, indeed, reduced to rubble by Allied bombs, but in a deeper sense Nuernberg had been destroyed a decade earlier, when it became the seat of the annual Nazi Party rallies, a focal point for the moral disintegration in Germany, and the private domain of Julius Streicher. The insane and malignant doctrines that Nuernberg spewed forth account alike for the crimes of these defendants and for the terrible fate of Germany under the Third Reich.

A nation which deliberately infects itself with poison will inevitably sicken and die. These defendants and others turned Germany into an infernal combination of a lunatic asylum and a charnel house. Neither science, nor industry, nor the arts could flourish in such a foul medium. The country could not live at peace and was fatally handicapped for war. I do not think the German people have as yet any conception of how deeply the criminal folly that was Nazism bit into every phase of German life, or of how utterly ravaging the consequences were. It will be our task to make these things clear.

These are the high purposes which justify the establishment of extraordinary courts to hear and determine this case and others of comparable importance. That murder should be punished goes without the saying, but the full performance of our task requires more than the just sentencing of these defendants. Their crimes were the inevitable result of the sinister doctrines which they espoused, and these same doctrines sealed the fate of Germany, shattered Europe, and left the world in ferment. Wherever those doctrines may emerge and prevail, the same terrible consequences will follow. That is why a bold and lucid consummation of these proceedings is of vital importance to all nations. That is why the United States has constituted this Tribunal.

I pass now to the facts of the case in hand. There are 23 defendants in the box. All but three of them—Rudolf Brandt, Sievers, and Brack—are doctors. Of the 20 doctors, all but one—Pokorny—held positions in the medical services of the Third Reich. To understand this case, it is necessary to understand the general structure of these state medical services, and how these services fitted into the over-all organization of the Nazi State. *[The material on the organization of the military medical personnel, and where the individual defendants fit into it, has been deleted.]*

CRIMES COMMITTED IN THE GUISE OF SCIENTIFIC RESEARCH

I turn now to the main part of the indictment and will outline at this point the prosecution's case relating to those crimes alleged to have been committed in the name of medical or scientific research. The charges with respect to "euthanasia" and the slaughter of tubercular Poles obviously have no relation to research or experimentation and will be dealt with later. What I will cover now comprehends all the experiments charged as war crimes in paragraph 6 and as crimes against humanity in paragraph 11 of the indictment, and the murders committed for the so-called anthropological purposes which are charged as war crimes in paragraph 7 and as crimes against humanity in paragraph 12 of the indictment.

Before taking up these experiments one by one, let us look at them as a whole. Are they a heterogeneous list of horrors, or is there a common denominator for the whole group?

A sort of rough pattern is apparent on the face of the indictment. Experiments concerning high altitude, the effect of cold, and the potability of processed sea water have an obvious relation to aeronautical and naval combat and rescue problems. The mustard gas and phosphorus burn experiments, as well as those relating to the healing value of sulfanilamide for wounds, can be related to air-raid and battlefield medical problems. It is well known that malaria, epidemic jaundice, and typhus were among the principal diseases which had to be combated by the German Armed Forces and by German authorities in occupied territories. To some degree, the therapeutic pattern outlined above is undoubtedly a valid one, and explains why the Wehrmacht, and especially the German Air Force, participated in these experiments. Fanatically bent upon conquest, utterly ruthless as to the means or instruments to be used in achieving victory, and callous to the sufferings of people whom they regarded as inferior, the German militarists were willing to gather whatever scientific fruit these experiments might yield.

But our proof will show that a quite different and even more sinister objective runs like a red thread through these hideous researches. We will show that in some instances the true object of these experiments was not how to rescue or to cure, but how to destroy and kill. The sterilization experiments were, it is clear, purely destructive in purpose. The prisoners at Buchenwald who were shot with poisoned bullets were not guinea pigs to test an antidote for the poison; their murderers really wanted to know how quickly the poison would kill. This destructive objective is not superficially as apparent in the other experiments, but we will show that it was often there.

Mankind has not heretofore felt the need of a word to denominate the science of how to kill prisoners most rapidly and subjugated people in large numbers. This case and these defendants have created this gruesome question for the lexicographer. For the moment we will christen this macabre science *thanatology*, the science of producing death. The thanatological knowledge, derived in part from these experiments, supplied the techniques for genocide, a policy of the Third Reich, exemplified in the "euthanasia" program and in the widespread slaughter of Jews, Gypsies, Poles, and Russians. This policy of mass extermination could not have been so effectively carried out without the active participation of German medical scientists.

* * *

The 20 physicians in the dock range from leaders of German scientific medicine, with excellent international reputations, down to the dregs of the German medical profession. All of them have in common a callous lack of consideration and human regard for, and an unprincipled willingness to abuse their power over, the poor, unfortunate, defenseless creatures who have been deprived of their rights by the ruthless and criminal government. All of them violated the Hippocratic commandments which they had solemnly sworn to uphold and abide by, including the fundamental principle never to do harm—"*primum non nocere.*"

Outstanding men of science, distinguished for their scientific ability in Germany and abroad, are the defendants Rostock and Rose. Both exemplify, in their training and practice alike, the highest traditions of German medicine. Rostock headed the Department of Surgery at the University of Berlin and served as dean of its medical school. Rose studied under the famous surgeon, Enderlen, at Heidelberg and then became a distinguished specialist in the fields of public health and tropical diseases. Handloser and Schroeder are outstanding medical administrators. Both of them made their careers in military medicine and reached the peak of their profession. Five more defendants are much younger men who are nevertheless already known as the possessors of considerable scientific ability, or capacity in medical administration. These include the defendants Karl Brandt, Ruff, Beiglboeck, Schaefer, and Becker-Freyseng.

A number of the others such as Romberg and Fischer, are well trained, and several of them attained high professional positions. But among the remainder few were known as outstanding scientific men. Among them at the foot of the list is Blome who has published his autobiography, entitled *Embattled Doctor*, in which he sets forth that he eventually decided to become a doctor because a medical career would enable him to become "master over life and death."

* * *

I intend to pass very briefly over matters of medical ethics, such as the conditions under which a physician may lawfully perform a medical experiment upon a person who has voluntarily subjected himself to it, or whether experiments may lawfully be performed upon criminals who have been condemned to death. This case does not present such problems. No refined questions confront us here.

None of the victims of the atrocities perpetrated by these defendants were volunteers, and this is true regardless of what these unfortunate people may have said or signed before their tortures began. Most of the victims had not been condemned to death, and those who had been were not criminals, unless it be a crime to be a Jew, or a Pole, or a Gypsy, or a Russian prisoner of war.

Whatever book or treatise on medical ethics we may examine, and whatever expert on forensic medicine we may question, will say that it is a fundamental and inescapable obligation of every physician under any known system of law not to perform a dangerous experiment without the subject's consent. In the tyranny that was Nazi Germany, no one could give such a consent to the medical agents of the State; everyone lived in fear and acted under duress. I fervently hope that none of us here in the courtroom will have to suffer in silence while it is said on the part of these defendants that the wretched and helpless people whom they froze and drowned and burned and poisoned were volunteers. If such a shameless lie is spoken here, we need only remember the four girls who were taken from the Ravensbrueck concentration camp and made to lie naked with the frozen and all-but-dead Jews who survived Dr. Rascher's tank of ice water. One of these women, whose hair and eyes and figure were pleasing to Dr. Rascher, when asked by him why she had volunteered for such a task, replied, "rather half a year in a brothel than half a year in a concentration camp."

Were it necessary, one could make a long list of the respects in which the experiments that these defendants performed departed from every known standard of medical ethics. But the gulf between these atrocities and serious research in the healing art is so patent that such a tabulation would be cynical.

We need look no further than the law which the Nazis themselves passed on the 24th of November 1933 for the protection of animals. This law states explicitly that it is designed to prevent cruelty and indifference of man towards animals and to awaken and develop sympathy and understanding for animals as one of the highest moral values of a people. The soul of the German people should abhor the principle of mere utility without consideration of the moral aspects. The law states further that all operations or treatments which are associated with pain or injury, especially experiments involving the use of cold, heat, or infection, are prohibited, and can be permitted only under special exceptional circumstances. Special written authorization by the head of the department is necessary in every case, and experimenters are prohibited from performing experiments according to their own free judgment. Experiments for the purpose of teaching must be reduced to a minimum. Medico-legal tests, vaccinations, withdrawal of blood for diagnostic purposes, and trial of vaccines prepared according to well-established scientific principles are permitted, but the animals have to be killed immediately and painlessly after such experiments. Individual physicians are not permitted to use dogs to increase their surgical skill by such practices. National Socialism regards it as a sacred duty of German science to keep down the number of painful animal experiments to a minimum.

If the principles announced in this law had been followed for human beings as well, this indictment would never have been filed. It is perhaps the deepest shame of the defendants that it probably never even occurred to them that human beings should be treated with at least equal humanity.

* * *

I said at the outset of this statement that the Third Reich died of its own poison. This case is a striking demonstration not only of the tremendous degradation of German medical ethics which Nazi doctrine brought about, but of the undermining of the medical art and thwarting of the techniques which the defendants sought to employ. The Nazis have, to a certain extent, succeeded in convincing the peoples of the world that the Nazi system, although ruthless, was absolutely efficient; that although savage, it was completely scientific; that although entirely devoid of humanity, it was highly systematic—that "it got things done." The evidence which this Tribunal will hear will explode this myth. The Nazi methods of investigation were inefficient and unscientific, and their techniques of research were unsystematic.

These experiments revealed nothing which civilized medicine can use. It was, indeed, ascertained that phenol or gasoline injected intravenously will kill a man inexpensively and within 60 seconds. This and a few other "advances" are all in the field of thanatology. There is no doubt that a number of these new methods may be useful to criminals everywhere, and there is no doubt that they may be useful to a criminal state. Certain advances in destructive methodology we cannot deny, and indeed from Himmler's standpoint this may well have been the principal objective.

Apart from these deadly fruits, the experiments were not only criminal but a scientific failure. It is indeed as if a just deity had shrouded the solutions which they attempted to reach with murderous means. The moral shortcomings of the defendants and the precipitous ease with which they decided to commit murder in quest of "scientific results" dulled also that scientific hesitancy, that thorough thinking-through, that responsible weighing of every single step which alone can ensure scientifically valid results. Even if they had merely been forced to pay as little as two dollars for human experimental subjects, such as American investigators may have to pay for a cat, they might have thought twice before wasting unnecessary numbers, and thought of simpler and better ways to solve their problems. The fact that these investigators had free and unrestricted access to human beings to be experimented upon misled them to the dangerous and fallacious conclusion that the results would thus be better and more quickly obtainable than if they had gone through the labor of preparation, thinking, and meticulous pre-investigation.

A particularly striking example is the sea-water experiment. I believe that three of the accused—Schaefer, Becker-Freyseng, and Beiglboeck—will today admit that this problem could have been solved simply and definitively within the space of one afternoon. On 20 May 1944 when these accused convened to discuss the problem, a thinking chemist could have solved it right in the presence of the assembly within the space of a few hours by the use of nothing more gruesome than a piece of jelly, a semipermeable membrane and a salt solution, and the German Armed Forces would have had the answer on 21 May 1944. But what happened instead? The vast armies of the disenfranchised slaves were at the beck and call of this sinister assembly; and instead of thinking, they simply relied on their power over human beings rendered rightless by a criminal state and government. What time, effort, and staff did it take to get that machinery in motion! Letters had to be written, physicians, of whom dire shortage existed in the German Armed Forces whose soldiers went poorly attended, had to be taken out of hospital positions and dispatched hundreds of miles away to obtain the answer which should have been known in a few hours, but which thus did not become available to the German Armed Forces until after the completion of the gruesome show, and until 42 people had been subjected to the tortures of the damned, the very tortures which Greek mythology had reserved for Tantalus.

In short, this conspiracy was a ghastly failure as well as a hideous crime. The creeping paralysis of Nazi superstition spread through the German medical profession and, just as it destroyed character and morals, it dulled the mind.

Guilt for the oppression and crimes of the Third Reich is widespread, but it is the guilt of the leaders that is deepest and most culpable. Who could German medicine look to to keep the profession true to its traditions and protect it from the ravaging inroads of Nazi pseudo-science? This was the supreme responsibility of the leaders of German medicine—men like Rostock and Rose and Schroeder and Handloser. That is why their guilt is greater than that of any of the other defendants in the dock. They are the men who utterly failed their country and their profession, who showed neither courage nor wisdom nor the vestiges of moral character. It is their failure, together with the failure of the leaders of Germany in other walks of life, that debauched Germany and led to her defeat. It is because of them and others like them that we all live in a stricken world.[1]

REFERENCE

1. *Trials of War Criminals Before the Nuremberg Military Tribunals Under Control Council Law 10,* Vol. 1 (Washington, D.C.: Superintendent of Documents, U.S. Government Printing Office, 1950); Military Tribunal, Case 1, *United States v. Karl Brandt et al.,* pp. 27–74.

(b) The Judgment, Aug. 20, 1947

Judges Harold Sebring, Walter Beals, and Johnson Crawford

Military Tribunal I was established on 25 October 1946 under General Orders No. 68 issued by command of the United States Military Government for Germany. It was the first of several military tribunals constituted in the United States Zone of Occupation pursuant to Military Government Ordinance No. 7, for the trial of offenses recognized as crimes by Law No. 10 of the Control Council for Germany.

* * *

The trial was conducted in two languages—English and German. It consumed 139 trial days, including 6 days allocated for final arguments and the personal statements of the defendants. During the 133 trial days used for the presentation of evidence 32 witnesses gave oral evidence for the prosecution, and 53 witnesses, including the 23 defendants, gave oral evidence for the defense. In addition, the prosecution put in evidence as exhibits a total of 570 affidavits, reports, and documents; the defense put in a total number of 901—making a grand total of 1,471 documents received in evidence.

* * *

COUNTS TWO AND THREE

War Crimes and Crimes Against Humanity. The second and third counts of the indictment charge the commission of war crimes and crimes against humanity. The counts are identical in content, except for the fact that in count two the acts which are made the basis for the charges are alleged to have been committed on "civilians and members of the armed forces [of nations] then at war with the German Reich . . . in the exercise of belligerent control," whereas in count three the criminal acts are alleged to have been committed against "German civilians and nationals of other countries."

With this distinction observed, both counts will be treated as one and discussed together.

Counts two and three allege, in substance, that between September 1939 and April 1945 all of the defendants "were principals in, accessories to, ordered, abetted, took a consenting part in, and were connected with plans and enterprises involving medical experiments without the subjects' consent . . . in the course of which experiments the defendants committed murders, brutalities, cruelties, tortures, atrocities, and other inhuman acts." It is averred that "such experiments included, but were not limited to" the following:

(A) *High-Altitude Experiments.* From about March 1942 to about August 1942 experiments were conducted at the Dachau concentration camp, for the benefit of the German Air Force, to investigate the limits of human endurance and existence at extremely high altitudes. The experiments were carried out in a low-pressure chamber in which the atmospheric conditions and pressures prevailing at high altitude (up to 68,000 feet) could be duplicated. The experimental subjects were placed in the low-pressure chamber and thereafter the simulated altitude therein was raised. Many victims died as a result of these experiments and others suffered grave injury, torture, and ill-treatment. The defendants Karl Brandt, Handloser, Schroeder, Gebhardt, Rudolf Brandt, Mrugowsky, Poppendick, Sievers, Ruff, Romberg, Becker-Freyseng, and Weltz are charged with special responsibility for and participation in these crimes.

(B) *Freezing Experiments.* From about August 1942 to about May 1943 experiments were conducted at the Dachau concentration camp, primarily for the benefit of the German Air Force, to investigate the most effective means of treating persons who had been severely chilled or frozen. In one series of experiments the subjects were forced to remain in a tank of ice water for periods up to 3 hours. Extreme rigor developed in a short time. Numerous victims died in the course of these experiments. After the survivors were severely chilled, rewarming was attempted by various means. In other series of experiments, the subjects were kept naked outdoors for many hours at temperatures below freezing. . . . The defendants Karl Brandt, Handloser, Schroeder, Gebhardt, Rudolf Brandt, Mrugowsky, Poppendick, Sievers, Becker-Freyseng, and Weltz are charged with special responsibility for and participation in these crimes.

(C) *Malaria Experiments.* From about February 1942 to about April 1945 experiments were conducted at the Dachau concentration camp in order to investigate immunization for treatment of malaria. Healthy concentration camp inmates were infected by mosquitoes or by injections of extracts of the mucous glands of mosquitoes. After having contracted malaria, the subjects were treated with various drugs to test their relative efficacy. Over 1,000 involuntary subjects were used in these experiments. Many of the victims died and others suffered severe pain and permanent disability. The defendants Karl Brandt, Handloser, Rostock, Gebhardt, Blome, Rudolf Brandt, Mrugowsky, Poppendick, and Sievers are charged with special responsibility for and participation in these crimes.

(D) *Lost (Mustard) Gas Experiments.* At various times between September 1939 and April 1945 experiments were conducted at Sachsenhausen, Natzweiler, and other concentration camps for the benefit of the German Armed Forces to investigate the most effective treatment of wounds caused by Lost gas. Lost is a poison gas which is commonly known as mustard gas. Wounds deliberately inflicted on the subjects were infected with Lost. Some of the subjects died as a result of these experiments and others suffered intense pain and injury. The defendants Karl Brandt, Handloser, Blome, Rostock, Gebhardt, Rudolf Brandt, and Sievers are charged with special responsibility for and participation in these crimes.

(E) *Sulfanilamide Experiments.* From about July 1942 to about September 1943 experiments to investigate the effectiveness of sulfanilamide were conducted at the Ravensbrueck concentration camp for the benefit of the German Armed Forces. Wounds deliberately inflicted on the experimental subjects were infected with bacteria such as streptococcus, gas gangrene, and tetanus. Circulation of blood was interrupted by tying off blood vessels at both ends of the wound to create a condition similar to that of a battlefield wound. Infection was aggravated by forcing wood shavings and ground glass into the wounds. The infection was treated with sulfanilamide and other drugs to determine their effectiveness. Some subjects died as a result of these experiments and others suffered serious injury and intense agony. The defendants Karl Brandt, Handloser, Rostock, Schroeder, Genzken, Gebhardt, Blome, Rudolf Brandt, Mrugowsky, Poppendick, Becker-Freyseng, Oberheuser, and Fischer are charged with special responsibility for and participation in these crimes.

(F) *Bone, Muscle, and Nerve Regeneration and Bone Transplantation Experiments.* From about September 1942 to about December 1943 experiments were conducted at the Ravensbrueck concentration camp, for the benefit of the German Armed Forces, to study bone, muscle, and nerve regeneration, and bone transplantation from one person to another. Sections of bones, muscles, and nerves were removed from the subjects. As a result of these operations, many victims suffered intense agony, mutilation, and permanent disability. The defendants Karl Brandt, Handloser, Rostock, Gebhardt, Rudolf Brandt, Oberheuser, and Fischer are charged with special responsibility for and participation in these crimes.

(G) *Sea-Water Experiments.* From about July 1944 to about September 1944 experiments were conducted at the Dachau concentration camp, for the benefit of the German Air Force and Navy, to study various methods of making sea water drinkable. The subjects were deprived of all food and given only chemically processed sea water. Such experiments caused great pain and suffering and resulted in serious bodily injury to the victims. The defendants Karl Brandt, Handloser, Rostock, Schroeder, Gebhardt, Rudolf Brandt, Mrugowsky, Poppendick, Sievers, Becker-Freyseng, Schaefer, and Beiglboeck are charged with special responsibility for and participation in these crimes.

(H) *Epidemic Jaundice Experiments.* From about June 1943 to about January 1945 experiments were conducted at the Sachsenhausen and Natzweiler concentration camps, for the benefit of the German Armed Forces, to investigate the causes of, and inoculations against, epidemic jaundice. Experimental subjects were deliberately infected with epidemic jaundice, some of whom died as a result, and others were caused great pain and suffering. The defendants Karl Brandt, Handloser, Rostock, Schroeder, Gebhardt, Rudolf Brandt, Mrugowsky, Poppendick, Sievers, Rose, and Becker-Freyseng are charged with special responsibility for and participation in these crimes.

(I) *Sterilization Experiments.* From about March 1941 to about January 1945 sterilization experiments were conducted at the Auschwitz and Ravensbrueck concentration camps, and other places. The purpose of these experiments was to develop a method of sterilization which would be suitable for sterilizing millions of people with a minimum of time and effort. These experiments were conducted by means of X ray, surgery, and various drugs. Thousands of victims were sterilized and thereby suffered great mental and physical anguish. The defendants Karl Brandt, Gebhardt, Rudolf Brandt, Mrugowsky, Poppendick, Brack, Pokorny, and Oberheuser are charged with special responsibility for and participation in these crimes.

(J) *Spotted Fever (Fleckfieber) Experiments.* From about December 1941 to about February 1945 experiments were conducted at the Buchenwald and Natzweiler concentration camps for the benefit of the German Armed Forces, to investigate the effectiveness of spotted fever and other vaccines. At Buchenwald, numerous healthy inmates were deliberately infected with spotted fever virus in order to keep the virus alive; over 90 percent of the victims died as a result. Other healthy inmates were used to determine the effectiveness of different spotted fever vaccines and of various chemical substances. In the course of these experiments 75 percent of the selected number of inmates were vaccinated with one of the vaccines or nourished with one of the chemical substances and, after a period of 3 to 4 weeks, were infected with spotted fever germs. The remaining 25 percent were infected without any previous protection in order to compare the effectiveness of the vaccines and the chemical substances. As a result, hundreds of the persons experimented upon died. Experiments with yellow fever, smallpox, typhus, para-typhus A and B, cholera, and diphtheria were also conducted. Similar experiments with like results were conducted at Natzweiler concentration camp. The defendants Karl Brandt, Handloser, Rostock, Schroeder, Genzken, Gebhardt, Rudolf Brandt, Mrugowsky, Poppendick, Sievers, Rose, Becker-Freyseng, and Hoven are charged with special responsibility for and participation in these crimes.

(K) *Experiments with Poison.* In or about December 1943 and in or about October 1944 experiments were conducted at the Buchenwald concentration camp to investigate the effect of various poisons upon human beings. The poisons were secretly administered to experimental subjects in their food. The victims died as a result of the poison or were killed immediately in order to permit autopsies. In or about September 1944 experimental subjects were shot with poison bullets and suffered torture and death. The defendants Genzken, Gebhardt, Mrugowsky, and Poppendick are charged with special responsibility for and participation in these crimes.

(L) *Incendiary Bomb Experiments.* From about November 1943 to about January 1944 experiments were conducted at the Buchenwald concentration camp to test the effect of various pharmaceutical preparations on phosphorus burns. These burns were inflicted on experimental subjects with phosphorus matter taken from incendiary bombs, and caused severe pain, suffering, and serious bodily injury. The defendants Genzken, Gebhardt, Mrugowsky, and Poppendick are charged with special responsibility for and participation in these crimes.

In addition to the medical experiments, the nature and purpose of which have been outlined as alleged, certain of the defendants are charged with criminal activities involving murder, torture, and ill-treatment of non-German nationals as follows:

7.   Between June 1943 and September 1944 the defendants Rudolf Brandt and Sievers . . . were principals in, accessories to, ordered, abetted, took a consenting part in, and were connected with plans and enterprises involving the murder of civilians and members of the armed forces of nations then at war with the German Reich and who were in the custody of the German Reich in exercise of belligerent control. One hundred twelve Jews were selected for the purpose of completing a skeleton collection for the Reich University of Strasbourg. Their photographs and anthropological measurements were taken. Then they were killed. Thereafter, comparison tests, anatomical research, studies regarding race, pathological features of the body, form and size of the brain, and other tests were made. The bodies were sent to Strasbourg and defleshed.

8.   Between May 1942 and January 1944 the defendants Blome and Rudolf Brandt . . . were principals in, accessories to, ordered, abetted, took a consenting part in, and were connected with plans and enterprises involving the murder and mistreatment of tens of thousands of Polish nationals who were civilians and members of the armed forces of a nation then at war with the German Reich in exercise of belligerent control. These people were alleged to be infected with incurable tuberculosis. On the ground of ensuring the health and welfare of Germans in Poland, many tubercular Poles were ruthlessly exterminated while others were isolated in death camps with inadequate medical facilities.

9.   Between September 1939 and April 1945 the defendants Karl Brandt, Blome,

Brack, and Hoven ... were principals in, accessories to, ordered, abetted, took a consenting part in, and were connected with plans and enterprises involving the execution of the so-called "euthanasia" program of the German Reich in the course of which the defendants herein murdered hundreds of thousands of human beings, including nationals of German-occupied countries. This program involved the systematic and secret execution of the aged, insane, incurably ill, of deformed children, and other persons, by gas, lethal injections, and diverse other means in nursing homes, hospitals, and asylums. Such persons were regarded as "useless eaters" and a burden to the German war machine. The relatives of these victims were informed that they died from natural causes, such as heart failure. Germans doctors involved in the "euthanasia" program were also sent to the eastern occupied countries to assist in the mass extermination of Jews.

* * *

Counts two and three of the indictment conclude with the averment that the crimes and atrocities which have been delineated "constitute violations of international conventions . . . , the laws and customs of war, the general principles of criminal law as derived from the criminal laws of all civilized nations, the internal penal laws of the countries in which such crimes were committed, and of Article II of Control Council Law No. 10."

* * *

THE PROOF AS TO WAR CRIMES AND CRIMES AGAINST HUMANITY

Judged by any standard of proof, the record clearly shows the commission of war crimes and crimes against humanity substantially as alleged in counts two and three of the indictment. Beginning with the outbreak of World War II criminal medical experiments on non-German nationals, both prisoners of war and civilians, including Jews and "asocial" persons, were carried out on a large scale in Germany and the occupied countries. These experiments were not the isolated and casual acts of individual doctors and scientists working solely on their own responsibility, but were the product of coordinated policy-making and planning at high governmental, military, and Nazi Party levels, conducted as an integral part of the total war effort. They were ordered, sanctioned, permitted, or approved by persons in positions of authority who under all principles of law were under the duty to know about these things and to take steps to terminate or prevent them.

PERMISSIBLE MEDICAL EXPERIMENTS

The great weight of the evidence before us is to the effect that certain types of medical experiments on human beings, when kept within reasonably well-defined bounds, conform to the ethics of the medical profession generally. The protagonists of the practice of human experimentation justify their views on the basis that such experiments yield results for the good of society that are unprocurable by other methods or means of study. All agree, however, that certain basic principles must be observed in order to satisfy moral, ethical and legal concepts:

1. The voluntary consent of the human subject is absolutely essential. This means that the person involved should have legal capacity to give consent; should be so situated as to be able to exercise free power of choice, without the intervention of any element of force, fraud, deceit, duress, over-reaching, or other ulterior form of constraint or coercion; and should have sufficient knowledge and comprehension of the elements of the subject matter involved as to enable him to make an understanding and enlightened decision. This latter element requires that before the acceptance of an affirmative decision by the experimental subject there should be made known to him the nature, duration, and purpose of the experiment; the method and means by which it is to be conducted; all inconveniences and hazards reasonably to be expected; and the effects upon his health or person which may possibly come from his participation in the experiment.

    The duty and responsibility for ascertaining the quality of the consent rests upon each individual who initiates, directs, or engages in the experiment. It is a personal duty and responsibility which may not be delegated to another with impunity.

2. The experiment should be such as to yield fruitful results for the good of society, unprocurable by other methods or means of study, and not random and unnecessary in nature.

3. The experiment should be so designed and based on the results of animal experimentation and a knowledge of the natural history of the disease or other problem under study that the anticipated results will justify the performance of the experiment.

4. The experiment should be so conducted as to avoid all unnecessary physical and mental suffering and injury.

5. No experiment should be conducted where there is an *a priori* reason to believe that death or disabling injury will occur; except, perhaps, in those experiments where the experimental physicians also serve as subjects.

6. The degree of risk to be taken should never exceed that determined by the humanitarian importance of the problem to be solved by the experiment.

7. Proper preparations should be made and adequate facilities provided to protect the experimental subject against even remote possibilities of injury, disability, or death.

8. The experiment should be conducted only by scientifically qualified persons. The highest degree of skill and care should be required through all stages of the experiment of those who conduct or engage in the experiment.

9. During the course of the experiment the human subject should be at liberty to bring the experiment to an end if he has reached the physical or mental state where continuation of the experiment seems to him to be impossible.

10. During the course of the experiment the scientist in charge must be prepared to terminate the experiment at any stage, if he has probable cause to believe, in the exercise of the good faith, superior skill and careful judgment required of him that a continuation of the experiment is likely to result in injury, disability, or death to the experimental subject.

Of the ten principles which have been enumerated, our judicial concern, of course, is with those requirements which are purely legal in nature—or which at least are so clearly related to matters legal that they assist us in determining criminal culpability and punishment. To go beyond that point would lead us into a field that would be beyond our sphere of competence. However, the point need not be labored. We find from the evidence that in the medical experiments which have been proved, these ten principles were much more frequently honored in their breach than in their observance. Many of the concentration camp inmates who were the victims of these atrocities were citizens of countries other than the German Reich. They were non-German nationals, including Jews and "asocial persons," both prisoners of war and civilians, who had been imprisoned and forced to submit to these tortures and barbarities without so much as a semblance of trial. In every single instance appearing in the record, subjects were used who did not consent to the experiments; indeed, as to some of the experiments, it is not even contended by the defendants that the subjects occupied the status of volunteers. In no case was the experimental subject at liberty of his own free choice to withdraw from any experiment. In many cases, experiments were performed by unqualified persons; were conducted at random for no adequate scientific reason, and under revolting physical conditions. All of the experiments were conducted with unnecessary suffering and injury and but very little, if any, precautions were taken to protect or safeguard the human subjects from the possibilities of injury, disability, or death. In every one of the experiments the subjects experienced extreme pain or torture, and in most of them they suffered permanent injury, mutilation, or death, either as a direct result of the experiments or because of lack of adequate follow-up care.

Obviously all of these experiments involving brutalities, tortures, disabling injury, and death were performed in complete disregard of international conventions, the laws and customs of war, the general principles of criminal law as derived from the criminal laws of all civilized nations, and Control Council Law No. 10. Manifestly human experiments under such conditions are contrary to "the principles of the law of nations as they result from the usages established among civilized peoples, from the laws of humanity, and from the dictates of public conscience."

Whether any of the defendants in the dock are guilty of these atrocities is, of course, another question.

Under the Anglo-Saxon system of jurisprudence every defendant in a criminal case is presumed to be innocent of an offense charged until the prosecution, by competent, credible proof, has shown his guilt to the exclusion of every reasonable doubt. And this presumption abides with a defendant through each stage of his trial until such degree of proof has been adduced. A "reasonable doubt," as the name implies, is one conformable to reason—a doubt which a reasonable man would entertain. Stated differently, it is that state of a case which, after a full and complete comparison and consideration of all the evidence, would leave an unbiased, unprejudiced, reflective person, charged with the responsibility for decision, in the state of mind that he could not say that he felt an abiding conviction amounting to a moral certainty of the truth of the charge.

If any of the defendants are to be found guilty under counts two or three of the indictment it must be because the evidence has shown beyond a reasonable doubt that such defendant, without regard to nationality or the capacity in which he acted, participated as a principal in, accessory to, ordered, abetted, took a consenting part in, or was connected with plans or enterprises involving the commission of at least some of the medical experiments and other atrocities that are the subject matter of these counts.

* * *

NOTE

The trial known as "The Case Against the Nazi Physicians" was completed on August 20, 1947. Fifteen of the 23 defendants were found guilty. Seven were found not guilty. One (Poppendick) was acquitted of the charges of having performed medical experiments but was found guilty of SS membership.

Sentence was pronounced the following day. Karl Brandt, Gebhardt, Mrugowsky, Rudolf Brandt, and three nonphysicians—Sievers, Brack, and Hoven—were sentenced to death by hanging. Life imprisonment sentences were imposed on Handloser, Schroeder, Genzken, Rose, and Fischer.

Herta Oberheuser, the only woman among the defendants, was sentenced to 20 years, as was Becker-Freysing. Beiglboeck was sentenced to 15 years, Poppendick to 10 years for SS membership. Rostock, Blome, Ruff, Romberg, Weltz, Schaefer, and Pokorny were acquitted and freed.

> The hangings took place on June 2, 1948. The scene was the prison at Landsberg, in the American zone. Here Hitler had been imprisoned while he wrote *Mein Kampf.*
>
> History records that the hangings took 62 minutes. Two black gallows were created in the prison courtyard. Karl Brandt was the only one of the seven who refused religious solace.
>
> The last words of the other murderers were not reported. In any event, 7 were hanged, only 4 of them physicians—7 out of the 23, and out of the many more who, as Dr. Mitscherlich's narrative makes clear, were involved in the Nazi medical crimes. It can never be said that the quality of American mercy had been strained. (A. Mitscherlich and F. Mielke, *Doctors of Infamy* [New York: Schuman, 1949], pp. 146–148)

Medicine and Human Rights: 20. Reflections on the Fiftieth Anniversary of the Doctors' Trial

George J. Annas and Michael A. Grodin

Many of our most important human rights documents are the product of the world's horror at the carnage of World War II. There are very broad and powerful announcements of human rights, such as the Universal Declaration of Human Rights, adopted by the United Nations in 1948. But there are also more specific statements of aspirations for all the world's inhabitants. In 1996 numerous observances marked the fiftieth anniversary of the commencement of the trial of Nazi physicians at Nuremberg, variously designated as the Doctors' Trial or the Medical Case.[1] In addition to documenting atrocities committed by physicians and scientists during the war, the most significant contribution of the trial has come to be known as the Nuremberg Code, a judicial codification of ten prerequisites for the moral and legal use of human beings in experiments. Some of the events that took place in 1996 and 1997 included international conferences in Nuremberg (sponsored by International Physicians for the Prevention of Nuclear War), in San Francisco (sponsored by the International Association of Bioethics), and in Washington, D.C. (sponsored by the United States Holocaust Memorial Museum). Anniversaries provide us with an opportunity to reflect upon the past, but they also enable us to renew our efforts to plan for the future. Have we learned the lessons of the Doctors' Trial? What can we do to make those lessons relevant for those practicing medicine fifty years later?

HISTORICAL CONTEXT

The trial of the Nazi doctors documented the most extreme examples of physician participation in human rights abuses, criminal activities, and murder. Hitler called upon physicians not only to help justify his policies of racial hatred with a "scientific" rationale (racial hygiene) but also to direct his euthanasia programs, experimentation programs and ultimately his death camps.[2] Almost half of all German physicians joined the Nazi Party.[3] In his opening statement at the Doctors' Trial, chief prosecutor Telford Taylor spoke of the watershed nature of the trial for the history of medical ethics and law:

> It is our deep obligation to all peoples of the world to show why and how these things happened. It is incumbent upon us to set forth with conspicuous clarity the ideas and motives which moved these defendants to treat their fellow men as less than beasts. The perverse thoughts and distorted concepts which brought about these savageries are not dead. They cannot be killed by force of arms. They must not become a spreading cancer in the breast of humanity. They must be cut out and exposed, for the reasons so well stated by Mr. Justice Jackson in the courtroom a year ago [before the International War Crimes Tribunal]: "The wrongs which we seek to condemn and punish have been so calculated, so malignant, and so devastating, that civilization cannot tolerate their being ignored because it cannot survive their being repeated."[4]

Fifteen defendants were found guilty of atrocities, of whom seven were executed. A universal standard of physician responsibility in human rights abuses involving experimentation on humans was articulated. The Nuremberg Code has been widely recognized by the world community, if not always followed.

The Nuremberg Code was a response to the horrors of Nazi experimentation in the death camps: wide-scale experimentation without consent, which often had the death of the prisoner-subject as its planned endpoint. The Nuremberg Code has ten provisions, two designed to protect the rights of subjects of human experimentation and eight designed to protect their welfare. The best known is its first, the consent requirement, which states in part:

> The voluntary consent of the human subject is absolutely essential. This means that the person involved should have legal capacity to give consent; should be so situated as to be able to exercise free power of choice, without the intervention of any element of force, fraud, deceit, duress, overreaching, or other ulterior form of constraint or coercion; and should have sufficient knowledge and comprehension of the elements of the subject matter involved as to enable him to make an understanding and enlightened decision.[5]

Although the Nuremberg Code has never been formally adopted as a whole by the United Nations, a statement related to torture appears as Article 5 of the Universal Declaration of Human Rights. A second sentence added to the text of Article 5, which further reflects the concerns of the Nuremberg Code, appears as Article 7 of the UN International Covenant on Civil and Political Rights. It states: "No one shall be subjected to torture or to cruel, inhuman or degrading treatment or punishment. In particular, no one shall be subjected without his free consent to medical or scientific experimentation."[6]

Most physicians would, of course, be shocked at having any assistance they give to patients considered "torture or ... cruel, inhuman or degrading treatment." They would thus view the Covenant's provisions in much the same way most physicians view the Nuremberg Code: as a legal document not applicable to actions taken by physicians. But this is a mistake, and only helps protect aberrant physicians by marginalizing their actions as nonmedical in nature and therefore of no concern to the medical profession. It is when a doctor disregards a person's bodily integrity that torture and involuntary human experimentation become virtually indistinguishable.[7]

THE WORLD MEDICAL ASSOCIATION

In late 1946, 100 delegates representing 32 national medical associations met in London to form the world's first international medical organization. The World Medical Association (WMA) was created to promote ties between national medical organizations and among doctors around the world. Its objectives are:

- To promote closer ties among national medical organizations and among the doctors of the world by personal contact and all other means available
- To maintain the honor and protect the interests of the medical profession
- To study and report on the professional problems which confront the medical profession in different countries
- To organize an exchange of information on matters of interest to the medical profession
- To establish relations with, and to present the views of the medical profession to the World Health Organization (WHO), the United Nations Education, Science and Culture Organization (UNESCO), and other appropriate bodies
- To assist all peoples of the world to attain the highest possible level of health
- To promote world peace[8]

In September 1947, shortly after the final judgment at the Doctors' Trial, the first official meeting of the WMA was held in Paris. The WMA formulated a new physician oath to promote and serve the health of humanity. This was followed by discussion of the "principles of social security." Key principles adopted included:

- Freedom of every physician to choose his location and type of practice
- All medical services to be controlled by physicians
- That it is not in the public's interest that doctors be full-time salaried servants of government or social-security bodies
- Remuneration of medical services ought not to depend directly on the financial condition of the insurance organization
- Freedom of choice of patient by doctor except in cases of emergency or humanitarian considerations[9]

Thus, one of the WMA's first acts was to protect the welfare of physicians themselves, which of course is perfectly consistent with the organizations' original objectives. The "principles of social security" were designed to support the personal and financial welfare of physicians rather than the security of their patients. The quest for a fee-for-service, private practice mode is in striking contrast to the social-obligation model that nearly all industrialized countries ultimately adopted: universal health care entitlements based on social welfare.

To the WMA's credit, however, one of the first issues discussed by its 1947 General Assembly was the "betrayal of the traditions of medicine" that occurred in Germany. The General Assembly asked, "Why did these doctors lack moral or professional conscience and forget or ignore the humanitarian motives and ideals of medical service [and] how can a repetition of such crimes be averted?" Also, it acknowledged the "widespread criminal conduct of the German medical profession since 1933."[10] The WMA endorsed "the judicial action taken to punish those members of the medical profession who shared in the crimes, and it solemnly condemned the crimes and inhumanity committed by doctors in Germany and elsewhere against human beings."[11] The General Assembly continued, "We undertake to expel from our organization those members who have been personally guilty of the crimes. . . . We will exact from all our members a standard of conduct that recognizes the sanctity, moral liberty and personal dignity of every human being."[12]

Nonetheless, consistent with its physician-protection goals, the WMA focused more on physicians' rights than patients' rights. Through its 1964 Declaration of Helsinki, for example, it endorsed shifting the focus of protection of human subjects in medical research toward the protection of patient welfare through physician responsibility away from the protection of the individual through informed consent. Further, the 1964 Declaration divided research into two types: research combined with professional care, and nontherapeutic research. Consent was required only for the latter. For the former, the individual serving as the subject of the research was identified as a patient, and consent merely urged: "If at all possible, consistent with patient psychology, the doctor *should* [emphasis added] obtain the patient's freely given consent after the patient has been given a full explanation."[13] The Declaration of Helsinki thereby undermined the primacy of subject consent as it appeared in the Nuremberg Code and replaced it with the paternalistic values of the traditional doctor-patient relationship.[14]

Although the WMA has also issued a number of noble statements condemning physician involvement in torture and capital punishment, it has largely acted like other professional trade associations. Its primary interest is the welfare of its members, with a secondary objective of issuing lofty ethical statements. With the exception of barring membership of Japanese and German medical professionals following World War II, the WMA has never sought to identify, monitor, or punish either physicians or medical societies who violate its ethical principles.[15]

BRITISH MEDICAL ASSOCIATION REPORT

The 1992 report of the British Medical Association's (BMA) Working Party on the Participation of Doctors in Human Rights Abuses documents continued physician involvement in crimes against humanity throughout the world.[16] Physicians have been directly involved in the torture of prisoners, as well as in indirect activities that facilitate torture. Physician involvement includes examination and assessment of fitness of prisoners to be tortured; monitoring of victims while being tortured; resuscitation and medical treatment of prisoners during torture; and falsification of medical records and death certificates after torture.

The BMA report documents cases of physician involvement in psychiatric diagnosis and commitment to mental institutions of political dissidents, forced sterilizations, force-feeding of hunger strikers, and supervision of amputation and other corporal punishments. Governments implicated span the globe, including the former Soviet Union, the United States, the United Kingdom, China, India, and South Africa, as well as countries in the Middle East and in Central and South America. The report notes the existence of international law and codes of ethics but acknowledges the lack of enforcement and inability to monitor compliance. The theme of the report is that neither medical associations nor international law has been effective in preventing physician involvement in human rights abuses.

CASE STUDY: PHYSICIAN PARTICIPATION IN HUNGER STRIKES

The increasing use of hunger strikes worldwide, especially by refugees and asylum seekers, creates situations urgently requiring physician attention to medical ethics. At the same time, it calls for effective international organizations to uphold and enforce standards relating to physician behavior. Within the past few years, there have been well-publicized hunger strikes for a variety of causes in many countries, including the United States, the former Soviet Union, China, South Africa, Sudan, Poland, the former Yugoslavia, Bangladesh, France, Egypt, Canada, Israel, and the Netherlands.[17]

For physicians, some of the most difficult situations involve individuals in the custody of the state, usually in prisons or other detention centers. In this context there have been deaths, most notably of ten Irish hunger strikers in Maze Prison in Northern Ireland in 1981.[18] Hunger strikes present two primary ethical questions for doctors: when is it ethical to force-feed a competent adult hunger striker, and when is it ethical to artificially provide nutrition to a hunger striker who has become incompetent or unconscious? Medical groups have offered conflicting ethical advice on the first issue, and virtually no guidance on the second. Thus, actual practice is mostly based on the personal beliefs of individual physicians rather than on professionally agreed upon ethical principles.

In the United Kingdom, the most definitive ethical statement remains the BMA's Central Ethical Committee's 1974 pronouncement that prison physicians must make the final decision with respect to intervention in prison hunger strikes.[19] The BMA's position seems to infer—wrongly, in our view—that force-feeding a competent adult should not always be viewed as torture. The WMA's point of view states that the doctor should act on behalf of the hunger striker as in any other doctor-patient relationship. However, the WMA avoids taking a position on the more difficult issue of what the physician should do after the hunger striker loses competence or consciousness, leaving to the individual physician to do what "he considers to be in the best interest of the patient."[20] The lack of definitive ethical standards caused consternation in the Netherlands in 1991 when a group of 180 Vietnamese refugees began a long hunger strike. The strike prompted the Johannes Wier Foundation for Health and Human Rights to organize a seminar in 1992 on assistance for hunger strikers, in cooperation with the Royal Dutch Medical Association.[21]

The seminar resulted in two concrete suggestions, both of which unfortunately raise more questions than they answer. The first is that the hunger striker be asked to fill out a document, modeled on the living will, called a Statement of Nonintervention. In this document, the striker sets forth his or her instructions regarding medical intervention in case there is a loss of competence. But does the living will model apply? Is the degradation of force-feeding eliminated by unconsciousness? Is the physician's role in accepting the written statement at face value more political than medical?

Second, the document suggests that an independent "doctor of confidence" be made available to prisoners who engage in hunger strikes. Of course prisoners should have access to physicians who can practice medicine free of state control, just as they must have access to their own lawyers; but what rules should this "doctor of confidence" follow? Moreover, what position should the prison physician take in countries where no such alternative physicians are available, and how can prison physicians who refuse to participate in torture or force-feeding be protected themselves?[22]

The lesson from the hunger strike example is that there is no credible international body capable of articulating universal medical-ethical standards, let alone any sort of plan to enforce them.[23] Until one is created, individual physicians will continue to muddle through these situations as best they can, using general ethical principles in settings in which these principles have little practical meaning.

A "PERMANENT NUREMBERG"

In light of these problems and many other ethical and human rights issues involving physicians, the authors, along with others, have argued that the world needs an international tribunal with authority to judge and punish those physicians who violate international norms of medical conduct, as well as an independent body to conduct ongoing surveillance and to develop a rapid response capacity. Without these, the world is as before Nuremberg—with international norms of medical conduct relegated solely to the domain of poorly defined medical ethics. In addition, the courts of individual countries, including the United States, have consistently proven incapable either of punishing those engaged in unlawful or unethical human experimentation or of compensating the victims of such experimentation. Primarily, this is because such experimentation is often justified on the basis of national security or military necessity.[24]

The International War Crimes Tribunal in 1946 declared that there were such things as war crimes and crimes against humanity, and that those who committed these crimes could be punished for them. The remaining trials at Nuremberg, including the Doctors' Trial, although based on the legal precedent articulated by the International War Crimes Tribunal (the so-called Nuremberg Principles), were held exclusively under the control and jurisdiction of the United States Army. M. Cherif Bassiouni, Robert Drinan, Telford Taylor, and others have argued eloquently and persuasively that a permanent international tribunal is needed to judge and punish those who commit war crimes and crimes against humanity.[25] Nonetheless, the international political will to form and support such a tribunal is lacking. There has even been difficulty in setting up ad hoc tribunals regarding Bosnia and Rwanda.

Arguments for a permanent international medical tribunal are every bit as compelling as those for a "permanent Nuremberg." Furthermore, establishment and support of a medical tribunal could also serve as a model for the broader international tribunal. The medical profession is perhaps the best entity to take a leading role in this regard. That is because it has an apolitical history, has consistently argued for at least some neutrality in wartime to aid the sick and wounded, has a basic humanitarian purpose for its existence and regards physician acts intended to destroy human health and life as a unique betrayal both of societal trust and of the profession itself. Moreover, it is much harder for governments to adopt inherently evil and destructive policies if they are denied the patina of legitimacy that physician approval provides.

AN INTERNATIONAL MEDICAL TRIBUNAL

Medicine and law are often viewed as opponents, but in the promotion of human rights regarding health they have a common agenda. In 1992, the world's physicians and lawyers were urged to work together to form and support an international medical tribunal.[26] Ideally, such a body would be established with the sanction and authority of the United Nations. However, given the competing political agendas of the member states, as evidenced by recent controversies at WHO, initial failure to win UN approval and support should not doom this project. Even if unable to punish with criminal sanctions, a tribunal could hear cases, develop an international code and publicly condemn actions of individual physicians who violate international standards of medical conduct. Establishment and support of such a tribunal is a worthy project for the world's physicians and lawyers.[27]

To move forward, establishment of such an international medical tribunal could become part of the advocacy efforts of medical and legal associations around the world. Because the tribunal must be both authoritative and politically neutral, no single country or political philosophy could be permitted to dominate it, either by having a disproportionate representation on the tribunal or by disproportionately funding it. The tribunal itself should be composed of a large panel of distinguished judges, the selective recruitment of which would be necessary for the tribunal's credibility. Governments would have to support the tribunal in a variety of ways, ranging from the funding of its infrastructure to permitting selected judges to take time off from their full-time judicial duties to hear cases.[28]

OTHER STEPS THE INTERNATIONAL COMMUNITY CAN TAKE

Steps should be taken at the level of national medical licensure boards (and state boards in countries in which political subdivisions have medical licensing authority) to articulate specific rules denouncing physicians who commit war crimes and crimes against humanity. Those found to have been involved in such crimes would lose their license to practice medicine, or be ineligible to obtain one if they were not yet physicians. Physicians who lost their license to practice medicine for war crimes or crimes against humanity in one jurisdiction would be prohibited from practicing medicine in all jurisdictions. Licensing agencies themselves could enter into a compact or agreement to adopt and enforce these rules and goals.

A central registry of physicians who have been found to have participated in war crimes or crimes against humanity could then be established. The registry could be kept by an independent nongovernmental organization of international physicians, lawyers, and jurists. The registry would also be a repository of evidence, such as affidavits and sworn testimony, that could be used by licensing agencies. Prior to licensing physicians, licensing agencies would query the central registry. The creation and use of such a registry is especially important in instances where countries authorize and use physicians to violate human rights, and where such violations would otherwise go unnoticed and unpunished. We, of course, realize that without an external investigating body and a functioning tribunal it will be difficult to identify these physicians, in that they are carrying out these violations in the name of the state. While this licensing sanction is not as strong as one might wish, it puts physicians on notice that should an investigation or adjudication reveal their involvement in human rights violations they would be unable to practice their profession outside of their own country.[29]

CONCLUSION

What lessons have we learned from the Doctors' Trial? Three stand out:

1. Statements, even authoritative statements, of medical ethics are not self-enforcing and require active promulgation, dissemination, and enforcement.

2. Human experimentation and torture are important areas in which violations of human rights and medical practice occur, but they merely represent

some of the broad range of physician involvement in human rights abuses around the world.

3. The world has no effective mechanism for promulgating and enforcing basic medical ethics and human rights principles.

An agenda for action flows naturally from these lessons: the world's physicians and lawyers should work together to develop and support worldwide mechanisms to articulate and enforce standards of medical ethics and human rights, including the establishment of an international organization dedicated to this cause, such as a permanent tribunal with the authority to punish relevant human rights abuses.

NOTES AND REFERENCES

1. G. J. Annas and M. A. Grodin (eds.), *The Nazi Doctors and the Nuremberg Code: Human Rights in Human Experimentation* (New York: Oxford University Press 1992); *Trials of War Criminals Before the Nuremberg Military Tribunal, Under Control Council 10*, vols. 1 and 2 (Washington, D.C. : Superintendent of Documents, U.S. Government Printing Office, 1950); Military Tribunal, Case 1, United States v. Karl Brandt et al., October 1946–April 1949.

2. R. Proctor, *Racial Hygiene: Medicine Under the Nazis* (Cambridge: Harvard University Press, 1987); J. R. Lifton, *The Nazi Doctors: Medical Killing and the Psychology of Genocide* (New York: Basic Books, 1986).

3. R. Proctor (see note 2), pp. 65–70.

4. Telford Taylor's opening statement, to *Trials of War Criminals* (see note 1), pp. 27–74.

5. The Nuremberg Code, ibid., Vol. 2, pp. 181–185. See pp. 298–299 in this book.

6. The International Covenant on Civil and Political Rights, GA Res. 2200 (XXI), 21 UN GAOR, Supp. (No. 16) 52, UN Doc. A/6316 (1966), art. 7.

7. J. Katz, "Human Experimentation and Human Rights," *Saint Louis University Law Journal* 38, 1 (Fall 1993): 7–54.

8. T. C. Routley, "Aims and Objects of the World Medical Association," *World Medical Association Bulletin* 1, 1 (1949): 18–19.

9. Ibid.

10. Editorial, *World Medical Association Bulletin* 1 (1949): 3–14.

11. Ibid.

12. Ibid.

13. *World Medical Association*, 1964 Declaration of Helsinki.

14. G. J. Annas, "The Changing Landscape of Human Experimentation: Nuremberg, Helsinki, and Beyond," *Health Matrix: Journal of Law-Medicine* 2 (1992): 119–140.

15. On the WMA election of a former member of the Nazi Party as president-elect, see M. A. Grodin, G. J. Annas and L. H. Glantz, "Medicine and Human Rights: A Proposal for International Action," *Hastings Center Report* 23, 4 (1993): 8–12.

16. Working Party, British Medical Association, *Medicine Betrayed: The Participation of Doctors in Human Rights Abuses* (London: Zed Books, 1992).

17. G. J. Annas, "Hunger Strikes," *British Medical Journal* 311 (October 1995): 1114–1115.

18. Some hospitalized patients, for example, may be as vulnerable to authoritarian

measures as prisoners. In the most famous case in the United States, a competent young woman, Elizabeth Bouvia, was continually force-fed in a California hospital after she threatened to starve herself to death. Although she was almost totally paralyzed from the neck down, four or more attendants were required to daily wrestle with her and restrain her while a nasogastric tube was forced through her nose and into her stomach. Her right to refuse such "treatment" was ultimately vindicated by the California courts, which have recently also ruled that prisoners retain this right of refusal as well. Legal authority is not the same thing as ethical conduct, but U.S. courts have held that a prisoner who is on a hunger strike to obtain a transfer or for better living conditions may legally be force-fed if necessary to preserve "order" in the prison setting. G. J. Annas, "When Suicide Prevention Becomes Brutality: The Case of Elizabeth Bouvia," *Hastings Center Report* 14, 2 (1984): 20–21; *Thor v. Superior Court*, 5 Cal. 4th 725, 855 P. 2d 375 (1993); G. J. Annas, "Prison Hunger Strikes: Why Motive Matters," *Hastings Center Report* 12, 6 (1982): 21–22.

19. Ethical statement: "Artificial Feeding of Prisoners," *British Medical Journal* (1974): 52–53.

20. World Medical Association, Declaration of Malta on Hunger Strikers (adopted by the 43rd World Medical Assembly in Malta in 1991 and revised at the 44th Assembly in Marbella in 1992).

21. This seminar was the basis for a pamphlet that has just been made available in English. The pamphlet itself relies heavily on the British Medical Association's 1992 Working Group report, *Medicine Betrayed: The Participation of Doctors in Human Rights Abuses*, and reprints the report's chapter on hunger strikes as its introduction. Johannes Wier Foundation for Health and Human Rights, *Assistance in Hunger Strikes: A Manual for Physicians and Other Health Personnel Dealing with Hunger Strikers* (Amersfoort: Johannes Wier Foundation for Health and Human Rights, 1995), pp. 5–12; British Medical Association (see note 16).

22. Perhaps the most arresting aspect of the Dutch document, representing as it does the philosophy of members of the only society to approve of physician killing, is what it leaves out. While the document was being prepared in early 1993, a sixty-five-year-old Dutch cancer patient went on a hunger strike after her physician refused to end her life through mercy killing. After twelve days of a highly publicized hunger strike, her request for euthanasia was agreed to by another physician. Who was this woman's physician and what role should her physician have played? Could (should) the second physician be considered a "doctor of confidence?" What is the relationship between the right to refuse treatment (including force-feeding) and "the right" to demand "treatment" (including medical killing)? "Hunger Striker Succeeds: Euthanasia for Dutch Woman," *Chicago Tribune*, March 23, 1993.

23. We will not find the "solution" to hunger strikes either by medicalizing them or by inventing new forms. Indeed, the Dutch suggestion simply highlights the physician's ethical dilemma, since a hunger striker could reasonably sign the Dutch form declining nutrition after incompetence, but privately instruct his doctor to ignore the signed form if treatment becomes necessary to save his life. This then makes the hunger striker look serious, while counting on the doctor not only to advertise his plight while conscious but to save his life should the hunger strike be unsuccessful. See G. J. Annas, "Hunger Strikes" (see note 17).

24. Grodin, Annas and Glantz (see note 15).

25. E.g., T Taylor, *The Anatomy of the Nuremberg Trials* (New York: Knopf, 1992); M. C. Bassiouni, *Crimes Against Humanity in International Criminal Law* (Dordrecht: Martinus Nijhoff, 1992).

26. Grodin, Annas, and Glantz (see note 15).

27. Such international nongovernmental organizations as Amnesty International and Physicians for Human Rights may have special roles to play in monitoring, reporting, and advocacy. The WMA has proven itself incapable of playing any meaningful role.

28. Ideally this tribunal should be under the jurisdiction of the United Nations and have criminal jurisdiction. But even without criminal jurisdiction, the tribunal could adjudicate cases based on international law, publicize the proceedings and results widely, and refer decisions for further action to relevant professional organizations and the board or agency responsible for licensing the physician or physicians involved. Accused physicians would be notified and given every opportunity to appear and present a defense. Without an international extradition agreement, however, physicians would not be compelled to attend. The trial should nonetheless proceed with appointed defense counsel if the defendant chooses not to appear, because a major goal is to deter war crimes and crimes against humanity through publication of their brutality and through international condemnation of them: punishment is not the only goal.

29. The advent of computer networks such as the Internet would facilitate universal access to search a central registry of physicians. Issues of privacy, confidentiality and the like would obviously have to be resolved. The World Wide Web is also a powerful tool for disseminating information about human rights. See, e.g., www.glphr.org.

21. Questing for Grails: Duplicity, Betrayal, and Self-Deception in Postmodern Medical Research

George J. Annas

Contemporary physicians and scientists often describe their experiments as part of a search for the "Holy Grail." Sometimes this quest is expressed more specifically, as when the Human Genome Project is described as a search for the "Holy Grail of biology."[1] This rhetoric suggests that experimental work is holy, God's work, and that the results will prove miraculous and good for everyone. But this type of blind devotion produces uncritical action that can ultimately destroy values essential to human dignity.

As Tennyson tells us in his poem, "The Holy Grail," "an excessively zealous pursuit after spiritual truth can be as destructive to social order as an indulgence in the materialistic qualities of life."[2] In Tennyson's poem, for example, a monk tells the questing Sir Percivale that forsaking his life at court for the hardship of the search for the Holy Grail was a choice he made at a time Percivale thought he could have both, a "double life," but that his dream of a better life was also a plague:

> but O the pity
> To find thine own first love once more—to hold,
> Hold her a wealthy bride within thine arms,
> Or all but hold, and then—cast her aside,
> Forgoing all her sweetness, like a weed!
> For we that want the warmth of a double life,
> We that are plagued with dreams of something sweet
> Beyond all sweetness in a life so rich,—[3]

Contemporary medical researchers often lead "double lives" in pursuit of their research goals, exhibiting the same determination and desperation as the questing knights of the Holy Grail. Like the knights of old, a medical researcher's quest of the good, whether that be progress in general or a cure for AIDS or cancer specifically, can lead to the destruction of human values we hold central to a civilized life, such as dignity and liberty.[4]

Doubling and duplicity in both language and action have become the hallmark of experimentation on humans in the United States and most of the developed world. We have come to this pass, like King Arthur's knights, with good intentions and worthy goals. Neither our intentions nor our goals, however, can justify the duplicitous use of language in human experimentation nor the betrayal of the Hippocratic ethic of "do no harm" in the physician/patient (researcher/subject) relationship.

This chapter explores the evolution of the rationales that physicians, from the Nazi doctors to contemporary experimenters, have used to justify experiments on their patient/subjects. The goal of this exploration is to articulate the destruction concealed by duplicitous language, including role ambiguity and overt deception. In conclusion, some remedial actions will be proposed. Although the scale and justification for research on humans is different when sponsored by the government or by private industry, language distortions and role ambiguities have infected both. This will be demonstrated by examining past government-sponsored, war-justified experiments (as exemplified by the radiation experiments), and current drug-company-sponsored, profit-justified experiments (as exemplified by cancer and AIDS experiments).

A POSTMODERN CRITIQUE

Most scholars date postmodernism from Hiroshima and the Holocaust, one an instantaneous annihilation and the other a systematic one. Together, they represent the death of our civilization's dream of moral and scientific progress that had characterized the modern age. The postmodern world is much more ambiguous and uncertain. Postmodern criticism seeks to subvert our culture and our beliefs. Nonetheless, by seeing culture and beliefs as subjects worthy of study and critique, it simultaneously legitimizes them. "It is . . . this doubleness that prevents any possible critical urge to ignore or trivialize historical-political questions."[5] The "double discourse" of the postmodern world is both illustrated and illuminated in our post–World War II discourse on human experimentation: a discourse that simultaneously condemns the Nazi experiments as barbaric, while demanding access to contemporary experiments as a human right. Use of a double discourse in this context obscures what should be illuminated and marginalizes what should be privileged. Exposing the pervasiveness of the double discourse at least gives us the option of confronting the ambiguities in our motivation and our actions and (re)forming, or at least (re)framing, current rules governing research on humans.

The concepts of doubling and "doublethink" live in contemporary human experimentation. For example, psychiatrist and author Robert Jay Lifton has suggested that the way in which the Nazi physicians at Auschwitz could continue to see themselves as healers while killing concentration camp inmates was through a process of "doubling." He describes it as "the division of the self into two functioning wholes, so that a part-self acts as an entire self."[6] Lifton's psychiatric assessment of the Nazi doctors need not be accepted. Nonetheless, there is a long history of the double in literature, including, for example, *Frankenstein* (between the creator and his creature) and *Dr. Jekyll and Mr. Hyde*. As Dr. Jekyll puts it:

> Though so profound a double-dealer, I was in no sense a hypocrite; both sides of me were in dead earnest; . . . With every day, and from both sides of my intelligence, the moral and the intellectual, I thus drew steadily nearer to that truth, by whose partial discovery I have been doomed to such a dreadful ship-wreck: that man is not truly one, but truly two.[7]

Doubling, of course, produces double standards; even "double thinking." This latter concept is well described in George Orwell's 1984, where power, "the capacity to inflict unlimited pain and suffering on another human being,"[8] is an end in itself. Orwell was writing primarily about totalitarian dictatorships, such as the Soviet Union under Stalin and Germany under Hitler. In Orwell's view, the key to a successful totalitarian system is abolishing truth as objective reality. When successful, "anyone who is a minority of one must be convinced that he is insane."[9] The dominant mode of thinking in this type of a society is denoted "doublethink," which means "'the power of holding two contradictory beliefs in one's mind simultaneously, and accepting both of them.'"[10]

The party's slogans in *1984* illustrate the concept of doublethink: "War is Peace, Freedom is Slavery, and Ignorance is Strength."[11] We tend to recognize these pairings as nonsensical, and think we could never be victims of such blatant propagandistic sloganeering. But even a cursory history of modern human experimentation demonstrates the pervasiveness of three doublespeak concepts: experimentation is treatment, researchers are physicians, and subjects are patients. Indeed, we have encapsulated all three into a "newspeak" word, "therapeuticresearch" (although we retain a space between the *c* and the *r*).

This doublespeak allows us to use double standards as they suit our purposes. It permits us to treat truth as negotiable and then allows us to act irrationally. We act in the best interest of patients. The experiment is justified as therapy or potential therapy. But if the experiment produces harm, it was after all, only an experiment and thus nonetheless a "success" because we learned something from it that could benefit others. It should be of only slight comfort that the term "therapeutic research" was invented not by a totalitarian government, but rather by physicians who were responding to a legal condemnation of experiments performed under the authority of a totalitarian government—the Nuremberg Code.

THE NUREMBERG CODE AND THE DECLARATION OF HELSINKI

The Nuremberg Code was formulated by United States judges at the end of the 1946–47 trial of twenty-three Nazi experimenters, twenty of them physicians. The Nazi experiments involved murder and torture: systematic and barbarous acts, with death often the planned endpoint. The subjects of these experiments were concentration camp prisoners, mostly Jews, Gypsies, and Slavs. The Nuremberg Code was articulated in response to horrendous nontherapeutic, nonconsensual concentration camp research. Nonetheless, the judges meant the application of the Code to be universal. After its fiftieth anniversary, the Nuremberg Code remains the most authoritative legal and ethical document governing international research standards and one of the premier human rights documents in world history.[12]

The judges based the Nuremberg Code on natural law theory. They derived it, with the help of expert witnesses from universal moral, ethical, and legal concepts. The Code protects individual subjects first by protecting their rights. Voluntary, informed, competent, and understanding consent is required by the first principle of the Code, and principle 9 gives the subject the right to withdraw from the experiment. The consent of the subject is necessary under the Nuremberg Code, but consent alone is *not sufficient*. The other eight principles of the Code are related to the welfare of subjects and must be satisfied *before* consent is even sought from the subject. The subject cannot waive these provisions. The requirements of these eight welfare provisions include a valid research design to procure information important for the good of society that cannot be obtained in other ways; the avoidance of unnecessary physical and mental suffering and injury; the absence of an *a priori* reason to believe that death or disabling injury will occur; risks that never exceed benefits; and the presence of a qualified researcher who is prepared to terminate the experiment if it "is likely to result in the injury, disability, or death" of the subject.[13]

Physician-researchers viewed the Nuremberg Code as constraining and inapplicable to their practices because (1) it was promulgated as a human rights document by judges at a criminal trial, and (2) the judges made no attempt to deal with clinical research on children, healthy volunteers, patients, or mentally impaired people. The Code, after all, applied only to Nazis. Moreover, the code has no explicit rules for many modern research agendas. The answer to the first concern is that the Code is universal; the response to the second lies in an interpretation of the Code, rather than in its abandonment. A reasonable analogy is the way we interpret the United States Constitution to apply to changes in technology.

The World Medical Association, nonetheless, has consistently tried to displace the Code with the Declaration of Helsinki, a more permissive alternative document, first promulgated in 1964 and amended three times since. The Declaration of Helsinki, is subtitled "Recommendations Guiding Doctors in Clinical Research" and is just that, recommendations by physicians to physicians. The declaration's goal is to replace the human rights-based agenda of the Nuremberg Code with a more lenient medical ethics model that permits paternalism.

U.S. researcher Henry Beecher probably best expressed medicine's delight with the Declaration of Helsinki's ascendancy when he said in 1970, "The Nuremberg Code presents a rigid act of legalistic demands. . . . The Declaration of Helsinki, on the other hand, presents a set of guides. It is an ethical as opposed to a legalistic document, and is thus a more broadly useful instrument than the one formulated at Nuremberg."[14]

The core of the Declaration of Helsinki is a doubling, dividing research into therapeutic ("Medical Research Combined with Professional Care") and nontherapeutic, thus blurring the line between treatment and research. The physician (researcher?) need not obtain the subject's (patient's?) informed consent to "medical research combined with professional care" if the physician submits the reasons for not obtaining consent to the independent review committee.[15] The current trend seems to seek to go even further, abolishing the distinctions between research and therapy, researcher and physician, and subject and patient altogether. In this new regime, research becomes treatment, the researcher become the healer, and the subject becomes a patient. The way language is use to obscure the truth and justify the unjustifiable can be illustrated by some cold war radiation experiments performed in the United States in the 1940s, 1950s, and 1960s, and contemporary experiments on terminally ill cancer and AIDS patients.

THE COLD WAR RADIATION EXPERIMENTS

In 1986, Representative Edward J. Markey (D-MA) released a report from the House Subcommittee on Energy Conservation and Power entitled "American Nuclear Guinea Pigs: Three Decades of Radiation Experiments on U.S. Citizens."[16] The report detailed thirty-one experiments conducted on more than seven hundred Americans by the federal government from the 1940s to the 1970s, most designed to test the effect on the human body of exposure to radiation. The experiments included injection of plutonium or uranium into terminally ill patients; irradiation of the testicles of prisoners to study the impact of radiation on fertility; exposure of nursing home residents to radium or thorium, either injected or ingested, to measure the passage of these radioactive substances through the body; and feeding of radioactive fallout to human subjects to see how the human body would excrete it. Although the 1986 report was carefully documented and cited specific published reports on the studies, it went virtually unrecognized and unheralded[17] primarily because the administration of President Ronald Reagan dismissed it as overblown.

Under the administration of President Bill Clinton, the reaction to similar disclosures, involving thousands of Americans, was dramatically different. In October 1993, reporter Eileen Welsome of the *Albuquerque Tribune* wrote a series of articles about five individuals who, without their knowledge or consent, had been injected with plutonium from 1945 to 1947 as part of an Atomic Energy Commission (AEC) study of the impact of plutonium on human beings.[18] The information was sought to help determine how to treat workers and scientists exposed to plutonium at weapons development and production plants. In one case, plutonium was injected into the leg of a thirty-six-year-old man who was thought to have bone cancer. The leg was then amputated for study. As a result of the amputation, the man could no longer work and was dependent upon his wife to support him. He died forty-five years later, in 1991. Another subject was misdiagnosed as having stomach cancer and was injected with plutonium in 1945. He lived to age seventy-nine, dying in 1966. The subjects were not told the purpose of the experiments, either at the time or when follow-up studies were conducted later.

When these stories became public, Hazel O'Leary, secretary of the U.S. Department of Energy (DOE),[19] said she was "appalled and shocked" by the plutonium experiments.[20] She took steps to begin an investigation of other radiation experiments conducted by the AEC and suggested that a way should be found to compensate the victims. This reaction was shared by President Clinton, who established an interagency task force to conduct a similar review of all federal agencies that might have been involved in radiation experiments during the cold war. The president also formed an advisory committee to the Task Force, which issued its final report in October 1995.[21]

The advisory committee's nine hundred-page report detailed a number of specific experiments and made recommendations regarding radiation experiments in particular, and research on human beings in general. Two specific experiments—one dealt with superficially by the advisory committee, the other in detail—illustrate the pervasive problems in the government-sponsored radiation experiments. The first was funded by the AEC and conducted at Boston's Massachusetts General Hospital in the mid-1950s. The experiment was designed to find the dose of uranium that could be tolerated by humans. The primary published report involved five terminally ill patients with brain tumors who were injected with uranium (U^{235}).[22] Four of the five were semicomatose or in a coma at the time; most died within two months, but one lived for seventeen months. There is no evidence of consent by anyone, although permission to perform an autopsy was refused by the family of the only woman in the study. The published report of the experiment (which indicated that the subjects had been exposed to a range of 10 percent to 30 percent of a lethal dose of uranium) concluded, "Of the common laboratory animals, man appears to correspond most closely to the rat in regard to intravenous tolerance to uranium."[23] Human subjects were used in the experiment because they were captive and available. No consent was sought or obtained, apparently because the researchers believed that terminally ill individuals could not be harmed. No disrespect to the subjects is intended by noting that they were treated no better than laboratory rats would have been. This was apparently not unusual in the 1950s. As one eminent physician, Louis Lasagna, told the advisory committee's investigators in an oral history interview, "Mostly, I'm ashamed to say, it was as if[,] and I'm putting this very crudely purposely[,] as if you'd ordered a bunch of rats from a laboratory and you had experimental subjects available to you."[24]

The advisory committee concluded that even if one of the purposes of the study had been to see if large doses of uranium localized in brain tumors, one of the patients had no such tumor.[25] "Even for the patient-subjects with brain cancer, there was no expectation on the part of investigators that the experiment would benefit the subjects themselves."[26] The committee concluded that although these patients were dying, and thus presumably were "not likely to live long enough to be harmed[,] it d[id] not justify failing to respect them as people."[27] Even though the committee found no evidence that informed consent was obtained from the subjects (it clearly could not be from those who were comatose), the committee nonetheless stopped short of condemning the experiment, saying simply, "Unless these patients [subjects?], or the families of comatose or incompetent patients, understood that the injections were not for their benefit and still agreed to the injections, this experiment . . . was unethical."[28]

But much more could (and should) have been said: Treating people like rats is unethical, even if relatives think it is acceptable. There are limits to what even dying patients can consent to if one takes the eight welfare principles of the Nuremberg Code seriously.[29]

The next experiment, the Cincinnati Whole Body Radiation Experiment, was conducted a decade later. By then, simply asserting that the patient was dying was no longer seen as sufficient justification for using patients for your own purposes. The Cincinnati Experiment, which involved eighty-eight subjects from 1960 to 1971, is described in a 1973 medical report by the investigators.[30] The study was financed by the U.S. Defense Project Support Agency "to determine whether amino acids or other biochemicals in the urine could 'serve as an indicator of the biological response of humans to irradiation.'"[31] Like the Massachusetts General Hospital study, this experiment was designed to test a hypothesis for the U.S. military on subjects selected primarily because they were available and thought to be terminally ill with cancer.

In the medical literature, the researchers attempted to transform this military research study into a civilian treatment series: "[t]he purpose of these investigations [was] to improve the treatment and general clinical management and if possible the length of survival of patients with advanced cancer."[32] It was alleged that, "[a]ll patients gave informed consent."[33] The patients were "eligible for this form of treatment if they ha[d] advanced cancer for which [a] cure could not be anticipated."[34] Later in the article, the experimental protocol itself is transformed into "the therapeutic regime."[35] Whether therapy or experimentation, however, serious problems were apparent even in this self-serving rendition: eight subjects (almost 10 percent) could have died directly from the radiation exposure; none were told of the risk of death nor of the common and devastating side effects of nausea and vomiting (56 percent experienced it); most patients were poor and black, and at least 12 percent had IQs under seventy.[36]

The principal investigator, noted radiologist Eugene Saenger, continues to defend this experiment as therapy. He has said that total body irradiation (TBI treatments) "were given as a 'palliative cancer therapy' for people for whom there was no better alternative."[37] This assertion is simply not credible.[38] The committee seems to have had considerable difficulty in deciding (1) whether these patients were subjects, (2) whether this intervention was innovative treatment (or experimental), and (3) whether the physicians were trying to help their patients. These are, of course, the ambiguities in research that are attenuated by duplicitous language. Nonetheless, the committee ultimately concluded:

> The impact of the research protocol on the care of the patient-subjects cannot be construed as beneficial to the patients; in addition, there is evidence of the subordination of the ends of medicine to the ends of research. The decisions to withhold information about possible acute side effects of TBI as well as to forgo pretreatment with antiemetics were irrefutably linked to advancing the research interests of the DOD. To the extent that this deviated from standard care, and caused unnecessary suffering and discomfort, it was morally unconscionable.[39]

The committee went on to raise, but not answer, a question at the core of our inquiry: "Whether the ends of research (understood as discovering new knowledge) and the ends of medicine (understood as serving the interests of the patient) necessarily conflict and how the conflict should be resolved when it occurs are still today open and vexing issues."[40]

Before the committee's *Final Report* was issued, a federal judge, relying on the Nuremberg Code, permitted a lawsuit by the families of these subjects against the researchers to proceed, stating:

> The allegations in this case indicate that the government of the United States, aided by officials of the City of Cincinnati, treated at least eighty-seven (87) of its citizens as though they were laboratory animals. If the Constitution has not clearly established a right under which these Plaintiffs may attempt to prove their case, then a gaping hole in that document has been exposed. The *subject of experimentation* who has not volunteered is merely an object.[41]

Because the committee recommended compensation for only a handful of injured subjects, the ultimate decision about monetary compensation for injury will be made in the courts.

CANCER AND AIDS

Writer Susan Sontag has noted that cancer and AIDS have become linked as perhaps the two most feared ways to die in the developed world. In her words, "AIDS, like cancer, leads to a hard death. . . . The most terrifying illnesses are those perceived not just as lethal but as dehumanizing, literally so."[42] Philosopher Michel Foucault was not speaking of the medicalization of death by cancer and AIDS when he chronicled the shift of power over life and death to government, but his words are equally applicable. "Now it is over life, throughout its unfolding, that power establishes its domination;

death is power's limit, the moment that escapes it."[43] In human experimentation on the terminally ill, we have Foucault's vision of public power played out in private; researchers take charge of the bodies of the dying in an attempt to take charge of the patient's lives and prevent their own personal deaths and death itself. One of the Nazi doctors' chief defenses at Nuremberg was that experimentation was necessary to support the war effort.[44] Now combating disease has itself become a "war" as we speak of a "war on cancer" and a "war on AIDS." And in that war, patients, especially terminally ill patients, are conscripted as soldiers. As former editor of the *New England Journal of Medicine* Franz Ingelfinger stated: "[T]he thumb screws of coercion are most relentlessly applied ... [to] the most used and useful of all experimental subjects, the patient with disease."[45] But as Sontag reminds us, war metaphors are dangerous in disease because they encourage authoritarianism, overmobilization, and stigmatization. In her words:

> No, it is not desirable for medicine, any more than for war, to be "total." Neither is the crisis created by AIDS a "total" anything. We are not being invaded. The body is not a battlefield. The ill are neither unavoidable casualties nor the enemy. We—medicine society—are not authorized to fight back by any means whatever.[46]

The self-deception inherent in seeing experimentation as treatment, especially in terminally ill cancer patients, is well illustrated by contemporary Phase I drug studies with anticancer agents. Are they research or therapy? Food and Drug Administration regulations state that Phase I studies are intended to have no therapeutic content, but are to determine "toxicity, metabolism, absorption, elimination, and other pharmacological action, preferred route of administration, and safe dosage range."[47] Nonetheless, National Cancer Institute researchers have insisted on calling them "potentially therapeutic."[48]

The self-deception problem is that in a terminally ill person, virtually any intervention, even a placebo, can be described as "potentially therapeutic." Once this misleading label is applied, the nonbeneficial Phase I study is *de facto* eliminated and transformed into therapy, now labeled "experimental therapy." Any distinction between experimentation and therapy is lost. This "Phase I doublespeak" has invaded even pediatric research, even though no cures or remissions for longer than a year have been documented in Phase I studies, and even though remissions occur less than 6 percent of the time and usually last less than two months.[49] Thus, the conclusion that "[a]dministration of chemotherapy in Phase I pediatric oncology trials should be considered a *therapeutic research* intervention because there is some likelihood of modest benefits accruing to *participating subjects*"[50] is untenable. Parents consenting on behalf of their dying children seem to be doing so because they are provided with false hope and unrealistic expectations. Moreover, 94 percent of investigators concede that patients (adults) enroll in Phase I studies "mostly for the possible medical benefit."[51]

Self-deception permits both researchers and subjects to "double" themselves: it permits researchers to see themselves as physicians and subjects to see themselves (and their children) as patients. When physician and researcher are merged into one person, it is unlikely that patients can ever draw the distinction between these two conflicting roles because most patients simply do not believe that their physician would knowingly harm them or would knowingly use them as a means for their own end. Because of the almost blind trust patients have in their physicians, the Helsinki Declaration's theoretical division between therapeutic and nontherapeutic research is meaningless. This is, of course, clearest for terminally ill patients who have "exhausted" all therapeutic options.

AIDS has always been perceived as the disease in which there literally is *no* distinction between treatment and experimentation. This is because, even though we are moving toward making AIDS a chronic condition, there is still no cure for AIDS. The disease primarily strikes the young, leading to a death that is premature. Existing treatments that can prolong life are far from satisfactory. ACT-UP's (AIDS Coalition to Unleash Power) political slogan, "A Drug Trial is Health Care Too," for example, serves to duplicitously conflate experimentation with therapy. It also encourages people with AIDS to seek out experimentation as treatment and physician-researchers to view AIDS patients as potential subjects who have "nothing to lose." Under this rationale, all types of experiments are performed under the guise of treatment. At the extreme are the experiments of Henry Heimlich in China, who used malaria infection to stimulate the immune system of AIDS patients. Anthony Fauci, director of the National Institute of Allergy and Infectious Disease and one of the nation's top authorities on AIDS, characterizes Heimlich's experiment as "quite dangerous and scientifically unsound."[52] Heimlich, on the other hand, says it is "'safe for patients,'" and he gets their consent.[53]

The most potentially far-reaching work in human experimentation is in the area of genetics. French Anderson, one of the leaders in the field, has argued that even the initial genetic experiments on humans should really be regarded as therapy:

> There exists a fundamental difference between the responses of clinicians [physicians] and basic scientists [researchers] to the question: Are we ready to carry out a human gene therapy clinical protocol?. . . .
>
> The basic scientist objectively analyzes the preclinical data and finds it wanting. . . .
>
> Clinicians look at the situation from a different perspective. Every day they are expected to provide their patients with the *best treatments for disease.* When they deal with incurable diseases, they must watch their patients die. . . . The urge to do something, anything, if it might help is very strong. . . .
>
> A clinician's reaction to a *new therapy protocol* tends to be: If it is relatively safe, and it might work better, then let's try it. Historically, much of medical innovation has resulted from trial and error experimentation. . . .

What's the rush? The rush is the daily necessity to help sick people. Their (our) illnesses will not wait for a more convenient time. We need help *when* we are sick.[54]

Anderson concludes his argument. "It will take many years of clinical studies before gene therapy can be a widely used treatment procedure. The sooner we begin, the sooner patients will be helped."[55] The distinction between experimentation and treatment is lost in this discussion, with the ethics of the inapplicable doctor-patient treatment model dominating the scientist-subject model. Likewise, the use of a baboon heart in the Baby Fae transplant was considered lifesaving therapy by the surgeon even though it was the first operation of its kind in the world.[56] It should be obvious that the fact that the patient is dying does not transform experimental interventions into standard treatment modalities and does not eliminate the necessity for informed consent. It is the nature of the intervention and the data that support its use, not the medical status of the patient or the intent of the physician-researcher, that determine the nature of the intervention. Likewise, consent can be asked for only after a justifiable research protocol has been developed. Just as consent is no justification for the torture, it is no justification for improper research. As I have put it previously:

> We must stop treating terminally ill cancer and AIDS patients as subhuman by [irrationally] offering them questionable experiments in the guise of treatment. We cannot justify this behavior on the basis of either their demand for it or our belief that the ultimate good of mankind will be served by it. Researchers who believe their subjects cannot be hurt by experimental interventions *should be disqualified* from doing research on human subjects on the basis that they cannot appropriately protect their subjects' welfare with such a view. Likewise, subjects who believe they have "nothing to lose" and are desperate because of their terminal illness should also be disqualified as potential research subjects because they are unable to provide voluntary, competent, informed or understanding consent to the experimental intervention with such a view. It should be emphasized that these are proposed *research* rules that would not necessarily apply to treatment in a doctor-patient relationship untainted by conflicts of interests.[57]

WHY LANGUAGE MATTERS

Language can clarify, but it can also obscure. The project of at least some leading medical researchers since Nuremberg seems to have been to use language to obscure—to blur or eliminate the distinctions between research and therapy, scientist and physician, and subject and patient. This doublethink is the essence of "therapeutic research," a concept that has been used to disguise the true nature of experimental protocols and to obscure the ideology of science (which follows a protocol to test a hypothesis) with the ideoogy of medicine (which uses treatments in the best interests of individual patients).[58] The motivation for disguising the distinction between interventions executed to test a hypothesis to gain generalizable knowledge and those performed for the benefit of the individual seems to be to lower the standards for obtaining informed consent. To the extent that physicians have been permitted to withhold certain risk information from patients under the "therapeutic privilege," this view has received at least some legal sanction. Modern informed consent doctrine, however, is meant to safeguard the patient's interest in both decision-making autonomy (liberty) and dignity. Thus, it is no longer appropriate to have separate disclosure requirements for therapy and research. Whatever differences currently exist in practice should be abolished because the rationale for information disclosure is identical in both cases.

There should be only one standard of informed consent, applying to both research and therapy, and it should be as set forth in article 1 of the Nuremberg Code: voluntary, competent, informed, and *understanding*. Courts have seemed to place the emphasis in the treatment arena on disclosure alone (i.e., the "informed" part of informed consent) rather than on the understanding of the information by the patient. Nonetheless, because the test of competence is the ability to understand and appreciate the information needed to give informed consent,[59] it is fair to conclude that the requirement of understanding the material information has always been an implicit part of the informed consent doctrine.

Consent requirements should also include all of the elements spelled out in the leading informed consent cases, such as *Cobbs v. Grant*[60] and their progeny,[61] and the federal rules for research on human subjects. Of course special rules can (and should) apply to those individuals who cannot consent for themselves, and these rules of substituted consent should be uniform (although there may be times when substitute consent is *not* permitted at all in the case of research because of its lack of benefit to the subject).[62] In this way, researchers should not be tempted to see their work as treatment so that they can avoid the requirements of informed consent—which in any event should be universal.

Informed consent is necessary in both contexts to protect the rights of the individual, but it is not sufficient. Consent, for example, has been transformed from a shield to protect subjects to a sword to be used against them in contemporary research. The consent (or demand) of the research subject is now often seen as sufficient justification in itself to perform the experiment on a human being.[63] But the consent of the research subject does not transform an experimental protocol into a therapeutic intervention. Consent speaks to liberty and dignity, not to reasonableness or risks and benefits. Choice, however, has been so reified in our society that we seldom ask "choice for what purpose?" Thus, Americans clamor for a "right to choose" virtually every consumer item and have already transformed medicine into a consumer commodity. Is it any wonder that Americans not only want to "choose" experimental, first-of-their-kind interventions, or that many have gone even further and insist on choosing death itself with the assistance of a physician?[64] Consent does not justify killing a person any more than it justifies an otherwise unjustifiable experiment. In the scientific research context, more safeguards are needed to protect the welfare of individual subjects. The "more" is, at minimum, the eight subject welfare precepts (updated as necessary) of the Nuremberg Code that the doublethink language seeks to obscure.

MARKET IDEOLOGY

Two ideologies have been explored: (1) the ideology of science, which puts the requirements of the research protocol designed to objectively test a hypothesis as the highest priority and (2) the ideology of medicine, which puts the best interests of the patient as the highest priority. Medicine, however, is currently faced with a new dominant ideology—the ideology of the marketplace, which puts profit-making (sometimes denoted by its method, cost containment) as its highest priority. For example, it has never been a secret that the pharmaceutical industry has been the most consistently profitable industry since World War II.[65] Now, however, as competition in this industry has heated up, and as the new biotechnology industry is emerging with great promises of future profits, the role of a successful clinical experiment has become central to the profitability of an entire industry. In this domain, both scientific truth and the best interests of patient-subjects can often find themselves sacrificed in the name of the bottom line. As one observer of the new biotechnology noted of the current state of medical science in the United States, "To do science you need money, but to raise money competitively you need to project illusions that are the antithesis of science."[66] Selling illusions to investors has replaced selling illusions to patients.[67]

A contemporary example combining cancer research and U.S. atomic research effectively illustrates the continuing pervasiveness of doublethink and its dangers to human subjects in an atmosphere governed not by war metaphors, but by market metaphors.[68] The Brookhaven National Laboratory is currently pursuing an experimental protocol to redo, in a more sophisticated manner, a radiation experiment conducted between 1951 and 1960. The experiment tests the use of a boron compound delivered to the brain in a stream of neutrons (generated by a nuclear reactor). The hope of this experiment is that the boron will become radioactive and deliver its radiation selectively to a brain tumor. This approach, termed "boron neutron capture therapy," proved either useless or fatal in the 1950s.[69]

The first subject, Joann Magnus, had a terminal brain tumor (a glioblastoma) and was admitted to the new experimental protocol before it was ready (in September 1994) because she had strong political connections. As Ms. Magnus herself said, "'I had nothing to lose.'"[70] Her physician said, "'I do what I think is best for each individual patient.... Without this treatment, she'd be dead.'"[71] Reporter Andrew Lawler's description of this first of its kind experiment in *Science* exemplifies the victory of doublethink. In his words, what happened involved "an improved version of a therapy," an "updated treatment," and simply, "the therapy."[72] Although only two subjects (of a planned protocol of twenty-eight) have undergone this experiment, Brookhaven National Laboratory is described as "bracing for a flood of requests from dying patients," having to devise "a lottery to choose from among those who meet stringent initial requirements for treatments."[73] "The procedure" is viewed as "a tremendous cash cow" for the laboratory.[74]

In our postmodern world, it seems to have struck no one as strange that DOE Secretary Hazel O'Leary, the very person who demanded (and received) a serious and sustained investigation into cold war radiation experiments, was also the person who sponsored the first subject for this U.S. government experiment.[75] In this case, Secretary O'Leary adopted the rationale of treatment of a terminally ill patient when she said, "There's a passion in the hearts of people who know they are terminal with a disease for which there seems to be no cure."[76] However, this particular experiment is about research, not treatment, and about giving the nuclear reactors made irrelevant by the end of the cold war a new lease on life (not "patients") by engaging them in, what O'Leary terms, "the positive side of nuclear technology."[77] Just how positive this procedure is remains to be seen. At least one critic, Princeton physicist and former head of the DOE's Office of Energy Research, William Happer, has noted that demand for experimentation with this procedure has existed for years and has been led by the "reactor mafia" who hope "to find some way to keep the reactors going."[78] What is obscured in this language is the experiment itself and that the "requirements" are those of science, not of medicine. This experiment is often viewed as a last-resort therapy, demonstrating the continuing ambiguity of postmodern experimentation on the terminally ill.[79]

Although the advisory committee decided not to explore contemporary radiation experiments like the one at Brookhaven, the committee did do the most comprehensive study to date on current research consent practices in the United States. Specifically, the advisory committee reviewed a random sample of eighty-four research protocols, consent forms, and institutional review board deliberations involving ionizing radiation funded from 1990 through 1993, and compared them with a sample of forty-one nonionizing radiation studies from the same period.[80] In a separate study, 1,900 patients at medical institutions across the country were interviewed.[81] Advisory committee member Professor Jay Katz of Yale conducted an independent review of ninety-three of these proposals.[82] No significant differences were found between radiation and nonradiation protocols or consent forms.[83] Of the 125 studies, 78 were rated as involving greater than minimal risk.[84] Of these, the committee concluded that about one-half raised serious or moderate ethical concerns, mostly affecting such things as the ability to understand the experiment, knowledge that participation is voluntary, and the ability to understand the potential risks involved. Professor Katz's separate study of the ninety-three proposals identified forty-one that posed greater than minimal risk. Of these, Katz identified thirty (or 75 percent) that raised serious ethical concerns, ten borderline, and twenty more serious.[85] In the committee's words:

> Katz found that the most striking element of the troublesome consent forms was the lack of a forthright and repeated acknowledgment that patient-subjects were *invited* to participate in human experimentation. All too quickly the language shifted to *treatment* and *therapy* when the latter was not the purpose and was only, at best, a by-product of the research.[86]

Katz described his own reaction to his study and the report in a "statement" in the body of the advisory committee's *Final Report*. On examining the informed consent process, Katz stated:

> I had expected to discover problems, but I was stunned by their extent. . . . The obfuscation of treatment and research, illustrated most strikingly in Phase I studies, but by no means limited to them; the lack of disclosure in randomized clinical trials about the different consequences to patient-subjects' well being if assigned to one research arm or the other; the administration of highly toxic agents, in the "scientific" belief that only the knowledge gained from "total therapy" will *eventually* lead to cures, but without disclosure of the impact of such radical interventions on quality of life or longevity.[87]

Katz concluded that although we all officially acknowledge that informed consent is central to the protection of subjects, we have "failed . . . to take responsibility for making these requirements meaningful ones."[88]

The message from this study is that the Institutional Review Board and informed consent mechanisms adopted to displace the Nuremberg Code's "rigid" requirements have failed. In almost half of all cases, this failure can be documented by a review of records alone—a review of actual consent discussions with the subjects would likely have been even more devastating. In its patient interview and survey, for example, the advisory committee found direct evidence of language choices used to deceive potential research subjects. The patients were asked to compare the terms "clinical trial," "clinical investigation," "medical study," and "medical experiment" with "medical research."[89] It will probably surprise no one that the term medical experiment "evoked the most striking and negative associations" and was the only term ranked worse than medical research.[90] "Clinical investigation" and "clinical trial" were somewhat better than "medical research," but the term "medical study" got the most favorable ratings of all.[91] Such studies were viewed as "less risky, as less likely to involve unproven treatments, and as offering a greater chance at medical benefit."[92] The study also indicated that many patients identify and conflate research with treatment.[93] In short, for many potential research subjects, deception or self-deception is inherent in our current research endeavors.

SOME SUGGESTIONS

It is no wonder that Americans demand experimentation as treatment and insist that their insurance companies and health care plans pay for experimental interventions. There is, of course, a continuum from (scientific) experiment to (therapeutic) treatment, but few interventions are in the gray zone, and an objective distinction can almost always be made between an experimental intervention and a treatment.[94] An experiment, for example, does not become therapy simply because no conventional (validated or invalidated) intervention exists any more than subjects become patients simply because they are given a terminal diagnosis. I have proposed elsewhere that we adopt special regulations to protect the rights and welfare of terminally ill patients from exploitative experimentation.[95] I continue to believe that this is necessary. Like the Nuremberg Code's consent requirement, however, it is not sufficient.

To confront not only our mortality, but also our morality, we must use language to clarify rather than obscure what we do to one another. Minimally, we must correctly identify and describe roles and responsibilities in human experimentation. In our postmodern world, it may not be realistic to think we can always distinguish research from therapy, physicians from scientists, or subjects from patients. Nonetheless, it is morally imperative to use language to clarify differences because ignoring these differences undermines the integrity of scientific research, the integrity of the medical profession, and the rights and welfare of patients and subjects.

This conclusion seems unremarkable and is not likely to be controversial. Putting it into practice, however, will require changes in the way we conduct contemporary experiments on humans that will likely cause controversy. Nonetheless, if we take the dignity, rights, and welfare of the subjects of human experimentation seriously in the clinical medicine arena, we should take at least the following minimal steps:

1. Research must always be identified as research, and its purpose (to gain generalizable knowledge) always spelled out and differentiated from medical treatment designed only to benefit the patient.

2. Patients should always continue to be patients, even if they also volunteer to serve as research subjects. It is unlikely that it will ever be possible—in our death-denying and death-defying world—for patients not to indulge in self-deception by imagining that research is really treatment and that they are patients, not research subjects. We cannot separate the subject into two persons. *But we can ensure that the subject-patient always has a physician whose only obligation is to look out for the best interests of the patient.* Thus, we can (and should) prohibit physicians from performing more than minimal-risk research on their patients, and as a corollary, only permit physician-researchers to recruit the patients of other physicians for their research protocols. In this way, at least the "doubling" of physician and researcher can be physically (and perhaps psychologically) eliminated.[96]

3. There should be strict disqualification rules for both subjects and researchers to engage in the research enterprise. At the extremes, for example, subjects who believe they have "nothing to lose" should be disqualified from participation because they are unable to give understanding (and perhaps voluntary) consent. Researchers who feel subjects have "nothing to lose" by participating should also be disqualified from doing research on them because they are not able to protect the dignity and welfare of their prospective research subjects with this attitude.[97]

4. The term "therapeutic research" and all of its progeny, such as "experimental treatment" and "invalidated treatment," should be abolished from research protocols and informed consent processes and forms. Research is research, designed to test a hypothesis and performed based on the rules of the protocol; treatment is something else, designed to benefit a patient, and subject to change whenever change is seen in the patient's best interest. Confusing research with treatment confuses both the researcher and subject and permits self-interested self-deception by both of them. The doubling and doublethink phenomena are difficult enough to control even when language itself is not used to disguise ambiguity.[98]

5. To help expose the new market ideology of experimentation, the researcher should be required to disclose any and all financial incentives involved in the research to both the IRB and to the potential subjects. This information should be presented to the subject in a separate written disclosure form so that the subject knows what financial incentives (i.e., conflicts of interest) may be affecting the scientific judgment or medical judgment of the researcher.[99]

6. Institutional review boards should be radically overhauled. We now have more than fifteen years experience with them, and they continue to support both doublethink and the double nature of the researcher physician. In this regard, they have primarily engaged in legitimizing ambiguity and deception and have betrayed the research subjects they are charged to protect. The explanation may be found in both the federal regulations that govern IRBs and the membership of these bodies. Reform on at least three levels is required. We need to (1) form a national human research agency to set the rules for research on humans, monitor their enforcement, and punish those who fail to follow them;[100] (2) rewrite current research rules to reflect the problems of doubling outlined in this chapter; and (3) restructure IRBs so that their role is to protect the subjects of research (not the researcher) and to hold researchers accountable to a national body (the proposed National Human Research Agency), not their own institution. At a minimum, this will require democratizing the IRBs by requiring a majority of members be community members and by opening all meetings to the public.

Changing our ways in our postmodern world will not be easy. Our quest for the Holy Grail of medicine (immortality?), as honorable as it is in theory, can become destructive in practice. As Bertolt Brecht has Galileo say in the version of his play he rewrote following Hiroshima:

I take it that the intent of science is to ease human existence. . . . Should you, then, in time, discover all there is to be discovered, your progress must become a progress away from the bulk of humanity. The gulf might even grow so wide that the sound of your cheering at some new achievement would be echoed by a universal howl of horror.[101]

NOTES AND REFERENCES

1. See, e.g., Those Who Forget Their History: Lessons for the Human Genome Quest, in *Gene Mapping: Using Law and Ethics as Guides*, pp. 46, 47–48 (George J. Annas and Sherman Elias, eds., 1992) (discussing this use of language by Judith P. Swazey).
2. *Tennyson's Poetry* 354 n.7 (Robert W. Hill Jr., ed., 1971).
3. Ibid., p. 368.
4. The most articulate, and most often quoted, statement of this principle is by Hans Jonas, and it deserves quotation here. Jonas understood that some of his suggested protections for human subjects might lead to slower medical progress, but nonetheless accepted this as a reasonable price to pay for the maintenance of important human values:

    > Let us not forget that progress is an optional goal, not an unconditional commitment, and that its tempo in particular, compulsive as it may become, has nothing sacred about it. Let us also remember that a slower progress in the conquest of disease would not threaten society, grievous as it is to those who have to deplore that their particular disease be not yet conquered, but that society would indeed be threatened by the erosion of those moral values whose loss, possibly caused by too ruthless a pursuit of scientific progress, would make its most dazzling triumphs not worth having.

    Hans Jonas, "Philosophical Reflections on Human Experimentation," 98 *Daedalus* (1969): 219, 245.
5. Linda Hutcheon, *The Politics of Postmodernism* (1989), p. 15.
6. Robert Jay Lifton, *The Nazi Doctors: Medical Killing and The Psychology of Genocide*, (1986), p. 418. Lifton also discusses the "healing-killing paradox" in which Nazi physicians kill for the sake of the health of the state, the "German biotic community." He goes on to explain:

    > Since the healing-killing paradox epitomized the overall function of the Nazi regime, there was some truth in the Nazi image of Auschwitz as the moral equivalent of war. War is the only accepted institution . . . in which there is a parallel healing-killing paradox. One has to kill the enemy in order to preserve—to "heal"—one's people, one's military unit, oneself (p. 431).
7. Robert L. Stevenson, *Dr. Jekyll and Mr. Hyde* (1891) (1989), p. 79.
8. George Orwell, *1984*, (Afterword by Erich Fromm), p. 263.
9. Ibid., p. 264.
10. Ibid.
11. Ibid., p. 7.
12. *The Nazi Doctors and the Nuremberg Code: Human Rights in Human Experimentation* (George J. Annas and Michael Grodin, eds., 1992) [hereinafter The Nazi Doctors and the Nuremberg Code].
13. See the Nuremberg Code in this book, pp. 298–99.
14. Sir William Refshauge, "The Place for International Standards in Conducting Research for Humans," *Bulletin of the World Health Organization* (Supp. 1977), 55, 133–135 (quoting H. K. Beecher, *Research and the Individual:*

Human Studies 279 (1970). The full text of all four versions of the Declaration of Helsinki appear in *The Nazi Doctors and Nuremberg Code* (see note 12).

15. *The Nazi Doctors and Nuremberg Code* (see note 12), p. 342.

16. Staff of House Subcomm. on Energy Conservation and Power of the Comm. on Energy and Commerce, 99th Cong., 2d Sess., *American Nuclear Guinea Pigs: Three Decades of Radiation Experiments On U.S. Citizens*, Comm. Print (1986).

17. A similar response greeted a later report of the Staff of Senate Comm. on Veterans' Affairs, 103d Cong., 2d Sess., *Is Military Research Hazardous to Veterans' Health? Lessons Spanning Half a Century*, Comm. Print (1994).

18. Eileen Welsome, "The Plutonium Experiment," *Albuquerque Tribune*, 1993 (a special reprint of a three-day series of articles originally published Nov. 15–17, 1993).

19. The Department of Energy is the successor to the Atomic Energy Commission.

20. Welsome (see note 18), p. 47.

21. Advisory Committee on Human Radiation Experiments, *Final Report* (1995) [hereinafter *Final Report*]. The president accepted the report in a White House ceremony on October 3, 1995; he also signed an executive order creating a National Bioethics Advisory Commission to advise the government on matters on research with human beings as well as other "bioethical issues." Executive Order No. 12,975, 60 Fed. Reg. 52,093 (1995).

22. A. J. Luessenhop et al., "The Toxicity in Man of Hexavalent Uranium Following Intravenous Administration," *American Journal of Roentgenology* 79 (1958): 83–100. There were eleven subjects altogether. See *Final Report* (see note 21), pp. 262–269.

23. Luessenhop, ibid., p. 100.

24. See Karen MacPherson, "Radiation Tests in Past Decades Broke Ethics Rules." *Sacramento Bee*, Jan. 23, 1995, p. A5 (quoting Dr. Louis Lasagna, reporting to the White House Advisory Committee on Human Radiation Experiments).

25. *Final Report* (see note 21), p. 263.

26. Ibid.

27. Ibid., p. 269.

28. Ibid.

29. The justification for treating human beings like rats was the same as one of the major justifications used by the Nazi doctors at Nuremberg: it was wartime (albeit a Cold War) and "extreme circumstances demand extreme action." In addition, these subjects were "already condemned to death" and thus were not harmed by the experiments. Michael A. Grodin, "Historical Origins of the Nuremberg Code," in *The Nazi Doctors and Nuremberg Code* (see note 12), p. 132.

30. *Final Report* (see note 21), pp. 385–406; Eugene L. Saenger et al., "Whole Body and Partial Body Radiotherapy of Advanced Cancer," *American Journal of Roentgenology Radium Therapy and Nuclear Medicine* 117 (1973): 670–685. The principal investigator, Eugene L. Saenger of the University of Cincinnati, wrote his first (and last) description of the study in the medical literature (yearly reports had been provided to the U.S. Defense Atomic Support Agency).

31. *Final Report* (see note 21), p. 386 (citation omitted).

32. Saenger (see note 30), p. 670.

33. Ibid., p. 671.

34. Ibid.

35. Ibid., p. 672.

36. Ibid., p. 680: *In re* Cincinnati Radiation Litig., 874 F. Supp. 796, 803 (S.D. Ohio 1995).

37. *Final Report* (see note 21), p. 387.

38. Nor should it, given the other types of studies that were conducted on these subjects. See, e.g., Louis A. Gottschalk et al., "Total and Half Body Irradiation: Effect on Cognitive and Emotional Process," *Archives of General Psychiatry* 31 (1969): 574–580. (discussing the effect of whole body radiation on their cognitive ability in a study done for the Defense Atomic Support Agency); Fred G. Medinger and Lloyd F. Craver, "Total Body Irradiation with Review of Cases," 48 *American Journal of Roentgenology Radium Therapy* 48 (1942): 651–671 (discussing a study, which Saenger himself cites in his 1973 article, indicating that whole-body radiation is useless for cancers that involve localized tumors).

　　Except for transient relief of pain in a few cases, the results in these generalized carcinoma cases were discouraging. The reason for this is quickly apparent. Carcinomas are much more radio resistant than the lymphomatoid tumors, and by total-body irradiation the dose cannot be nearly large enough to alter these tumors appreciably [without killing the patient]. Ibid., p. 668.

39. *Final Report* (see note 21), p. 405.

40. Ibid.

41. In re Cincinnati Radiation Litig., 874 F. Supp. 796. 822 (S.D. Ohio 1995) (emphasis added). It is heartening that the judge relied heavily on the Nuremberg Code as a basic human rights document in reaching her decision and was not swayed by the doublethink in the 1973 article. Ibid., p. 820. This case, however, is most noteworthy for its uniqueness. Usually, experimentation is successfully disguised as therapy. For example, immediately prior to the Gulf War, the U.S. Department of Defense sought and received permission from the Food and Drug Administration not to obtain informed consent from soldiers who were to be given drugs and vaccines under an "investigational new drug" protocol. The justification for this exemption was that consent was "not feasible," although no objective evidence was presented to support this assertion. Instead, it was simply alleged that these investigational agents were really "preventative or therapeutic treatment[s] that might save" lives. Request for Exemption from Informed Consent Requirements for Operation Desert Shield. Department of Defense, 55 Fed. Reg. 52, 813–17 (1990). *See generally,* George J. Annas, *Changing the Consent Rules for Desert Storm, New England Journal of Medicine* 326 (1992): 770–73 (discussing the rule and the legal challenges to it and recommending that it be withdrawn by the FDA).

42. Susan Sontag, *Illness as Metaphor and AIDS and Its Metaphors* (1990), p. 126.

43. Michel Foucault, *The History of Sexuality* 138 (Robert Hurley trans. 1990)

44. Grodin (see note 29), p. 132.

45. Franz J. Ingelfinger. "Informed (but Uneducated) Consent" *New England Journal of Medicine* 287 (1972): 465–466.

46. Sontag (see note 42), pp. 182–183.

47. President's Commission for the Study of Ethical Problems in Medicine and Biomedical and Behavioral Research, *Protecting Human Subjects* 65 (1981).

48. Ibid. (quoting letter from Edward N. Brandt, Jr., Assistant Sec. for Health, Dept. of Health and Environment (Nov. 20, 1981, pp. 3–4).

49. Wayne L. Furman et al., "Mortality in Pediatric Phase I Clinical Trials," *Journal of the National Cancer Institute* 81 (1989): 1193. This review of thirty-one Phase I clinical trials in children involving 577 "patients" found "34 objective

responses (11 complete and 23 partial) to . . . 27 Phase I agents, yielding an overall response rate of 5.9 percent. . . . The duration of the 11 complete responses
ranged from 12 to 300 days, with a median of 60 days." Ibid., p. 1193.

50. Terrence F. Ackerman. *The Ethics of Phase I Pediatric Oncology Trials,* IRB,
Jan.–Feb. 1995, pp. 1, 5 (emphasis added).

51. Eric Kodish et al., "Ethical Issues in Phase I Oncology Research: A Compari-
son of Investigators and Institutional Review Board Chairpersons," *Journal of
Clinical Oncology* 10 (1992): 1810, 1812; Mortimer B. Lipsett, *On the
Nature and Ethics of Phase I Clinical Trials of Cancer Chemotherapies,* 248
Journal of the American Medical Association 941–42 (1982). For a discussion
of the limits of parental authority to consent on behalf of their children, see
Catherine L. Annas, Irreversible Error: The Power and Prejudice of Female
Genital Mutilation, *Journal of Contemporary Health Law and Policy* 12
(1996): 325 (next chapter in this book).

52. Tim Bonfield, "Heimlich Uses Malaria in Research on AIDS," *Cincinnati
Enquirer,* Nov. 7, 1994.

53. Ibid. This "treatment" was also used in an episode of *Chicago Hope.* See
George J. Annas, "Sex, Violence and Bioethics: Watching *ER* and *Chicago
Hope,*" *Hastings Center Report,* Sept.–Oct. 1995), pp. 40, 42.

54. French Anderson, "What's the Rush?" *Human Gene Therapy* 1 (1990): 109,
110 (emphasis added); see also "New Zealand's Leap into Gene Therapy,"
Science 271 (1996): 1489 (describing a first of its kind genetic experiment as
"therapy"): Larry Thompson, "Should Dying Patients Receive Untested
Genetic Methods?" *Science* 259 (1993): 452.

55. Ibid. That genetic therapy (experimentation) has been oversold was recognized
by an NIH review panel set up by Director Harold Varmus to study the current
state of the technology. In December 1995 report, the panel concluded that
"gene therapists and their sponsors are 'overselling' the technology, promoting
the idea that 'gene therapy is further developed and more successful than it actually is.'" Eliot Marshall, "Less Hype, More Biology Needed for Gene Therapy,"
Science 270 (1995): 1752. In fact, the panel concluded that "[c]linical efficacy
has not been definitively demonstrated at this time in any gene therapy protocol . . . despite anectdotal claims of successful therapy." Ibid., see also Mered-
ith Wadam, Hyping Results 'Could Damage' Gene Therapy *Nature* 378 (1995):
655 (discussing view by a panel at the National Institute of Health that U.S.
biomedical researchers have been "overselling" the result of somatic gene therapy trials).

56. George J. Annas, "Baby Fae: The Anything Goes School of Human Experimentation," *Hastings Center Report,* Feb. 1985, p. 15.

57. George J. Annas, "The Changing Landscape of Human Experimentation:
Nuremberg, Helsinki and Beyond," *Health Matrix* 2 (1992): 119, 135.

58. See Alexander Capron, "Informed Consent in Catastrophic Disease Research,"
U. Penn L. Rev. 123 (1974): 340, 350; Jay Katz, "Human Experimentation
and Human Rights," *St. Louis University Law Journal* 12 (1993); Nancy King,
"Experimental Treatment: Oxymoron or Aspiration?" *Hastings Center Report,*
July–Aug. 1995), p. 6.

59. George J. Annas and Joan Densberger, "Competence to Refuse Medical Treatment: Autonomy vs. Paternalism," *Toledo Law Review* 15 (1984): 561, 578.

60. 502 P.2d 1 (Cal. 1972).

61. For a discussion of these cases, see George J. Annas and Frances H. Miller,
"The Empire of Death: How Culture and Economics Affect Informed Consent
in the U.S., the U.K., and Japan," *American Journal of Law and Medicine* 20

(1994): 357; and Heather Goodare and Richard Smith, "The Rights of Patients in Research," *British Medical Journal* 310 (1995): 1277.

62. See, e.g., *Children as Research Subjects: Science, Ethics and Law* (Michael Grodin and Leonard Glantz, eds., 1994); see also note 95 and accompanying text (providing recommended rules for terminally ill research subjects).

63. This seems to be especially true in AIDS research. See, e.g., George J. Annas, "Faith (Healing) Hope and Charity at the FDA: The Politics of AIDS Drug Trials," *Villanova Law Review* 34 (1989): 771 (providing examples of FDA actions in the AIDS area that were politically motivated).

64. See, e.g., *Vacco v. Quill*, 117 S.Ct. 2293 (1997) (reversing a lower court decision that there is no distinction between refusing life-sustaining treatment and committing suicide). George J. Annas, "The Bell Tolls for a Constitutional Right to Physician-Assisted Suicide," *New England Journal of Medicine* 337 (1997): 1098; Margaret Sommerville, "The Song of Death: The Lyrics of Euthanasia," *Journal of Contemporary Health Law and Policy* 9 (1993): 1 (on the use of language in the euthanasia debate).

65. Brian O'Reilly, "Drugmakers under Attack," *Fortune*, July 29, 1991, p. 48.

66. Barry Werth, *The Billion Dollar Molecule* (1994), p. 355.

67. Of course, illusions may be protected by both parties in the human experimentation context. As Christopher Hitchens notes in his iconoclastic biography of Mother Teresa, he is more interested in understanding the public's reaction to her alleged sainthood than Mother Teresa's own views of herself. In his words,

> What follows here is an argument not with a deceiver but with the deceived. If Mother Teresa is the adored object of many credulous and uncritical observers, then the blame is not hers, or hers alone. In the gradual manufacture of an illusion, the conjurer is only the instrument of the audience. He may even announce himself as a trickster and a clever prestidigitator and yet gull the crowd. *Populus vult decipi—ergo decipiatur.*

Christopher Hitchens, *The Missionary Position* (1995), p. 15.

68. See, e.g., George J. Annas, "Reframing the Debate on Health Care Reform by Replacing Our Metaphors," *New England Journal of Medicine* 332 (1995): 744.

69. See, e.g., L. E. Farr et al., "Neutron Capture Therapy of Gliomas Using Boron," in *Transactions of the American Neurological Association* (1954): 110–13; W. H. Sweet et al., "Boron-Slow Neutron Capture Therapy of Gliomas," *Acta Radiological* 1 (1963): 114; Scott Allen, "Radiation Experiments Coming Back to Haunt Researches," *Boston Globe*, May 29, 1995, pp. 27, 28.

70. Faye Flam, "Atomic Medicine's Second Chance: Brain Cancer Case Revives Boron Radiation Therapy Method Using Nuclear Reactor," *Washington Post*, Dec. 13, 1994 (Health Magazine), p. 9.

71. Ibid. A parallel example involves the use of genetic experiments for glioblastoma. See Larry Thompson, "Should Dying Patients Receive Untested Genetic Methods?" *Science* 259 (1993): 452.

72. Andrew Lawler, "Brookhaven Prepares for Boron Trials," *Science* 267 (1995): 956.

73. Ibid.

74. Ibid.

75. Ibid.

76. James Warren, "Positive Side of Nuclear Science: Energy Officials Find Them-

selves Playing in Life and Death Dramas," *Chicago Tribune*, Apr. 23, 1995, Sec. 5, p. 2.

77. Ibid.
78. Earl Lane, "A Treatment Before Its Time," *Newsday*, Sept. 4, 1994, at A7, A67.
79. Nor should it surprise us that even before her death, when Ms. Magnus suffered her first setback the medical director at Brookhaven announced: "None of us view this a failure in any sense." Arguing that what was going on was research, not treatment, he continued by noting that "the initial goals of the research are to show that treatment is safe and has no unintended side effects. 'Hopefully we get some information as to the effectiveness' as well." Earl Lane, "Pioneer Patient Hospitalized, Setback for Women in Neutron Therapy," *Newsday*, May 3, 1995.
80. *Final Report* (see note 21), pp. 695–697.
81. Ibid., pp. 724–25.
82. Ibid., p. 711.
83. Ibid., p. 701.
84. Ibid., p. 700.
85. Ibid., p. 712.
86. Ibid., p. 713.
87. Ibid., p. 853.
88. Ibid., p. 854.
89. Ibid., p. 734 (emphasis omitted).
90. Ibid.
91. Ibid.
92. Ibid.
93. Ibid., pp. 747–750
94. See, e.g., Renée Fox and Judith Swazey, *The Courage to Fail* (1974).
95. Proposed Regulations Governing Research on Terminally Ill Patients:
    (1) For the purpose of these regulations a "terminally ill patient" is one whose death is reasonably expected to occur within six months even if currently accepted and available medical treatment is used.
    (2) In addition to all other legal and ethical requirements for the approval of a research protocol by national and local scientific and ethical review boards (including IRBs), research in which terminally ill patients participate as research subjects shall be approved only if the review board specifically finds that:
       (a) The research, if it carries any risk, has the intent and reasonable probability (based on scientific data) of improving the health or well-being of the subject, or of significantly increasing the subject's length of life without significantly decreasing its quality;
       (b) There is no a *priori* reason to believe that the research intervention will significantly decrease the subject's quality of life because of suffering, pain, or indignity attributable to the research; and
       (c) Written informed consent will be required of all research participants over the age of 16 in research involving any risk, and such consent may be solicited only by a physician acting as a patient rights advocate who is appointed by the review committee, is independent of the researcher, and whose duty it is to fully and objectively inform the potential subject of all reasonably foreseeable risks and benefits inherent in the research protocol. The patient rights advocate will also be empowered to monitor the actual research itself.
    (3) The vote and basis for each of the findings in subpart (2) shall be set forth

in writing by the review board and be available to all potential subjects and the public.

(4) All research protocols (including the financial arrangements between the sponsor and the researcher) involving terminally ill subject shall be available to the public, and the meetings of the scientific and ethical review boards on these protocols shall be open to the public. Annas (see note 57), p. 138.

96. This suggestion has been made many times in the past. The primary objections to it have not been philosophical but practical. In major cancer centers, for example, virtually every patient has been referred for "new" or experimental protocols because conventional therapy has failed. Their primary care physician may be from another city or state. Who is to be the patient's physician (with only the patient's best interests in mind)? Simply appointing someone at the cancer research hospital may not be sufficient because it can be assumed that this person will share the general research/science ideology of the institution itself. But the logistics can be mastered if the goal is taken to be one of high priority—and in this setting, there can be no higher priority than protection of the patient's welfare. One approach, for example, is to use retired or semi-retired physicians as patient advocates whose only job is to look out for the patient's welfare. See the *Final Report* (note 21), pp. 140–41.

97. It is not just the use of the magic words "nothing to lose" that would trigger the disqualification (since both researchers and subjects would quickly learn not to use them), but an objective evaluation of the experiment and the researchers and/or subject's evaluation of it. The example of inducing malaria to treat AIDS necessarily requires both a researcher who thinks the patient has nothing to lose and a patient-subject who agrees with this assessment (see note 52).

98. See King (note 58).

99. Cf. *Moore v. Regents of the University of California,* 793 P.2d 479 (Cal. 1990). This case is discussed in George J. Annas, *Standard of Care: The Law of American Bioethics* (1993): 167–180; see also Harold Edgar and David J. Rothman, "The Institutional Review Board and Beyond: Future Challenges to the Ethics of Human Experimentation," *Milbank. Q.* 73 (1995): 489, 501 (recommending the preclusion of research on patients of a product in which the researcher has a commercial stake).

100. See, e.g., *Final Report* (note 21), pp. 855–856; and the Final Report of the Tuskegee Syphilis Study Ad Hoc Advisory Panel, U.S. Dept. of Health Education and Welfare(1973), pp. 23–24 (recommending a national review panel).

101. Bertolt Brecht, *Galileo* 18 (Charles Laughton, trans., and Eric Bentley, ed., 1992).

22. Irreversible Error: The Power and Prejudice of Female Genital Mutilation

Catherine L. Annas

During the 1994 Population Conference in Cairo, CNN showed a child being tortured in Egypt.[1] The child, a ten-year-old girl, was "circumcised"[2] by a barber while several men held her down.[3] Though four men were later arrested in connection with the act,[4] many believe the arrests were directly related to the publicity surrounding this United Nations conference.[5] In fact, after the media attention dissipated, Egypt's health minister withdrew his promise to pursue a legislative ban on the practice of female circumcision.[6] Instead, under pressure from Islamic fundamentalists, the Egyptian government lifted an existing thirty-five-year-old ban on performing the procedure in government hospitals.[7] However, the government again reversed its position in October 1995 and reimposed the ban.[8]

This practice, known as female circumcision, sometimes referred to as "cutting," is routine in many countries.[9] But because "female genital mutilation" is the more accurate phrase, I will use it for this chapter. Many political leaders and physicians throughout the world condemn the practice of female genital mutilation, and its prevalence has led some human rights organizations to respond with legal action against both government and religious leaders who support this practice.[10]

Why are fifty-five hundred females each day subjected to genital mutilation?[11] The answer is complex, intertwining issues of politics, gender, culture, nationalism, medical ethics, and law. Although the legal treatment of this procedure differs from country to country, its human rights implications transcend national boundaries and cultural beliefs.[12]

In the United States, the principles of familial privacy and personal autonomy are respected and protected, but how would these principles address a tradition such as female genital mutilation? While many human rights organizations and individual governments have condemned female genital mutilation, its practice has yet to be specifically condemned by international human rights laws. [13] This article will explain the medical procedures associated with female genital mutilation, explore the legal theories and problems raised by this practice, and conclude with recommendations designed to prohibit the continued practice of female genital mutilation.

INTRODUCTION

Female genital mutilation is usually performed on girls three to ten years of age.[14] In some countries, it is practiced upon newborns; in other countries, upon adolescents.[15] Female genital mutilation in no way resembles male circumcision.[16] While male circumcision involves the removal of the outer skin of the penis without damaging the organ itself,[17] female genital mutilation involves the actual removal of parts of the vulva. Female circumcision produces no health benefits.[18] Rather, it produces many damaging physical and psychological consequences.[19]

Forty countries around the world,[20] including more than twenty-six countries in Africa alone,[21] are home to the ritual of genital mutilation upon young girls. It has been estimated that the practice itself is six thousand years old,[22] and as many as a hundred million women in the world have endured some form of genital mutilation.[23] This is not a dying ritual. Each year, two million girls are subjected to genital mutilation.[24] Although perceived as a "religious necessity" by many Muslims,[25] it is neither mentioned in the Holy Koran[26] nor in the modern theological texts of Islam.[27]

Although female genital mutilation takes a variety of forms, there are three basic types: sunna circumcision, excision, and infibulation.[28] Sunna circumcision is the least destructive form and involves the removal of the prepuce and the tip of the clitoris.[29] Excision, the most common of the procedures,[30] involves the removal of the clitoris and the labia minora.[31] At times, this procedure also includes the removal of all external genitalia.[32] Finally, the most invasive of the three procedures is infibulation, where the clitoris, labia minora, and parts of the labia majora are all removed.[33] The two sides of the vulva are then stitched over the vagina, making intercourse impossible.[34] Although excision itself does not involve stitching, the vulvae often adhere to one another during the healing of the wound, which effectively results in infibulation.[35] Since excision is the most common form of genital mutilation[36] and infibulation is the most severe,[37] these two forms cause the most concern among health professionals. Female sexual pleasure occurs with stimulation of the clitoris. Its removal causes the genital area to become insensitive to touch,[38] making it virtually impossible for a woman to experience an orgasm.[39] Although there is much disagreement about whether or not a woman's sex drive is reduced by this procedure,[40] it dramatically reduces the sexual pleasure a woman may experience.

When exploring the subject of female genital mutilation, it is important to examine both the permanent medical and psychological effects of the procedure and the methods by which the procedure is performed. In Africa and the Middle East, an elder woman, often referred to as the "midwife," performs the operation.[41] The woman is not a doctor and, in most cases, has no medical training.[42] The midwife does the cutting, while two or three women (often the girl's mother and aunts) hold the child down and force her legs apart.[43] No anesthetic is used,[44] and the cutting instrument varies from a sharp razor to a knife or a sharp stone.[45] In many cases, the midwife circumcises a number of girls, one after another, without sterilizing the blade.[46] In some cultures, dirt and ashes are thrown on the wound to stop bleeding.[47] Barring any complications, the procedure may take only six minutes.[48] The child's legs are then bound together to allow the wound to heal.[49] In an infibulation procedure, thorns or a sticky paste are used to fasten together the bleeding sides of the labia majora,[50] leaving an opening about the size of a "matchstick or fingertip" for the passage of urine and menstrual blood.[51] The girl's legs remain tied together until the wound heals, which may take several weeks to more than a month.[52] The psychological wounds, however, may never heal.[53]

On her wedding night, the infibulated woman's vagina must be cut open by her new husband, often with the aid of a knife.[54] Repeated and prolonged sexual intercourse is then necessary to ensure the reopening of the vulva.[55] Reinfibulation is usually performed after childbirth, divorce, and widowhood.[56]

The risks associated with female genital mutilation are numerous and severe. The child experiences severe pain and shock.[57] Medical risks include the risk of exposure to HIV and other blood-borne diseases from unsterile instruments used during the procedure,[58] as well as the risk of death caused by infection and hemorrhaging.[59] Septicemia (blood poisoning) can also occur.[60]

With infibulation, women almost always experience difficulties in urination[61] and menstruation.[62] Sexual intercourse can be very painful, and penetration is difficult.[63] In addition, dermoid cysts often form in the line of a scar, and can grow "as large as grapefruits."[64] Increased infertility and infant mortality are also consequences of this procedure.[65] Difficulties during childbirth are frequent and lead to an increase in the number of children born with brain damage because of anoxia during delivery.[66] The highest infant mortality rates in the world occur in areas where female genital mutilation is practiced.[67] In addition, 25 percent of infertility is attributable to female genital mutilation.[68]

The justifications advanced by the cultures that practice female genital mutilation include tradition,[69] religion,[70] the sexual control of women,[71] and social acceptance.[72] While the use of "tradition" to justify an inhuman practice is not a novel concept, tradition is unpersuasive as a reasonable rationale for female genital mutilation. Slavery, for instance, is an example of a pernicious "tradition" eventually abolished in the United States by government action.[73] Another unpersuasive reason for permitting female genital mutilation is religion. No established religion in the world requires, or even suggests, that this procedure should be inflicted upon women.[74] Nonetheless, religion seems to be used as a pretext in some cultures by local religious leaders[75] to perpetuate the practice of female genital mutilation through generation after generation.[76]

Another justification advanced for female genital mutilation is control, or suppression, of the sexual behavior of women.[77] Infibulation, in particular, is used to ensure the "closed bride" that men in some cultures often require as the price for marriage.[78] Sexual suppression of women is the primary purpose of female genital mutilation.[79] The practice is used to ensure the virginity of girls prior to marriage[80] and to control promiscuity after and sometimes during marriage.[81] This explains why some women who are infibulated are restitched after they are divorced, widowed, or even during long periods of separation from their husbands.[82] Sexual control of women is a worldwide reality, but institutionalized gender inequality cannot justify female genital mutilation.

One of the most difficult justifications to address is social acceptance. Female genital mutilation occurs most frequently in societies where women have a one-dimensional presence and purpose.[83] In a society where girls are brought up to fulfill the role of wife and mother, female genital mutilation can become a prerequisite for achieving this goal. If a girl does not undergo some form of genital mutilation, she is deemed unfit to marry and has no other societal role. In areas where female genital mutilation is practiced, most men will not marry uncircumcised women,[84] and other women will not associate with them. They are social outcasts,[85] perceived as dirty, different, and even dangerous.[86]

BRINGING FEMALE GENITAL MUTILATION TO THE WEST: THE UNITED STATES, CANADA, AND FRANCE

The extent of American society's experience with female genital mutilation has been recent and limited.[87] In 1994, Lydia Oluloro attempted to halt deportation proceedings[88] against her by raising the defense of "cultural asylum."[89] Oluloro was born in Nigeria and claimed that her country's cultural tradition of female genital mutilation was a threat to her daughters. Although Oluloro herself underwent the ritual in Nigeria when she was four years old,[90] her daughters, Shade, age six, and Lara, age five, had not undergone the ritual.[91] On March 23, 1994, United States Immigration Judge Kendall Warren granted Oluloro's request for the suspension of her deportation.[92] Finding that the threat of female genital mutilation to Oluloro's daughters established the "extreme hardship"[93] required to establish residency status, Judge Warren concluded that female genital mutilation is "cruel and serves no known medical purpose."[94]

Unlike the United States, Canada and France have dealt with the issue of female genital mutilation in their societies for some time.[95] On May 10, 1994, in a case similar to that of Lydia Oluloro's, the Refugee Division of the Canadian Immigration and Refugee Board granted convention refugee status to a Somalia woman, Khadra Hassan Farah,[96] and her ten-year-old daughter and seven-year-old son.[97] The board found that the trauma Farah would experience as a result of losing custody of her children[98] (as would be almost certain if she was returned to Somalia) and the trauma that her son would experience as a result of being separated from his mother[99] were sufficiently "well-founded fear[s] of persecution."[100] The basis for Farah's claims stemmed from the fear that her daughter would be subjected to female genital mutilation if she was forced to return to Somalia.[101] The board determined that such gender-based persecution[102] would result in a gross infringement upon personal security,[103] thereby making the family eligible for convention refugee status.[104]

Canadian Deputy Prime Minister Sheila Copps has argued that assault and child abuse laws render female genital mutilation a crime in Canada.[105] However, Canadian criminal law makes no specific reference to it.[106] Some have called upon the Canadian government to specify female genital mutilation as a crime.[107] In 1992, the College of Physicians and Surgeons of Ontario warned its members against participation in female genital mutilation.[108]

In Paris, France, an estimated four thousand girls per year are subjected to female genital mutilation.[109] Recently, three young females died as a result of hemorrhaging after being circumcised.[110] In the recent criminal case of a woman from Mali who was performing the procedure in France, a judge suspended her one-year prison sentence.[111] She was the nineteenth person in France to be tried for participation in the procedure; however, very few judges have imposed prison sentences.[112]

Unlike Canada and the United States, France has established female genital mutilation as a form of persecution sufficient for refugee status.[113] Yet, unlike in Canada, no person has been granted such status in France.[114] With its increasing multicultural composition, including immigrants from countries where female genital mutilation is practiced, the United States should execute a preemptive attack upon female genital mutilation by using both legal tools and professional standards.

UNITED STATES LAW

The Rights of Children

American society is sympathetic to personal privacy, and the United States as a nation is built upon the idea of individualism. Exactly how far this doctrine extends in the context of the parent-child relationship is difficult to assess.[115] Nevertheless, one must come to some conclusions about the right of privacy in the parent-child relationship to understand how far the government may go in criminalizing the practice of female genital mutilation.

Individuals who immigrate to the United States bring with them many different cultural traditions. In the case of female genital mutilation, immigrant mothers may ask their American physicians to perform the ritual on their daughters.[116] The practice of female genital mutilation raises questions concerning the point where a state may constitutionally interfere with a parent's decision concerning his or her child. At what point does the state's interest in a child's health and well-being warrant interference with the parent's decision?

Parents are obligated to provide their children with necessities, including food, clothing, shelter, and necessary medical care.[117] Courts have permitted parents to refuse to have children treated for medical conditions in those cases where treatment may be deferred until the child is old enough to give consent.[118] However, parents must provide lifesaving treatment for their children, such as blood transfusions, even if such treatment violates their religious beliefs.[119] Where a child's life is in danger, courts have allowed the state to intervene and require treatment, often appointing guardians to protect the child's interest.[120]

More recently, child abuse and neglect statutes have been enacted with the express purpose of preventing parents from physically injuring their children.[121] These statutes do not prohibit spanking, corporal punishment, or discipline, but do prohibit permanent physical injury to children.[122] Therefore, child abuse laws can be construed as prohibiting the practice of female genital mutilation by parents or at the request of parents, because the practice results in permanent physical injury, is dangerous, and confers no medical benefit on the child.

Parents are also generally obligated to act in the best interests of their children; what this means, however, is often unclear.[123] Some cultural practices that were initially suspect in the United States because of their departure from established American culture have now been accepted in certain areas of the country. One example is "coining,"[124] a common healing method practiced by members of the Indochinese community to relieve fevers and other minor ailments. Coining, also called *cao gio*, involves passing a heated coin across the skin of the ailing person, thereby drawing the person's blood to the surface of the skin.[125] This procedure allegedly aids in treating colds by inducing the person to perspire.[126] Coining often leaves red marks on one's skin, which teachers sometimes assume are marks of child abuse.[127] Although some contend that coining constitutes a form of child abuse, most authorities refrain from filing child abuse charges against parents who engage in this practice.[128] This is because, unlike female genital mutilation, coining is relatively harmless and has no permanent effects, at least as long as it is performed in conjunction with (not instead of) appropriate medical treatment.

A state's *parens patriae* obligation to protect children is broad.[129] A state, for example, may prohibit parents from authorizing a sterilization procedure for their child, even if the parents believe "the child's adulthood would benefit therefrom."[130] The cutting required for female genital mutilation makes it more analogous to sterilization than coining, in that a permanent decision concerning a child's sexual future is made for the child. In fact, female genital mutilation may be considered more abusive than sterilization because of the fear and manipulation involved. In addition, female genital mutilation is always irreversible, while some sterilizations are not. Female genital mutilation can also be analogized to nonbeneficial, risky experimentation, which parents cannot consent to on behalf of their children because these procedures harm the child without the prospect of an offsetting benefit.[131]

Adults: Privacy and Consent

Female genital mutilation almost exclusively involves young girls, but some adult women who move to the United States after having been infibulated as a child in another country may seek reinfibulation following childbirth. Many would argue that because reinfibulation is so debilitating, a complete prohibition would have few negative effects. Legal prohibition of reinfibulation, however, raises potential problems, including whether such a restriction unconstitutionally limits a woman's personal autonomy.

There are many nontherapeutic operations performed on adults in the United States. Although some are socially condemned, they remain legal.[132] This is largely because of the high value Americans place on bodily autonomy and privacy. Although not specifically mentioned in the Constitution, a right of privacy has been recognized by the Supreme Court for almost thirty years. In the landmark case of *Griswold v. Connecticut*,[133] Justice William Douglas recognized a "zone of privacy" established by the Ninth and Fourteenth Amendments to the Constitution which extends to reproductive decisions.[134] This right to privacy was held broad enough to encompass a woman's right to terminate a pregnancy in *Roe v. Wade*.[135] In *Cruzan v. Director, Missouri Department of Health*, the Supreme Court also assumed that there is a strong right to bodily autonomy, a "constitutionally protected right to refuse life-sustaining hydration and nutrition,"[136] although the Court labeled this a liberty rather than privacy right.

Informed consent to reinfibulation is central to bodily autonomy. A patient must know and understand the risks of a procedure before entering into an agreement to undergo it.[137] Informed consent is extremely difficult to obtain with a practice such as female genital mutilation because of the misinformation surrounding the procedure. For example, myths are sometimes used to frighten girls into agreeing to be mutilated, and many women who are infibulated continue to believe such myths through their adult lives.[138] Due to the physical and psychological risks to the patient, doctors should refuse to participate in the reinfibulation of women because participation would tend to legitimize the procedure. The American Medical Association (AMA) seems to agree with this position. In a recently adopted policy report, the AMA House of Delegates urged Congress to pass legislation prohibiting female genital mutilation as a medically unnecessary practice.[139] Such legislation, however, is not necessary to permit physicians to lawfully refuse to perform reinfibulation since reinfibulation is not a medically necessary procedure.

States have nonetheless limited the actions that physicians may take, regardless of adult consent.[140] Examples include human experimentation,[141] actions considered to constitute assisted suicide, and maiming.[142] Consent is necessary before human experimentation may take place. However, consent alone is not sufficient.[143] In addition, eight other provisions of the Nuremburg Code must also be present,[144] including a reasonable hypothesis. However, reinfibulation does not fall under the category of human experimentation because it is sought by patients, rather than doctors, and it is not practiced to further medical knowledge.

Doctors are prohibited in some states from participating in activities that effectively amount to assisting suicide. Michigan, for example, passed a temporary statute forbidding physician-assisted suicide in response to Jack Kevorkian's ongoing crusade to aid those suffering from terminal illness,[145] and Michigan's highest court has declared that statute constitutional, even as applied to competent adults.[146]

In a 1992 California case, a man was denied the legal right to have his doctor assist him in cryogenically preserving his body.[147] In that case, Thomas Donaldson wanted to freeze his body while he was still alive and then be "reanimated" when a cure for brain cancer was found.[148] Donaldson wanted to undergo cryopreservation before he died or progressed into a persistent vegetative state.[149] The California Court of Appeals ruled that cryopreservation would be the equivalent of inducing death, which is defined in California to include "[a]n individual who has sustained . . . irreversible cessation of all functions of the entire brain."[150] That is exactly what would happen to Donaldson's body after being frozen. Characterizing the issue as a legislative one, the court refused to hold that Donaldson had a constitutional right to what it characterized as "state-assisted death,"[151] even though Donaldson's expressed desire was to live longer and not to die. Reinfibulation, however, does not approach the threshold of death the way cryopreservation does. While the risk of death certainly accompanies the initial removal of genitalia,[152] reinfibulation is sought long after the original mutilation has occurred.

Reinfibulation may, however, be considered a maiming, and it has been held that even an adult cannot consent to being maimed.[153] In *State v. Bass*[154] a physician was found guilty of the crime of mayhem for helping to amputate the healthy hand of an adult male so that the patient could collect disability benefits.[155] This case, however, was decided prior to the Supreme Court's decision in *Roe v. Wade* and did not concern an operation affecting reproductive organs. Since *Roe,* reproductive decision-making has been honored as a personal matter protected by the individual's privacy rights. Reinfibulation may be seen as required by the woman to resume sexual relations with her husband, and thus might be constitutionally protected.

Medical standards can and should be established to educate both doctors and patients about reinfibulation and to discourage its practice. Courts and legislatures, however, may be appropriately reluctant to forbid a procedure involving the reproductive organs of consenting adults that may be more benign than other legal operations. Although female genital mutilation is medically unethical, there are far more physically complex sexual operations performed on adults every day.

For instance, female-to-male sex-change operations involve a series of major surgery and hormone injections, including a double mastectomy and genital surgery occurring anywhere from a year to ten years later.[156] Reinfibulation, of course, is a much less invasive procedure than female-to-male sex-change operations. In addition, reinfibulation does not remove previously healthy tissue (as do double mastectomies), but instead is performed on tissue that has been previously altered. Female-to-male sex-change operations differ from reinfibulation in that doctors recognize sex-change operations as necessary when one's psychological gender differs from one's physiological gender. The changes made upon the body by sex-change operations are extreme and invasive. One's reaction to the idea of legally restricting female-to-male sex-change operations may be that so long as the individual involved fully understands the risks and consequences of the procedure, then it should be a decision for her to make with the assistance of her physician. Female genital mutilation is different from a female-to-male sex-change operation because it has no medical or psychological purpose. Reinfibulation, however, could be regarded as a personal choice because the procedure is less intrusive and does not destroy healthy tissue.

Plastic surgery is big business in America.[157] It is used to repair, to reduce and to enhance the human body. In addition, body piercing, tattooing, and branding are all popular ways to make individual statements and decorate one's body. Breast implants may be the most controversial plastic surgery procedure of all. Between two hundred thousand and one million American women have had breast implants inserted into their bodies.[158] Silicone gel implants have had many adverse health consequences, causing the manufacturing companies to discontinue their sale and to try to settle the potential legal claims of women who have been injured.[159] Among the proven side effects of silicone breast implants is an increased difficulty in cancer detection.[160] In addition, at least 20 percent of breast implants require repeat surgery to remedy the "ensuing pain, infection, blood clots or implant ruptures."[161] Twenty percent of breast implants follow breast cancer surgery, but the other 80 percent are undergone for purely cosmetic reasons.[162] Although there are ethical questions concerning the replacement of healthy tissue with potentially debilitating silicone merely for enhancement purposes, such operations have not been completely outlawed.[163] Again, the principle of bodily autonomy has trumped protectionist impulses and has led the FDA to refrain from prohibiting educated decisions by consenting adult women simply because those decisions may be thought too dangerous for the women involved.[164] Nonetheless, such regulatory action would not be unconstitutional if supported by a health and safety rationale and implemented under the authority of the commerce clause.[165]

While breast implants are still considered acceptable to mainstream society, branding, body piercing, and tattooing are all less acceptable to this "mainstream." However, they are outlawed for adults in only a few states.[166] "Branding" is the practice of making a burn design on one's skin by holding hot metal against it.[167] The scars that are formed as a result of the branding can take more that six weeks to heal.[168] In the cases of tattooing and body piercing, infections are common. Many more risks are associated with breast implants than any of these other procedures, but implants may be more acceptable because they make women look more like the supposed social ideal. Tattooing (at least facial tattooing) or branding, on the other hand, may be considered a departure from that ideal, used more to allow an individual to stand out as unique.[169] Nonetheless, decisions to undergo any of these procedures are left to the individual. Whether to be part of the "ideal" or rebel against it is seen as an expression of one's individuality and thus of autonomy. Although there are more severe risks associated with adult reinfibulation, education about those risks and rejection of the "benefits" involved may better serve to eradicate this practice than legal prohibition which could call into question other procedures that have been, until now, accepted in the legal arena.

Proposed Legislation to Outlaw Female Genital Mutilation

Although exposure to the issue of female genital mutilation in this country is recent, politicians and journalists have begun to express their concern and outrage against it. In 1992, Senator Edward Kennedy wrote a letter to the World Health Organization expressing his objection to this practice.[170] Geraldine Ferraro, the United States representative to the United Nations Commission on Human Rights, stated that "tradition and culture can no longer be cited to justify repression of half the world's population."[171] In addition, numerous journalists have attempted to bring the subject of female genital mutilation into the mainstream.[172] In what has been perhaps the strongest effort thus far to ensure that this practice is not undertaken in the United States, Congresswoman Patricia Schroeder[173] introduced a bill in Congress to outlaw female genital mutilation upon girls under the age of eighteen.[174]

On February 14, 1995, Congresswoman Schroeder introduced the Federal Prohibition of Female Genital Mutilation Act of 1995 in Congress.[175] This bill would make acts of female genital mutilation performed upon girls under the age of eighteen criminal assaults under federal law.[176] In the text of the bill, Schroeder specifies the age of eighteen as the time for possible consent to such operations. Although she and others working in this area do not condone reinfibulation, Congresswoman Schroeder's proposed bill recognizes the danger of restricting personal privacy in reproductive matters and is supported by the analysis of this chapter. Her bill also includes a "medically necessary" exception[177] and a section relating to educating the public on the practice.[178] Although the bill has not yet been passed, the House of Representatives has passed a resolution proposed by Congresswoman Schroeder urging President Clinton to encourage other countries to impose and enforce laws against female genital mutilation and to educate people about its dangers.[179]

The Schroeder bill was introduced to fulfill obligations of the United States under the International Covenant on Civil and Political Rights.[180] However, it is important for both the public and physicians that this practice be specifically condemned by American law as well as by international law. The law should be based on the exercise of Congress's commerce clause power so that it reaches all American physicians.[181]

Enforcement of the proposed ban on female genital mutilation on girls under the age of eighteen raises many questions. One question is whether to impose criminal penalties on parents who request that their daughters be "circumcised." Though female genital mutilation is not acceptable in the United States, criminal sanctions on parents who perform or request performance of the act may be somewhat undeserved. Many of these parents would eradicate the practice if given the choice. However, they feel as if they do *not* have a choice in the matter.[182] Though they may be subjecting their daughters to unfair and brutal physical pain, they are presumably attempting to protect them from cultural and social judgments that also can be painful and isolating.

The problem with extending the scope of criminal sanctions beyond the physicians performing such operations is that it is the child who is ultimately punished if her parents are prosecuted. Furthermore, if parents know that they are subject to criminal sanctions, they may be less likely to contact medical personnel when their child becomes ill as a result of the procedure.[183] Where parents are concerned, education would likely have a more positive impact than criminal punishment. However, while it can be assumed that some parents may not know better than to have this done to their daughters, such assumptions cannot be made about physicians.[184]

A Legitimate Medical Procedure?

To be accepted by the medical community, female genital mutilation would have to be recognized as a legitimate medical procedure. Clearly, it is not.[185] It offers no health benefits, imposes many risks, and perpetuates ideas of gender inequality. Female genital mutilation may be necessary for acceptance as a bride in some cultures, but it is not consistent with the values of American society. The medical community should not condone female genital mutilation and should actively discourage it.

Guidelines for dealing with reinfibulation should be set within the medical community. In particular, the American College of Obstetrics and Gynecology (ACOG) should supply its physicians with written information concerning reinfibulation.[186] Such information should explain the medical consequences and the harmful effects of reinfibulation. Physicians should be required to provide any patient who requests reinfibulation with such information. If a woman still insists on undergoing reinfibulation, the decision to participate must be left to the individual physician. No physician can be forced to perform a procedure he or she believes to be morally wrong. Doctors should not participate in unethical procedures such as female genital mutilation; for women over the age of eighteen, however, restrictions should stop short of legal prohibition.

Although reinfibulation is not the ideal in this situation, it seems to be the lesser of the evils. If outlawed in adult cases, women could be placed at physical risk, and other unwanted legal restrictions could follow. If guidelines are established within the medical profession to discourage this practice through education, autonomy in private matters will be retained, and people will be able to learn that there is no need, nor should there be a desire, to have female genital mutilation performed on their daughters.

INTERNATIONAL LAW: DOCTORS, GOVERNMENTS, AND HUMAN RIGHTS

The statement from the 1994 United Nations Population Conference in Cairo included the sentence "Governments are urged to prohibit female genital mutilation wherever it exists and to give vigorous support to efforts among non-government and community organizations and religious institutions to eliminate such practices."[187] As noted at the beginning of this article, the airing of an actual act of female genital mutilation on CNN received so much criticism[188] that at the conclusion of the conference Egypt's population minister and health minister promised the introduction of a law that would ban female genital mutilation in Egypt.[189] This is an example of why *constant* pressure must be applied to governments to ensure the eradication of female genital mutilation.[190]

The medical profession has repeatedly denounced female genital mutilation on the international stage. In 1982, the World Health Organization (WHO) released a statement noting that "female circumcision should never be performed by doctors in health establishments."[191] This statement recognizes the reality that the medical profession often stands as the judge of societal acceptance concerning physical interventions in the world today. The presence or involvement of a physician tends to make an activity appear more benign and credible since physicians are expected to act in the best interests of their patients.[192] This is the main reason why higher ethical standards are placed upon physicians and why their involvement in torture and human experimentation, as in Germany during World War II, is seen as much more horrific than the involvement of nonphysicians.[193]

In addition to WHO, other health organizations, as well as individual bioethicists, have voiced strong opposition to the practice of female genital mutilation. In 1994, the General Assembly of the International Federation of Gynecology and Obstetrics passed a resolution directing doctors to refuse to perform female genital mutilation.[194] The resolution directed doctors to

"oppose any attempt to medicalize the procedure or to allow its performance, under any circumstances, in health establishments or by health
professionals."[195] This resolution directly opposes the recent action of the
Egyptian government allowing female genital mutilation to be performed in
government hospitals. The 1993 Vienna Declaration of the World Conference on Human Rights also held that female genital mutilation is a human
rights violation.[196] Bioethicist Eike-Henner Kluge of the University of Victo-
ria has described doctors who perform such procedures as being "co-respon-
sible for participating in something that could only be described as barbaric,
unethical, and an abuse of persons."[197]

In the international forum, female genital mutilation has been recognized
as a human rights violation. It is a violation of the Geneva Convention[198]
and has been denounced by numerous international tribunals, including the
U.N. Commission on Human Rights[199] and WHO.[200] It has also been
specifically outlawed by many countries. In 1985, for example, Great Britain
enacted the Prohibition of Female Circumcision Act,[201] and in 1992 the
Dutch government expressed its opposition to all forms of "female circumcision."[202] Just as the binding of women's feet in China both injured them
and symbolized their subservience to men,[203] female genital mutilation has
been recognized as a weapon of sexual dominance and social conformity
against women.[204] Other gender-specific crimes are also used as instruments
to reinforce male dominance.[205]

Fran P. Hosken, a leading American expert on female genital mutilation,
has stated, "The same ideology that rape cannot be controlled . . . to keep
women in fear and dependent upon 'male protection' supplies the rationale
for genital mutilation."[206] Rape has a history of being considered a "crime
against humanity,"[207] but female genital mutilation would have to be considered under the "other inhuman acts committed against any civilian population" category of the definition of crimes against humanity.[208] It is more
difficult to have the international community recognize an act as a crime
against humanity if it is included only within the "other" category and not
specifically referred to, as "murder" and "enslavement" are. It is important
to have the "other" category for crimes that would not fall under the defined
categories. But when a crime is as widespread as female genital mutilation,
it should be recognized specifically by name.

In 1982, WHO recommended that governments "adopt clear national
policies to abolish the practice, and . . . inform and educate the public about
its harmfulness."[209] Some countries do have laws against female genital
mutilation, but they are generally not enforced.[210] Female genital mutilation has been outlawed in the Sudan since 1946, yet today 80 percent of the
women there have been subjected to the procedure.[211] Education and
understanding, in addition to legal prohibition, are imperative to realize the
beginning of the end of this practice. Therefore, individual countries, especially countries where women have a minimal voice in their political system,

cannot be left alone to deal with this issue. For international law to play an effective role in eradicating this practice, it must do so unequivocally.

International human rights law currently exists primarily as an ethical ideal by exposing morally inhuman practices in the world. Similarly, natural law principles provide guidelines for human rights, which are important in the search for justice and equality.

Female genital mutilation may violate both Article 3 and Article 5 of the Universal Declaration of Human Rights.[212] Female genital mutilation constitutes "inhuman" treatment under Article 5, which has been interpreted by the European Commission on Human Rights as "at least such treatment as deliberately causes severe suffering, mental or physical."[213] Female genital mutilation causes *both* mental and physical pain. Although it may be argued that such pain is not inflicted deliberately, the fact that no anesthetic is used during the procedure to reduce pain shows that some level of pain is intentionally inflicted. However, because of the permanent consequences of mutilation, the use of an anesthetic would not make female genital mutilation any more acceptable.

Female genital mutilation could also be considered "torture" under Article 5, where the "consent or acquiescence of a public official" is required.[214] Even if government inaction in enforcing laws against female genital mutilation will not be interpreted as "acquiescence or consent" (thus classifying it as "torture" under Article 5),[215] female genital mutilation can clearly be seen to constitute "inhuman treatment," and thus a violation of Article 3's guarantee of "security of person."[216]

The Convention on the Rights of the Child, which was adopted by the U.N. General Assembly on November 20, 1989, and went into effect on September 2, 1990, also provides specific protections for children. While female genital mutilation can arguably be a violation of the broader protections provided by Article 19 (protecting of the child from "all forms of physical or mental violence, injury or abuse"), Article 24 (recognizing the child's right to enjoy "the highest attainable standard of health") and Article 37 (ensuring that no child be subject to "torture or other cruel, inhuman or degrading treatment or punishment"), more specific references could be used to protect girls from female genital mutilation. For example, Article 34 provides that "States Parties undertake to protect the child from all forms of sexual exploitation and sexual abuse." Even if rejected as a form of "sexual abuse" for purposes of Article 34, female genital mutilation would still be included under Section 3 of Article 24's recognition of the child's right to enjoy "the highest attainable standard of health," which provides that "States Parties shall take all effective and appropriate measures with a view to abolishing traditional practices prejudicial to the health of children." Nonetheless, countries that have adopted or will adopt the convention should add the phrase "including female genital mutilation" to the end of Section 3 of Article 24.

CONCLUSION

Because female genital mutilation involves cultural, religious, and gender issues, debates often escalate to characterize Western "outsiders" as paternalistically judging the cultural practices of others.[217] Those who practice female genital mutilation condemn and dismiss criticisms without attempting to understand them. It is time to abandon the debate over the justifications for this practice and focus instead on its effects. Female genital mutilation has been ignored and allowed for many reasons. One reason is that many cultures consider a young girl to be the property of her nation or her tribe. On a more personal level, she is treated as the property of her parents, who dictate what will happen to her. The focus of this debate should not be on culture or nationalism, but on the subjects of this practice: the young girls who are routinely violated.

Throughout history there have been groups of people who have been treated as subordinates to the ruling race, gender, or class. The practice of female genital mutilation has continued as a sexist suppression of women in society. It continues almost unquestioned because it is practiced primarily upon women of color. It is also overlooked because it is imposed upon children and not adults. While all of these reasons are unacceptable, arguing about whether such oppression and discrimination exists will not protect the girls at risk.

Congresswoman Schroeder's proposal is a useful step and should be adopted. Nevertheless, we need not wait for passage of her proposal to condemn female genital mutilation. The practice of female genital mutilation is illegal in the United States because it violates child abuse laws that prohibit parents from mutilating their child's genitalia or encouraging or permitting others to do so. It also violates laws regarding maiming. For doctors, female genital mutilation is not a necessary medical practice, and therefore doctors are not protected from criminal prosecution for performing this act. Finally, any doctor who engages in the practice is civilly liable to the child for battery because the parent's consent in this instance is invalid. In addition, the doctor is liable for negligence because the procedure does not accord with reasonable medical practice given the widespread condemnation of the practice by medical organizations.

Because female genital mutilation is widespread, international action is appropriate to condemn it by specifically declaring it a human rights violation. Section 3 of Article 24 of the Convention of the Rights of the Child should be amended to specifically provide that "States Parties shall take all effective and appropriate measures with a view to abolishing traditional practices prejudicial to the health of children, *including female genital mutilation.*" Although adopting this proposal would not end the practice, it would be a concrete symbol of condemnation by the international community.

Unless the practice of female genital mutilation is addressed, it will continue because people fear rejecting the status quo. "Inalienable rights" is a beautiful phrase. However, for it to have true meaning, an attempt must be made to apply it to all people equally. The young girls who are at risk of female genital mutilation have the right to experience an adolescence and adulthood free of physical and psychological brutality. When the effects of female genital mutilation are honestly faced, nothing can justify it. Not culture. Not tradition. Not parental rights. Nothing.

REFERENCES

1. Eileen A. Powell, "Publicity on Taboo in Egypt May Reduce Number of Female Genital Mutilations," *Rocky Mountain News*, Oct. 9, 1994.
2. Although some countries continue to use the term "circumcision" to describe this practice, the term "genital mutilation" more accurately describes it. Fran Hosken, *The Hosken Report. Genital and Sexual Mutilation of Females* 32 (4th ed. 1993), established the term "female genital mutilation"); see also Phillipa Rispin, "It's Female Mutilation," *The Gazette* (Montreal), June 15, 1995, p. B2 (denouncing the use of the phrase "female circumcision").

   Since some African and Arab traditionalists still object to calling these female genital operations a "mutilation," the definition of the word should be examined. According to *Webster's*, to mutilate (from *mutilus*—maimed) means "to cripple, to injure, to damage, or otherwise make imperfect, especially by removing an essential part or parts." The term "mutilation" quite correctly describes what is done by [these] operations— which remove the most sensitive organ of the female body—and irrevocably injure and damage the female person.

   The equivalent procedure performed on men, excision of part or all of the penis, could be termed a "penisectomy," Rispin notes. Such a procedure would remove the possibility of orgasm for a man (as genital mutilation does for a woman). See Marlise Simons, "Mutilation of Girls' Genitals: Ethnic Gulf in French Court," *N.Y. Times* (Late Edition), Nov. 23, 1993.
3. "Government Prepares Law Banning Female Circumcision," *Agence France Presse*, Sept. 26, 1994.
4. "Four Men Arrested in Circumcision of 10-Year-Old Girl," *Wash. Post*, Sept. 13, 1994, p. A12.
5. "The Fight Against Female Genital Mutilation: Once-Taboo Subject Faces Criticism," *Toronto Star*, Sept. 27, 1994, p. B5.
6. After the Population Conference, Egypt's Health Minister Minster Dr. Ali Abdul Fatah Omaar stated that the Egyptian government has "no plans to ban [female circumcision] by introducing legislation." Peter Kandela, "Egypt Sees U Turn on Female Circumcision," *Brit. Med. J.* 310 (1995): 12.
7. John Donnelly, "Female Circumcision Draws New Scrutiny in Mideast," *Dallas Morning News* (Bulldog Edition), June 18, 1995, available in LEXIS, News Library, DALNWS File. The lifting of the ban has been attributed to increased pressure on the Egyptian government by the Islamic fundamentalist movement. Specifically, a recent Fatwa (religious decree) issued by Gad El-Haq Ali Gad El-Haq, theologian and grand sheik at Al Alzhar University, characterized female circumcision as a religious duty.
8. "Egypt Restores Limits on Female Circumcisions," *Boston Globe*, Dec. 30, 1995, p. 12.
9. Although most documentation on female genital mutilation focuses on the exis-

tence of the practice in Africa, female genital mutilation also occurs in Malaysia and Indonesia. See Hosken (note 2), pp. 45–46.

10. The Egyptian Organization of Human Rights ("EOHR") has filed a lawsuit against Sheik Gad Al Haq Ali Gad Al Haq for declaring female circumcision to be an Islamic duty. Shyam Bhatia, "Women Battle for Ban on Mutilation in Name of God," *The Observer*, July 30, 1995, available in LEXIS, News Library, OBSRVR File. As part of its case, the organization is citing the death of a fourteen-year-old girl, Amira Kamil, who died in September 1994 from massive hemorrhaging just days after being circumcised.

11. *Stats Quo, The Weekend Sun* (British Columbia), Oct. 1, 1994, p. B3.

12. In 1959, an Egyptian decree ordered that only doctors may perform the procedure. See *Four Men Arrested* (note 4), A12. In 1985, Great Britain passed a law banning female circumcision. Hosken, (see note 2), p. 35. In 1982, Sweden passed a law making all forms of female genital mutilation illegal. Nahid Toubia, "Female Circumcision as a Public Health Issue," *New Eng. J. Med.* 331 (1994): 715.

13. Hosken (see note 2), p. 36. For example, the U.N. Commission on Human Rights, as well as the *Country Reports on Human Rights Practices*, published annually by the United States Department of State, have deemed female genital mutilation a human rights violation.

14. Asim Z. Mustafa, "Female Circumcision and Infibulation in the Sudan." 73 *J. Obstetrics Gynaecology Brit. Cwlth.* 73 (1966): 303.

15. Hosken (see note 2), pp. 35, 40.

16. Toubia, (see note 12), p. 712.

17. Edgar J. Schoen, "Correspondence: Female Circumcision," *New Eng. J. Med.* 332 (1995): 188 (letter to the editor).

18. Toubia (see note 12), p. 713.

19. Robyn C. Smith, "Female Circumcision: Bringing Women's Perspectives into the International Debate," *S. Cal. L. Rev.* 65 (1992): 2451.

20. *Stats Quo* (see note 11).

21. Hosken (see note 2), p. 42. The practice of female genital mutilation is widespread globally, occurring in Mexico, Peru, and Brazil, as well as in parts of Australia and Russia. See Mustafa (note 14), p. 303.

22. Alice Walker and Pratibha Parmar, *Warrior Marks: Female Genital Mutilation and the Sexual Binding of Women* (New York: Harcourt Brace, 1993), p. 82.

23. Barbara Crossette, "Female Genital Mutilation by Immigrants Is Becoming Cause for Concern in the U.S." *N.Y. Times* (Late Edition), Dec. 10, 1995, p. 18.

24. Ellen Goodman, "Rescued from a Cruel Ritual," *Boston Globe*, Mar. 27, 1994, p. 75; "Two Million Women a Year Subjected to Sexual Mutilation," Agence France Presse. Oct. 2, 1994.

25. See Salman Rushdie, "Simple Truths and Apostles of Death." *N.Y. Times*, July 14, 1994, p. A23.

26. Walker and Parmar (see note 22), p. 327; Bhatia (see note 10), p. 14.

27. Walker and Parmar ibid.

28. Hosken (see note 2), p. 33.

29. Ibid. "Sunna" means "tradition" in Arabic.

30. Ibid.

31. Ibid.

32. Fran P. Hosken, "Genital Mutilation of Women in Africa," *Munger Africana Library Notes* 36, no. 7 (1976): 7.

33. Ibid.

34. Hosken, (see note 2), p. 34.
35. Ibid.
36. Fran P. Hosken, "Female Genital Mutilation in the World Today: A Global Review," *Int'l J. Health Services* 11 (1981): 422.
37. "Female Genital Mutilation Presents Array of Medical and Cultural Challenges," *ACOG Newsletter*, Jan. 1995, p. 10; J. A. Black, G. D. Debelle, "Female Genital Mutilation in Britain," *Brit. Med. J.* (1995).
38. Hosken (see note 2), p. 40.
39. Ibid., p. 37.
40. Some argue that female genital mutilation cannot curb sexual desire because such desire originates in one's brain. "Attack on Female Circumcision," *Sacramento Bee* (Metro), Sept. 4, 1994, available in LEXIS, News Library, SACBEE File. Others argue that the pain associated with the act of female genital mutilation has the effect of reducing one's desire to engage in sexual intercourse. Caryle Murphy, "'Mother This Isn't Fair of You'; In Egypt, Female Circumcision Is an Unyielding Tradition," *Wash. Post*, Aug. 28, 1994.
41. Ibid., p. 33.
42. Hosken (see note 2), p. 33. The decision whether and when to "circumcise" a girl is sometimes made by a barber. For example, one circumcisor in Egypt, Mohammed Abdel Fattah, has been quoted as saying, "First I examine them intimately. If their clitoris hangs out and arouses them sexually by rubbing against their underwear, then that's the time it should be cut. The operation is not necessary for those women whose clitoris is concealed." Bhatia, (see note 10), p. 14.
43. Council on Scientific Affairs, American Medical Association, "Female Genital Mutilation," *JAMA* 274 (1995): 1714.
44. Hosken (note 2), p. 33.
45. Lawrence P. Cutner, "Female Genital Mutilation," 40 *Obstetrical and Gynecological Surv.* 440 (1985); Mustafa (see note 14), p. 303.
46. Walker and Parmar (see note 22), p. 212.
47. Hosken (see note 2), p. 37.
48. Donnelly (see note 7).
49. Hosken (see note 2), p. 33.
50. Ibid.
51. Smith (see note 19), p. 2450 (citation omitted).
52. Hosken (see note 2), p. 33; "A Traditional Practice That Threatens Health— Female Circumcision," *WHO Chron.* 40 (1986): 31, 32.
53. Cutner (see note 45), p. 441.
54. *Female Circumcision* (see note 52), p. 32.
55. Hosken (see note 2), p. 15.
56. *Female Circumcision* (see note 52), p. 32.
57. Hosken (see note 2), p. 37.
58. Laurel Fletcher et al., "Human Rights Violations Against Women," *Whittier L. Rev.* 15 (1994): 331; Leslie H. Gise, "Women's Mental Health, Africa," *JAMA* 268 (1992): 1941 (reviewing *Women's Mental Health in Africa* [Esther D. Rothblum and Ellen Cole, eds., 1990]).
59. Hosken (see note 2), p. 37. In England, at least four girls have bled to death from botched circumcisions since 1978. "Female Genital Mutilation," *Am. Med. News*, March 13, 1995, p. 15.
60. Hosken (see note 2), p. 37.

61. Dottie Lamm, "Egypt: Land of Contrasts, Contradictions," *Denver Post*, Oct. 2, 1994, p. F4.
62. Hosken (see note 2), p. 37.
63. Smith (see note 19), p. 2451.
64. Toubia (see note 12), p. 713. A dermoid cyst is "a congenital cyst filled with sebaceous material and containing primary germ-cell layers and, perhaps, fetal remains. Upon removal the cysts are often found to contain hair, bone, teeth, and cartilage." Benjamin F. Miller and Claire Brackman Keane, *Encyclopedia and Dictionary of Medicine and Nursing* 263 (1972).
65. Hosken (see note 2), p. 37.
66. *Female Circumcision* (see note 52), p. 32. The rate of death of women in North America from pregnancy-related causes has been documented as 1 in every 4,000. "AIDS Growing Faster Among Women Than Men, U.N. Report Says," *Deutsche Presse-Agentur*, Aug. 2, 1995, available in LEXIS, News Library, Curnws File. This ratio is as high as 1 in 23 for women in African countries. Ibid.
67. Hosken (see note 2), p. 37.
68. Hosken (see note 32), p. 16.
69. Hosken (see note 2), p. 18.
70. Ibid., p. 40.
71. Ibid.
72. Ibid.
73. In addition to slavery, other immoral traditions include foot binding (China) and the burning of widows (India). Ibid., p. 18.
74. "What's Culture Got to Do With It? Excising the Harmful Tradition of Female Circumcision," *Harv. L. Rev.* 106 (1993): 1951 n. 57.
75. Ibid., p. 1950.
76. Cutner (see note 45), p. 439.
77. Lamm (see note 61), p. F4.
78. Hosken (see note 2), p. 15.
79. Ibid. at 32.
80. Ibid.
81. L. F. Lowenstein. "Attitudes and Attitude Differences to Female Genital Mutilation in the Sudan: Is There a Change on the Horizon?, *Soc. Sci. and Med.* 12 (1978): 417.
82. Hosken (see note 2), p. 34.
83. Toni Y. Joseph, "Scarring Ritual; Ancient African Custom of Female Circumcision Destines Women to Life of Subservience, Critics Say," *Dallas Morning News*, Apr. 18, 1993.
84. Hosken (see note 2), p. 34.
85. Kay Boulware-Miller, "Female Circumcision: Challenges to the Practice as a Human Rights Violation," *Harv. Women's L.J.* 8 (1985): 157–58.
86. Hosken (see note, 2), p. 40. This prejudice will not likely change until the practice of female genital mutilation is abolished.
87. Ibid., p. 36. However, female genital mutilation is documented to have occurred in the United States between 1890 and the late 1930s. Alison T. Slack, "Female Circumcision: A Critical Appraisal," *Human Rts. Q.* 10 (1988): 437, 461. Minnesota is one state that recently encountered the practice. Ellen R. Anderson, "Legislating Cultural Change: Female Genital Mutilation in Minnesota," *Hennepin Law.* 64 (1994): 16, 16. Once young girls started arriving at emergency rooms with severe hemorrhaging, the Minnesota

legislature moved quickly to enact a law that criminalized female genital mutilation. Ibid. The Minnesota law is broader than the federal bill introduced by
Congresswoman Patricia Schroeder (see notes 173–180) and accompanying
text, in that the Minnesota law criminalizes *all* acts of female genital mutilation that take place within the state, including those performed upon adult
women. See Anderson, p. 16. It should be noted that those few legislators
opposed to the Minnesota law dissented on the ground that restricting the
personal autonomy of women could serve as a negative precedent and could
be used to limit abortion rights. Anderson, p. 17.

88. *In re* Oluloro, No. A72 147 491 (Exec. Off. Immig. Rev., March 23., 1994).
Ms. Oluloro entered the United States to live with her husband who was a
lawful permanent resident of the United States, but he elected not to file for a
visa on Ms. Oluloro's behalf. When they divorced, and she was granted
custody of their two daughters. Mr. Oluloro informed the INS of her illegal
status in the United States. Ms. Oluloro claimed that her ex-husband was
abusive and that she feared leaving her daughters with him if she was deported.

89. Sophfronia S. Gregory, "At Risk of Mutilation," *Time,* Mar. 21, 1994, p. 45.

90. *In re Oluloro,* No. A72 147 491, oral dec., p. 7.

91. Timothy Egan, "An Ancient Ritual and a Mother's Asylum Plea," *N. Y. Times,*
Mar. 4, 1994, p. A25.

92. *In re Oluloro,* No. A72 147 491, oral dec., p. 20.

93. Ibid., p. 17.

94. Ibid., p. 16. Although Lydia Oluloro was successful in suspending her deportation, it is probable that she would have failed to establish grounds for asylum
or for an order withholding deportation without recognition of gender-based
prosecution as a basis because of the higher burdens these two other categories
require. See Patricia D. Rudloff, "Oluloro: Risk of Female Genital Mutilation
as 'Extreme Hardship'" in "Immigration Proceedings," *St. Mary's L.J.* 26
(1995): 899. to gain asylum, the person seeking such remedy is required to
have "a well-founded fear of persecution"(p. 889). In order to be granted a
declaration withholding deportation, the alien must prove that a clear probability of persecution exists—a higher burden than that for asylum (p. 890)
(citations omitted). Some courts have denied other sexually-related categories
of persecution. See, e.g., *Gao v. Waters,* 869 F. Supp. 1474, 1476 (N.D. Cal.
1994) (denying an alien's attempt at asylum from China's policies of coerced
sterilization and abortion).

95. Hosken (see note 2), p. 2.

96. Clyde H. Farnsworth, "Canada Gives a Somali Mother Refugee Status," *N. Y.
Times* (Late Edition), July 21, 1994.

97. *Immigration and Refugee Board Decision 193–12198* (May 10, 1994), p. 4.

98. Ibid., p. 6.

99. Ibid., p. 11.

100. Ibid., p. 1.

101. Ibid., p. 3.

102. Ibid., p. 8.

103. Ibid., p. 10.

104. Ibid., p. 11.

105. Allan Thompson, "Genital Mutilation Illegal, Copps Says," *Toronto Star*
(Metro Edition), Oct. 4,. 1994, p. A10.

106. Ibid.

107. Melissa Arasim, "Make Genital Mutilation a Criminal Act," *Toronto Star* (Metro Edition, Editorials and Letters), Oct. 13, 1994, p. A26.
108. Hosken (see note 2), p. 36 (citation omitted).
109. Kathryn Hone, "Tackling Africa's Ritual of Female Circumcision," *Irish Times*, Oct. 12, 1994, available in LEXIS, News Library, NON-US File. It has been estimated that 25,000 young girls from countries that practice female genital mutilation were living in France in 1993. Collette Gallard, "Female Genital Mutilation in France," *Brit. Med. J. 310* (1995): 1593.
110. Hosken (see note 2), p. 36.
111. Alexander Dorozynski, "French Court Rules in Female Circumcision Case," *Brit. Med. J.* 301 (1994); Andrew Gumbel, "Leniency in Female Circumcision Case Decried," *The Gazette* (Montreal), Sept. 17, 1994, p. A19.
112. Dorozynski (see note 111), p. 831.
113. Farnsworth (see note 96), p. A14.
114. Ibid.
115. See, e.g., *Roe v. Wade*, 410 U.S. 113, 116 (1973) (recognizing the constitutional right to privacy to include a woman's right to terminate a pregnancy); *Prince v. Massachusetts*, 321 U.S. 158, 166 (1944) (upholding child labor laws).
116. Hosken (see note 2), p. 36.
117. See George J. Annas, *The Rights of Patients*, 211 (2d ed. 1989).
118. Ibid., p. 112.
119. See generally *Jehovah's Witnesses v. King County Hosp.*, Unit Number 1, 278 F. Supp. 488 (W.D. Wash. 1967) (holding that Washington statutes granting judges the power to declare children dependent for the purpose of authorizing blood transfusions against objection of parents were constitutional).
120. See Annas (see note 117), p. 212.
121. Ibid., pp. 213–214.
122. See Leonard H. Glantz, "The Law of Human Experimentation," in *Children As Research Subjects: Science, Ethics and Law*, Ed. Michael A. Grodin and Leonard H. Glantz (New York: Oxford University Press, 1994), pp. 103, 106.
123. The subjective doctrine of substituted judgment is sometimes referred to in cases where children are not legally competent to make medical decisions. See Dan W. Brock, "Ethical Issues in Exposing Children to Risks in Research," in *Children as Research Subjects*, ibid., 84–85. Nonetheless, what is really at stake is the *objective* best interests standard because there is no reason to believe immature children will grow up to make idiosyncratic decisions (i.e., decisions objective observers would say were not in their best interests). Because society believes parents will usually act in the best interests of their children, parents are allowed to make certain decisions for their minor children. However, where particularly sensitive personal issues are involved, legislatures and courts often grant minors the legal right to consent for themselves. See Glantz (note 122), p. 112. State legislatures also recognize the constitutional protection of a right to privacy (including the right of a minor to consent to an abortion with or without parental notification). Sometimes parental authority itself is restricted. In one case, a court ordered a surgical operation to be performed on a child despite the objection of the child's mother. Annas (see note 117), pp. 112–113 (citation omitted).
124. Mary A. Perez, "Amazing ESL Stories Ring True; Adjustments to a New Land Can Be Traumatic, Book by Cal State Student Shows," *L.A. Times*, May 30, 1993, available in LEXIS, News Library, LATIMES File; Andy Rose,

"Breaking Down Cultural Barners; Police and Asian Community Learn Each Other's Customs," *L.A. Times* (Orange County), May 20, 1986.

125. Leslie Berger, "Learning to Tell Custom From Abuse," *L.A. Times*, Aug. 24, 1994, p. A1; Anne M. Lipinski, "Clinic Refugees Ease into Society," *Chi. Trib.*, Aug. 4, 1985, p. 8; Myrna Oliver, "Immigrant Crimes; Cultural Defense—A Legal Tactic," *L.A. Times*, July 15, 1988, pp. 13, 28.

126. Rose (see note 124.

127. Denise Hamilton, "Drawing the Line Between Love and Abuse," *L.A. Times*, Sept. 15, 1994.

128. Berger (see note 125), p. A1: Rose (see note 124.

129. *Prince v. Massachusetts*, 321 U.S. 158, 167 (1994). The *Prince* Court noted that "the state has a wide range of power for limiting parental freedom and authority in things affecting the child's welfare." Ibid. While this case addressed the issue of child labor laws, courts have noted other areas in which parental rights over a child may be restricted. For example, in *Wisconsin v. Yoder*, 406 U.S. 205 (1972), while upholding parental rights to remove children from school after the eighth grade on religious grounds, the Court noted that "the power of the parent . . . may be subject to limitation under Prince if it appears that parental decisions will jeopardize the health or safety of the child." *Yoder*, 406 U.S., p. 233. In addition, the "mature minor" rule has been used by states to "apply the law of competence to minors." Glantz (see note 122), pp. 112–113.

130. *A.L. v. G.R.H.*, 325 N. E.2d 501, 502 (Ind. Ct. App. 1975), *cert. denied*, 425 U.S. 936 (1976).

131. See *In re Sampson*, 278 N. E.2d 918 (N.Y. 1972); *In re Seiferth*, 127 N. E.2d 820 (N.Y. 1955).

132. For example, breast implants cause many medical complications. See Susan Faludi, *Backlash: The Undeclared War Against American Women* 219 (New York: Doubleday, 1991), p. 219.

133. 381 U.S . 479 (1965).

134. Ibid., p. 484.

135. In *Roe*, a leading case in the law of privacy, Justice Harry Blackmun wrote, "[T]his right of privacy . . . is broad enough to encompass a woman's decision whether or not to terminate a pregnancy" (*Roe*, 410 U.S., p. 153). However, Justice Blackmun further stated that "only personal rights that can be deemed 'fundamental' or 'implicit in the concept of ordered liberty' are included in this guarantee of personal privacy" (p. 152). These fundamental rights include marriage, *Loving v. Virginia*, 388 U.S. 1, 12 (1967), procreation, *Skinner v. Oklahoma*, 316 U.S. 535, 536 (1942), contraception, *Griswold*, 381 U.S., p. 479, and may even include, as Chief Justice William Rehnquist assumed in 1990 without deciding, the right of a "competent person . . . to refuse lifesaving hydration and nutrition" *Cruzan v. Director, Missouri Dep't of Health*, 497 U.S. 261, 279 (1990).

136. *Cruzan*, 497 U.S., p. 279; see also Walter Wadlington, "Medical Decision Making for and by Children: Tensions Between Parent, State, and Child," *U. Ill. L. Rev.* 311, 311 (1994) (analyzing the conflict between parental autonomy and the government's interest in protecting children as it arises in the context of refusing medical treatment).

137. George J. Annas et al., *Informed Consent to Human Experimentation: The Subjects Dilemma* (1994): 21.

138. Young women are sometimes told that if they are not "circumcised" their vaginas will grow teeth. Walker and Parmar (see note 22), p. 110.

139. Wayne Hearn, "Ban Sought on Genital Mutilation," *Am. Med News*, Dec. 26, 1994, p. 6.

140. Annas et al. (see note 137), p. 38.

141. Ibid., p. 21.

142. *State v. Bass*, 120 S. E.2d 580, 583 (N.C. 1961).

143. Annas et al. (see note 137), p. 20.

144. George J. Annas, "The Changing Landscape of Human Experimentation: Nuremburg Helsinki, and Beyond," *Health Matrix J. L. and Med.* 2 (1992): 119, 121.

145. George J. Annas, "Physician Assisted Suicide—Michigan's Temporary Solution," *New Eng. J. Med.* 328 (1993): 1574.

146. *People v. Kevorkian*, 527 N.W.2d 714 (Mich. 1994), *cert. denied, Hobbins v. Kelley*, 115 S.Ct. 1795 (1995) (holding that the United States Constitution does not prohibit a state from imposing criminal penalties on one who assists another in committing suicide). Kervorkian was found not guilty of violating this statute in March 1996. Carol J. Castaneda, "Suicide Ruling Sends a Message," *USA Today*, March 8, 1996, p. 3A.

147. *Donaldson v. Van De Kamp*, 4 Cal. Rptr. 2d 59 (1992).

148. Ibid., p. 61.

149. Ibid., p. 59.

150. Ibid.

151. Ibid., p. 64.

152. Hosken (see note 2), p. 35.

153. *State v. Bass*, 120 S. E.2d 580, 583 (N.C. 1961).

154. 120 S. E.2d 580 (N.C. 1961).

155. Ibid., p. 583.

156. Amy Bloom, "The Body Lies," *The New Yorker*, July 18, 1994, p. 38.

157. Profits from breast implant surgery in America have been estimated at between $168 million and $374 million. Faludi (see note 132), p. 218.

158. Naomi Wolf, *The Beauty Myth: How Images of Beauty Are Used Against Women* (New York: Doubleday, 1992), p. 241.

159. "Revisited Offer on Implants," *Chic. Sun-Times*, Nov. 15, 1995, p. 56; Mark Corriden, "Lawyers Advise Implant Clients to Reject Offer," *A.B.A. J.*, Jan. 1996, p. 18.

160. Wolf (see note 158), p. 229.

161. Faludi (see note 132), p. 219.

162. Marcia Angell, "Breast Implants—Protection or Paternalism?" 326 *New Eng. J. Med.* 1695 (1992).

163. They have been, however, stringently restricted. The FDA has required that when used for enhancement purposes only, breast implants be performed as part of an experiment so that safety data can be collected. Kim Painter, "Rheumatologists Find No Implant, Disease Link," *USA Today*, Oct. 25, 1995, p. 4D.

164. For example, other controversial genital operations, such as "vaginal-angle" surgery, have been performed in the United States. "Dr. Burt: Vaginal Surgery Patients 'Fully Informed'," *Am. Med. News*, Oct. 17, 1994, p. 32. Such operations, arguably, increase the sexual responsiveness of females. Ibid. Some may argue that an adult woman's right to be reinfibulated is no different than her right to have cosmetic surgery. See Slack (note 87), p. 463.

165. *United States v. Rutherford*, 442 U.S. 544 (1979) (upholding FDA regulation of Laetrile).
166. In Illinois, for example, tattooing is illegal only for minors (Phillip J. O'Conner, "South Suburb Is Needled By Tattoo Loophole," *Chic. Sun-Times*, Sept. 8, 1995), p. 9, and there are no laws against body branding in that state (Greg Beaubien, "Burning Question; Branding Makes Its Mark as the Latest Fad in Body Modification, but Is It Art or Selfmutilation?" *Chic. Sun-Times*, Feb. 17, 1995, p. 1).
167. Richard Cole, "Body Branding—Scarring—Is the New Thing to Do," *The Day*, Dec. 10, 1994, p. A2.
168. Ibid.
169. Matthew McAllester, "New Rules for Tatoos, Piercing?" *Newsday*, Oct. 29, 1995, p. A25.
170. 13 *Inter-African Committee on Traditional Practices Affecting the Health of Women and Children* 14 (1992).
171. 15 *Inter-African Committee on Traditional Practices Affecting the Health of Women and Children* 9 (1993).
172. Particularly, Ellen Goodman of the *Boston Globe*, A. M. Rosenthal of the *New York Times*, and various television news shows such as *Day One, Nightline, and Dateline* have aired major stories on the subject. Alice Walker brought this subject into American literature with her novel *Possessing the Secret of Joy* and continued its discussion in *Warrior Marks*, a book she co-authored about the making of a documentary film on female genital mutilation in Africa.
173. Congresswoman Schroeder is a Democratic representative from Colorado.
174. See H.R. 941, 104th Cong., 1st Sess. (1995). The bill was originally introduced by Representative Schroeder in the 103d Congress. The Senate's version of the bill, S. 1030, 104th Cong., 1st Sess. (1995), is sponsored by Senator Reid (D-Nev.). In September 1995, the Senate approved the bill, but the House of Representatives has yet to do so. "This Gruesome CustomIs a Crime," *Chic. Trib.*, Dec. 23, 1995.
175. S. 1030, 104th Cong., 1st Sess. (1995).
176. Ibid.
177. H.R. 3247, 3d Cong., 1st Sess. 2(a)(a) (1993).
178. H.R. 3247, 3d Cong., 1st Sess. 3 (1993).
179. Congressional Press Releases, *House Passes Schroeder Resolution on Female Genital Mutilation*, Federal Document Clearing House, Inc., June 7, 1995.
180. Ibid.
181. Recently, the Supreme Court made it clear that it is not sufficient for Congress to simply state that an activity is involved with interstate commerce for the court to approve congressional jurisdiction. In *United States v. Lopez*, 115 S. Ct. 1624 (1995), the court struck down the Gun-Free School Zones Act of 1990 on the basis that:

    > The possession of a gun in a local school zone is in no sense an economic activity that might, through repetition elsewhere, substantially affect any sort of interstate commerce. Respondent was a local student at a local school; there is no indication that he had recently moved in interstate commerce, and there is no requirement that his possession of the firearm have any concrete tie to interstate commerce. (1634)

    Even after *Lopez*, however, courts have found the Freedom of Access to Clinic Entrances Act of 1994, which prohibits the use of force or threat of force to intimidate individuals from obtaining or providing reproductive services, to be within Congress's commerce clause authority. See *Cheffer v. Reno*, 55 F.3d 1517 (11th Cir. 1995). This is because reproductive health services are a "commercial activity" and were so found by Congress, which noted that "doctors and patients often travel across state lines to provide and receive services. . . . In addition, clinics receive supplies through interstate commerce."

182. Murphy (see note 40), p. A1.

183. For example, judges in France have been reluctant to extend criminal sanctions to parents because parents have no "criminal motivation" or intent. "French Court Rules in Female Circumcision Case," *Brit. Med. J.* 309 (1994): 832.

184. The American Medical Association has made recommendations concerning female genital mutilation and the medical profession. One recommendation is to support legislation aimed at eliminating the practice in the United States. Council on Scientific Affairs, American Medical Association, "Council Report: Female Genital Mutilation," *JAMA* 274 (1995): 1716.

185. See "Female Genital Mutilation," *ACOG Committee Opinion* (The American College of Obstretricians and Gynecologists, Washington, D.C.) (Jan. 1995) [hereinafter ACOG Committee Opinion].

186. Ibid. The committee recommends education on the issue of female genital mutilation by "promoting awareness among the public and health-care workers and by developing methods for educating physicians regarding the gynecologic and obstetric care of women who have undergone this procedure".

187. A. M. Rosenthal, "A Victory in Cairo," *N.Y. Times*, Sept. 6, 1994, p. A19.

188. Judy Mann, "When Journalists Witness Atrocities," *Wash. Post*, Sept. 23, 1994, p. E3.

189. *Law Banning Circumcision* (see note 3); Powell (see note 1).

190. Donnelly (see note 7).

191. Female Circumcision, 1982 Statement of WHO Position [hereinafter *WHO Statement*].

192. Annas et al. (see note 137), p. 20–21.

193. A doctor places herself in a higher ethical category than the average person when she takes the Hippocratic Oath, which states, "I will prescribe regiment for the good of my patients according to my ability and judgment and never to harm anyone."

194. Carolyn Adolph, "Doctors Must Become Advocates for Women, Conference Is Told," *The Gazette* (Montreal), Oct. 1, 1994, p. A3.

195. Deborah Charles, "Medical Group Calls for Ban on Female Circumcision," *Reuters World Service*, Sept. 30, 1994.

196. Toubia (see note 12), p. 715.

197. Lisa Priest, "Our MDs 'Involved' in Genital Mutilation," *Toronto Star*, Oct. 3, 1994, p. A9.

198. The Universal Declaration on Human Rights: A Commentary 103 (Asbjorn Eide et al., eds., 1992).

199. Hosken (see note 2), p. 36.

200. WHO Statement (see note 191).

201. See 12 Hasbury's Statutes of England and Wales 969 (4th ed. 1989).

202. 14 *Inter-African Committee on Traditional Practices Affecting the Health of Women and Children* (1993).

203. Jonathan E. Berman, "Understand Female Genital Mutilation, Yes, But Don't Condone It," *N.Y. Times*, Nov. 30, 1993, p. A24.

204. See Nahid Toubia, "Female Genital Mutilation," in *Women's Rights, Human*

Rights: International Feminist Perspectives, Ed. (Julie Peters and Andrea Wolper) (New York: Routledge, 1994), p. 224.

205. For example, it is estimated that even today up to fifteen thousand deaths in India per year are the result of murder because of "dowry disputes." Kathleen Koman, "India's Burning Brides," *Harvard Magazine*, Jan.–Feb. 1996, pp. 18–19.

206. Hosken (see note 2), p. 84. Although this may seem an overstatement, rape itself has been used as a war strategy. See The Center for Reproductive Law and Policy, *Recognizing Forced Impregnation as a War Crime Under International Law* 4–5 (1993). For example, in Bosnia Herzegovina, Serbian soldiers have used rape camps and forced pregnancy as a strategy of war. While there are also reports of Serbian women who have been raped by Bosnian Muslim soldiers, Serbian soldiers have practiced "systematic rape." Fletcher et al. (see note 58), p. 322. Forced pregnancies occur when female prisoners are raped by Serbian soldiers and then detained until their pregnancies have advanced to the stage where abortions can no longer be legally obtained. Sherry Ricchiardi, "Bosnian Rape Victims Tell of Terror: Relief Workers Documenting Women's Stories," *St. Louis Post Dispatch* (Five Star), Feb. 8, 1993, 3. Like female genital mutilation, rape as a strategy of war is not a recent phenomenon; mass rapes have been documented during battles as far back as Ancient Greece. See Dianna Marder, "Once Again, Rape Becomes a Weapon of War," *Atlanta J. and Const.*, Feb. 17, 1993. In Japanese prisons during World War II, Korean women were held and repeatedly raped by Japanese soldiers up to 100 times per day. Ibid. These women were inaccurately described as "comfort women," implying that they had willingly become prostitutes. Ibid. In the 1970s and 1980s, rape was often used as a tool for oppressing women in Central America. Fletcher et al. (see note 58), p. 319. More recently, during the conflict in Haiti, both rape and female genital mutilation have been used by the military to threaten and frighten supporters of ousted President Aristide. See Clare Kittredge, "For Haitian Women, A Matter Of Justice," *Boston Globe*, Sept. 26, 1994, pp. 13, 14. For a discussion on the prevalence of Serbian rape camps in Bosnia, see Grace Haskell, "From U.S., Too Little, Too Late?" *Orlando Sentinel Trib.*, Mar. 7, 1993.

207. Benjamin B. Ferencz, *An International Criminal Court a Step Toward World Peace*, vol. 1 (1980), 489. Article II of the Allied Control Council Law No. 10 defines "Crimes against Humanity" as "Atrocities and offences, including but not limited to murder, extermination, enslavement, deportation, imprisonment, torture, rape, or other inhuman acts committed against any civilian population."

208. Ibid.

209. (See note 191).

210. Julie Flint, "The First Cut," *The Guardian* (London), Apr. 25, 1994, p. 11. For example, England, Sweden, and Switzerland all have laws against female genital mutilation that are not enforced. Ibid.

211. Hosken (see note 2), p. 89.

212. Universal Declaration (see note 198), pp. 77, 101.

213. Ibid., p. 103 (quoting European Commission on Human Rights).

214. Hurst Hannum, Ed., *Guide to International Human Rights Practice* 2d ed. (Philadelphia: University of Pennsylvania Press, 1992), p. 282.

215. Ibid.

216. Unlike human rights violations, for an act to be considered a "crime against humanity," government approval is required. See Stephen A. James, "Recon-

ciling International Human Rights and Cultural Relativism: The Case of
Female Circumcision," *Bioethics* 8, no. 1 (1994): 16.

217. Walker and Parmar (see note 22), p. 109. Supporters of the tradition of female
circumcision contend that the abolition of this practice would represent the
imposition of "outside values" that might result in the disruption of the
balance of complex cultural systems. Slack (see note 87), p. 463.

Research and Informed Consent 23.
in Africa—Another Look

Carel Ijsselmuiden and Ruth Faden

The current practice of requiring the informed consent of research subjects is relatively new. The emphasis on a person's right to accept or refuse participation in biomedical research stems directly from the atrocities committed by Nazi scientists—an extreme instance of ignoring the value of individual human beings allegedly in the pursuit of knowledge.[1] Similar but less dramatic disrespect for the subjects of medical research was common just after the Second World War and reflected the paternalistic atmosphere that pervaded medical practice at that time.[2] More recent examples of unethical research, which stimulated the development of the current theory and practice of informed consent, include the study of immune reactions to live cancer cells injected into mentally disabled persons in New York in 1963[3] and the Tuskegee study of the natural history of untreated syphilis, which continued until 1973.[4]

Although both the Nuremberg Code of 1948 and the Declaration of Helsinki of 1964 made the consent of subjects a central requirement of ethical research, it was not until the mid-1970s that the practice of requiring informed consent for medical research became conventional in the West. (In this chapter, "the West" and "Western" are used to indicate the United States, Canada, and Western Europe.) Given the relatively recent advent of consent requirements, it is not surprising that many questions about the scope and the specifics of these requirements have not yet been satisfactorily answered. Nevertheless, there seems to be considerable consensus about the moral importance of informed consent in medical research.[5] The fundamental justification for requiring consent from human subjects as a matter of U.S. public policy is best stated in the Belmont Report of 1978, which bases the obligation to obtain consent on the ethical principle of respect for persons."[6] The Belmont Report, which resulted from years of public debate and the deliberations of a national commission, made the protection of the autonomy and personal dignity of research subjects the focus of the informed-consent process.[7]

This strong emphasis on respect for autonomy is, however, neither unchallenged in the United States itself,[8] nor necessarily accepted elsewhere in the world, including Western Europe and Africa.[9] The challenge centers on the validity of applying ethical guidelines for research that are accepted in one part of the world to a different cultural setting.[10] It is in this context that the appropriateness of first-person informed consent (i.e., informed consent given by the subjects themselves), as practiced in the West, is being questioned.[11] The debate has given rise to such concepts as the "culturally relevant" or "culturally sensitive" application of Western medical ethics to research in developing countries.[12] These concerns are fueled by fear of "medical-ethical imperialism" and almost antithetical doubts about the use of double standards by Western researchers conducting studies in other countries, where different practices are common.[13] The ethical guidelines provided by the World Health Organization (WHO) and the Council for International Organizations of Medical Sciences (CIOMS), which were drafted to facilitate the formulation of ethical principles in "transcultural" research, are not helpful in resolving this dilemma, since they are sufficiently vague to allow for virtually any method of obtaining consent.[14]

The most fundamental argument against modifying the obligation of researchers to obtain informed consent from individual subjects is that such an obligation expresses important and basic moral values that are universally applicable, regardless of variations in cultural practice. Although we are sympathetic to this position, our arguments in this chapter do not turn on claims about universal morality or criticism of cultural relativism. Instead, our aim is to argue the inapplicability of such arguments on moral grounds that appeal to cultural relativism on factual grounds, rather than the unjustifiability of such arguments on moral grounds. Broadly speaking, the appropriateness of first-person informed consent in developing countries has been questioned on three grounds: that it is culturally or anthropologically inappropriate; that potential subjects have questionable competence to give informed consent or that there are insurmountable communication problems; and that the need for immediate research findings makes informed-consent requirements unreasonable. We shall consider these arguments in turn.

CULTURAL AND ANTHROPOLOGIC ARGUMENTS

In discussions of biomedical ethics, the anthropologic literature on Africa is often represented as indicating that in African culture[15] a person typically perceives himself or herself as an extension of the family and as an intermediary between ancestors and future generations, rather than as an individual person in his or her own right.[16] In terms of social structures, it is argued that authority is located in the leader of a village or tribe and in the head of the household, who is usually a man.[17] In response to these observations, it is argued that insistence on first-person informed consent in group-oriented cultures is a form of medical-ethical imperialism that is morally unacceptable.[18]

There are, however, major problems with this cultural argument for waiving the requirement for first-person informed consent in Africa. Although cultures in Africa have changed greatly in recent history, the anthropologic data on which the arguments about informed consent practice in Africa are based have not kept pace with these changes. Furthermore, the generalizability of these studies is limited, and the same dated studies are used repeatedly. We argue instead that African societies are changing in ways that make informed consent requirements more rather than less appropriate.

The medical ethics literature on research in Africa leaves the impression that there is only one culture on the African continent and that this culture is static. For example, a 1988 discussion by Christakis of the ethics of designing a trial of a vaccine against the acquired immunodeficiency syndrome (AIDS) in Africa used five review papers published between 1969 and 1986 as the sources for its anthropologic claims: each of these papers was based on original research conducted at least a decade earlier, primarily in rural settings or in relation to particular situations and subpopulations. Barry, also writing in 1988,[19] based her consideration of alternatives to individual informed consent in AIDS research in the developing world on only two review articles, one from Central Africa[20] and one from South Africa,[21] both of which summarized studies that were conducted primarily in traditional, rural settings before 1970. One of these articles[22] was also used in the paper by Christakis on the ethics of AIDS vaccine trials.[23]

In fact, there is no single African culture. More than 900 different contemporary or historical ethnic and cultural groups have been described in Africa,[24] and these cultures have not been static. The colonial history of Africa is characterized by prolonged civil warfare and large-scale disruption of traditional patterns of life,[25] including the notorious "forced removal" of 10 to 15 percent of South African blacks for ideological reasons.[26] Probably the most extensive changes in traditional lifestyles have been caused by urbanization, education, and industrialization.[27] Forty percent of Africa's population is already urbanized, and this number is projected to grow by 5 percent per year in the future.[28] More recently, the AIDS epidemic itself has become a leading cause of change in mores and traditions in Africa.[29] In view of such major social changes, there is no justification for accepting as accurate any but the most recent assessments of social structures, perceptions, and conceptualizations.

Consider, for example, the suggestion that in addition to, or even instead of, first-person informed consent, researchers should obtain consent on behalf of otherwise competent adults from a "trusted village leader."[30] Besides the dwindling number of such persons as a result of urbanization and development,[31] there are serious problems in identifying who they are[32] and in assessing whether or not they are genuinely trusted.[33] It is also far from obvious that village leaders speak for all the inhabitants of a village—which may include recent immigrants, the landless, or those outside the leaders' clan.[34] Tribal heads in South Africa's homelands are appointed directly or indirectly by the white minority government,[35] and their credibility with the people they govern is therefore low.[36] In other African countries traditional leaders have been replaced by party officials or cell leaders.[37] Some countries have dictatorships, whereas in others civil wars have wiped out almost all traces of traditional life. Furthermore, many African governments have become infamous for civil rights abuses and corruption.[38] Under these circumstances, it cannot be automatically assumed that consent obtained from tribal leaders or government officials has been given in the best interest of the study participants. Certainly, there are still trusted village leaders in Africa as well as honest officials and health professionals. In many contexts, however, it may be difficult to identify these people, especially for foreign researchers who are unfamiliar with the intricacies of local power structures.

A similar argument applies to consent given by heads of household on behalf of women. Migrant labor often takes the male heads of household to urban areas for the greater part of the year. Physical and sexual abuse, alcoholism, and child abuse, although less well documented than in the West, are certainly not rare in Africa. At the same time, women's educational status and the number of households headed by women are increasing, and demands for an end to discriminatory practices against women are being voiced.[39] How, then, can one justify asking heads of households for consent on behalf of competent adults, a practice that would be morally unacceptable in the West? It is certainly out of step with the movement in many African countries toward structural changes to enhance the emancipation of women, exemplified by the Women's League of the African National Congress and many other developments.

This is not to say that customs such as informing village leaders and heads of households of intended research should be omitted. What we challenge is the validity of obtaining their consent instead of or even in addition to that of individual research subjects.

PROBLEMS OF COMPETENCY AND COMMUNICATION

The term "incompetence" is used confusingly in the literature on consent practices in a cross-cultural situation; it may be used to indicate a state of mental incompetence or difficulties in communication and comprehension arising from differences in language, from nonscientific conceptions of health and illness, or from poor education.[40] Researchers have been urged to adapt the information ordinarily disclosed in the process of obtaining informed consent to local concepts of disease and health[41] and even to lie in describing the nature of their study.[42] Implicit in the arguments based on the problem of competency is the view that it is time-consuming and difficult, if not impossible, to obtain valid consent from subjects in developing countries. This position is obvious in the Proposed International Guidelines for Biomedical Research Involving Human Subjects of the WHO and the CIOMS, which state:

> Ideally, each potential research subject should possess the intellectual capacity and insight to provide valid informed consent, and enjoy the independence to exercise absolute freedom of choice over the extent of the collaboration without fear of discrimination. However, many investigations, and particularly those intended to subserve the interests of underprivileged communities and vulnerable minorities including children and the mentally ill, would be debarred if these preconditions were accepted as mandatory criteria for recruitment.

Although doubtless unintentionally, the WHO-CIOMS guidelines leave the impression that socially disadvantaged research subjects, presumably. including most subjects in developing countries, demonstrate a lack of competency or cognitive capacity analogous to that of children and the mentally ill.[43] The assumption that adults in developing countries are mentally incompetent to give informed consent to participation in research is false if not downright insulting.[44] Indeed, one of the main outcomes of the Nuremberg trials was the explicit requirement that the autonomy of adults who do not suffer from mental deficiency be respected.[45]

The argument that, because investigators and subjects do not share a common understanding of health and illness or of the scientific enterprise, true informed consent cannot be obtained may be slightly more defensible. This argument, however, applies equally well to research in the West, with its great variety of subcultures.[46] There is no compelling reason to conclude that the cultural differences between Africa and the West are so much greater than those between Western researchers and their Western subjects that Africans should be subjected to consent practices that are substantially different from those accepted in the West. The sociological literature on doctor-patient and scientist-subject interactions in Western countries has often noted the differences in culture and class between doctors and their patients and subjects and has documented the limited effectiveness of communication between people from different social classes or cultures.[47] The causes of such miscommunication include differences in language and culture and the lack of a shared understanding of health and disease. Yet no one has argued that different consent practices should be implemented within the same Western country on the basis of social class or culture.

Instead, we argue that, with extra effort, researchers can effectively communicate with subjects whose cultural backgrounds are different from their own and that claims about cultural or communication gaps overstate what is required for persons to have an adequate understanding of the implications of participation in a research project. Potential subjects can, for example, make valid decisions about participating in research without understanding the underlying pathophysiology of the disease to be studied or the physics of the test to be performed.[48] Although the ethical requirements of conducting research in cross-cultural contexts, including Third World societies, "may be more, rather than less, exacting"[49] than in settings where investigator and subject share a common culture, cultural differences do not constitute insurmountable barriers to obtaining valid consent or refusal.

THE URGENCY OF RESEARCH IN THE DEVELOPING WORLD

That the process of obtaining valid informed consent in Africa may require considerable time and resources leads to a third argument for waiving or relaxing the obligation to obtain first-person informed consent. This is the argument that the need for data is so immediate and important in Africa that the time required to obtain informed consent cannot be justified.[50]

This sense of urgency in clinical trials and public health research, as in the case of the development of an AIDS vaccine, is often not warranted, however. No rapid response to positive research findings is likely in the resource-starved developing countries. Although there are many urgent health problems to be solved in the developing world, the crucial question is whether such urgency precludes researchers from obtaining adequate first-person informed consent and from possibly spending additional funds, time, and effort to ensure that the consent is indeed voluntary and based on adequate understanding of the research to be conducted. The pace with which research findings have so far been implemented in Africa does not support this contention.

A case in point is the hepatitis B vaccine, which was shown to be safe and effective in the West as early as the late 1970s and early 1980s.[51] Replication of vaccine trials in Africa in the 1980s was important, since there could have been differences in host response from that documented in the Western trials.[52] It could not have been successfully argued, however that the urgency was so great that researchers should be excused from undertaking the additional efforts that might be required to ensure that meaningful informed consent was obtained from subjects, since there was no reason to believe that a finding of efficacy would be translated rapidly into widespread distribution of the vaccine. The cost of the vaccine[53] exceeds the per capita health expenditure of many African countries, yet there was no commitment by governments, the international community, or the producers to begin a vaccination program should the studies provide conclusive evidence of efficacy and safety. Consequently, a decade later, after many studies, Africa is still not benefiting substantially from hepatitis B vaccine. Although cheap vaccines may now become available, the lag between research findings and action in Africa is almost always so long that the argument that urgency requires ethical shortcuts is simply not sustainable; this is true not only for the hepatitis B vaccine but also for most urgent health problems in Africa.

THE REQUIREMENTS FOR ETHICAL RESEARCH IN AFRICA

The concept of cultural sensitivity in research[54] is appealing. It suggests the sophistication of the researcher, an absence of ethnocentricity, and an appreciation of the values of other cultures. Appeals to cultural sensitivity, however, are no substitute for careful moral analysis. We see no convincing arguments for a general policy of dispensing with, or substantially modifying, the researcher's obligation to obtain first-person consent in biomedical research conducted in Africa. Those who defend such a policy have relied on limited and often dated anthropologic literature that does not reflect the rapid cultural changes brought about by colonialism and independence, warfare, and urbanization. Their position is also based on confusing and confused appeals to problems of competence and communication and on an exaggerated sense of the role of biomedical research in solving Africa's pressing health problems.

Proposals to modify informed consent requirements must take account of the complex motivation behind decisions to conduct research in the developing world rather than in the West. Among the reasons for carrying out studies in Africa are such questionable factors as lower costs, lower risks of litigation, less stringent ethical review, the availability of populations prepared to cooperate with almost any study that appears curative in nature, anticipated underreporting of side effects because of low consumer awareness, the desire for personal advancement, and the desire to create new markets for pharmaceutical agents and other products.[55] None of these reasons is necessarily common among investigators, and most biomedical research in Africa is doubtless conducted with good intentions. Nevertheless, the existence of such an array of reasons, generally antithetical to the interests of research subjects, provides further justification for regarding with suspicion any suggestions to replace or modify requirements for first-person informed consent.

Although careful reflection by Western scientists about the ethics of conducting research in Africa is essential, it is no substitute for the establishment of standards and practices by Africans themselves. To encourage the development of ethical theory and practice in medical research in Africa, local experts, medical and nonmedical, must become more actively involved in screening transcultural research proposals. A mechanism for ethical review was proposed in Nigeria in 1980[56] but has not been fully implemented. Expertise and interest in medical ethics in Africa is already considerable, however. Perhaps it is time to bring together this African expertise to help redefine research ethics on the continent. The years of public debate and governmental consultation that led to the Belmont Report in the United States are an example waiting to be emulated elsewhere.

REFERENCES

1. Faden, R. R., and Beauchamp, T.L. *A History and Theory of Informed Consent.* New York: Oxford University Press, 1986; Beauchamp, T.L., and Childress, J.

F. *Principles of Biomedical Ethics,* 3rd ed. New York: Oxford University Press, 1989; Smith H. L. "Ethical Considerations in Research Involving Human Subjects." *Ethics Set. Med.* 6 (1979): 167–175.

2. Faden and Beauchamp (see note 1); Beecher, H. K. "Ethics and Clinical Research." *New Eng. J. Med.* 274 (1966): 1354–1360.

3. Ibid.

4. Faden and Beauchamp (see note 1); Jones, J. H. *Bad Blood.* New York: Free Press, 1981.

5. Faden and Beauchamp (see note 1); Beecher (see note 2); the National Commission for the Protection of Human Subjects of Biomedical and Behavioral Research. "The Belmont Report: Ethical Guidelines for the Protection of Human Subjects of Research." Washington, DC: Department of Health, Education, and Welfare, 1978 (DHEW publication no. [OS] 3–0012).

6. National Commission for the Protection of Human Subjects (see note 5).

7. Ibid.

8. Veatch, R. M. "Autonomy Temporary Triumph." *Hastings Center Rep.* 5 (1984): 38–40.

9. Smith (see note 1); Jones (see note 4); National Commission for the Protection of Human Subjects (see note 5); Veatch (see note 8); Christakis, N. A. "The Ethical Design of an AIDS Vaccine Trial in Africa," *Hastings Center Rep.* 18, no. 3 (1988): 31–37; Barry, M., "Ethical Considerations of Human Investigation in Developing Countries: the AIDS Dilemma." *New Eng. J. Med.* 319 (1988): 1083–1086; Beauchamp, TL. *Philosophical Ethics.* New York: McGraw-Hill, 1982, pp. 39–80; Taylor, C. E. "Clinical Trials and International Health Research." *Am. J. Public Health* 69 (1979): 981–998; Smith, H. L. "Medical Ethics in the Primary Care Setting." *Soc. Sci. Med.* 25 (1987): 705–709.

10. Christakis (see note 9); Barry (see note 9); Taylor (see note 9); Angell, M. "Ethical Imperialism? Ethics in International Collaborative Clinic Research." *New Eng. J. Med.* 319 (1988): 1081–1083.

11. Christakis (see note 9); Barry (see note 9); Taylor (see note 9); Willett, W. C., Kilama, W. L. and Kihamia, C. M. "Ascaris and Growth Rates: A Randomized Trial of Treatment." *Am. J. Public Health* 69 (1979): 987–991; Ekunwe, E. O., and Kessel, R. "Informed Consent in the Developing World." *Hastings Center Rep.* 14, no. 3 (1984): 22–24.

12. Christakis (see note 9); Barry (see note 9); Durojarye, M.O.A. "Ethics of Cross-Cultural Research Viewed from Third World Perspective. *Int. J. Psychol.* 14 (1979): 137–141.

13. Barry (see note 9); Taylor (see note 9).

14. Ekunwe and Kessel (see note 11); Durojarye (see note 12).

15. Smith (see note 1); Barry (see note 9).

16. Christakis (see note 9); Barry (see note 9); Taylor (see note 9); Willett, Kilama and Kihamia (see note 11); Ekunwe and Kessel (see note 11); Durojarye (see note 12); De Craemer, W. A. "Cross-Cultural Perspective on Personhood." *Milbank Mem. Fund Q.* 61 (1983): 19–34.

17. Christakis (see note 9); Barry (see note 9); Taylor (see note 9); Willett, Kilama, and Kihamia (see note 11); De Creamer (see note 16).

18. Christakis (see note 9); Barry (see note 9); Taylor (see note 9); Durojarye (see note 12).

19. Barry (see note 9).

20. De Craemer (see note 16).

21. Setiloane, G. M. "African Traditional Views." In *Ethical and Moral Issues in*

Contemporary Medical Practice, ed. S. R. Benatar. Cape Town: South Africa University of Cape Town Printing Department, 1986, pp. 32–35.

22. De Craemer (see note 16).
23. Ibid.
24. Price, D. H. *Atlas of World Cultures: A Geographical Guide to Ethnographic Literature.* Newbury Park, CA: Sage, 1989.
25. Oyugi, W. O., Atieno Odhiambo, E. S., Chege, M., Gitonja, A. D., eds. *Democracy Theory and Practice in Africa.* Portsmouth, England: Heinemann, 1988.
26. World Health Organization. *Apartheid and Health.* Geneva: WHO, 1983.
27. Ankrah, E. M. "AIDS: Methodological Problems in Studying Its Prevention and Spread." *Soc. Sci. Med.* 29 (1989): 265–276; Cleland, J. G., Van Ginneken, J. K. "Maternal Education and Child Survival in Developing Countries: The Search for Pathways of Influence." *Soc. Sci. Med.* 27 (1988): 1357–1368.
28. Grant, J. P. *The State of the World's Children.* Oxford, UK: Oxford University Press, 1989.
29. Ankrah, E. M. "AIDS and the Social Side of Health." *Soc. Sci. Med.* 32 (1991): 967–980.
30. Christakis (see note 9); Barry (see note 9); Taylor (see note 9); World Health Organization, "Proposed International Guidelines for Biomedical Research Involving Human Subjects." Geneva: WHO and Council for International Organizations of Medical Sciences, 1982.
31. Ankrah, "AIDS: Methodological Problems" (see note 27).
32. Christakis (see note 9).
33. Ankrah, "AIDS and the Social Side of Health" (see note 29); Chambers, R. *Rural Development: Putting the Last First,* 4th ed. New York: Longman, 1985, pp. 18–19, 133–134, 160–167; Zulu, P. "Socio-Political Structures in Rural Areas, and Their Potential Contribution to Community Development in KwaZulu." In *Second Carnegie Inquiry Into Poverty and Development in Southern Africa.* Cape Town: University of Cape Town Press, 1984.
34. Ibid.
35. De Beer, C. *The South African Disease: Apartheid Health and Health Service.* Johannesburg: South African Research Service, 1984.
36. Zulu (see note 33).
37. Naipaul, S. *North of South: An African Journey.* New York: Penguin Books, 1980.
38. Ibid.
39. Ankrah, "AIDS and the Social Side of Health" (see note 29); Raikes, A. "Women's Health in East Africa." *Soc. Sci. Med.* 28 (1989): 447–459.
40. Christakis (see note 9); Barry (see note 9); Taylor (see note 9); Angell (see note 10); Willett, Kilama and Kihamia (see note 11); Ekunwe and Kessel (see note 11); Durojarye (see note 12); WHO, "Proposed International Guidelines" (see note 30); Ankrah, "AIDS: Methodological Problems" (see note 27).
41. Christakis (see note 9); Barry (see note 9); Ekunwe and Kessel (see note 11).
42. Ekunwe and Kessel (see note 11).
43. WHO, "Proposed International Guidelines" (see note 30).
44. Faden and Beauchamp (see note 1); Beauchamp and Childress (see note 1); Beecher (see note 2); Ekunwe and Kessel (see note 11).
45. Faden and Beauchamp (see note 1).
46. Susser, M., Watson, W. and Hopper, K. *Sociology in Medicine,* 3rd ed. New York: Oxford University Press, 1985; Bergh, K. D., Asp, S., and Culhane-Pera, K. A. "Sociocultural Influences on Medicine and Health." In *Textbook of*

Family Practice, 4th ed., ed. R. E. Rakel. Philadelphia: W. B. Saunders, 1990, pp. 285–296.

47. Ibid.; Angell (see note 10); Gillick, M. R. "Commonsense Models of Health and Disease." *New Eng. J. Med.* 313 (1985): 700–703; Ingelfinger, F. J. "Informed (But Uneducated) Consent." *New Eng. J. Med.* 287 (1972): 465–466; Katz, R. L. "Informed Consent: Is It Bad Medicine?" *West J. Med.* 126 (1977): 426–428; Ajayi, O. O. "Taboos and Clinical Research in West Africa." *J. Med. Ethics* 6 (1980): 61–63.

48. Beecher (see note 2); Beauchamp, *Philosophical Ethics* (see note 9).

49. Angell (see note 10).

50. WHO, "Proposed International Guidelines" (see note 30).

51. Maynard, J. E., Kare, M. A. and Hadler, S. C. "Global Control of Hepatitis B Through Vaccination: Role of Hepatitis B Vaccine in the Expanded Programme on Immunization." Rev. Infect. Dis. 11, Suppl. 3 (1989): S574-S578.

52. Ibid.; Schoub, B. D., Johnson, S., McAnemey, J. M., et al. "Integration of Hepatitis B Vaccination Into Rural African Primary Health Care Programmes." Brit. Med. J. 302 (1991): 313–320; Yvonnet, B., Coursaget, P., Chotard, J., et al. "Serve-Year Study of Hepatitis B. Vaccine Efficacy in Infants From an Endemic Area (Senegal)." Lancet 2 (1986): 1143–1145; Gamora Hepatitis Study Group, "Hepatitis B Vaccine in the Expanded Programme of Immunisation: the Gambian Experience." Lancet 1 (1989): 1057).

53. Maynard, Kare and Hadler (see note 51); Schoub, Johnson, and McAnemey (see note 52).

54. Christakis (see note 9), Barry (see note 9); Taylor (see note 9); Durojarye (see note 12).

55. Ankrah, "AIDS: Methodological Problems" (see note 27) and "AIDS and the Social Side of Health" (see note 29); Chambers (see note 33); Kurpooea, P. and Rienter, J. "Unethical Trials of Dipyrone in Thailand." *Lancet* 2 (1988): 1491; Serwadda, D. and Katongole-Mbudde, E. "AIDS in Africa: Problems for Research and Researchers." *Lancet* 335 (1990): 842–843.

56. Ajayi (see note 47).

Human Rights and Maternal-Fetal HIV Transmission Prevention Trials in Africa

24.

George J. Annas and Michael A. Grodin

Since the adoption of the Universal Declaration of Human Rights by the United Nations General Assembly in 1948, the countries of the world have agreed that all humans have dignity and rights. In 1998, the fiftieth anniversary of the Universal Declaration of Human Rights, this document's aspirations have yet to be realized, and poverty, racism and sexism continue to conspire to frustrate the worldwide human rights movement. The human rights and public health issues of maternal-fetal human immunodeficiency virus (HIV) transmission prevention trials in Africa, Asia, and the Caribbean are not unique to acquired immunodeficiency syndrome (AIDS) or to those countries. Open discussion of these issues provides an opportunity to move the real human rights agenda forward.[1] This is why Global Lawyers and Physicians (GLP), a transnational organization dedicated to promoting and protecting the health-related provisions of the Universal Declaration of Human Rights, joined with Ralph Nader's Public Citizen organization to challenge the conduct of a series of AIDS clinical trials in these developing countries.[2]

THE CLINICAL TRIALS

In 1994, the first effective intervention to reduce the perinatal transmission of HIV was developed in the United States in AIDS Clinical Trials Group (ACTG) Study 076. In that trial, use of zidovudine administered orally to HIV-positive pregnant women as early as the second trimester of pregnancy, intravenously during labor, and orally to their newborns for six weeks reduced the incidence of HIV infection by two-thirds (from about 25 percent to about 8 percent).[3] Six months after stopping the study, the U.S. Public Health Service recommended the ACTG 076 regimen as the standard of care in the United States.[4] In June 1994, the World Health Organization (WHO) convened a meeting in Geneva at which it was concluded (in an unpublished report) that the 076 regime was not feasible in the developing world. At least sixteen randomized clinical trials (fifteen using placebos as controls) were subsequently approved for conduct in developing countries, primarily in Africa. These trials involve more than 17,000 pregnant women. Nine of the studies, most of them comparing shorter courses of zidovudine, vitamin A or HIV immunoglobulin to placebo, are funded by the Centers for Disease Control and Prevention (CDC) or the National Institutes of Health (NIH).[5]

Most of the public discussion about these trials has centered on the use of placebos.[6] The question of placebo use is a central one in determining how a study should be conducted. But we believe the more important issue these trials raise is the question of whether they should be done at all. Specifically, when is medical research ethically justified in developing countries that do not have adequate health services (or on U.S. populations that have no access to basic health care)? This question is especially pertinent because CDC, NIH, and UNAIDS officials announced in February 1998 that, on the basis of a Thailand study in which a short course of zidovudine reduced HIV transmission by 50 percent, they would recommend that the use of placebos be halted in all mother-to-fetus transmission studies.[7]

RESEARCH ON IMPOVERISHED POPULATIONS

The central issue involved in doing research with impoverished populations is exploitation. Harold Varmus, speaking for the NIH, and David Satcher, speaking for the CDC, both seem to realize this. They wrote in the *New England Journal of Medicine* last year that "trials that make use of impoverished populations to test drugs for use solely in developed countries violate our most basic understanding of ethical behavior."[8] However, instead of trying to demonstrate how the study interventions, such as a shorter course of zidovudine (AZT), could actually be delivered to the populations of the countries in the studies, they assert that the studies can be justified because they will provide information that the host country can use to "make a sound judgment about the appropriateness and financial feasibility of providing the intervention."[9] However, what these countries require is not good intentions, but a real plan to deliver the intervention, should it prove beneficial.

Unless the interventions being tested will actually be made available to the impoverished populations that are being used as research subjects, developed countries are simply exploiting these subjects in order to use the knowledge gained from the clinical trials for the developed countries' own benefit. If the research reveals regimens of equal efficacy at less cost these regimens will surely be implemented in the developed world. If the research reveals the regimens to be less efficacious, these results will be added to the scientific literature, and the developed world will not conduct those studies. Ethics and basic human rights principles require not a thin promise, but a real plan as to how the intervention will actually be delivered. Actual delivery is also, of course, required to support even the utilitarian justification for the trials, which is to find a simple, inexpensive, and feasible intervention in as short a time frame as possible because so many people are dying of AIDS. No justification is supportable unless the intervention is actually made widely available to the relevant populations.

Neither NIH nor CDC (nor the host countries) has a plan that would make the interventions they are studying available in Africa, which is where more than two-thirds of all people who are infected with HIV reside. As an example, Varmus and Satcher point out that the wholesale cost of zidovudine in the 076 protocol is estimated to be in excess of $800 per mother and infant and that this amount is far greater than what most developing countries can pay for standard care.[10] The CDC estimates that the cost of the "short course" zidovudine regimens being investigated to be roughly $50 per person. The cost of merely screening for HIV disease, a precondition for any course of therapy, is approximately $10, and all pregnant women must be screened to find the cases to treat. These costs must be compared with the total per capita health care expenditures of the countries where this research is being conducted (see Table 1). Given this fact, African countries involved in the clinical trials (or some other funder) must make realistic assurances that if a research regimen proves effective in reducing mother-to-fetus transmission of HIV, resources will be made available so that the HIV-positive pregnant women in their countries will receive this regimen.

However, the mere assertion that the interventions will be feasible for use in the developing countries is simply not good enough given our experience and knowledge of what happens in Africa now. For example, we already know that treating sexually transmitted diseases such as syphilis, gonorrhea and chancroid with the simple and effective treatments that are now available can drastically lower the incidence of HIV infection. Yet these inexpensive and effective treatments are not delivered to poor Africans. For example, a recent study showed that improving the treatment of sexually

Table 1.   Health Care Expenditures of African Countries Involved in Mother-to-Fetus HIV Transmission Prevention Trials

Country (Year)	Per Capita (U.S. dollars)	As % of GDP*
Burkina Faso (1992)	22	5.5
Cote d'Ivoire (1995)	22	3.4
Ethiopia (1990)	5	3.9
Kenya (1992)	13	2.5
Malawi (1990	11	5.0
Tanzania (1990)	5	5.0
Uganda (1994)	10	3.9
Zimbabwe (1991)	86	6.5

Data from World Bank Sector Strategy, Health, Nutrition, and Population, 1997.
*GDP = gross domestic product

transmitted diseases in rural Tanzania could reduce HIV infections by 40 percent.[11] Nonetheless, this relatively inexpensive and effective intervention is not delivered. Vaccines against devastating diseases have also been developed with sub-Saharan African populations as test subjects. Nonetheless, even though vaccines such as the group A meningococcal meningitis vaccine are inexpensive and effective, they are not adequately delivered to the relevant sub-Saharan African populations.[12]

CULTURAL RELATIVISM OR UNIVERSAL HUMAN RIGHTS?

In their article in the *New England Journal of Medicine,* Varmus and Satcher sought to bolster their ethical position by quoting the chair of the AIDS Research Committee of the Uganda Cancer Institute, who wrote in a letter to Dr. Varmus:

> These are Ugandan studies conducted by Ugandan investigators on Ugandans. . . . It is not NIH conducting the studies in Uganda, but Ugandans conducting their study on their people for the good of their people.[13]

Two points are especially striking about Varmus and Satcher using this justification. First, their justification is simply not accurate. If the NIH and the CDC were not involved in these studies, these agencies would not have to justify them; indeed, the studies would not have been undertaken. These U.S. agencies *are* involved—these trials are not just Ugandans doing research on other Ugandans. Second, and more important, the use of this quotation implies support for an outdated and dangerous view of cultural relativism.

Even if it were true that the studies in question were done by Ugandans on Ugandans, this would not mean that the United States or the international community could conclude that they should not be criticized. (This rationale did not inhibit criticism of apartheid in South Africa, genocide in Rwanda, or torture and murder in the Congo). Human Rights Watch, referring to repression in Central Africa, said in its December 1997 review of the year on the issue of human rights that the slogan "African solutions to African problems" is now used as a "thin cover" for abusing citizens.[14] That observation can be applicable to experimentation on citizens as well.

The other major justification both the NIH and the CDC use for the trials is the consensus reached at the June 1994 meeting of researchers at WHO. Of the many analogies that have been drawn with the U.S. Public Health Service's Tuskegee syphilis study, perhaps the most telling is the reliance on professional consensus instead of ethical principle to justify research on poor. As historian James Jones wrote in his book *Bad Blood,* which was written about the Public Health Service's Tuskegee experiment: "The consensus was that the experiment was worth doing, and in a profession whose members did not have a well-developed system of normative ethics, consensus formed the functional equivalent of moral sanction."[15]

Neither researcher consensus nor host country agreement is ethically sufficient justification for choosing a research population. As the National Research Council's Committee on Human Genome Diversity properly put it in the context of international research on human subjects: "Sensitivity to the specific practices and beliefs of a community cannot be used as a justification for violating universal human rights."[16] Justice and equity questions are also important to the ability of the individual research subjects to give informed consent.

INFORMED CONSENT

Research subjects should not be drawn from populations who are especially vulnerable (e.g., the poor, children, or mentally impaired persons) unless the population is the only group in which the research can be conducted and the group itself will derive benefits from the research. Even when these conditions are met, informed consent must also be obtained.[17] In most settings in Africa, voluntary, informed consent will be problematic and difficult, and it may even preclude ethical research. This is because in the absence of health care, virtually any offer of medical assistance (even in the guise of research) will be accepted as "better than nothing," and research will almost inevitably be confused with treatment, making informed consent difficult.

Interviews with women subjects of the placebo-controlled trial in the Ivory Coast support this conclusion. For example, one subject, Cécile Guede, a twenty-three-year-old HIV-infected mother participating in a U.S.-financed trial, told the *New York Times,* "They gave me a bunch of pills to take, and told me how to take them. Some were for malaria, some were for fevers, and some were supposed to be for the virus. I knew that there were different kinds, but I figured that if one of them didn't work against AIDS, then one of the others would."[18] The *Times* reporter who wrote the front-page story, Howard W. French, said, "For Ms. Guede, the reason to enroll in the study last year was clear: it offered her and her infant free health care and a hope to shield her baby from deadly infection. . . . The prospect of help as she brought her baby into the world made taking part in the experiment all but irresistible."[19]

Persons can make a gift of themselves by volunteering for research. However, it is extremely unlikely that poor African women would knowingly volunteer to participate in research that offered no benefit to their communities (because the intervention would not be made available) and would only serve to enrich the multinational drug companies and the developed world.[20] Thus, a good ethical working rule is that researchers should presume that valid consent cannot be obtained from impoverished populations in the absence of a realistic plan to deliver the intervention to the population. Informed consent, by itself, can protect many subjects of research in developed countries, but its protective power is much more compromised in impoverished populations who are being offered what looks like medical care that is otherwise unavailable to them.

THE INTERNATIONAL COMMUNITY AND THE AIDS PANDEMIC

If the goal the of clinical trials is to reduce the spread of HIV infection in developing countries, what strategy should public health adopt to achieve this end? It is not obvious that the answer is to conduct clinical trials of short-term zidovudine treatment. In the developed world, for example, HIV-infected women are advised not to breast-feed their infants because 8 percent to 18 percent of them will be infected with HIV from breast milk.[21] However, in much of the developing world, including in most African countries, WHO continues to recommend breast-feeding because the lack of clean water still makes formula-feeding more dangerous. As long as this recommendation stays in effect and is followed, even universal use of the ACTG 076 regime, which would lower the overall newborn infection rate by about 16 percent, would likely serve only to reduce the incidence of HIV infection in infants by about the same amount that it is increased by breast-feeding (8 percent to 18 percent). A more effective public health intervention to improve the health of women and their children may be to put more efforts into providing clean water and sanitation. This will help not only to deal with HIV, but also to alleviate many other problems, including diarrheal diseases.

President Jacques Chirac of France was on target in his December 1997 speech to the 10th International Conference on Sexually Transmitted Disease and AIDS in Africa, which was held in the Ivory Coast. Chirac proposed creating an international "therapy support fund" funded primarily by European countries (the former colonial powers in Africa).[22] Although he put emphasis on the new drugs available for AIDS treatments, it would be more useful to consider the public health priorities of the countries themselves, for example, prevention—especially in areas such as sanitation, water supply, nutrition, education—and the delivery of simple and effective vaccines and medical treatments for sexually transmitted diseases.

CONCLUSION

Actual delivery of health care requires more than just paying lip service to the principles of the Universal Declaration of Human Rights; it requires a real commitment to human rights and a willingness on the part of the developed countries to take economic, social, and cultural rights as seriously as they do political and civil rights.

REFERENCES

1. Mann, J. M. "Medicine and Public Health, Ethics and Human Rights," *Hastings Center Report* 27, 3 (1997): 6–13; Letter to HHS Sec. Donna Shalala, April 27, 1997.
2. Lurie P., Wolfe, S. M. "Unethical Trials of Interventions to Reduce Perinatal Transmission of Human Immunodeficiency Virus in Developing Countries," *New England Journal of Medicine* 331 (1994): 1173–1180.
3. Connor, E. M., Sperling, R. S., Gelber, R. et al. "Reduction of Maternal-Infant

Transmission of Human Immunodeficiency Virus Type 1 with Zidovudine Treatment," *New England Journal of Medicine* 331 (1994): 1173–1180.

4. "Recommendations of the U.S. Public Health Service Task Force on the Use of Zidovudine to Reduce Perinatal Transmission of Human Immunodeficiency Virus," *MMWR Morb. Mort. Wkly. Rpt.* 43 (RR-11) 1994): 1–20.

5. Lurie and Wolfe (see note 2).

6. Ibid.; Angell, M. "The Ethics of Clinical Research in the Third World," *New England Journal of Medicine* 337 (1997): 847–849; Varmus, H. and Satcher, D. "Ethical Complexities of Conducting Research in Developing Countries." *New England Journal of Medicine* 337 (1997): 1003–1005.

7. Brown, D. "AZT's Success in Pregnancy May Help Expand AIDS Treatment for Poor," *Washington Post* (Feb. 19, 1998), p. A10.

8. Varmus and Satcher (see note 6).

9. Ibid.

10. Ibid.

11. Grosskurth, H., Mosha, F., Todd, J. et al., "Impact of Improved Treatment of Sexually Transmitted Diseases on HIV Infection in Rural Tanzania: Randomized Control Trial." *Lancet* 346 (1995): 530–536.

12. Robbins, J. B., Towne, D. W., Gotschlich, E. C. and Schneerson, R. "'Love's Labours Lost': Failure to Implement Mass Vaccination Against Group A Meningococcal Meningitis in Sub-Saharan Africa," *Lancet* 350 (1995): 880–882.

13. Varmus and Satcher (see note 6).

14. Clines, F. X. "Rights Group Assails U.S. on Land Mines and Ties with China," *New York Times* (Dec. 5, 1997), p. A13.

15. Jones, J. H. *Bad Blood: The Tuskegee Syphilis Experiment* (New York: Free Press, 1981), p. 112.

16. Committee on Human Genome Diversity. *Evaluating Human Genetic Diversity* (Washington, DC: National Academy Press, 1997), p. 65.

17. Annas, G. J. and Grodin, M. A. (eds.). *The Nazi Doctors and the Nuremberg Code: Human Rights in Human Experimentation* (New York: Oxford University Press, 1992); also see Ijsselmuiden, C. and Faden, R. "Research and Informed Consent in Africa – Another Look," *New England Journal of Medicines* 326 (1992): 830–834, and Chapter 23 in this book.

18. French, H. W. "AIDS Research in Africa: Juggling Risks and Hopes," *New York Times* (Oct. 9, 1997), p. A1.

19. Ibid.

20. Committee on Human Genome Diversity (see note 16).

21. Van de Perre, P. "Postnatal Transmission of Human Immunodeficiency Virus Type 1: The Breast-Feeding Dilemma." *American Journal of Obstetrics & Gynecology* 173 (1995): 483–487.

22. Bunce, M. "Chirac Seeks Worldwide Relief for AIDS in Africa." *Boston Globe* (December 8, 1997), p. A2.

25. Human Rights and Human Genetic Variation Research

Committee on Human Genetic Diversity,
National Research Council

As science advances, new insights into the methods of science emerge. In human genetic research, one important insight has been the recognition of ethical issues in the design of basic research on human genetic variation. In short, as the scientific community seeks to conduct genetic variation studies with people from an ever-wider variety of populations, it increasingly faces the challenge of respecting the rights and interests of research subjects who participate in the research both as individuals and as representatives of groups.

The research-design questions that this challenge provokes are not new to human biology or peculiar to the study of human genetic variation; they have been encountered many times in the contexts of human population genetics, biologic anthropology, and epidemiology. However, as the scope and depth of genetic variation research expand, the stakes for both individual research subjects and the groups that they represent will increase. Moreover, as representatives of groups, the individuals who provide DNA for genetic variation research are playing a role in science that our individual-oriented norms of research ethics are ill equipped to address. It will be increasingly important for new investigators to appreciate the ethical issues that they encounter and to be able to adapt how they approach such issues to the cultural circumstances in which they would like to work. The goal of this chapter is to address that need by describing the major lessons of the scientific community's experience with ethical issues and the research-design considerations that have emerged from them.

Proposals for human genome diversity research that do not adequately anticipate the issues raised by the proposers' population focus have already proved capable of generating a remarkable amount of public controversy. One prominent call to begin a systematic collection of human genetic samples for study (Cavalli-Sforza et al. 1991) produced an unprecedented international reaction, including cautionary statements from UNESCO's Bioethics Committee (UNESCO 1995), the UN Commission on Human Rights (UN Commission on Human Rights 1996), the U.S. Human Genome Project (U.S. Congress 1993), and numerous public-advocacy organizations (Amazanga Institute et al. 1996; Mead 1996; RAFI 1993). Because a final statement of the goals and methods of such a project does not exist, it is difficult to determine what concerns are justified and even harder to suggest how the scientific community might resolve them. However, it is not difficult to understand the sources of the concerns; they flow from the convergence of several sets of public experiences that all accentute the risks posed by genetic-variation research.

This suggests an approach for our analysis. Different kinds of genetic-variation research will engage the concerns expressed by the public in different ways and to different degrees. Examining each of the DNA-sampling strategies from the perspectives of the controversies that serve as background to the current debate should allow us to identify the issues that are most likely to be raised by different strategies and to assess the extent of their challenges to the design and conduct of human genetic variation studies.

CONTEXT OF CONCERNS ABOUT STUDYING HUMAN GENETIC VARIATION
Human Genetics and the Misuse of Scientific Information

One of the concerns expressed by public reaction to the call for genetic diversity research is that such research could inadvertently exacerbate, rather than lessen, the habit of assigning people to socially defined ethnic categories for political and economic purposes. This habit, of course, long predates scientific thinking about human genetics. In some forms—such as racism, tribalism, and nationalism—it is likely to continue to flourish even in the absence of any additional research on human genetic variation. But the short history of the scientific study of human biology shows that where science can be interpreted to support socially defined categories, it is often used to give authority to the social policies that the categorization is designed to support (Caplan 1994; Rex and Mason 1988). That is not the intention of the scientists involved. Often, scientists sort people into socially defined groups simply for methodological convenience, using the groups as rough markers of human biologic lineages. Sometimes, they begin with such categories to falsify them by showing that biology belies our social classification of humanity. Most contemporary proponents of human genome-diversity research, in fact, use both of those contradictory rationales (HUGO 1993). Nevertheless, when the research is designed in terms of the problematic social categories, it becomes difficult for investigators to escape the accusation that they have participated in perpetuating, rather than confronting, the social problems that the categorization creates.

The danger is illustrated by an early episode in human population genetics: the 1920–1950 study of genetic variation underlying the global distribution of human blood types. That research contributed much to our scientific understanding of blood type genetics, but it was framed by many in the scientific community in terms of the taxonomy of human "races" that was influential in U.S. and European cultures at the time. The research was understood by many to provide an objective biological underpinning for the culture's prevalent concept of "races" and scientific support for the variety of discriminatory social policies that had been built on racial classifications (Marks 1996; Schneider 1996). As the history of blood-group genetics suggests, scientific studies that accept and use socially defined human taxonomies as biologically based can give inappropriate substance to those categories and lend credibility to the policies that they suggest (Barkan 1992).

The Rio de Janeiro Biodiversity Summit and Genetic Exploitation

A second common theme in the international reaction to calls for human genome-diversity research is concern over potential commercial exploitation of the participating individuals and social groups. The concern is extrapolated from the experiences of indigenous peoples with expatriate pharmaceutical and agricultural research efforts that led to commercially profitable discoveries for the sponsors but not for the peoples whose natural resources were used. The Rio de Janeiro Earth Summit on Biodiversity of 1992 highlighted international public concern over this trend and the resulting development, in many nations, of public policies governing the ownership and control of their indigenous biologic materials (Friedlander 1996). The coincidence between the language of biodiversity in these international public-policy debates and the call for studies of human genome-diversity has now provoked public concern that international efforts to study human genetic variation might result in an analogous commercial exploitation of human genetic "resources" (Friedlander 1996). This concern has been exacerbated recently by international reactions to episodes such as the U.S. government's attempt to patent a cell line from a native of Papua New Guinea (Taube 1995).

The Human Genome Project and Genetic Discrimination

The third important backdrop to the current discussion of human genomic-diversity research is the international Human Genome Project itself. In its efforts to anticipate and address the ethical implications of its genetic-mapping and sequencing work, the Human Genome Project has succeeded in raising the awareness of both the scientific community and the public of how personal genetic information can be used by social institutions against the interests of individuals and families (Juengst 1994). The Human Genome Project's documentation of the deterministic and reductionistic interpretations of personal genetic information by health professionals, insurers, employers, governments, and the public at large has, for example, already influenced the rules by which genetic research with individuals and families is conducted.

Numerous studies in which large families and linkage analysis were used to isolate and identify human genes have been conducted over the last several decades; they developed relatively seamlessly out of older traditions of Mendelian and medical family-history studies. The accelerated pace of that research and its increasing successes have resulted in increased scrutiny of the standards of practice in genetic family studies because such studies can inadvertently reveal genetic characteristics of individuals who have not given consent in the research. Past genetic family studies often recruited subjects opportunistically and dealt with issues concerning the recording of research data on nonparticipant family members and the publication of identifiable pedigrees only as they arose (Frankel and Teich 1993). Now they are required to address such concerns in advance to ensure that participation of all those affected by a study is voluntary and informed, that families are aware of the full array of possible risks, and that privacy of genetic information is protected (OPRR 1993).

The risks associated with "genetic discrimination" are real enough at the individual and family levels to justify serious consideration of the practices of medical genetics researchers (Geller et al. 1996; Hudson et al. 1995). Risks are likely to be even more substantial at the level of social groups. However, translating the kinds of protections that medical geneticists have adopted for individuals and family-research subjects into protections for entire social groups might require more radical changes in the traditional professional practices of biologic anthropologists and population geneticists than the ones that medical geneticists had to face.

ETHICAL CONSIDERATIONS IN THE DESIGN OF HUMAN GENETIC VARIATION RESEARCH

The extent to which the issues raised above become challenges in research on human genetic variation will depend heavily on the goals of the research and the sampling strategy used to achieve them. However, two basic principles will always be relevant in research involving humans: (1) a scientifically valid research design in which the risks to human subjects are outweighed by the expected benefits is necessary, and (2) for any project that involves collecting DNA samples from individual human beings (as opposed to other sources, such as anonymized blood banks), the free and informed consent of the persons from whom the DNA is collected must be obtained.

There has been some renewed interest in cultural relativism and in requiring researchers to be culturally sensitive in carrying out research in countries and communities other than their own. Such awareness is appropriate, but sensitivity to the specific practices and beliefs of a community cannot be used as a justification for violating universal human rights. These rights must be respected by all researchers, regardless of the research rules or customs in their own countries or the countries in which the research is performed. Fundamental human-rights documents that require respect for the human rights and dignity of all people include the Nuremberg Code (1947), the International Declaration of Human Rights (1948), and the International

Covenant on Civil and Political Rights (1976); these documents support the "equal and inalienable rights of all members of the human family" to choose for themselves whether and how to contribute to scientific knowledge by participating in research (Steiner and Alston 1996).

Those international documents derive the rights that they enumerate from the "inherent dignity of the human person" (Preamble, ICCPR). Not only must people's dignity and welfare be respected, but so must their individual rights. Thus, Article 7 of the International Covenant on Civil and Political Rights specifically provides that "no one shall be subjected without his free consent to medical or scientific experimentation." The requirement to obtain people's informed consent to participate in research ensures that they have enough information about a given project to weigh the benefits and risks associated with becoming involved in the research before they agree to participate. It is a recognized principle of research ethics that research involving risks should not be conducted on populations who will not be able to benefit from the research if it is successful (CIOMS 1993). Consent alone cannot justify research on populations that will not be able to benefit from it because such research violates basic principles of social justice and equality. Research subjects can make a gift to researchers or humanity, but the validity of such a gift in the context of studying genetic diversity, especially of isolated populations, is too problematic to provide the sole justification for the research. Nonetheless, the most important ethical question in research is always whether the research is worth doing. Only after that question and the risk-benefit question are answered favorably is it ethical to approach human subjects to solicit their participation in research.

Therefore, it is crucial to have a complete research protocol for review before the actual consent form and process for obtaining consent can be designed and evaluated. For any specific goal-oriented protocol, it should be possible to anticipate the risks and benefits to the subjects and pursue informed consent accordingly. For projects that are not able to specify goals in sufficient detail to quantify risks and benefits reasonably, the worst-case scenario should be assumed: the benefits will be at the lowest anticipated level, and the risks at the highest. That means that the burden of proof for any DNA-sampling project that does not have a well-defined hypothesis will be high. It also underlines the most basic starting point for all ethical analyses of genetic-variation research, regardless of which model is pursued: defining a hypothesis and determining the benefit of knowing whether it is true.

Studies Involving Geographic, Nonpopulation Sampling

The collection and storage of random samples of human DNA (sampling strategy I) that cannot be linked to identifiable persons, geographical areas, or populations would pose the fewest ethical concerns for genetic-variation research. The absence of identifiers that could be used to associate specific genomic variations with specific human populations avoids the risks of inappropriately treating socially defined groups as biological lineages and exacerbating existing social problems. By the same token, the collection of samples with this strategy need not be organized in terms of and in consultation with recognized social groups. No identifying correlations would be made, so negotiation of terms of participation with the individuals who are the sources of DNA would also be avoided because no direct benefits or risks to the individuals would flow from their participation. Finally, because no individuals would be identifiable through such a collection, protection of the rights and interests of identified individual human subjects in the later control of sample uses would be obviated.

Studies Involving Geographic-Grid-Based Sampling

Sampling strategy II also avoids the need to address many of the ethical considerations discussed earlier in this chapter. The fact that the samples cannot be linked to identifiable individuals or populations allows researchers to avoid the complexity of human-subject protections and social-group interests that are involved in strategies that require more identification. However, the extent to which these issues can be avoided depends on the size of the grid used. Grids whose resolution makes it possible to isolate individual nations or populations would result in associating the geographic location of a DNA sample's source with a particular people. The ethical and social dynamics of the research would then change considerably, in ways that are best illustrated by considering the next sampling strategy, in which populations are explicitly identified.

Studies Involving Population-Identification-Based Sampling

The ethical challenges of genetic-variation research increase with sampling strategy III and are exacerbated with sampling strategies IV and V. In these sampling strategies, specific human groups are identified as sample sources, and the subjects assume the role of representing the group. The social categories that define them might often be artificial from the biologist's point of view, but social groups are real human entities with both rights and interests to be respected and protected. Two issues of research design are particularly important in this respect: identifying groups to be sampled and obtaining group concurrence and involvement.

Identifying Populations to Be Sampled

Using social identities as the basis for defining populations for the study of genetic variation is probably the most controversial and problematic aspect of genetic-variation research. The reasons are both scientific and political. From a scientific perspective, some genetic variation studies seek populations that function as demes: endogamous (interbreeding) populations that are substantially reproductively isolated from other populations. Intergroup comparisons and intragroup comparisons typically require identifying human populations that function as demes. Many socially defined groups can satisfy that criterion from small geographically isolated communities to ethnically heterogeneous (but still largely endogamous) nations such as the United States. But many cannot, and identifying them for scientific purposes can be difficult without an adequate understanding of the social and political structures of the areas being studied. Some human demes have fewer internal barriers to gene flow—created by stratification by class, caste, ethnic group, or clan affiliation—within the population than others.

The fact that a group name exists for political purposes can be scientifically misleading. Centralized authorities, whether concerned with the overall unity of a people or with the dominance of a particular group, can affect how humans are grouped despite their biological connections. They can emphasize the homogeneity of the people that they recognize officially as groups. They can discount other claims to "peoplehood" in a country's body politic, or they can foster a particular process of national unification or self-interested differentiation in a country on the basis of hopes for the future more than present (or past) circumstances (Dominguez 1986, 1989; Gladney 1991; Handler 1988). Surveys of self-identified minority groups in given locales typically reveal greater heterogeneity than that recognized by central government authorities unless it benefits the central government to declare that a group of people claiming "peoplehood" is too heterogeneous to be considered a group for political purposes. Regional-level, such as state, governments might give people the name of the administrative center under whose jurisdiction they fall. Or people in a region might be referred to collectively by a name given to them by people with whom they trade. For example, the so-called Nakanai of New Britain were named by the people from the Rabaul area who traded with them; they now refer to themselves as Nakanai. In fact, however, the Nakanai comprise several linguistically distinct groups of villages with different histories. Individuals identify themselves to one another not by cultural or linguistic group names, but by village and clan, the socially important (and not biologically irrelevant) units in their lives. If a sample drawn from an area does not account for language groups, village locations and the clans of the DNA sources, the information essential for both intragroup and intergroup comparisons will be lost.

Another challenge in identifying populations for study is that, as the case of the Nakanai illustrates, the socially defined groups that we use to identify ourselves are always internally differentiated. Investigators will have to decide in advance what level within a given hierarchy of human organization to use to identify groups relevant to a particular study of human genetic variation and by which criteria. Some have suggested that perhaps the fairest and most revealing approach would be to solicit the advice of local populations to identify level of analysis and the group identifications that would make the most sense to them. In theory, that approach could be used to protect the autonomy and interests of self-identified human groups and to avoid the use of distorting labels. However, as the Nakanai example suggests, it is not always a solution for accurately defining groups. Much will depend on from whom advice is sought on the composition and identification of human social groups. Multiple interviews should be conducted to avoid relying exclusively on one or two sources.

Accurate identification of population units for sampling purposes requires extensive knowledge of the social, political and linguistic composition of the region to be sampled. Published ethnographic studies can provide some of this knowledge, as can anthropologists who work with the peoples. If this information is not available, researchers are advised to study the local situation in consultation with local leaders, experts, and other researchers before designing the sampling strategy.

Group Concurrence and Involvement

Many in the field believe that it is necessary to involve the social group itself in the design and implementation of a local sampling plan. This requirement challenges standard research practices at two distinct stages in the research process. The first stage, which we will call consultation, involves the initial invitation of a potentially participating group. Investigators should involve appropriate commmunity representatives in the design of their sampling strategies, collection methods, and reciprocity agreements before any plan to sample a particular group is considered final or any individual is approached for consent. This process could take different forms with different populations: meeting first with local scientists in one context, with community leaders in another or with lay groups devoted to particular genetic diseases in a third.

The next stage of community involvement is obtaining approval of the group to participate in the study that the first stage of consultation generates. This requires activating the process that the group uses to make collective decisions on issues related to their corporate identity and interests. The process is analogous to the informed consent obtained from the individuals providing samples, and it requires the same forms of information disclosure by the investigators.

The concept of community approval is not well articulated in contemporary research policies, but it is similar to some forms of community consultation already used in some population-level research. The communication processes between the researcher and the group and the community decision-making processes that will be required to achieve group concurrence will necessarily vary from group to group. But to the extent that the research has the potential to affect the social interests of the group as a whole, any research on members of groups or communities (as defined by themselves or the researchers) must develop a protocol for community consultation and a mechanism for community input into how the research is designed, how the research itself will be conducted, and how the results will be used.

The concept of group approval has limits. Recently, the World Health Organization and the Council for International Organizations of Medical Sciences updated their International Ethical Guidelines for Biomedical

Research Involving Human Subjects (1993). Those guidelines, which are based on the Nuremberg Code (1947), the World Medical Association's Declaration of Helsinki (1964), the Universal Declaration (1948), and the International Covenants (1976), articulate specific requirements. Even when community consent is obtained as a prerequisite for conducting research with group members, investigators must obtain the informed consent of individual prospective subjects (guideline 1). The information needed to obtain informed consent must be conveyed by the investigator in language that the subject is capable of understanding, including the research, its duration, reasonably expected benefits, foreseeable risks, alternative procedures, the extent of confidentiality, the availability of compensation, and the facts that participation is voluntary and that the subject may withdraw at any time without penalty (guideline 2). If the investigator has difficulty in communicating with the prospective subjects "to make prospective subjects sufficiently aware of the implications of participation to give adequately informed consent, the decision of each prospective subject on whether to consent should be elicited through a reliable intermediary such as a trusted community leader." However consent is obtained, all prospective subjects must be clearly informed that their participation is entirely voluntary and that they are free to refuse to participate or to cease to participate at any time without loss of any entitlement (commentary on guideline 8). In locations where women's rights to self-determination are not recognized (and thus their informed consent not possible), "women should not normally be involved in the research" (commentary on guideline 11 of the International Ethical Guidelines for Biomedical Research Involving Human Subjects), because it is likely that they will not have the freedom and power to choose whether to participate. While it is obviously wrong to exclude women from participation in a study that could lead to results from which they could benefit, it is equally important to insist on informed consent that is freely given.

Current international policy does not address whether a community should be able to veto the voluntary participation of individual members in legitimate research. If the group has decided not to participate, should individual volunteers who identify themselves as group members continue to be recruited and enrolled as representatives of the group? This conflict is particularly likely to occur in situations in which, for example, expatriate or immigrant communities of some social group's location have caused it to think about participation in research in a different way from members of their group who live elsewhere. We think that it too extreme a position to require both group and individual consent to DNA collection for genetic variation research. Nonetheless, researchers will have to make sure that their participants understand both the objections of their community and the rationale for them as part of the informed consent process and, when doing research that is opposed by a specific community, will also have to take into account the possible impact of doing such research on the likelihood that other communities will cooperate with other genetic variation researchers in the future.

Individually Identified DNA Sampling

Any sampling strategy that collects enough phenotypic, genealogical, or other ethnographic data to identify individual human sources of the DNA has the potential to put individual subjects and families at risk for confusion, intrafamilial disruption, stigmatization, and discrimination (Juengst 1996). That reinforces the need to have both individuals and families participate actively in the consent process and gives them rights and interests in controlling the use of their DNA samples and results that should override the claims of their communities or groups. Consequently, agreements regarding the research to be conducted on individually identified and population-representative samples should be negotiatd at three levels: community, familial and individual. At each successive level, potential research participants should be afforded the right to decline or further qualify their participation in the study, within the limits of the agreements established by the larger groups that they represent. The potential for individual and familial identification has other implications that are not as important in other sampling strategies.

First, adequate confidentiality protections must be ensured. Studies that simply collect group-identification data about their sample sources cannot reasonably promise to protect the confidentiality of their findings about the group if group identification is integral to the point of the study, and they should not attempt to do so. However, when information about individuals and families is collected, a promise of confidentiality is important to offer and honor. Steps must be taken to ensure that other individuals do not learn of the information derived from the sample if the sample can be linked to an identifiable individual. That is a basic concept in all genetics research, and it requires strict data management, oversight of data storage, rules for coding and disclosing data, rules regarding redisclosure and basic data security and monitoring. It is especially important to institute measures that will prevent unauthorized access to individually identifiable genetic information, so as to protect individual research participants from stigmatization and discrimination. That will require a continuing monitoring mechanism to prevent breaches of confidentiality and to permit appropriate action to be taken against those who participate in such breaches. The degree of potential breaches of confidentiality and invasion of privacy might be so high that ethical conduct of such research will be impossible unless only DNA samples that cannot be linked to identifiable individuals are stored.

Second, studies that collect individually identifiable DNA must include mechanisms for follow-up about the results of the studies conducted on collected samples. In initial consultations with the communities to be sampled, investigators should agree on what information and follow-up services will be available to individuals or families who are found to have specific illnesses or a genetic predisposition to specific illnesses. In most cases of medically relevant genetic findings, arrangements involve a comprehensive protocol for the genetic screening and counseling of individuals, including mechanisms for dealing with findings, such as misidentified paternity, ambiguous or uncertain results, and the reproductive-risk implications of the information collected.

CONTROL

The extent of continuing involvement in the research by the group being sampled must be addressed. This includes whether groups or group spokespersons will be involved in monitoring the research conducted on DNA samples taken from their people, in granting permission for new uses of those samples if they are identifiable, in determining whether the group can withdraw from the research and in determining how to share financial or other benefits.

With a DNA-databank research resource, the responsibility of the collection managers to monitor research conducted by external investigators is especially strong. Systems should be in place that aid the collection managers in anticipating the social consequences of particular research findings and help the public and the groups involved to prepare for those consequences. The collection manager in effect, must assume the role of the genetic counselor for the participating groups, and administrators must be prepared to disclose the results of the testing in a responsible manner. To be consistent with practice in other fields of human genetics, the disclosure of the results of the research to the general public through scientific publications should be negotiated with the representatives of the donor groups (Powers 1993).

It is not ethically or legally acceptable to ask research participants to "consent" to future but as-yet-unknown uses of their identifiable DNA samples. Consent in such a case is a waiver of rights, and such waivers are explicitly prohibited by federal research regulations.

People have the right to withdraw their consent to research at any time, including the right to have identifiable samples destroyed or withdrawn. But how does that work on the community level? Should the population itself be able to withdraw from the project? The answer might be that "community withdrawal" is not possible; if that is the case, it should be spelled out in both the protocol and the individual consent processes, as well as in the discussion of the protocol with community representatives. In general, consent and withdrawal are rights of individual research subjects and should not depend on the approval or disapproval of government authorities, however defined. Some studies of American Indians have used the relevant tribal council both to give approval of proposed research and to review and have right of refusal to publish all research findings. That procedural protection might seem extreme to scientists, but such agreements are reported to have worked well in a variety of medical research projects. It is a way for genetic variation projects to respond to the legitimate interests of subjects and groups in the research.

COMMERCIALIZATION AND RECIPROCITY AGREEMENTS

Some proponents of human genetic-variation research argue that it will be essential to negotiate arrangements regarding possible commercial benefits with the subject groups in advance of research, to make the participating groups "partners" with scientists in the research (North American Committee). Such a partnership implies that the subject groups will be given some role in determining the uses to which research results will be put.

Arrangements regarding financial interests in the products or outcomes of the research should be negotiated as part of the original project review and informed-consent process. In addition, a monitoring and enforcement mechanism, with representation of the affected groups, should be in place. One of the major lessons from the Rio de Janeiro Biodiversity Summit is the importance of economic and political considerations in negotiating research participation with identified human groups. That should not be surprising, inasmuch as social groups are usually created and sustained as a means of pursuing their members' economic and political interests. However, this adds a dimension to informed consent negotiations that is foreign to most social and biomedical scientists: negotiating over what the participating group receives in return for participation.

Perhaps the most contentious issue in the short history of human genetic diversity research is the growing practice of patenting cell lines and gene sequences. Some indigenous populations are so averse to patenting that many researchers not only state that they will refuse commercial funding for genetic diversity research, but also explicitly promise not to patent or profit from any potentially profitable discoveries that might be made. Of course, researchers can speak only for themselves. As long as it is legal to patent human genes and gene sequences, others might obtain patents on them. Prohibiting the patenting of genes and gene sequences would require an international agreement binding at least all the major industrialized countries. Debate on this issue continues in Europe; only France has explicitly stated it will not permit patenting of genes and gene sequences. Nonetheless, much or most of the international controversy over collecting genes to study human genetic variation would disappear if the patenting of genes and gene sequences was outlawed.

Outlawing the patenting of human genes and gene sequences would solve one immediate problem, but it would not address the controversy over patenting human cell lines. The committee heard testimony from John Moore, whose spleen was used as a source of a cell line that was immortalized and patented without his knowledge or permission. When Moore discovered what had occurred, he sued his physician and the biotechnology companies that obtained the patent for his cell line. The California Supreme Court ultimately ruled that other people and companies could own John Moore's cell line and could patent it but that he himself could not assert an ownership interest in his own cells (*Moore v. Regents* 1990). The court stated that that result was necessary to protect the biotechnology industry, which might falter if individual ownership of cells (and DNA) were permitted (Annas 1993; Knoppers et al. 1996). After Moore briefed the committee, another witness, Abadio Green Stocel, from a Colombian group, said "If this can happen to a U.S. businessman, what chance do we have?" These arguments raised a second possible approach that assumes at least some patenting will continue; the committee considered this argument in its deliberations.

A less comprehensive, mutually agreeable strategy would be to require that all such patent applications include an agreement to share a set proportion of the resulting net proceeds or profits with the person whose body was the source of the DNA or, at that person's election, with the community of which he or she is a member. Or such "royalty" payments could be made to an international body such as UNESCO or WHO, for the benefit of the participating populations (Knoppers et al. 1996).

A more sophisticated and more-complicated approach would be to form an international organization to serve as a trustee and fundholder for all the sampled populations. Patents would be issued in the name of this trustee organization, which would license anyone who signs an agreement to share a portion of the net proceeds from products made from any patented gene, gene sequences, or cell line with the trustee organization. The trustee organization, in turn, would be required to ensure that the revenue benefited the participating populations, which would be represented in the trustee organization. Such an organization not only could ensure that financial fairness is observed in genetic diversity research but also could develop, monitor and enforce universal rules for protocol review and informed consent in such research.

CONCLUSION

Collecting biological samples from specific individuals and families to extrapolate information about the social groups to which they belong is not a new scientific practice. However, as one research team put it, "The day of informal donations of DNA samples is past" (Hannig et al. 1993). The confluence of several sets of ethical considerations gives that practice greater risks that human genetic-variation researchers must recognize. Continued use of outmoded social categories to structure biomedical research (Osborne and Feit 1992), emerging possibilities for commercializing biomedical knowledge and heightened awareness of the stigmatizing potential of genetic information all increase public concern about human genetic-variation research. To the extent that human genetic-variation research must continue to rely on socially defined human groups as surrogates for human demes (until technology to infer deme membership exists), the process of managing any coordinated effort to survey human diversity will be increasingly complex. For each socially identified set of samples, protocols for group consultation, consent and control will have to be negotiated and balanced against the researchers' fundamental ethical obligations to protect the freedom, privacy, and welfare of the individuals involved, including the right not to participate in a study.

REFERENCES

Amazanga Institute and others. 1996. Declaration of indigenous peoples of the western hemisphere regarding the human genome diversity project. *Cultural*

Survival 20: listed in Mead ATP. Genealogy, sacredness and the commodities market: 15 statements by regional indigenous people's organizations. *Cultural Survival* 20 (Summer): 50.

Annas, G. J. 1993. *Standard of care: The law of American bioethics.* New York: Oxford University Press, pp. 167–177.

Barkan, E. 1992. *The retreat of scientific racism: changing concepts of race in Britain and the United States between the World Wars.* Cambridge, England: Cambridge University Press.

Caplan, A. 1994. Handle with care: race, class and genetics. In Murphy, T. F., Lappe, M., editors. *Justice and the Human Genome Project.* Berkeley: University of California Press, pp. 30–45.

Cavalli-Sforza, L. L., Wilson, A. C., Cantor, C. R., Cook-Deegan, R. M., King, M. C. 1991. Call for a world-wide survey of human genetic diversity: a vanishing opportunity for the human genome project.

[CIOMS] Council for International Organizations of Medical Sciences. 1993 International ethical guidelines for biomedical research involving human subjects. Available from: CIOMS, pp. 1–63.

Dominguez, V. 1986. *White by definition: social classification in creole Louisiana.* New Brunswick, N.J.: Rutgers University Press.

Dominguez, V. 1989. *People as subject, people as object: selfhood and peoplehood in contemporary Israel.* Madison: University of Wisconsin Press.

Frankel, M., Teich, E., editors. 1993. *Ethical and legal issues in pedigree research.* Washington, D.C.: AAAS.

Friedlander, J. 1996. Genes, people and property. *Cultural Survival Quarterly* 20 (Summer): 22–24.

Geller, L., Alper, J., Billings, P., Barash, C., Beckwith, J., Natowicz, M. 1996. individual, family and societal dimensions of genetic discrimination: a case study analysis. *Sci. Eng. Ethics* 29: 71–88.

Gladney, D. C. 1991. *Muslim Chinese: ethnic nationalism in the People's Republic of China.* Cambridge, Mass.: Harvard University Press.

Handler, R. 1988. *Nationalism and the politic of culture in Quebec.* Madison: University of Wisconsin Press.

Hannig, V., Clayton, E., Edwards, K. 1993. Whose DNA is it, anyway? Relationships between families and researchers. *Genetics* 47: 257–60.

[HUGO] Human Genome Organization. 1993. The Human Genome Diversity, (HGD) Project: summary document. Available from HUGO Europe. One Park Square West, London, England, pp. 1–8.

Hudson, K., Rothenberg, K., Andrews, L., Kahn, M., Collins, F. 1995. Genetic discrimination and health insurance: an urgent need for reform. *Science* 270: 391–93.

Juengst, E. 1994. Human genome research and the public interest: progress notes from an American science policy experiment. *Hum Genet* 54: 121–128.

Juengst, E. 1996. Respecting human subjects in genome research: a preliminary policy agenda. In Vanderpool, H., editor. *The ethics of research involving human subjects: facing the 21st century.* Frederick, Md.: University Publishing Group, pp. 401–429.

Knoppers, B. M., Hirtie, M., Lormeau, S. 1996. Ethical issues in international collaborative research on the human genome: the HGP and the HGDP. *Genomic* 34: 271–282.

Marks, J. 1996. The legacy of serological studies in American physical anthropology. *History and Philosophy of the Life Sciences.* 18: 75–91.

Mead, A.T.P. 1966. Genealogy, sacredness, and the commodities market. *Cultural Survival Q.* 20.

Moore v. Regents of the University of California 793 P.2d 479, 271 Cal Rptr 146. (1990).

North American Committee of the Human Genome Diversity Project. 1993. Model ethical protocol. Available from the Morrison Institute for Population and Resource Studies, Stanford University, Stanford, Calif.

[OPRR] Office of Protection from Research Risk, Department of Human Health Services. 1993. Human genetic research. In *Protecting human research subjects: institutional review board guidebook*, Chapter H. Bethesda, Md.: OPRR.

Osborne, N., Feit, M. 1992. The use of race in medical research. *JAMA* 267: 275–279.

Powers, M. 1993. Publication-related risks to privacy: empirical implications of pedigree studies. *IRB: A review of human subjects research* 15: 17–22.

[RAFI] Rural Advancement Foundation International. 1993. Patents, indigenous peoples, and human genetic diversity. RAFI Communique: May.

Rex, J., Mason, D., editors. 1988. *Theories of race and ethnic relations*. Cambridge, England: Cambridge University Press.

Schneider, W. H. 1996. The history of research on blood group genetics: initial discovery and diffusion. *History and Philosophy of the Life Sciences*, 18: 7–33.

Steiner, H., Alston, P., editors. 1996. *International human rights in context: law, politics and morals*. Oxford, England: Oxford University Press.

Taube, G. 1995. Scientists attacked for "patenting" Pacific tribe. *Science* 270: 1112.

UNESCO. 1995. Subcommittee on Bioethics and Populations Genetics of the UNESCO International Bioethics Committee. Nov. 15, 1995 Report.

United Nations Commission on Human Rights. 1995. Mataatua declaration on cultural and intellectual property rights of indigenous peoples. *Cultural Survival* 20 (Summer): 52–53.

United States Congress. 1993. Testimony of Francis Collins, NIH, and David Galas, DOE. Human Genome Diversity Project. Hearings before the Senate Committee on Governmental Affairs, U.S. Senate, 103 Congress, first session, April 26, 1993. Washington, D.C.: U.S. Government Printing Office, pp. 6–15.

PART VI

How to Proceed From Concept to Action

The field of health and human rights was developed in the context of advocacy and action. If the field is to flourish, it must continue to grapple with not only the conceptual framework of the health and human rights interplay but also with their practical and effective application to the real world. The final section is devoted to such advocacy and action.

The first chapter, "Common Strategies for Health and Human Rights: Moving from Theory to Practice," by Stephen Marks, comes from the Second International Conference on Health and Human Rights. It focuses on the five major partners working for health and human rights: health professionals and the human rights community, public institutions, nongovernmental organizations, intergovernmental organizations, and the public citizen. Ways must be found for these partners to work together. Marks identifies points of entry for a common strategy that includes the political process, norm-setting environments, service delivery areas, the research arena, and the education system. Finally, Marks focuses on planning and funding strategies to bring these transformative strategies into reality.

The Marks' chapter is followed by chapters that focus on the work of health and human rights nongovernmental organizations (NGOs). The first of these chapters describes Physicians for Human Rights. This organization mobilizes health professionals to work toward human rights. Activities include investigation and documentation of human rights abuses, medical assistance, legislative action, advocacy education and training. While much of the work of Physicians for Human Rights has been reactive to abuses, this chapter also considers ways for the organization to protect and promote health and human rights before the abuses occur.

The chapter by Renée Fox focuses on the link between medical humanitarianism and human rights actions within the context of a structured response. The goal of the physician organizations she describes is to provide urgent medical care anywhere in the world there is suffering, particularly when such suffering occurs as the consequence of violence, torture, persecution, warfare, disenfranchisement, oppression, abandonment, exile or exodus. This rapid, emergency- and rescue-oriented in-the-field response is but one way these organizations bear public witness to violations of human rights and dignity.

As another example of moving theory to action, we have included "A Call to Action," which was published in the *Journal of the American Medical Association*. This is a policy perspective written by a group of U.S. physicians and nurses calling themselves the Ad Hoc Committee to Defend Health Care. This group of health professionals criticizes the growing trend in U.S. health care to transform healing from a covenant to a contract and the increasing corporatization of medicine. These health care providers state unequivocally that access to health care must be the right of all. In transforming concept to action, the group has petitioned legislators, called for a moratorium on for-profit takeovers of health care institutions, initiated demonstrations, and organized teach-ins and meetings. Their final call to action is to provide humane, comprehensive, and equitable health care for all.

Finally, we close this section and the book with an exploration of health and human rights by Jonathan Mann, who discusses how human rights thinking and action have become closely integrated with public health and medical work. This chapter focuses on the potential burden on human rights created by medical and public health policies, programs and practices as well as on how violations of human rights have adverse health effects on physical, mental and social well-being. This chapter brings together many of the themes developed in this book and is a call for action.

Common Strategies for Health and Human Rights: From Theory to Practice

26.

Stephen P. Marks

My task is to encourage both health workers and human rights workers to think about the ways forward, to devise a strategy to move from theory to practice. In offering some thoughts about a common strategy for health and human rights, I am starting from two assumptions. The first assumption is that the health and human rights communities that the François-Xavier Bagnoud Center has brought together at its two conferences share a growing awareness of a common agenda. There are numerous indicators of this trend. One is the increase in the number of participants from the first conference to the second. It is truly extraordinary that five hundred people came to explore a theme that, a few short years ago, might have appeared esoteric and marginal. A second indicator is the spectacular growth in subscriptions to *Health and Human Rights*, truly remarkable for a scholarly journal. Something is capturing the attention of people. A third sign of this shared perception is the extraordinary number of relevant projects under way around the world.

The second assumption behind a strategy for the future is that the problems of violence and disease along with other health- and-related society-issues to which we would apply a common strategy of action are both numerous and urgent. Such a list is itself an agenda calling for a common strategy.

It is not enough to acknowledge the need for a common strategy; we need to move from thought to action. To do so I propose to focus on (1) the actors or the partners who are going to join in a common strategy, (2) the points of entry for such a strategy to be put into practice, and (3) the resources that can be marshalled to make it possible to carry out such a strategy.

PARTNERS FOR A COMMON STRATEGY

If our ideas are to have a wider impact, we need to work with partners. Approximately five categories of potential partners can be mentioned as able to contribute, in one way or another, to this common strategy. The first are, of course, the professional categories, subdivided into two. The health professionals include *both* health professionals and the medical professionals, each with different professional backgrounds and approaches but working together in a remarkable way. The human rights community includes those professionals who focus, to a large extent, on the application of law and on the use of advocacy. These two professional groups—of health and human rights—are the core partners in our common strategy.

The second category of actors are public institutions. The notion of the state itself has frequently been challenged, and yet we are constantly reminded that some of our best partners work for and represent the state. Some of those who have put together the most forward-looking programs belong to state institutions. For example, the Swiss government has a new three-part policy of health and development that draws explicitly on the essential linkages between health and human rights. The Swiss officials who elaborated and who implement this program are ahead of us. They are putting our theory into practice already. Of the billions of dollars being spent on official development assistance (ODA), most goes through government channels. That is where the resources are; that is where policies can have an impact on a vast scale. Those who are in charge of implementing those policies need to be partners in this enterprise. I have learned from talking to some of the people in government that to mobilize their institutions will require sort of a pincer movement. You have to deal at the programmatic level with the midlevel professionals, and, at the same time you have to deal with their bosses and their bosses' bosses. If you work only from the top down or the bottom up, the lead time between proposing a bold new idea and seeing it implemented is about ten years in the best scenario. If you work from both directions at the same time, you cut the lead time in half or less. We therefore need to reach both midlevel bureaucrats and assistant secretaries or vice ministers with human-rights-sensitive health policies.

The third category of partners is the nongovernmental (NGO) community. Two major categories are: the advocacy NGOs and the service-delivery NGOs. Amnesty International, Human Rights Watch, and Physicians for Human Rights, for example, belong to the first category, while Médecins Sans Frontières (MSF), Oxfam, and the International Committee of the Red Cross belong to the second category. We have heard of some of the training courses that MSF is carrying out and wants to expand to all humanitarian organizations dealing precisely with the human rights dimensions of health policy and action. This effort appears exemplary of the strategy we are attempting to design.

The fourth category of potential actors in this common strategy are the intergovernmental organizations (IGOs). They are sometimes also criticized as being part of the problem, but we all know that they are also an important part of the solution. I would suggest that we need to utilize two of the ways in which IGOs operate in our common strategy: norm setting and field operations. Regarding norm setting, Stephen Lewis has eloquently described the impact an international convention can have in moving from theory into action affecting the lives of millions of children. At the operational level, IGOs are spending billions of dollars in ODA resources. The message to our friends in IGOs is that they must spend these funds in ways that advance the health and human rights agenda.

The fifth category consists of the bystanders, ordinary people who are not directly involved in health or human rights policy but who are indirectly engaged as citizens and taxpayers. These people need to be mobilized through the media and other means and made aware of the benefits to the public of wise policies of health and human rights. They vote; they join voluntary organizations; they write letters to public officials and the media. This is an untapped resource for the movement we are promoting today.

To engage these five categories of potential partners in a common strategy, we need to consider ways of mobilizing them more fruitfully. One proposal is to establish a roster of persons in each of these categories who could be called upon, for example, to be a speaker at an event or to join a task force on a health policy issue at the local level. Such a roster would be a source of volunteer talent to implement the strategy.

POINTS OF ENTRY FOR A COMMON STRATEGY

Now I come to the second element: points of entry for a common strategy. The first is the policy-making process. Specifically, the time has come to implement the health and human rights policy optimization model outlined in chapters 5 and 6 of this book. This concept should move from theory to practice as soon as possible. Both preventive and curative health policies are being devised at the community, national, regional, and international levels all over the world without the application of this very insightful approach. We must generalize the practice of human rights people and health specialists working together to critique a public health policy from both the human rights and health policy perspectives in order to optimize both sets of concerns. I became convinced two years ago of the soundness of this approach, and yet we have not moved very far from the theory to the practice of this model. The time has come.

The second point of entry is the norm-setting environment. Norm-setting environments are pertinent in three main areas relevant to people drafting standards relevant to health and human rights. Professional associations are engaged in this process, but efforts could be broadened and deepened. For example, the American College of Physicians recently adopted a policy on sanctions and health and human rights after being convinced of the need to do so by the International Association of Bioethics and Physicians for Human Rights. This is what I mean by intervening in the norm-setting arena.

A second norm-setting environment is the legislature. Parliaments draft laws and elaborate principles that affect health and human rights. A magnificent example is happening in South Africa, where legislation that draws upon these principles is being drafted. Parliamentarians and their staffs are not likely to reinvent these ideason their own; we need to bring the ideas to them. We need to create opportunities to discuss our strategic objectives with members of parliaments and their staffs.

Intergovernmental organizations constitute a third norm-setting environment where the principles we are elaborating can be adopted in the form of resolutions and normative instruments (i.e., conventions and recommendations). Many opportunities have been discussed, such as sessions of the World Health Assembly and the Commission on Human Rights. We have heard about the African Commission on Human Rights, the Sub-Commission on the Prevention of Discrimination and Protection of Minorities, the Committee on Economic, Social and Cultural Rights, and other human rights treaty bodies. We have learned about the technique of counter-reports or shadow reports submitted to the Committee on Economic, Social and Cultural Rights. A complaints procedure would also be useful. Draft optional protocols allowing individual complaints are in preparation for both the Covenant on Economic, Social and Cultural Rights and the International Convention on the Elimination of All Forms of Discrimination Against Women. These procedures would put some teeth into the standards that are basic to health and human rights concerns. Lobbying efforts within the intergovernmental organizations will be increasingly valuable as we move from theory to practice.

The third point of entry is the service delivery area, covering such issues as refugee relief, vaccination programs and humanitarian actions, which are taking place on a vast scale around the world. With few exceptions, these programs function without a conscious policy of integrating health and human rights. It is an urgent and vital point of entry.

The research agenda is the fourth point of entry. There is no need to give any examples, for this book provides a rich list of research themes that can be taken up by any number of our partners willing to focus on the intersection of health and human rights, as well as their application to the policy agenda.

And the fifth point of entry for this strategy, I would argue, is education. Jacqueline Pitanguy reminds us that we cannot educate politicians. They are "hopeless." This reminds me of experiences I have had with programs to teach human rights to military and police officers. A two-week seminar will not create a new value system nor alter the thought and behavior of adults already socialized in their political, military, or correctional environment. It is a slow process, the crucial moments of which exist much earlier in the individual's psychological development. Before education can change the behavior of those individuals who may participate in torture and other acts that violate human rights or who might be inclined to adopt an unsound health policy or practice violative of human rights, it is essential to obtain firm directive at the top of the hierarchical structures in which those individuals operate. The order comes from the top down, from the commander of the troops, the commissioner of police or the top of the party structure or bureaucracy. As a result of the political pressures brought upon the person issuing the order, those who execute the top-down orders tend to obey, assuming the system of rewards and negative inducements with which they are familiar is operative. A politician who knows there is a constituency that believes that health is a human right does not need to be educated about human rights texts; that politician wants to be reelected and will begin to believe that health is a human right. Without such inducements where they count, the politician will not budge. This is also true for the torturing police officer. If his superior will be out of a job if torture occurs, and may even be prosecuted, the order is given in a way that the torturing police officer understands. An education program can reinforce and direct the behavior of officials who already have an objective motivation to observe sound health and human rights practices. With this proviso, an education program directed at officials belongs in our common strategy.

A second observation about education applies particularly to the United States. This month, October, is Roosevelt History Month. Instead of Roosevelt history, we are fed lengthy articles about the death of liberalism and how being tainted with the "L-word" means political suicide. However, this country has a political tradition of believing that, even after a devastating war, freedom from want is a fundamental human right, is a part of human rights, and should attain a normative level beyond that of merely "desirable" governmental programs. That heritage, that legacy, needs to be reclaimed.

There has also been considerable discussion about the forms of mass education and about the relationship between the health and human rights agenda, on one hand, and the human rights education agenda on the other. Our common strategy should place a priority on issues linking health and human rights within the framework of the Plan of Action of the UN Decade for Human Rights Education.

PLANNING AND FUNDING THE COMMON STRATEGY

Let me make a specific proposal for the implementation of the strategy I have outlined. What is needed to transform these ideas into action is a plan of action for implementing a common health and human rights strategy. I am proposing a plan of action based on the premise that the most likely groups to carry them out would be able to incorporate them into their respective budgets and planning for the future. There are plenty of organizations who could put in a small project here, a small mission there, a trip to Geneva here, a pilot task force for a policy project there.

The costs of such a plan of action are not excessive. The budget should be adequate to cover the following four types of expenditure:

(1) Costs of travel and incidentals for task forces to implement the health and human rights policy optimization program. If participating experts volunteer their time, the cost could be kept to between $1,000 and $5,000 per task force. The costs would obviously increase if in-depth impact or other studies needed to be commissioned.

(2) Costs of travel and incidentals for brief missions by people on the roster mentioned earlier to accept speaking engagements, engage in advocacy, and other opportunities to have an impact. These activities would cost between $500 and $3,000.

(3) Legal expenses for a litigation program where lawyers could put into practice the theories we have been discussing by challenging destructive policies. A modest program of two or three cases per year could utilize pro bono attorneys and cost about $10,000 per case or less, depending on whether the project lawyers act as amicus or as counsel.

(4) Fees and staff time for research projects on key issues. If partners collaborate, several studies could be carried out with a contribution of about $20,000 per study, assuming similar contributions from other partners.

Those four sets of activities might amount to $100,000 to 200,000 per year. That is a modest level to start implementing our common strategy. Three sources of funding could be tapped: governments, including ministries of health; intergovernmental organizations; and foundations. With a coherent plan of action and involvement of relevant partners, the common strategy can be transformed into fundable projects.

POLITICAL REALITIES

The common strategy outlined here has generally stayed away from discussion of political realities. However, power relations are fundamental to the causes and cures of most health and human rights emergencies. Health professionals tend, I believe, to be less comfortable than human rights workers with the politics of action, but the existing power structures favor three "elites," and this affects what we are trying to accomplish with this strategy. First, those who benefit from exploitation, inequality and repression, including patriarchal structures, have no motivation to seek a human rights policy in the health field. Second, those who do not need improvements in health delivery also have no such motivation. You do not need to ask the authors of the "personal responsibility legislation," the so-called welfare reform in the United States, whether health is a human right. They have no reason to believe that health is a human right. Ask the people who are denied health care if health is a human right, and they will give you a different answer. The third category of those who lack motivation to seek a human rights policy regarding health are the lawyers and doctors themselves, the vast majority of our professional colleagues who are conservative by tradition and by interest.

If we take these political realities into account, we need to adjust our strategy for mobilizing partners around health and human rights issues to give it both a reformist and a transformative orientation. It should be reformist insofar as it seeks to operate within the system, within the current power structures. What this means is developing approaches that are sensitive to human rights-related causes of injury and illness and the human rights consequences of health policies. Land mines are a good example of this orientation. The case for their elimination is urgent and compelling and can be pursued without challenging any basic structures of power, although there are plenty of interests resisting their elimination. This reformist motivation applies to much of our agenda and is appealing to most of our partners.

But there are numerous participants who are willing to go further, to develop a transformative strategy that challenges the prevailing power structures and attitudes, that pursues the pedagogies of liberation and hope. Both human rights education and liberation medicine are relevant to this more radical strategy. This strategy flows from the awareness that the governments, corporations and financial institutions responsible for practices contrary to health and human rights are structurally incapable of overcoming injustice. Numerous references have been made in this regard to the processes of globalization of the world economy. The role of a health and human rights strategy is to delegitimize policies and practices that favor the powerful at the expense of those whose health is regarded as expendable for corporate and national material wealth. This transformative strategy requires new forms of accountability of governments, of corporations, and of health and legal professionals.

This politically charged agenda within the common strategy is not for all of us, however. Some believe that realism and professional responsibility dictate caution in challenging existing structures. I call on them to join in the innumerable components of our common strategy that seek the application of existing norms and procedures for a human rights-sensitive health policy. I conclude, therefore, with a call to action addressed to everyone, so that we will not remain bystanders while millions upon millions of children, women, and men continue to live in ignorance, poverty, and deprivation of their fundamental dignity and integrity. Ideas do change the world, and the linkage of human rights and health work is one of those ideas.

27. The Health Professional as Human Rights Promoter: Ten Years of Physicians for Human Rights (USA)

Kari Hannibal and Robert Lawrence

Health professionals have been on the front lines of the struggle for protection of international human rights, often being the first witnesses of the physical and psychological harm that human rights violations cause to individuals and communities. In the past three decades, the health care community has mobilized itself to act to protest violations, to document their health consequences, and to examine its own role in perpetrating or ending these abuses. This article examines the role of one activist organization, the U.S.-based Physicians for Human Rights (PHR), in the international human rights movement.

ORIGINS

Like most human rights organizations, the mandate of PHR is largely defined by the rights enunciated in the Universal Declaration of Human Rights, adopted by the United Nations in 1948 in response to the Nazi atrocities of World War II. Other standards that PHR uses in its work are the Geneva Conventions of 1949 and the Additional Protocols of 1977. These further define the protections and guarantees of medical neutrality during armed conflict, and mandate the protection of patients and health professionals, the right to access to care and the humane treatment of civilians living in war zones.

Recognition of human rights became an important element of U.S. foreign policy during the Carter administration (1977–1981), at the same time that the world learned of large-scale political repression in Argentina, the Soviet Union, and Cambodia. In the former Soviet Union, leading scientists such as Andrei Sakharov and Yuri Orlov were sent into internal exile, stripped of their scientific duties or banished to labor camps. Groups such as Amnesty International, Helsinki Watch, the Committee on Scientific Freedom and Responsibility of the American Association for the Advancement of Science (AAAS) and the Human Rights Committee of the National Academy of Sciences (NAS) denounced the human rights abuses directed against these dissident scientists, and organized efforts within the scientific and medical communities to secure the protection of colleagues.

Attention to human rights in U.S. foreign policy diminished in the 1980s due to political changes in the administration and the intensification of the cold war. As a result, repressive régimes were often rewarded for their staunch anti-Communist policies despite flagrant human rights abuses. Increasingly, U.S. military assistance provided the means to suppress civilian populations in such countries as El Salvador, the Philippines, and South Korea. Violations of medical neutrality were reported with alarming frequency. Indigenous groups of human rights activists documented tortures, assassination, and disappearances. The abuse of psychiatry in the Soviet Union, where diagnoses of mental disorders were used to suppress dissent, and the collaboration of physicians in the monitoring of torture victims in Chile, Uruguay and elsewhere added new and disturbing dimensions to the linkage between health and human rights. The Colegio Medico in Chile, the Medical Action Group (MAG) in the Philippines and Tutela Legal in El Salvador requested assistance from U.S. human rights groups to help document abuses, expose official complicity, and break down the walls of impunity.

Early in 1983, two U.S. scientific and medical delegations conducted human rights missions of inquiry to El Salvador. One represented the Institute of Medicine (of the NAS), the International League for Human Rights, and the AAAS Committee on Scientific Freedom and Responsibility. The other team consisted of health professionals representing the American Public Health Association. On their return to the United States, both groups testified before congressional committees, gave grand rounds at teaching hospitals, and spoke to professional colleagues at conferences about their findings, as well as about the role that concerned health professionals could play in the politics of the United States' assistance to government security forces in El Salvador. In the professional community, interest in the public health consequences of human rights abuses and the application of public health and medical skills to curtail these abuses was beginning.

At about the same time, Dr. Jonathan E. Fine, long active with Physicians for Social Responsibility (PSR) and International Physicians for the Prevention of Nuclear War (IPPNW), was visiting the Philippines at the request of MAG, to discuss the work of IPPNW. MAG leaders told him of the harassment experienced by some of their colleagues trying to deliver health care in contested zones. This harassment was conducted by the Marcos security forces. MAG and the Task Force Detainees, a group of Franciscan nuns monitoring human rights, invited Dr. Fine to return to conduct a medical fact-finding mission. The assassinations of two Filipino physicians added urgency to the MAG request.

The November 1983 mission was funded and sponsored by the AAAS Committee on Scientific Freedom and Responsibility, along with the American College of Physicians and the American Nurses Association, in order to provide broad, mainstream support and to enhance the delegation's political influence. The delegation, which included Dr. Fine, another physician, and a staff member of the AAAS Committee, spent three weeks traveling throughout the Philippines and established a pattern of activity that influenced many subsequent missions. The team contacted government officials, opposition groups who had invited the team, family members, professional colleagues, and local officials. Team members interviewed and medically examined victims of human rights abuses and obtained forensic materials such as X rays and copies of medical records when possible. After the Justice Department denied a request by the team to visit political prisoners in the detention centers, the team divided itself up. Accompanied by a nun from the Task Force Detainees, individual team members were able to present themselves as concerned colleagues from the United States and to enter detention centers to obtain testimony and examine prisoners directly.

Dr. Fine returned to Boston committed to forming a human rights group that could respond to groups such as MAG and intervene on behalf of victims of human rights violations. He created the American Committee for Human Rights (ACHR) and invited a small group of colleagues to serve as members of its board of directors. Supported largely by Dr. Fine's personal savings and the pro bono work of the board members, the ACHR struggled in 1984 and 1985 to define a coherent mission statement, raise funds, and respond to crises in South Korea, Chile, and Central America. Slowly it became clear that the ACHR's unique contribution lay in its capacity to mobilize physicians to work for human rights. At the urging of board members, the name of the organization was changed in 1986 to Physicians for Human Rights, reflecting the focus of their mission. Dr. Jane Green Schaller, chair of the Department of Pediatrics at Tufts University, had joined PHR after returning from a profoundly disturbing trip to assess child health in South Africa. That summer, she convened a meeting of board members and interested health professionals to plan the future of the new organization and the recruitment of a broad base of member support from the health professions. She was elected PHR's first president.

METHODS OF WORK

The philosophy behind the decision to create an organization of health professionals to work on behalf of human rights arose from two insights, best described by PHR members Drs. H. Jack Geiger and Robert Cook-Deegan:

> First was the recognition that many human rights violations had significant health consequences. These include the physical and psychological trauma of individual victims of violence, torture, and rape, but also stem from breaches

of medical neutrality, forced deportations, the use of indiscriminate weapons, mass executions, and other violent acts that affect entire populations. The purposeful destruction of health facilities and essential civilian infrastructures also leads to slower forms of death—from epidemic infectious disease, untreated chronic disease, or starvation.[1]

The second insight was that health professionals are uniquely situated to collect the medical documentation that provides concrete evidence of human rights violations. PHR members are internists, nurses, pathologists, social workers, epidemiologists, toxicologists, burn specialists, orthopedic surgeons, psychiatrists, psychologists and forensic scientists, among others. These specialists contribute "many relevant medical tasks, ranging from physical examinations of individuals to forensic exhumations of mass graves. . . . These can often produce evidence of abuse more credible and less vulnerable to challenge than traditional methods of case reporting. Such medical documentation is far more difficult to refute than oral or written testimonies of abuse, no matter how well corroborated by witnesses."[2]

Because PHR organizes its responses to human rights violations based on these two premises, it has adopted three interdependent and complementary strategies in its work: direct documentation, advocacy, and education and training.

Direct Documentation

PHR's most visible and effective method of investigating human rights violations affecting health is the fact-finding mission. PHR brings both the prestige of the medical profession and high-level medical documentation and evaluation skills to its investigations. Health professionals have led or participated in virtually all of the seventy-five missions PHR has undertaken to more than forty-three countries in the past decade. Mission delegates not only document the health consequences of human rights violations, but examine the ethical obligations and responses of the local health community when faced with these violations.

PHR's first missions were highly visible investigations of specific incidents involving allegations of systematic torture, disappearances, extrajudicial killings, and political imprisonment. Typical of its early missions were interventions on behalf of a Malaysian medical colleague imprisoned without charge or trial, of detained leaders of the Chilean Medical Association, and of the suspicious death in custody of a political prisoner in Czechoslovakia.

As PHR gained experience and began to receive requests for help from other countries, it started investigating the dire health consequences of the systematic use of indiscriminate weapons of mass destruction on civilian populations. In response to reports of the South Korean government's excessive use of tear gas to quell demonstrations, PHR sent a delegation to study the chemicals' health effects. Subsequent PHR missions investigated the reported use of toxic chemicals as a method of crowd control in Soviet Georgia, and the Iraqi government's use of poison gas against its Kurdish population. PHR's systematic epidemiological studies of the medical consequences of land mines in Cambodia and northern Somalia were the first of their kind.

In the late 1980s with the waning of the cold war, regional and ethnic conflicts erupted that deprived whole populations of basic human rights and means of survival. PHR attempted to respond selectively to these massive humanitarian emergencies. For example, following the complete collapse of Somalia with the fall of Siad Barre, PHR and Africa Watch visited hospitals and spoke with international relief staff in Mogadishu in February 1992. The delegation documented substantially larger civilian casualties than media reports had suggested at the time, and warned the international community of an approaching famine of unprecedented proportion. PHR also conducted epidemiological studies on the effects of war, conflict and forced relocation on civilian populations in Iraqi and Turkish Kurdistan, and in Panama. Accompanying many of these large-scale attacks on civilians were assaults on medical personnel, interruption of medical care to civilians and other violations of medical neutrality. PHR found that armed groups were purposely disrupting the ability of health professionals to carry out their tasks. It became apparent that procedures for the protection of medical neutrality in all conflicts were inadequately defined by international codes, and not protected on the ground.

Many of PHR's missions in recent years have investigated acts of genocide and extrajudicial executions. PHR forensic experts have introduced medico-legal evidence from their investigations into court cases in Honduras, Brazil, Israel, Guatemala and the former Yugoslavia. They have also worked with the families of victims to lay to rest their uncertainties about the fates of their loved ones, as well as to set the historical record straight.

PHR frequently receives requests for assistance from local human rights or medical organizations, as well as governments and intergovernmental organizations. With the Salvadoran-based Association in Search of Disappeared Children, PHR is using genetic testing to assist their efforts to prove family relationships in order to reunite children kidnapped from their parents during the military assaults on civilians in the early 1980s. Today, PHR is under contract with the International Criminal Tribunal for the former Yugoslavia and the International Tribunal for Rwanda to provide technical assistance in the investigation of extrajudicial executions and other massive human rights violations in those regions.

Fact-finding missions are powerful mechanisms for exposing violations and alerting governments and health professionals to their destructive health impacts. Original data collected on missions, including medical documentation of physical and psychological trauma, supplemented by firsthand testimonies collected by PHR and other groups, are powerful evidence to convince policy-makers, the health professional community, the media, and the public about often unreported or clandestine abuses.

Advocacy

PHR's documentation efforts are only as successful as the use that is made of the data. With the help of its board, staff, and members, PHR has developed a variety of techniques to advocate for the protection of human rights.

PHR's primary method of disseminating the findings of a mission is through published reports or articles in peer-reviewed scientific journals. In the past five years, conclusions and recommendations from more than twelve PHR-sponsored missions have appeared in medical journals. Dozens of print and radio journalists in the United States and overseas have done stories based on PHR press releases or position statements. Substantive pressure is also brought to bear through meetings of PHR mission delegates with foreign government officials and embassy staff, and within the United States in meetings with officials at the State Department, members of Congress and representatives of the administration. Because offending governments do not always welcome PHR's findings, sustained attention through ongoing dialogue with government officials, local human rights and medical organizations, and the media is often necessary to press for resolution of human rights problems.

Letter-writing, long a tactic of international and national human rights organizations, remains a standard method of response to many reports of human rights violations. The organization and its members regularly send letters to government leaders on behalf of individual health professionals whose human rights have been violated or political prisoners who need immediate medical attention.

While sometimes effective, letter-writing strategies do not always yield significant results and may not be fulfilling to health professionals who want to make use of their medical skills to protect human rights. Many human rights organizations are reevaluating their use of letter-writing campaigns and are designing new tactics to exert pressure on governments to change behaviors that cause or condone human rights violations.

PHR has found that coordinated efforts from the health care community are a vital means of exerting pressure for change. Collective appeals from prominent health organizations, medical schools, hospitals, and individual health care providers will often force policy-makers in the targeted country to take notice. For example, widespread and prolonged pressure from the health and scientific communities in the United States and Europe certainly helped to secure the release of prominent Soviet dissident and psychiatrist Anatoly Koryagin in 1987. Certain issues, such as the worldwide problem of land mines, require the mobilization of the medical community and collaboration with human rights, legal, and other professional organizations operating as nongovernmental or governmental entities, as well as inter-governmental organizations.

PHR's role in introducing a medical focus to the international campaign against the production, sale, use and export of land mines is a good example of such cooperation. The international campaign estimates that a hundred million land mines lie unexploded in at least sixty-two countries, with some five hundred injuries or deaths from land mines occurring each week.[3] Through investigative missions to Cambodia, Mozambique and Somalia, where medical teams examined hospital records and interviewed communities affected by land mines, PHR was among the first organizations to document and publicize the devastating health effects of mines on civilian populations and on the health care systems of countries recovering from war and displacement. PHR has hosted symposia, press conferences and briefings for governments officials, and has encouraged groups (such as the American College of Physicians, the American Nurses Association, the American Fracture Association, and the American Public Health Association) to join the international campaign to ban land mines.[4] With more than four hundred participating organizations, including hundreds of human rights, humanitarian, arms control, professional, civic, and religious organizations around the world, the campaign is mounting a concerted effort to convince government experts reviewing the Conventional Weapons Convention to adopt a total ban on land mines, just as chemical weapons were banned in the past.

Education and Training

PHR's membership is a fraction of the health professional population in the United States. While the mission of PHR may be immediately attractive to only a few health professionals, the organization also realizes that the human rights message needs to reach many more health care providers in the United States. Today's challenge is to make international human rights relevant and obvious to the American health professional.

One method is to provide opportunities for clinicians to use their medical skills to help victims of human rights violations in their own country. For example, thousands of people attempt to emigrate to or receive asylum in the United States every year, having fled war, civil conflict, torture or persecution in their native countries. In response, PHR has established a network of 260 volunteer physicians and psychologists who conduct medical evaluations of asylum seekers in the United States. Network volunteers receive orientation materials on evaluating evidence of physical or psychological trauma, preparing written reports and testifying before officials of the Immigration and Naturalization Service. In 1995 PHR's asylum network evaluated more than a hundred asylum seekers from thirty-six countries—a fourfold increase from 1994. Of cases completed over the last five years of the program, more than 90 percent of applicants evaluated by PHR members have been granted asylum.

LESSONS LEARNED

Early PHR missions were often single investigations into a critical situation in a country, as the organization searched for a balanced response to worldwide reports of oppression. In recent years, PHR has made long-term commitments to work intensively with local health and human rights groups in several countries, including Turkey, Cambodia, the former Yugoslavia, Israel and the Occupied Territories.

PHR has learned in its work that the most effective investigations are coordinated with local groups, provided that such groups exist. Together, the visiting delegation and local groups can plan strategies for exposing and ending violations in ways that are most productive and culturally sensitive. Collaborative planning and publicity about human rights violations also strengthen the international human rights movement, and avoid enhancing one organization's reputation at the expense of another's.[5] In addition, visits from foreign delegations can lend support and prestige to local organizations, which are often under suspicion or attack by their own governments. Due respect must be given to the political constraints under which local organizations operate.

It follows that people who are sent on missions should have a solid understanding of international human rights and humanitarian law and be prepared for adverse circumstances. They need to be politically astute, quick-thinking, sensitive to cultural and legal differences, resilient in the face of physical and psychological obstacles and able to gather information with minimal retraumatization of the population they are trying to assist. Solid premission preparation and postmission debriefings are now a priority at PHR (and at many other organizations), particularly for individuals sent to volatile situations or those who are new at human rights fact-finding.

Human rights as a theoretical issue involving laws or codes of ethics has little appeal for many health professionals. But with exposure to a real situation, especially one involving their peers, human rights becomes a reality for health professionals. For instance, many health professionals around the world were inspired to speak out in support of a medical colleague in South Africa who was being pressured by her medical superiors under the apartheid government not to report torture-related injuries in a prison population.[6] Those who participate in human rights missions, who volunteer for the asylum program or who have met with government leaders for PHR on human rights issues are excellent advocates for international human rights because of these experiences.

As PHR increases its membership, it is challenged to put to good use all of the individuals who volunteer to help. A recent survey of PHR's 5,500 members revealed that of those who responded, primarily health professionals, 79 percent expressed interest in participating on fact-finding missions. Forty-four percent volunteered to use their medical skills to care for victims of humanitarian or human rights violations by participating in PHR's program to provide medical evaluations to asylum applicants.

Because of timing, money matters, and the language and professional skills needed, PHR has not yet been able to meet the needs of all its volunteer members. As a first step, it hopes to create a critical mass of health professionals who are well informed about international human rights. Through its educational events, PHR trains health professionals on the application of their skills to the documentation and promotion of human rights. Armed with such knowledge, PHR next expects health professionals to identify for themselves areas of research, advocacy, public policy, and medical education where the health and human rights intersections deserve greater attention from the medical community (and also need little PHR staff support).

FUTURE PLANS

PHR's work has generally been reactive to reports of human rights violations. Such work is frequently frustrating. New crises arise each week, and one is daunted in the face of so much human-made catastrophe. PHR and many other human rights organizations are searching for ways to protect human rights and not merely report on violations and their consequences. PHR missions to Somalia in 1992 and to Burundi in 1994 warned the international community of impending violence and of the desperate need for immediate international humanitarian assistance for the civilian populations. But the crises were not averted.

International and national courts of inquiry or investigation, which are also able to try those accused of crimes of war, crimes against humanity, and massive human rights abuses, can have a preventive effect. Truth commissions, tribunals, international courts, and other legal and quasi-legal proceedings not only publicly air and recognize past crimes but work toward ensuring that criminal actions not go unpunished. PHR contributes to these processes by providing medical and scientific documentation on specific and often large-scale human rights violations.

Education about human rights has been adopted as a prevention strategy by PHR and many other human rights groups. Health professionals knowledgeable about human rights can provide better care to patients who have suffered from traumatic physical and psychological persecution due to political violence. They are also best suited to move forward the dialogue concerning the scope of a health professional's obligations in the face of human rights violations.[7] Health professionals need to know when to report abuses, to whom they should report them, how to stop them, and how to balance that obligation with the personal risks they may assume for reporting abuses.

Human rights should be incorporated into the medical and nursing education of future health professionals. Courses taught at the public health and medical schools of the University of California-Berkeley and Harvard University can serve as models for educators interested in human rights education for health care providers.[8] Measures to evaluate the effectiveness and usefulness of human rights education for the health professional still need to be developed and systematically reviewed.

The staff and directors of PHR acknowledge that human rights is best approached from a holistic point of view—with full realization of the interplay of economic, social, cultural, civil, and political rights in promoting good health and in respecting the dignity and well-being of the individual. Nevertheless, PHR's board has voted repeatedly to limit the projects that the organization undertakes and to move slowly in introducing new issues that will expand its mandate into areas related to social, economic, and cultural rights. However, PHR joined John Snow, Inc., in a 1995 mission to examine the environmental and health effects of industrial pollution from a government-owned petrochemical plant in the Lake Maracaibo region of Venezuela. Based on the mission's findings, a Venezuelan court ruled that residents were entitled to immediate relocation to housing away from contaminants and to medical exams and treatment—all at the expense of the plant.

PHR has made a conscious effort to expose health and human rights problems not only overseas but also in the United States. It has examined abusive restraint practices in a Syracuse, New York, prison, is currently researching the health care given to unaccompanied minors held in detention facilities of the Immigration and Naturalization Service and has repeatedly spoken out against physician participation in state-sponsored executions as a violation of medical ethics. The PHR board and staff will continue to balance PHR's overseas activities with its work in the United States.

Today, many organizations—and the United Nations itself—rely on the expert opinions of those who can provide physical evidence of human rights abuses to corroborate witness testimony. The factual evidence these organizations offer can provide incontrovertible proof that human rights violations have taken place and make it impossible for governments to deny them. Through this documentation, the objectives of many human rights organizations, including PHR, are to hold violators accountable, promote the rule of law, seek justice and relief for victims of abuse, pressure the perpetrators to change their behavior and urge other governments and/or the international community to respond effectively to stop human rights abuses. Health professionals constitute a powerful international community that can help achieve the goals of the UN Charter, to affirm "fundamental human rights [and] the dignity and worth of the human person."[9]

SELECTED ACTIVITIES OF PHYSICIANS FOR HUMAN RIGHTS 1994–1996
Investigations and Research

Cambodia (1994)

PHR recommended specific procedures to protect prisoners from abuses in Cambodian prisons and to improve sanitary conditions and access to health care. In response, Cambodian authorities moved inmates from an over-crowded prison.

El Salvador (1995–1996)

PHR worked to locate children abducted by military personnel during counterinsurgency operations in El Salvador in the early 1980s. Through genetic family tracing and training of local health professionals in blood-collection protocols for DNA testing, PHR helped to establish the family identity of these children.

Israel (1995)

PHR participated in the autopsy of a Palestinian prisoner who died in 1995 shortly after his arrest by Israeli security forces, helping to establish that the man had died because he was shaken violently while in custody. PHR submitted an opinion to the Israeli High Court of Justice, bringing further attention to Israel's controversial policy of allowing security forces to use "moderate physical pressure" on detainees.

Mozambique (1994)

PHR conducted an epidemiological study of land mine injuries in Mozambique in March 1994, later published in *The Lancet*.

Rwanda (1995–1996)

PHR provided forensic expertise to the International War Crimes Tribunal in Rwanda in late 1995 and early 1996, and conducted the largest excavation of a mass grave in history.

Turkey (1994–1995)

PHR sent several missions to investigate and report on the role of health professionals called on to care for patients who have been victims of state-sanctioned torture. It is also examining violations of medical neutrality and the health consequences of the conflict in southeast Turkey.

Venezuela (1994–1995)

PHR joined with other groups on a mission to investigate allegations that a state-owned petrochemical company had contaminated the town's environment and nearby water supply. Team members presented their findings in a civil case brought before the Venezuelan courts.

Former Yugoslavia (1995)

Forensic evidence collected and documented by a PHR international team at a mass grave found in Vukovar was critical to securing indictments against three senior Yugoslav People's Army officers on charges of war crimes and crimes against humanity in connection with the alleged killings of more than two hundred civilians in 1991.

Medical Assistance

Asylum Network (ongoing since early 1990s)

In the United States, volunteers conducted physical or psychological evaluations of a hundred asylum seekers from thirty-six countries. In the last five years, 90 percent of the applicants evaluated have been granted asylum.

Legislative Action

Asylum (1995–1996)

PHR joined a broad-based coalition effort to preserve the right to seek asylum in the United States. PHR opposed proposed restrictions in immigration legislation that would drastically limit the time to apply for asylum, effectively excluding survivors of torture.

International Campaign to Ban Land Mines (1995)

PHR members wrote to their congressional representatives urging them to support U.S. legislation aimed at ending the U.S. military's use of land mines. By year's end, that legislation passed both the House and Senate, and President Clinton signed the bill in 1996.

Campaign Against Medical Participation in Capital Punishment in the United States (1994)

PHR was party to a legal complaint filed in the state of Illinois seeking disclosure of the identities of physicians who had participated in an Illinois execution, and an injunction against such involvement. The suit became legally moot.

Education and Training

Course at the University of California, Berkeley (1995–1996)

The PHR Western regional director taught graduate-level courses on health and human rights.

Course on Medical Documentation of Human Rights Abuses (May 1995)

More than sixty health professionals attended a one-day continuing medical education course entitled "Human Rights and the Health Professional: Medical Documentation of Human Rights Abuses and Political Asylum" cosponsored by PHR, the Columbia University College of Physicians and Surgeons, and the New York Academy of Sciences.

Human Rights and Humanitarian Assistance (February 1995)

PHR organized a daylong conference on human rights and humanitarian assistance at Tufts University, one of the first interagency discussions of the links and tensions between the humanitarian and human rights responses to ethnic cleansing and genocide.

Turkey (January 1995)

More than one hundred and fifty Turkish doctors participated in a two-day conference entitled "Human Rights and Physician Responsibility," sponsored by PHR, the Turkish Medical Association, and the Human Rights Foundation of Turkey.

Case Advocacy

Alerts (1995)

PHR issued six Medical Action Alerts (letter-writing actions for PHR members) for cases in Ethiopia, Vietnam, and Nigeria and to support U.S. action to ban land mines, passage of the Torture Victims Relief Act and intervention to stop the killing in Bosnia.

Individual Case Advocacy Letters (1995)

PHR researched dozens of cases of health professionals and others who experienced violations of their human rights or were in need of medical care, and sent letters to government officials in twenty-six countries on their behalf.

REFERENCES

1. H. J. Geiger and R. M. Cook-Deegan. "The Role of Physicians in Conflicts and Humanitarian Crises: Case Studies from the Field Missions of Physicians for Human Rights, 1988–1993." *Journal of the American Medical Association* 270 (1993): 616–620.
2. Ibid.
3. "International Campaign to Ban Landmines," brochure (Boston: PHR, 1995).
4. To date, twenty-two countries have called for a comprehensive ban on mines (the United States has not), and forty-three countries have issued moratoria or other restrictions on the export of land mines. Belgium and Norway have enacted a total ban, while France has banned production and trade of land mines.
5. The authors thank Virginia Sherry, Human Rights Watch/Middle East, for her insights on these issues.
6. For more information on this doctor, Wendy Orr, see M. Rayner. *Turning a Blind Eye: Medical Accountability and the Prevention of Torture in South Africa*. (Washington, D.C.: American Association for the Advancement of Science, 1987).
7. Conversation with Robert Cook-Deegan, January 1996.
8. See J. Brenner. "Human Rights Education in Public Health Graduate Schools: 1996 Survey." *Health and Human Rights* 2 (1996): 129–139.
9. See Preamble, *Universal Declaration of Human Rights*, adopted and proclaimed by UN General Assembly Resolution 217A (December 10, 1948).

Medical Humanitarianism and Human Rights: Reflections on Doctors Without Borders and Doctors of the World

28.

Renée Fox

I have been doing exploratory research on Doctors Without Borders (Médecins Sans Frontières), and Doctors of the World (Médecins du Monde), two historically connected international organizations of French origin that, since the 1970s, have played a generative role in linking medical humanitarian and human rights action, within the larger framework of what has been termed a *"sans frontièrisme"* movement.[1] I am preparing for what I hope will be a firsthand study of the precepts and values on which these associations and their projects are founded; their leaders, members, and supporters; the missions they undertake; the social systems and models of operation they have developed; and the short- and long-term impact of their ventures.

But my interest lies as much in what Doctors Without Borders and Doctors of the World represent as in what they concretely do—in the societal, cultural, civilizational, and global developments of our profoundly changed and changing, late-twentieth-century world from which such organizations emanate, and to which they constitute a particular kind of structured response. In the address that he delivered on July 4 1994, when he received the Philadelphia Liberty Medal at Independence Hall, Václav Havel, president of the Czech Republic, described the "transitional," "postmodern world" we now inhabit as one in which "everything is possible and nothing is certain. This state of affairs has its social and political consequences," he continued:

> The planetary civilization to which we all belong confronts us with global challenges. We stand helpless before them because our civilization has essentially globalized only the surface of our lives. But our inner self continues to have a life of its own. And the fewer answers the era of rational knowledge provides

to the basic questions of human being, the more deeply it would seem that people, behind its back as it were, cling to the ancient certainties of the tribe.

Because of this, individual cultures, increasingly lumped together by contemporary civilization, are realizing with new urgency their own inner autonomy and the inner differences of others. Cultural conflicts are increasing and are more dangerous today than at any time in history. Politicians are rightly worried by the problem of finding the key to insure the survival of a civilization that is global and multicultural. . . .

These questions have been highlighted with particular urgency by the most important political events in the second half of the 20th century: the collapse of colonial hegemony and the fall of Communism.

"The central political task of the final years of this century," Havel declared, "is the creation of a new model of coexistence among the various cultures, peoples, races and religious spheres, within a single interconnected civilization." It involves "the awareness" that "we are rooted in the Earth and, at the same time, the cosmos"—an awareness that "endows us with the capacity for self-transcendence."[2]

This chapter focuses on the way that Doctors Without Borders and Doctors of the World are approaching these *fin-de-siècle* questions and challenges of our individual and collective being, how they are grappling with them, and what kinds of issues and dilemmas they are encountering in doing so. For the most part, I will deal with the common origins and attributes of the two organizations, deferring discussions of their dissimilarities to future research and analysis.

HISTORICAL ROOTS OF DOCTORS WITHOUT BORDERS AND DOCTORS OF THE WORLD

According to its historically grounded myth of origin, Médecins Sans Frontières (Doctors Without Borders) was founded in 1971 by a small group of French physicians, headed by Bernard Kouchner, upon their return from Biafra. In the context of the civil war in Nigeria, under the joint aegis of the French and the International Red Cross, these young physicians had served as volunteers in Biafra doing medical relief work among the Ibo. Their presence in Biafra and subsequent creation of Doctors Without Borders were not only shaped by their personal biographies and motivation, but also by the effects that certain post–World War II events and currents of thought in France had upon the generation of French intellectuals to which they belonged. Primary among these influences were:

- The continuing aftermath of the German occupation of France during World War II, the Vichy régime, and the French Resistance.
- The growing realization of the magnitude and meaning of the crimes against humanity that the Nazi concentration camps and the Holocaust entailed.
- The grip of Soviet Communism on the utopian imagination of the French intelligentsia from the liberation of France in 1994 until the watershed

speech made by Khrushchev in 1956 denouncing Stalin, and the totalitarian terror and failure of Stalinism.

- The subsequent shift in attention of French intellectuals from Communism and Europe to issues of decolonization in Third World countries. What historian Tony Judt calls this *tiers-mondisime*³ of the 1960s was precipitated by the widespread occurrence of anticolonialist movements in Africa, Asia, and Latin America—especially by the Algerian war for independence, and the questions about France's colonial policy, presence, and military role in North Africa that it raised.

- The development of a post-Stalinist, "New Left" movement in France in the late 1950s, led by middle-class students, with its concepts of total revolution and liberation, and its heroization of African, Latin American, and Asian political figures as the incarnations of true revolutionaries. The movement reached its climax with the eruption of the May 1968 "Student Revolution" in French universities.⁴ (Bernard Kouchner and some of his friends were involved in this movement and these events through their membership in the Union des étudiants communistes. They later expressed discontent with what they described as the "armchair warriors" nature of the meetings and activities in which it engaged them.)

- Médecins du Monde (Doctors of the World), founded in 1980, was the product of a split within Médecins Sans Frontières between members of its founding and its second generations. The split took place in 1979, in connection with the so-called Vietnamese boat people, trying to flee their embattled country by ship, who were drowning and dying by the thousands in the South China Sea. Bernard Kouchner decided that Médecins Sans Frontières should invest its resources and reputation in chartering a boat *(L'île de Lumière)* to rescue some of these shipwrecked refugees, joining their efforts with a number of France's most prominent intellectuals, and mobilizing the media to support and publicly dramatize their action.

Although he was backed by most of his peers, younger members of Doctors Without Borders took the position that the predicament of the "boat people" surpassed the competence and capacities of a medical humanitarian organization like theirs. Nor were they happy with what they regarded as the undemocratic and publicity-seeking style in which Kouchner had proceeded. A vote was taken and the majority rejected the "boat for Vietnam" project. According to Kouchner he was "expelled" and "betrayed" by the organization of which he was a founder-leader; according to the "anti-boat" members who remained within the organization, he staged a coup d'état. Whatever the interpretation, as a consequence of this episode, Kouchner, along with the majority of his "elders of Biafra" companions, left Doctors Without Borders, and established Doctors of the World. The schism between them notwithstanding, the two organizations continue to share the same goals.

Since their founding in 1971 and 1980 respectively, Doctors Without Borders and Doctors of the World have developed in parallel ways to become international organizations with branches in a number of countries and missions on every continent. Doctors Without Borders, the larger of the two, now the best known and most generously supported voluntary association in France, has sections in Belgium, Holland, Luxembourg, Spain, Switzerland, and the United States. According to its own publications, as of February 1, 1994, it was conducting projects in some seventy countries. Doctors of the World presently has affiliates in Greece, Hungary, Poland, Spain, Sweden, Switzerland, and the United States, with projects in at least forty countries. Although Doctors Without Borders has established a permanent international secretariat to coordinate the actions of its European sections, Paris, France, continues to be the locale of its central headquarters—and in a real sense, its summit—which is true for Doctors of the World as well.

Thus, the genesis of both Doctors Without Borders and Doctors of the World is rooted in contemporary French history, society, and intellectual culture. From the outset, the universalistic vision of the human condition and of "the rights of man" on which they were based was conceived of as inherent to French civilization, and as a "message (and initiative) of France."[5] Yet the scope of these organizations has become international, their outreach worldwide; and the significance of the events that brought them into being— World War II, the Holocaust, the crises of colonialism and decolonization, the rise and fall of Communism, and the increasingly tribal nature of the cultural strife occurring within (rather than between) nations—transcends any particularistic societal, political, or cultural claim. In this respect, on a microscale, Doctors Without Borders and Doctors of the World embody the tension-ridden duality that Václav Havel identified as the key problem facing our postmodern world: how to reconcile and integrate "the global and multi-cultural . . . within a single interconnected civilization."[6]

PRINCIPLES AND VALUE-COMMITMENTS UNDERLYING THE ACTION OF DOCTORS WITHOUT BORDERS AND DOCTORS OF THE WORLD

Doctors Without Borders and Doctors of the World are both premised on the conviction that the provision of medical care, service, and relief is a humane form of moral action, with the capacity to bind up wounds that are more than physical, to "heal the body politic" as well as the human body,[7] and to further reconciliation and peace, even between enemies locked in combat. Their vision of medicine is transcendentally universalistic as well as militantly pacific. Illness and injury "do not respect borders," they aver, nor should medical care. Rather, it should be rendered to all who need it, regardless of their social backgrounds, their life histories, or "the values they defend or attack."[8]

The core concept on which the medical and the human rights action of Doctors Without Borders and Doctors of the World is premised was first articulated by Bernard Kouchner as *"le droit d'ingérence"*—the right to interfere—which, over time, has evolved into what is frequently expressed as *"le devoir d'ingérence,"* the duty to interfere. This notion of justified and, beyond that, mandatory interference is anchored in the belief that there is an "ardent obligation to act"[9] to alleviate the suffering of people urgently in need of medical care and succor, wherever on the face of the earth that suffering exists, particularly when it is a consequence of violence, torture, persecution, warfare, disenfranchisement, oppression, abandonment, exile or exodus. Such interference entails what the French term *engagement*—an involvement and commitment (in the words of Jean-Christophe Rufin, a vice president of Doctors Without Borders/France) that are the antitheses of "withdrawing from reality, [or] of dedicating one's self to a distant future." It calls for "plunging into the arena . . . dashing headlong into the midst of wars . . . being in the fray . . . in order to reach the victims . . . breaking whatever rules are used against [them and] humankind," and making enough "noise" in the process to be "heard."[10] A director of Doctors of the World/France whom I interviewed expressed this notion of interference more laconically: "Act always! Speak always!" he declared, coining a double aphorism for what he characterized as "real, direct, immediate, and fervid action" (*"action vécue"*).

The kind of action espoused by Doctors Without Borders and Doctors of the World, especially in early phases of their development, calls for rapid, first-hand, emergency- and rescue-oriented immersion in the field where a human catastrophe is taking place. It is passionately committed, heroically aggressive, warriorlike medical action that is also masculine and doctor-centered in its ethos and self-presentation (even though many of the organizations' largely volunteer participants are women, and female nurses seem to play as large a role as physicians in the front-line care undertaken and delivered). As originally conceived, the principal type of disaster to which this medical humanitarian action was geared to respond were the "multitude of jungle conflicts, civil wars, [and] ethnic rebellions" pervading the Third World.[1]

The form and spirit of the action in which Doctors Without Borders and Doctors of the World mobilized themselves to engage was intended to break through, and stand above what they critically view as the constraints, compromises, and vested interests of the "classical humanitarian aid" dispensed by more traditional, bureaucratized, and partisan voluntary agencies and "charities"—most notably, by the Red Cross, on one hand, and by religious missionary groups, on the other. In fact, one of Doctors Without Borders and Doctors of the World's most fundamental principles of action—their resolve to bear public witness to the violations of human rights and dignity that they encounter in the field—grew directly out of their reaction to the fact that the International Committee of the Red Cross, which was allowed by Nazi Germany to deliver food and medicine to people in concentration camps during World War II, did not speak out against the atrocities taking place in those camps. Rather, the Red Cross maintained an established policy of silence to protect what they defined as their neutrality and their permission to continue doing relief work in that holocaust setting. The conception of action under which Doctors Without Borders and Doctors of the World operate vehemently rejects such a rule of silence and the accommodation that it represents. They are not only committed to rupturing that silence, but also to informing a vast, world-scale public about the human rights abuses that they encounter in the milieux they enter, and to evoking public indignation about them, making sophisticated use of the mass media to do so.

While it is not neutrality that Doctors Without Borders and Doctors of the World profess, what might be called their "nonideological ideology" disavows any political or religious identification or affiliation. Furthermore, in the name of their nonsectarian "without borders," humanitarian commitment, they do more than assert their independence of political and governmental bodies. They also challenge what they refer to as the "sacred principle" of the sovereignty of the state: the idea that a nation should be free to determine its own destiny, integral to the emergence, development and the very definition of nation-states throughout the nineteenth and twentieth centuries, and to the phenomenon of nationalism. Doctors Without Borders and Doctors of the World share a global vision of a new world order governed by the principles of the Universal Declaration of Human Rights (set forth by the General Assembly of the United Nations on December 10, 1948), and by an international tribunal that is "above nation-states." While acknowledging the limitations and imperfections of the United Nations, they see it as the closest approximation to this kind of tribunal. But they are less inclined to recognize the degree to which the "rights of man" stated in the UN Charter are imprinted with Western culture.

Over time, the perspective, principles, and commitments of Doctors Without Borders and Doctors of the World have become progressively institutionalized, both within these organizations and on a much broader scale. "The right to interfere, in spite of frontiers and in spite of States, if suffering persons need aid" has been incorporated into several resolutions passed by the General Assembly of the United Nations. Invoking the vision of a "new humanitarian order," these resolutions legitimate the role of nongovernmental organizations such as Doctors Without Borders and Doctors of the World, along with nation-states, in providing *in situ* aid wherever situations of natural catastrophe or manmade emergency occur—including under circumstances of civil war. They emphasize the necessity of free access to the victims of these events, and they support the creation of "corridors of emergency" to enable aid to be transported directly to the scenes of such disasters.[12] In France, under the presidency of François Mitterand, the right and duty to interfere across borders was woven into what the national government calls its "humanitarianism of the State" policies, and the functions of the Secretariat for Humanitarian Health that it established.* Those two organizations' suprafrontiers, global outlook and concept of justified humanitarian intervention have also been approvingly sanctioned by religious and secular world leaders ranging from the President of the Czech Republic to the Pope and the Dalai Lama. The "without borders" concept is now so appreciated that a plethora of professional and voluntary associations have made it a part of their mission statements, and of their names. During the twenty-year period that their existence spans, Doctors Without Borders and Doctors of the World have grown in size, scale, range of activities, numbers of projects undertaken, theaters of operation, staff and volunteer personnel, budget and financial resources, matériel and logistical capacities, means of print and electronic communication, public saliency and support, and in the complexity of their organizations. Their expansion has also involved widening their original conception of action and engagement to include some less emergency-oriented, more long-term medical and public health projects, in modern as well as developing society settings, and in domestic as well as overseas locations.

In all these respects, as the sociologist Max Weber would have observed, they have moved beyond their early, small-scale, face-to-face, charismatic stage of development, and "succeeded in the world." Their internal and external institutional success has not only enhanced their work, however; it has also accentuated some of the problems and dilemmas that their committed action and advocacy entail.

THE ALLOCATION OF COMMITMENTS AND OF HUMAN AND MATERIAL RESOURCES

Even if Doctors Without Borders and Doctors of the World had strictly confined themselves to their foundational goals—providing medical humanitarian assistance, relief, and succor to the imperiled and suffering victims of natural and human catastrophes in developing countries, and giving public testimony to the misery and human rights violations witnessed in the field — they would have been overwhelmed by the escalating number and scale of the disasters taking place in the Third World: murderous civil wars in Afghanistan, Angola, Mozambique, El Salvador, and Nicaragua; clanic blood feuds and famine in Somalia; a war of all against all and life-threatening hunger in southern Sudan; starvation in Ethiopia; unending consequences of the "Killing Fields" in Cambodia, and of the abuse and torture of the Khmer Rouge and of the Pol Pot regime; civil strife between the army and Tamil rebels in Sri Lanka; peasant (Zapatista) rebellion and guerrilla warfare in Mexico's southern state of Chiapas; the forcible expulsion of all persons of BaLuba/South Kasa ethnic origins from the "Katangese" Shaba province of Zaire; and the intertribal massacre of Tutsi and Hutu in Burundi and in Rwanda, where the genocidal slaughter has resulted in the largest and worst humanitarian crisis in a generation—these are only some of the calamities that have erupted in Third World countries on nearly every continent of the globe. Most of them are caused by internal cultural conflicts, accompanied by massive violence (killing, wounding, and rape); the loss of basic personal security; a lack of food, safe water, fuel for heating and transport, medical supplies, and health services; the threatened or the actual outbreak and spread of epidemic disease (cholera, dysentery, malaria, typhoid fever, pneumonic and bubonic plague, and HIV/AIDS); the displacement, exodus and isolation of whole populations; and the relegation of refugees to huge incarceration camps. (According to the United Nations High Commissioner for Refugees, the number of refugees and "internally displaced" persons has reached the staggering level of 49 million, which means that one out of every 114 people in the world has been uprooted by war and famine).

"[T]he members of various tribal cults are at war with one another," Václav Havel has stated in his description of these pervasive conflicts.[13] How can organizations such as Doctors Without Borders and Doctors of the World respond to all these tragic happenings? Should they try? Or must they choose between them? And if so, on what grounds ought they make such a choice? "But how many times. . .," asked Joelle Tanguy, an executive director of Doctors Without Borders, her voice dying in her throat, when she was interviewed by journalists about the terrible events in Rwanda. What she meant, *New York Times* columnist Anna Quindlen explained, "is that the volunteer doctors have been ricocheting from crisis to crisis," from one "great disaster" to another.[14]

Nor are these disasters restricted to the Third World. The ethnic conflicts that have broken out in republics that were once part of the Soviet Union (Georgia, Tajikistan, Armenia, and Azerbaijan), and the civil war in former Yugoslavia, especially the ethnic, religious, and territorial combat between Serbs, Muslims, and Croats in Bosnia, with its atrocities of "ethnic cleansing," have dramatized the fact that such primordial conflicts not only can take place, but are doing so in European settings even in certain supposedly modern, industrialized countries. Historian Tony Judt writes:

> That Europeans might come to blows over such traditional matters as borders, nationality, or ethnic territorial claims seemed unthinkable; that they might do so in ways uncannily redolent of earlier conflicts hitherto assigned to history books would have seemed horrific and absurd five years ago. . . . [T]he events in Yugoslavia reveal . . . the extent to which Europe has been unable to escape its past. . . . We have not come to the end of intra-European wars, and it is now clear that there is little that a place called "Europe" can do about them.[15]

Doctors Without Borders and Doctors of the World have not only undertaken a number of medical humanitarian projects in former Yugoslavia, but also in other "intra-European" war situations, such as those in Albania and Romania. They have moved beyond their original Third World commitment, stretching their organizational, logistical, financial, material and human means to do so. The difficult allocation of scarce resources and questions confronting them are made all the more painful by the fact that in spite of their heroic emergency action, there seems to be no end to the crises with which they are attempting to deal. Rather, the conflicts keep coming and coming back.

DILEMMAS OF THE MILITARIZATION OF HUMANITARIAN ACTION AND OF SECURITY

One of the most serious moral dilemmas that Doctors Without Borders and Doctors of the World face in the field stems from the militarization of humanitarian action: the use of United Nations and national military forces to help with emergency medical care in devastated areas; move large quantities of supplies, materials and personnel to these locations; develop transportation and communication systems there; establish safe havens; and provide sufficient security in the midst of ongoing warfare, violence, and rampant disorder for relief activities to proceed. United Nations Resolution 688, passed by the Security Council on April 5, 1991, set into motion such a mission—"Operation Provide Comfort"—along the Turkey-Iraq border, following the Persian Gulf War. Coalition military forces air-dropped emergency supplies to the hundreds of thousands of ethnic Kurds who had fled northern Iraq after a failed revolt, were stranded in remote and freezing mountain passes between Iraq and Turkey and were besieged by the Iraqi army. "Provide Comfort" forces then created a safe haven, furnished ground-based security and logistical support for relief organizations, and gave direct medical assistance to the Kurds. In "Operation Restore Hope", military personnel from a number of countries were sent to Somalia in mid-December 1992, to support and create security for relief organizations already at work there in the midst of civil war, clanic strife, widespread famine, and the collapse of the indigenous medical and public health systems. More recently, during the summer of 1994, a contingent of French troops was deployed to Rwanda to create a safety zone insulated from the Hutu-Tutsi massacres, and a U.S. Pentagon airlift was organized to funnel relief supplies to the massive exodus of refugees from Rwanda to bordering communities in Zaire, to install modern airfield equipment in the area for this purpose, and to help set up portable water and sanitation facilities in the swarming refugee camps.

In the view of Doctors Without Borders and Doctors of the World, there is an inherent contradiction between such military interventions, on the one hand, and their mandate of political neutrality and "vocation of healing action," on the other. For not only are military forces directed by government policy, but especially in situations where armed conflict is involved, their presence and interests are likely to be perceived as more adversarial than humanitarian. Under these circumstances, military events can ensure that former president of Doctors Without Borders, Dr. Rony Brauman, has deemed the "humanitarian crime" of "killing under the banner of humanitarianism" can occur.[16] Such was the case during Operation Restore Hope in Somalia, where military actions were taken "that appeared to favor one local faction over another, [which] resulted in hostilities against relief workers and . . . [a number of] deaths."[17] When this occurred, Doctors Without Borders decided to leave Somalia, whereas Doctors of the World opted to stay in the field, affirming their continuing belief that "the specificity" of their role would protect them, and that the situation "precluded their departure" before their public health rehabilitation work, in collaboration with Somalians, had advanced to a further stage.[18]

Despite their apprehensiveness about the militarization of humanitarianism, and the different ways they have responded to the paradoxes and perils it entails, both Doctors Without Borders and Doctors of the World acknowledge that many of the catastrophes with which they are dealing are of such epic proportions that they cannot be handled solely by nongovernmental agencies, using traditional humanitarian means. "This is a humanitarian crime without any humanitarian solution," exclaimed Dr. Jacques de Milliano, the current president of Doctors Without Borders, in July 1994, in the midst of desperate efforts of volunteer medical workers from his organization to deal with severe cholera and dysentery epidemics that had erupted among the one million Rwandese refugees who had fled from the Hutu-Tutsi carnage in their country to the small border town of Goma in Zaïre. "There has to be a political solution" that goes hand in hand with the humanitarian dimensions, he said, adding his voice to those from other relief agencies who were calling for "a substantial United Nations force" to be sent to Rwanda to ensure protection for the largely Hutu refugees, terrified of the possibility of retaliatory persecution and slaughter by the Tutsi-dominated Rwandan Patriotic Front, which had declared a new government. Only if the refugees felt it was safe to return to Rwanda, representatives of the humanitarian organizations ministering to them urgently insisted, could the ravages of disease, malnutrition, thirst, and lack of sanitation in the overcrowded, filthy, death-ridden refugee camps be brought under control, and the sorghum crop, one of Rwanda's two main subsistence economy sources of food, be harvested in time to keep it from rotting in the fields and setting off still another cycle of starvation. Military contingents would be needed to help make that possible, relief workers contended.[19]

As the violence and physical danger surrounding the missions in which Doctors Without Borders and Doctors of the World are involved have grown greater, the question of the security of their volunteer workers, with or without the protection of military forces, has also become more acute and ethically complex. "How far will we dare to, must we, push humanitarian duty and personal sacrifice . . . ? Where is the boundary between courage and temerity, between the morality of extreme emergency and the reckless gesture?" What kind of balance should be struck between "presence," "security," and "efficacy"?[20] These issues were central themes in the presentations made at the Fifteenth General Assembly of Doctors Without Borders, held in Brussels on May 7 and 8, 1994. Although they were identified by the president and board of directors as major dilemmas, which should be discussed "between headquarters and the field . . . with serenity and realism," it was acknowledged that no policy consensus about these difficult problems had been reached:

> Certain [volunteers] have expressed weariness about not being able to fully accomplish their mission in the surrounding climate of insecurity [it was said]. When one cannot reach a hospital as in Kigali, when one must evacuate a

hospital which is bombed as in Gorazde, when one cannot get into the regions where famine and epidemics threaten, in Somalia, when one must establish contracts for transportation or reconstruction with corrupt local entrepreneurs under the threat of death, we are outraged by the narrowing of our mandate.[21]

But "we cannot become an army without arms," volunteers were cautioned. And so, it was recommended that in "the triple equation 'presence-security-efficacy,'" the "efficiency of the medical act" be given the highest priority, rather than "being present at any cost," including "the possible cost in human lives." This advice notwithstanding, volunteers were exhorted never to cease to be "indignant" and to continue to be "combatants against the inadmissible," as they and the organizations of which the are a part struggle to achieve a rightful balance between effective competence, on the one hand, and ardent action that is tenacious, on the other.[22]

DILEMMAS OF THE ROLE OF THE MASS MEDIA IN MEDICAL HUMANITARIAN ACTION

There is a certain analogy between the dilemmas of military involvement in humanitarian relief and those presented by the role of mass media and of high-tech communication in the work of Doctors Without Borders and Doctors of the World. For their overseas logistics, the transmission of information in and from the field, their human rights witnessing, their recruitment of volunteers, and their fund-raising, the two organizations are highly dependent on the extensive and sophisticated use of these means. It might even be said that conveying their experiences and their messages to an international public through the print and electronic media is a principle as well as an instrument of their action—one that could be conceptualized as "the duty to give testimony and to inform." They consider the "mediaization" of their missions to be an essential element in what they call their "new humanitarianism."

Nevertheless, the two organizations are cognizant of the moral conflicts and pitfalls that are also associated with their employement of the media. Above all, media coverage creates a kind of theatricalization of human disaster and tragedy that it creates—particularly through the way that omnipresent television cameras bring into our homes, "at once so immediate and distant," scenes of people dying, and starving, and engaging in acts of violence. One of the ironic consequences of seeing such disasters "writ large on our television screens," as journalist Anna Quindlen eloquently points out, is that it can dehumanize the victims and the spectators, rather than "enlarg[ing] . . . understanding of the essential tie of humanity" they share:

> Tragedy on a monumental, perhaps historic scale, as in Rwanda, lends itself
> . . . to depersonalization. So does the television coverage, which is at once so
> immediate and so distant. Who ever imagined that we would be able to watch

as the light of life passed from the eyes of a stranger thousands of miles away? Who ever imagined that we would be as close to a newly minted orphan, tears a swath of patent leather on his dusty face, as to our own children? Who knew we would become so accustomed to the image of corpses in a mass grave that it would lose not only the power to shock, but the power to move?[23]

"Numbing" humanity in the name of humanitarianism is not the only danger that Doctors Without Borders' and Doctors of the World's use of the media carries with it. Because of their continuous, professionalized relationship to the media, and their own newsworthiness, they have the ability to use these means in influential, self-serving, as well as disinterested ways— to grandstand, for example, to propagandize, to compete with other relief agencies for funds, recognition, and prestige, or to stage-manage their activities for media coverage. There have been incidents of this sort in the history of both organizations, and self-searching debate about them.

Irrespective of the moral questions and policy issues it may raise for them, however, "mediatization," like militarization, is indispensable to their operation, and to the accomplishment of their humanitarian action and goals.

ISSUES CONCERNING THE BACKGROUNDS, MOTIVATIONS, AND TRAINING OF THE VOLUNTEERS

What about the persons who are front-line participants in this action—the individuals who undertake volunteer stints under Doctors Without Borders and Doctors of the World? Who are they? And how well prepared are they, medically and technically, psychologically and culturally, for their assignments? Perhaps there is no adequate way to ready persons for what they will see, feel, and be asked to do in situations as physically threatening and emotionally devastating as Rwanda, Somalia, and Bosnia. But what kind of training do these organizations try to give to the relatively young and professionally inexperienced women and men who make up a large portion of their volunteer cohorts?

At this stage of my research, I have the impression that most of the volunteers' learning takes place on the job after, rather than before, they enter the field, buttressed by reliance on more experienced staff who have gone on previous missions and who are accustomed to operating within the organizations' logistical framework of action. The unforeseeable nature of the emergency situations that Doctors Without Borders and Doctors of the World enter, their geographical dispersion, the rapidly shifting array of societies and sites that they involve, the immediate response they require, and their relatively short duration—all make it difficult to give volunteers advance instruction about the sorts of injuries, diseases, and psychic distress they are likely to encounter, or to acquaint them with the language, history, and culture of the areas into which they are catapulted. However, even in connection with the less crisis-oriented, more long-term development projects that Doctors Without Borders and Doctors of the World undertake to improve or rebuild health services, not much organized attention seems to be directed toward equipping volunteers with medical and cultural knowledge that might help them to work effectively and cooperatively in the disadvantaged, impoverished, or decimated foreign milieux in which these projects are traditionally located.

The organizations seem to rely heavily on what they assume to be the idealism of most of their volunteers, their youthful adventuresomeness, courage, and resiliency, their desire to use their medical and technical skills productively, and on the power of those qualities to help the volunteers cope with the unknown, the danger, and the suffering they will encounter in the field.[24] Although on the application forms they fill out, and in the intake interviews they undergo, volunteers supply information about their social backgrounds and life histories, neither Doctors Without Borders nor Doctors of the World appears to make systematic use of this information to characterize their volunteer pool, or to screen, assign, or teach them. If anything, there is a tendency to play down the volunteers' social and cultural attributes, along with those of the persons whom they go on mission to aid. The universalistic value systems of the two organizations, with their emphasis on a transcendent conception of human worth, and on the oneness of the human condition, contribute to their ideological reluctance to attach undue importance to particular social and cultural factors. One of the consequences of this outlook has been their structured disinclination to seriously consider and systematically analyze the relevance of knowledge about the "otherness" of others or, to use Havel's language, about "what we ourselves are not," and "what seems distant to us in time and space."[25] For example, how might understanding of the traditional clan structure and the blood feud in Somalia, or a historical perspective on tribal and ethnic relations between Hutu and Tutsi in Rwanda and Burundi, or between Serbs, Croats, Muslims and Albanians in the former Yugoslavia be brought to bear upon the humanitarian action of Doctors Without Borders and Doctors of the World in those countries? How pertinent is such knowledge, in what concrete ways? Could it be mobilized and conveyed to volunteers in emergency situations quickly enough and with sufficient detail and depth to be useful to them, or is it only applicable to longer-term development projects—if at all? At this point in my exploratory research, I do not have the impression that such questions are high on the agendas of Doctors Without Borders and Doctors of the World.

OVERSEAS VERSUS DOMESTIC MISSIONS

Not only has the outreach of Doctors Without Borders and Doctors of the World expanded to include projects of greater duration as well as emergency and rescue interventions, in both developed and developing countries; their national branches have also increasingly turned their attention to situations of socio-medical deprivation in their own countries. In turn, this has added to the complexity of issues concerning how best to allocate human and material resources that the two organizations face.

In the late 1980s, as the repercussions of severe economic recession and of structural unemployment deepened and spread in Western Europe, Doctors of the World in France, for example, and Doctors Without Borders in France and Belgium organized domestic projects to help persons to whom they referred as "those excluded from the system of social security" in their countries, or simply as *les exclus*. These are young men, women, children, and entire families of French, Belgian, and foreign immigrant origins, who are poor, hungry, homeless, abandoned, vulnerable to illness, and without access to work, or to decent medical care. "Must we accept, in this rich country which is France, in the homeland of the rights of man and of the citizen, the ineluctable spiral of poverty which results in what more and more resembles professional and social apartheid?" Dr. Bernard Granjon, president of Doctors of the World/France, has asked rhetorically. He answered his own question with an affirmation about the role that humanitarian associations like his own are now ready to play in aiding the *exclus*.[26] "The duty to assist all human beings, whatever their race, religion or the country in which they live, remains fundamental," affirms a Doctors Without Borders/Belgium fund-raising brochure. "Belgium is not an exception," it continues. "While thousands of kilometers from us, men, women and children suffer from not being helped, one also meets them, alas, in our own cities, on the streets or even on our doorstep. . . . Whether it concerns Belgium or any other place on the planet, it is your solidarity above all of which the teams of Doctors Without Borders have need. . . . They work in our country uniquely thanks to the financial support that you contribute to them."

In Brussels, Belgium, since the end of the 1980s, Doctors Without Borders teams provide basic medical services in a traveling bus. They have also established two stationary medical centers in Antwerp and Verviers. Care and prescribed medications are given without charge. Unpaid, volunteer physicians act as consultants. Agreements have been established with hospitals and laboratories that make it possible to hospitalize patients who are seriously ill and to carry out whatever supplementary medical tests are necessary. In addition, Doctors Without Borders collaborates with the so-called Brussels Forum of agencies that are organized to fight against poverty and that take charge of the social problems of the persons who come for medical consultations. In France, since 1987, in cooperation with the government, both Doctors of the World and Doctors Without Borders are active participants in what is known as "Mission France" or "Mission Solidarité France." This began as an effort to alert French public authorities to the situation of the *exclus,* and developed into a network of centers in as many as twenty-six cities, where persons receive free medical care and social service assistance, including help in being "inserted" or "reinserted" into the social security system. "Mission France" also collects data on the men and women who come to the centers, as part of a concerted attempt to analyze the causes and mechanisms of the societal phenomenon of *exclusion* that they represent.

The national sections of Doctors Without Borders and Doctors of the

World vary in the degree and kind of importance that they attach to their "domestic" projects—in the conviction and energy, personnel, and resources that they invest in their "home" mission compared to their "overseas" undertakings. For example, Doctors of the World/USA is intensely committed to its New York City-based work. The organization's headquarters is located there and since the group's establishment in 1990, it has been heavily involved in what members call their "streetside" project in Harlem, on the Lower East Side and in the South Bronx. Some twenty physicians are among the volunteers who literally go into the streets to address the health needs of underserved populations in these areas of the city, providing medical and social services directly to people living with HIV/AIDS, to drug users, to the homeless and to other poor and marginalized people, for whom they also help to arrange access to the hospital system. From its starting point in these deprived milieux of New York, Doctors of the World/USA has radiated out to include other projects in its orbit that are located abroad. Most prominent among these are its rural community health program in the villages of the former civil war zone of Morazon, El Salvador; its children's immunization program and pediatric clinic and day hospital in Kosovo, an ethnic Albanian province in the most impoverished part of former Yugoslavia; its participation in shelters and clinics in St. Petersburg, Russia, that treat homeless children and children living in poor or troubled households; and its project in the Gaza Strip and on the West Bank, which focuses on the mental health needs of Palestinian women who have suffered domestic abuse, incest, and trauma due to confrontations with the police and military. These overseas endeavors do not alter the fact that the origins and roots of Doctors of the World/USA are in the streets of New York among the American equivalents of *les exclus*. In contrast, the starting points and original commitments of Doctors of the World/France (like those of Doctors Without Borders/France) were located in developing Third World countries. Their involvements in their own country came later, and were assumed only after dissensus within their ranks about opening a first Mission France center in Paris was resolved, and it came to be seen as more than a temporary, consciousness-raising venture.

FRENCH/NON-FRENCH TENSIONS

The *engagé* notion of immediate, emergency-oriented, interventionist action with which both Doctors of the World and Doctors Without Borders in France began still predominates in the French milieux of these organizations. The American branches respect this *action vécue* outlook of their French colleagues; and Doctors of the World/USA has participated in a number of joint missions with them.[27] The Americans' view of action entails a stronger commitment to sustained rehabilitation, and to long-term development projects than their French associates; more emphasis on cooperation with indigenous medical organizations and personnel in their work abroad and at home, and on mobilizing local communities; greater stress on teaching as a

form of action, particularly on "the exchange of information and training
so that communities are fundamentally strengthened after Doctors of the
World's work ends";[28] and more openness to examining their philosophical
assumptions, policies, and field operations through a process of inquiry and
research.

As the work of the various branches of both Doctors Without Borders
and Doctors of the World has evolved, what kind of balance to strike
between emergency, rehabilitation, and development projects has not only
become a more pressing issue. It has also become an element in the strains
that have arisen between the French and non-French branches of the organizations. A major focus of these tensions concerns whether the Paris offices
have superordinate authority over the action of the non-French divisions,
and the spirit and style in which they conduct them. It is not clear how independent the non-French branches are considered to be, either in their own
eyes or as viewed by the French, or how their national differences are recon-
ciled within the ideological and structural framework that they share. A
telling indicator of this uncertainty can be found in the variety of terms that
Doctors of the World and Doctors Without Borders use to refer to what I
have been calling their branches. These terms include "sections," "coordi-
nates," "affiliates," "antennae," and "nationally based missions."

Below the surface of these ostensibly organizational matters lie deeper historical and cultural factors. Doctors Without Borders and Doctors of the
World were founded by French physicians despite their internationalization,
they continue to be profoundly French in their culture and in the centralized
and hierarchical way that their Paris headquarters tend to view their relationship to other national affiliates. A steadfast inclination to regard Paris as
the command post of the organizations, to define the "right to interfere"
principle as a French creation, and to consider France "the homeland of
human rights" prevails in the Paris offices. These attitudes are felt throughout the branches of Doctors Without Borders and Doctors of the World. Not
only are they a source of difficulty in negotiating certain joint policy decisions, and in relations between French and non-French volunteers in the field;
they also curtail the overall internationalism of the two organizations. As
Bernard Granjon has stated, for these organizations to become truly international involves more than being present, rendering care, and witnessing in
many "spots of the globe." It requires changing the perspective and behavior
of their members so that "globalization" (*mondialisation*) of "the interven-
ers along with their interventions" is progressively achieved.[29]

METAQUESTIONS: HOW TO BE "GLOBAL" AND "MULTICULTURAL"?

These frictions and challenges are connected with the largest, most fundamental set of questions that Doctors Without Borders and Doctors of the
World face. Inside their own organizations, they are grappling with a micro-
version of the world problem that lies at the heart of many of their missions.
It is the problem of how to be "global and at the same time clearly multi-

cultural" that Václav Havel identified as the supreme political, moral, and spiritual challenge of our era.[30]

In their philosophical outlook, Doctors of the World and Doctors Without Borders seem to attach greater weight to a "global" than to a "multicultural" perspective. They are cognizant of societal and cultural differences, and they deal with them constantly, both in their domestic and their overseas work. But as previously mentioned, they are inclined to play down the importance and the overt recognition of such distinctions. They are not "clearly multicultural" either in the training they give volunteers for working abroad or in the insights they bring to resolving conflicts between their national branches. The transnational, "without borders" precepts to which they are dedicated contribute to this tendency, along with their espousal of "total independence from governments, and all political, economic or religious powers."** Their commitment to human rights and freedoms, to human dignity and social justice is also integral to their globalism. They regard these values not only as generally held universal principles to which people in all societies and cultures aspire, but as constituent elements of a fully human person.

The transocietal and transcultural vision of Doctors Without Borders and Doctors of the World is a noble one. But it flies in the face of the fact that the so-called "universal rights of man" are rooted in certain assumptions about freedom, equality, justice, democracy and the individuality of a person that are more congruent with some of the basic tenets and the cosmic view of Western cultures than of other civilizations. Even within the framework of the West, as Tony Judt points out, there has been difficulty in grounding and translating such concepts as human rights and social justice—which are regarded as "crucial building blocks of international moral institutions"—into "universally acknowledged propositions that are equally acceptable in the terrains of Continental Europe, Great Britain, and North America."[31]

No matter how exalted their mission, how strong their commitment, or how impressive the human and material resources they are able to mobilize, it is not within the purview of organizations like Doctors Without Borders and Doctors of the World to create and implement a model of multicultural and global coexistence and action that can remedy the maladies of our times. But from the ways that they are confronting them—from the problems, dilemmas, and limitations, as well as the accomplishments of their medical humanitarian work and their public witnessing—there is much to learn that is relevant to the progressive realization of a more healthy, humane, and peaceful world. It is for this reason, more than any other, that I hope to have the opportunity and the privilege of pursuing the study of Doctors Without Borders and Doctors of the World that I have only begun.

ACKNOWLEDGMENTS

I am grateful to Nicholas A. Christakis, Willy De Craemer, Robert Klitzman, Michael Lotke, and Jan Vansina for their critical yet encouraging comments on this essay.

ENDNOTES

 * Bernard Kouchner was initially named to head the Secretariat.
 ** This phrase is excerpted from the Charter of Doctors without Borders.

REFERENCES

1. Rufin, J. *Le Piege humanitaire, suivi de Humanitaire et Politique depuis la chute du Mur,* pp. 62–66. Editions Jean-Claude Lattes, Paris, 1986. (Collections Pluriel, 2nd ed., 1992).
2. Havel, V. Verbatim text of his address on receiving the Liberty Medal at Independence Hall in Philadelphia on July 4, 1994.
3. Judt, T. *Past Imperfect: French Intellectuals, 1944–1956,* pp. 284–286. Los Angeles: University of California Press, 1992.
4. For a penetrating analysis of the attributes of the New Left, see L. Kolakowski, *Main Currents of Marxism: Its Origins, Growth and Dissolution. Vol. 3: The Breakdown,* pp. 487–494. Oxford, England: Oxford University Press, 1981.
5. Pierre, A. and Kouchner, B. *Dieu et: Les Hommes (Dialogues et propos receueillis par M.-A. Burnier),* pp. 118, 123. Editions Robert Laffont, Paris, 1963.
6. Havel (see note 2).
7. Kaplan, R. "Getting Involved." *The New Physician,* July 17, 1993.
8. Rufin (see note 1).
9. Granjon, B. "Bosnie: denoncer encore et toujours." Editorial, *Les Nouvelles,* No. 33 (March 1994), p. 2.
10. Rufin (see note 1).
11. Ibid.
12. See Resolution 43/131 of the General Assembly of the United Nations (December 8, 1988) and Resolution 45/100 (December 14, 1990).
13. Havel (see note 2).
14. Quindlen, A. "The Numbness Factor," *New York Times,* July 23, 1994, p. 19.
15. Judt, T. "Nineteen Eighty-Nine: The End of *Which* European Era?" *Daedalus* 123, 3 (1994): 7.
16. Quoted in "Somalie: Pourquoi Partir, Pourquoi Rester? Le Depart de MSF." Commentaires, *Les Nouvelles* 32 (December 1993): 20.
17. Sharp, T. W., Yip, R., and Malone, J. D. "U.S. Military Forces and Emergency International Humanitarian Assistance: Observations and Recommendations From Three Recent Missions." *J. Amer. Med. Assoc.* 272, 5 (1994): 389. This article (pp. 386–390) presents an intelligent and perceptive analysis of observed advantages, limitations, and dilemmas of the role of armed forces in humanitarian assistance.
18. Hirtz, P. "Medecins du Monde: 'Nous Restons,'" *Les Nouvelles.* (See note 16).
19. Bonner, R. "Rwanda Relief Workers Fear Cholera Epidemic," *New York Times,* July 21, 1994, pp. A1, A8.
20. Moreels, R. (Au nom du Conseil D'Administration de Medecins Sans Frontieres), "Rapport Moral 93–94" (Assemblee Generale Extraits). *Medecins San Frontieres* 53 (June 1994): 19.
21. Ibid.

22. Ibid.

23. Quindlen (see note 14).

24. Although there is informal recognition of the range of motivations that bring volunteers to these organizations, including motives other than the desire to be of service to others (such as the need to test one's self under adversity, and a way to get away from problems in one's daily personal and professional life), there is an overall tendency to regard the reasons for volunteering as primarily altruistic and noble.

25. Havel (see note 2).

26. Granjon, B. "Mission France existe encore." Editorial, *Les Nouvelles,* No. 32, December 1993, p. 2.

27. Doctors Without Borders/U.S.A. is largely confined to fund-raising and the recruitment of volunteers. It does not undertake field missions. One of the more recent joint ventures of Doctors of the World/France and Doctors of the World/U.S.A. (which began on February 1, 1994) has involved providing physicians for the San Carlos Hospital in Altamirano, Chiapas, Mexico, in response to the fact that eight of the hospital's nine doctors abandoned their work there due to the Zapatista rebellion and its repercussions. Normally, this hospital serves more than 60,000 indigenous people in 600 communities in the area.

28. This quote is taken from the covering letter of response that Doctors of the World in New York sends to prospective volunteers, along with materials about the organization, a volunteer application form, and a request for copies of the applicant's curriculum vitae, medical degree (if applicable), licensing certificate, board certification papers, and for the names and telephone numbers of three professional references.

29. Granjon, B. "Medecins du Monde International." Editorial, Les Nouvelles, No. 34, June 1994, p. 2.

30. Havel (see note 2).

31. Judt, "Nineteen Eighty-Nine" (see note 15).

29. For Our Patients, Not for Profits: A Call to Action

The Ad Hoc Committee to Defend Health Care

We are Massachusetts physicians and nurses from across the spectrum of our professions. We serve patients rich and poor, in hospitals and clinics, private offices and health maintenance organizations (HMOs), public agencies, community settings and academia. Mounting shadows darken our calling and threaten to transform healing from a covenant into a business contract. Canons of commerce are displacing dictates of healing, trampling our professions' most sacred values.[1] Market medicine treats patients as profit centers. The time we are allowed to spend with the sick shrinks under the pressure to increase throughput, as though we were dealing with industrial commodities rather than afflicted human beings in need of compassion and caring. The right to choose and change one's physician, the foundation of patient autonomy and a central tenet of American medicine, is rapidly eroding.

Physicians and nurses are being prodded by threats and bribes to abdicate allegiance to patients, and to shun the sickest, who may be unprofitable. Some of us risk being fired or "delisted" for giving, or even discussing, expensive services, and many are offered bonuses for minimizing care. Listening, learning, and caring give way to deal-making, managing, and marketing. The primacy of the patient yields to a perverse accountability to investors, to bureaucrats, to insurers, and to employers. And patients worry that their physician's judgment and advice are guided by the corporate bottom line.

Public resources of enormous worth—nonprofit hospitals, visiting nurse agencies, even hospices—built over decades by taxes, charity, and devoted volunteers are being taken over by companies responsive to Wall Street and indifferent to Main Street. Communities find vital services closed by remote executives; savings are committed not to more pressing health needs, but to shareholders' profits. Not-for-profit institutions, forced to compete, must also curtail unprofitable activities such as research, teaching, and charity or face bankruptcy. Hospital chains' profits reach $100 per patient per day;[2] a single HMO president nets $990 million in a takeover deal;[3] and insurers' overhead consumes $46 billion annually.[4]

At the same time, the ranks of the uninsured continue to grow, while safety-net public hospitals and clinics shrink and public health programs erode. Even many with insurance find coverage deficient when they need it most; care or payment are too often denied for emergencies or expensive illnesses. The sick are denied skilled nursing care, rushed out of hospital beds, and hurried through office visits. Increasingly, patient comfort and the special needs of the elderly, infirm, or disabled are ignored if they conflict with the calculus of profit.

The shift to profit-driven care is at a gallop. For nurses and physicians, the space for good work in a bad system rapidly narrows. For the public, who are mostly healthy and use little care, awareness of the degradation of medicine builds slowly; it is mainly those who are expensively ill who encounter the dark side of market-driven health care.

We criticize market medicine not to obscure or excuse the failings of the past, but to warn that the changes afoot push nursing and medicine further from caring, fairness, and efficiency. We differ on many aspects of reform, but on the following we find common ground:

1. Medicine and nursing must not be diverted from their primary tasks: the relief of suffering, the prevention and treatment of illness, and the promotion of health. The efficient deployment of resources is critical but must not detract from these goals.
2. Pursuit of corporate profit and personal fortune has no place in caregiving.
3. Potent financial incentives that reward overcare or undercare weaken patient-physician and patient-nurse bonds and should be prohibited. Similarly, business arrangements that allow corporations and employers to control the care of patients should be proscribed.
4. A patient's right to a physician of choice must not be curtailed.
5. Access to health care must be the right of all.

Before the values we cherish are irretrievably lost, we invite members of the health professions and the public to join in a dialogue on health care's future. The headlong rush to profit-driven care has occurred without the assent of patients or practitioners, through a process largely hidden from public scrutiny and closed to citizen participation. This must be replaced by an open and inclusive process that is not dominated by the loudest voices— those amplified by money and political influence.

America's history is replete with examples of powerful social movements kindled by initially unimposing moral voices: in the eighteenth century, the Boston Tea Party; in the nineteenth century, abolitionism; and in the twentieth century, appeals for civil rights and nuclear disarmament. Only a comparable public outcry can reclaim medicine. We believe that our professions' voices can gain extraordinary resonance when we speak selflessly in patients' interests. From Massachusetts we pledge the following initial steps:

1. We have petitioned our governor, legislature, and attorney general for a moratorium on for-profit takeovers of hospitals, insurance plans, HMOs, physicians' practices, and other health care institutions. We expect public officials to oppose such takeovers and not to abrogate their duty to safeguard indispensable community resources. We urge colleagues in other states to join in the call for a moratorium, pending the development of comprehensive state and national policies addressing these issues.

2. On the publication date of this Call to Action, physicians and nurses will convene in the historic heart of Boston. This open meeting will call the public's attention to the deterioration of care and caring and initiate a colloquy on a future for health care guided by science and compassion rather than greed. We have invited colleagues across the nation to gather simultaneously at similar meetings.

3. These events will launch an ongoing series of teach-ins and meetings in hospitals, clinics, HMOs, offices, and nursing and medical schools to discuss the health care crisis. We ask that each health institution throughout the nation devote a major conference such as grand rounds to the moral crisis facing our professions. These conferences should review national and local data and draw on each group's clinical experience to assess the impact of the corporate takeover, the fundamental values that are at risk, elements of reform necessary to meet the needs of patients and communities, and strategies to resist and reverse the onrush of for-profit systems. Such discussions must acknowledge the realities of funding as well as caring. Our group is prepared to assist in the preparation of these conferences by offering evidence-based syllabi, slides, and other materials.

4. We invite public endorsement of this Call to Action by additional colleagues and by medical, nursing and lay groups. The Harvard Medical School Class of 1997, voting at a convocation held on "Internship Match Day," was the first group to offer its formal endorsement.

Our goal is not endorsement of a prespecified program for medical reform. Indeed, we believe that a number of programmatic solutions could provide the humane, comprehensive, and equitable care that our nation deserves. We seek an inclusive and empowering dialogue with patients and the public to formulate a caring vision true to the community roots and Good Samaritan traditions of American medicine and nursing.

REFERENCES

1. R. Crawshaw, D. E. Rogers, E. D. Pellegrino et al. "Patient-physician Covenant." *Journal of the American Medical Association* 273 (1995): 1553.
2. Columbia HCA Healthcare Corp. *10Q Report Filed with the Securities and Exchange Commission.* (Nashville, Tenn: Columbia HCA Healthcare Corp., November 19, 1995).
3. "Abramson to Get $35 Million Plus A Jet." *Managed Healthcare Market Report* June 30, 1996, p. 1.
4. K. R. Levit, H. C. Lazenby and L. Sivarajan. "Health Care Spending in 1994: Slowest in Decades." *Health Affairs (Millwood)* 15 (1996): 130–144.

Medicine and Public Health, Ethics and Human Rights

30.

Jonathan M. Mann

The relationships among medicine, public health, ethics, and human rights are now evolving rapidly, in response to a series of events, experiences, and struggles. These include the shock of the worldwide epidemic of human immunodeficiency virus and AIDS, continuing work on diverse aspects of women's health, and challenges exemplified by the complex humanitarian emergencies of Somalia, Iraq, Bosnia, Rwanda, and Zaire.

From among the many impacts of these experiences, three seem particularly salient. First, human rights thinking and action have become much more closely allied to, and even integrated with public health work. Second, the long-standing absence of an ethics of public health has been highlighted. Third, the human rights-related roles and responsibilities of physicians and other medical workers are receiving increased attention.

PUBLIC HEALTH AND MEDICINE

To explore the first of these issues—the connections between human rights and public health—it is essential to review several central elements of modern public health.

Medicine and public health are two complementary and interacting approaches for promoting and protecting health—defined by the World Health Organization (WHO) as a state of physical, mental, and social well-being. Yet medicine and public health can and also must be differentiated, because in several important ways they are not the same. The fundamental difference involves the population emphasis of public health, which contrasts with the essentially individual focus of medical care. Public health identifies and measures threats to the health of populations, develops governmental policies in response to these concerns, and seeks to assure certain health and related services. In contrast, medical care focuses upon individuals—diagnosis, treatment, relief of suffering, and rehabilitation.

Several specific points follow from this essential difference. For example, different instruments are called for. While public health measures population health status through epidemiological, survey, and other statistically based methods, medicine examines biophysical and psychological status using a combination of techniques including dialogue, physical examination and laboratory study of the individual. Public health generally values most highly (or at least is supposed to) primary prevention, that is, preventing the adverse health event in the first place, such as helping to prevent the automobile accident or the lead poisoning from happening at all. In contrast, medicine generally responds to existing health conditions, in the context of either secondary or tertiary prevention. Secondary prevention involves avoiding or delaying the adverse impact of a health condition such as hypertension or diabetes. Thus, while the hypertension or insulin deficiency exists, its effects, such as heart disease, kidney failure, or blindness, can be avoided or delayed. So-called tertiary prevention involves those efforts to help sustain maximal functional and psychological capacity despite the presence of both the disease, such as hypertension, and its outcomes, such as heart disease, stroke, or kidney failure.

Accordingly, the skills and expertise needed in public health include epidemiology, biostatistics, policy analysis, economics, sociology and other behavioral sciences. In contrast, medical skills and expertise center on the exploration, analysis, and response to the biophysical status of individuals, based principally on an understanding of biology, biochemistry, immunology, pharmacology, pathology, pathophysiology, anatomy, and psychology.

Naturally, the settings in which public health and medicine operate also differ. Governmental organizations, large-scale public programs, and various fora associated with developing and implementing public policy are inherently part of public health, while private medical offices, clinics, and medical care facilities of varying complexity and sophistication are the settings in which medical care is generally provided.

Finally, the relationship between the profession and the people with whom it deals differs: in a sense, public health comes to you, while you go to the doctor. And expectations associated with each domain differ: from medicine, individual care and treatment are sought; from public health, protection against broad health threats such as epidemic disease, unsafe water, or chemical pollution is expected.

Therefore, public health and medicine are principally distinguished by their focus on collectivities or on individuals, respectively, with a series of subsidiary differences involving methods of work, systems of analysis and measurement, emphasis on primary versus secondary or tertiary prevention, types of expertise and relevant skill, settings in which work is conducted, and client/public relationships and expectations.

Yet obviously there is substantial overlap. Public health requires a sound biomedical basis, and involves many medical practitioners, whose services are organized in settings such as maternal and child health clinics or immunization programs. Also, medical practice operates within a context highly influenced and governed by law and public policy. The potentially fluid relationship between public health and medicine is further suggested by recent proposals in this country that certain traditional public health functions be delegated to the private medical sector.

Despite these many differences, people equate medical care with health. Certainly this basic confusion has informed the recent discussions of health care in the United States; and coverage of health issues in the popular press around the world reflects this perspective, in which access to medical care and the quality of that care are seen as the principal health needs of individuals and populations.

MEDICINE AND HEALTH

Yet the contribution of medicine to health, while undeniably important (and vital in certain situations), is actually quite limited. For example, it is estimated that only about one-sixth of the years of life expectancy gained in this country during this century can be attributed to the beneficial impact of medicine, medical care, and medical research. And it has been estimated that only about 10 percent of preventable premature deaths are associated with a lack of medical care. Similarly, the World Bank has estimated that a lack of essential clinical services is responsible for between 11 and 24 percent of the global burden of disease. Of course, none of these data, including also the notable decline in diseases such as tuberculosis well before antimycobacterial therapy became available, suggest that medical care is irrelevant; rather, they suggest its limits.

In 1988, the United States Institute of Medicine defined the mission of public health as "ensuring the conditions in which people can be healthy." This profound definition begs the most vital question for public health, namely, what are these essential conditions in which people can best achieve the highest possible level of physical, mental, and social well-being? If not medical care—its availability and quality—then what?

The vast majority of research into the health of populations identifies so-called societal factors as the major determinants of health status. Most of the work in this area has focused on socioeconomic status as the key variable, for it is clear, throughout history and in all societies, that the rich live generally longer and healthier lives than the poor. Thus, in the United Kingdom in 1911, the age-adjusted standardized mortality rate among members of the lowest social class was 1.6 times higher than for the highest social class. Interestingly, following creation of the National Health Services to ensure full access to medical care, and despite a dramatic change in major causes of death (from mainly infectious to mainly chronic diseases), in 1981 this societal gradient not only persisted but increased, to a 2.1-fold higher standardized mortality rate among the lowest compared with the highest social class.

A major question arising from the socioeconomic status–health gradient is why there is a gradient. For example, among more than ten thousand

British civil servants followed for many years, health status and longevity were better for each successive category of civil servants, from lowest to highest. This raises two issues: first, while we believe we can—at least intuitively—explain poor health among the destitute when compared with the rich, associated with a lack of good food, poor housing, and poor sanitary conditions, even the lowest class of British civil servants cannot be considered poor. Secondly, why should the civil servants in the next-to-highest group, living in quite comfortable circumstances, experience poorer health than the highest group?

Beyond these unanswered issues, many recent studies have pointed to the limited explanatory power of socioeconomic status, generally measured in terms of current income, years of education, and job classification. Other measures, such as the extent of socioeconomic inequality within a community; the nature, level and temporal pattern of unemployment; societal connectedness and the extent or involvement in social networks; marital status; early childhood experiences and exposure to dignity-denying situations, have all been suggested as powerful potential components of a "black box" of societal factors whose dominant role in determining levels of preventable disease, disability, and premature death is beyond dispute.[1]

AN ETHICS FOR PUBLIC HEALTH

Public health, although it began as a social movement, has—at least in recent years—responded relatively little to this most profound and vital knowledge about the dominant impact of society on health. To illustrate: we all know that certain behaviors have an enormous impact on health, such as cigarette smoking, excess alcohol intake, dietary choices, or levels of exercise and physical fitness. How these behaviors are conceptualized determines how they will be addressed by public health. The basic question is whether and to what extent these behaviors can be considered, and therefore responded to, as isolated individual choices.

The curve represented in Figure 1 (replicable among public health practitioners in at least three countries) reflects a strong belief that important health-related behaviors are substantially influenced by societal factors and context. Yet examining public health programs designed to address the health problems associated with these same behaviors reveals that they generally consist of activities that assume individuals have essentially complete control over their health-related behaviors. Traditional public health seeks to pro-

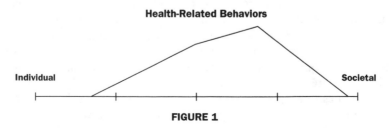

Health-Related Behaviors

Individual   Societal

FIGURE 1

vide individuals with information and education about risks associated with diet or lack of exercise, along with various clinic-based services such as counseling or distribution of condoms and other contraceptives. However, while public health may cite, blame or otherwise identify the societal-level or contextual issues—which it acknowledges to be of dominant importance, both in influencing individual behavior and for determining health status more broadly—it does not deal directly with these societal factors.

At least three reasons for this paradoxical inaction may be proposed. First, public health has lacked a conceptual framework for identifying and analyzing the essential societal factors that represent the conditions in which people can be healthy. Second is a related problem public health lacks a vocabulary with which to speak about and identify commonalities among health problems experienced by very different populations. Third, there is no consensus about the nature or direction of societal change that would be necessary to address the societal conditions involved. Lacking a coherent conceptual framework, a consistent vocabulary, and consensus about societal change, public health assembles and then tries valiantly to assimilate a wide variety of disciplinary perspectives from economists, political scientists, social and behavioral scientists, health systems analysts, and a range of medical practitioners. Yet while each of these perspectives provides some useful insight, public health becomes thereby a little bit of everything and not enough of anything.

With this background in mind, it would be expected that in the domains of public health and medicine, different yet complementary languages for describing and incorporating values would be developed. For even when values are shared at a higher level of abstraction, the forms in which they are expressed, the settings in which they are evoked and their practical application may differ widely.

Not surprisingly, medicine has chosen the language of ethics, as ethics has been developed in a context of individual relationships and is well adapted to the nature, practice, settings and expectations of medical care. The language of medical ethics has also been applied when medicine seeks to deal with issues such as the organization of medical care or the allocation of societal resources. However, the contribution of medical ethics to these societal issues has been less powerful when compared, for example, with its engagement in the behavior of individual medical practitioners.

Public health, at least in its contemporary form, is struggling to define and articulate its core values. In this context, the usefulness of the language and structure of ethics as we know it today has been questioned. Given its population focus and its interest in the underlying conditions upon which health is predicated (and that these major determinants of health status are societal in nature), it seems evident that a framework that expresses fundamental values in societal terms, and a vocabulary of values that links directly with societal structure and function, may be better adapted to the work of public health than a more individually oriented ethical framework.

For this reason, modern human rights, precisely because they were initially developed entirely outside the health domain and seek to articulate the societal preconditions for human well-being, seem a far more useful framework, vocabulary, and form of guidance for public health efforts to analyze and respond directly to the societal determinants of health than any inherited from the biomedical or public health tradition.

PUBLIC HEALTH AND HUMAN RIGHTS

The linkage between public health and human rights can be explored further by considering three relationships. The first focuses on the potential burden on human rights created by public health policies, programs, and practices. As public health generally involves direct or indirect state action, public health officials represent the state power toward which classical human rights concerns are traditionally addressed. Thus, in the modern world, public health officials have, for the first time, two fundamental responsibilities to the public: to protect and promote public health, and to protect and promote human rights. While public health officials may be unlikely to seek deliberately to violate human rights, there is great unawareness of human rights concepts and norms among public health practitioners. In stark contrast to the large number of bioethics courses available in medical education settings, a recent survey of all twenty-eight accredited schools of public health in the United States and schools of public health in thirty-four other countries identified only seven formal courses in human rights for the presumed future leaders of public health.

Public health practice is heavily burdened by the problem of inadvertent discrimination. For example, outreach activities may "assume" that all populations are reached equally by a single, dominant-language message on television; or analysis "forgets" to include health problems uniquely relevant to certain groups, such as breast cancer or sickle-cell disease; or a program "ignores" the actual response capability of different population groups, as when lead poisoning warnings are given without concern for financial ability to ensure lead abatement. Indeed, inadvertent discrimination is so prevalent that all public health policies and programs should be considered discriminatory until proven otherwise, placing the burden on public health to affirm and ensure its respect for human rights.

In addition, in public health circles there is often an unspoken sense that public health and human rights concerns are inherently confrontational. At times this has been true. In the early years of the HIV epidemic, the knee-jerk response of various public health officials to invoke mandatory testing, quarantine, and isolation did create a major clash with protectors of human rights.

However, while modern human rights explicitly acknowledges that public health is a legitimate reason for limiting rights, more recently the underlying complementarity rather than inherent confrontation between public health and human rights has been emphasized. Again in the context of AIDS, public health has learned that discrimination toward HIV-infected people and people with AIDS is counterproductive. Specifically, when people found to be infected were deprived of employment, education, or ability to marry and travel, participation in prevention programs diminished. Thus, recent attention has been directed to a negotiation process for optimizing both the achievement of complementary public health goals and respect for human rights norms.

A second relationship between public health and human rights derives from the observation that human rights violations have health impacts, that is, adverse effects on physical, mental, and social well-being. For some rights, such as the right not to be tortured or imprisoned under inhumane conditions, the health damage seems evident, indeed inherent in the rights violation. However, even for torture, only more recently has the extensive, lifelong, family and communitywide, and transgenerational impact of torture been recognized.

For many other rights, such as the right to information, to assembly or to association, health impacts resulting from violation may not be initially so apparent. The violation of any right has measurable impacts on physical, mental and social well-being; yet these health effects still remain, in large part, to be discovered and documented. Yet gradually the connection is being established.

The right to association provides a useful example of this relationship. Public health benefits substantially from—even requires—involvement of people in addressing problems that affect them. Because the ability of people concerned about a health problem to get together, talk, and search for effective solutions is so essential to public health, wherever the right to association is restricted, public health suffers. Taking a positive example from the history of HIV/AIDS: needle exchange—the trading in of needles used for drug injection for clean needles, so as to avoid needle sharing with consequent risk of HIV transmission—was invented by a union of drug users in Amsterdam. Needle exchange was a classic example of an innovative local response to a pressing local problem. Needle exchange was not and would have been highly unlikely to have been developed by academics, government officials, or hired consultants! Yet the creative solution of needle exchange and respect for the right of association are closely linked. Thus, in societies in which people generally, or specific population groups, cannot associate around health or other issues, such as injection drug users in the United States, or sex workers, or gay and lesbian people in many countries, local solutions are less able to emerge or be applied, and public health is correspondingly compromised.

A third relationship between health and human rights has already been suggested: namely, that promoting and protecting human rights is inextricably linked with promoting and protecting health. Once again, this is because human rights offers a societal-level framework for identifying and responding to the underlying—societal—determinants of health. It is important to emphasize that human rights are respected not only for their instrumental value in contributing to public health goals, but for themselves, as societal goods of preeminent importance.

For example, a cluster of rights, including the rights to health, bodily integrity, privacy, information, education, and equal rights in marriage and divorce, have been called "reproductive rights," insofar as their realization (or violation) is now understood to play a major role in determining reproductive health. From an early focus on demographic targets for population control to an emphasis on ensuring "informed consent" of women to various contraceptive methods, a new paradigm for population policies *and* reproductive health has recently emerged. Articulated most forcefully at the United Nations Conference on Population and Development in 1994 in Cairo, the focus has shifted to ensuring that women can make and effectuate real and informed choices about reproduction. And in turn, this is widely acknowledged to depend on realization of human rights.

Similarly, in the context of HIV/AIDS, vulnerability to the epidemic has now been associated with the extent of realization of human rights. For as the HIV epidemic matures and evolves within each community and country, it focuses inexorably on those groups that, before HIV/AIDS arrived, were already discriminated against, marginalized and stigmatized within each society. Thus, in the United States the brunt of the epidemic today is among racial and ethnic minority populations, inner-city poor and injection drug users, especially women in these communities. In Brazil, an epidemic that started among the jet-set of Rio and São Paulo with time has become a major epidemic among the slum-dwellers in the *favelas* of Brazil's cities. The French, with characteristic linguistic precision, identify the major burden of HIV/AIDS to exist among *les exclus,* those living at the margins of society. Now that a lack of respect for human rights has been identified as a societal-level risk factor for HIV/AIDS vulnerability, HIV prevention efforts—for example, for women—are starting to go beyond traditional educational and service-based efforts to address the rights issues that will be a precondition for greater progress against the epidemic.

Ultimately, ethics and human rights derive from a set of quite similar, if not identical, core values. As with medicine and public health, rather than seeing human rights and ethics as conflicting domains, it seems more appropriate to consider a continuum on which human rights is a language most useful for guiding societal-level analysis and work, while ethics is a language most useful for guiding individual behavior. From this perspective, and precisely because public health must be centrally concerned with the structure and function of society, the language of human rights is extremely useful for expressing, considering, and incorporating values into public health analysis and response.

Thus, public health work requires both ethics applicable to the individual public health practitioner and a human rights framework to guide public health in its societal analysis and response.

These relationships between medicine and public health, and between ethics and human rights, can be provisionally diagrammed as in Figure 2.

At the hypothetical extreme of individual medical care, ethics would be the most useful language. However, to the extent that the individual practitioner is cognizant of the societal forces acting upon the individual patient, societal-level considerations may also be articulated in human rights terms. At the other extreme of public health, human rights is the most useful language, speaking as it does directly to the societal-level determinants of well-being. Nevertheless, the ethical framework remains critical, for public health is carried out by individuals within specific professional roles and competencies. In practice, of course, positions between the hypothetical extremes of medicine and public health are more common, calling for mixtures of human rights and ethical concepts and language.

PROFESSIONAL ROLES AND RESPONSIBILITIES

The placement of both human rights and ethics, and public health and medicine at ends of a continuum suggests also that the interest domains of individuals and organizations can be "mapped" (as in Figure 3), and areas calling for additional attention can be highlighted.

According to this mapping approach, the "French doctors" movement (Médecins Sans Frontières, Médecins du Monde) can be seen as primarily medical, primarily ethics-based, yet with growing involvement in the public health dimensions of health emergencies and in human rights issues raised by these complex humanitarian crises. Similarly, many traditional, medical ethics-based institutes and centers can be placed on this map. At the Harvard School of Public Health, the François-Xavier Bagnoud Center for Health and Human Rights, along with several others, is now focusing on the health–human rights territory. This map also suggests two major gaps in current work: on the ethics of public health, and on the relationships between medicine and human rights.

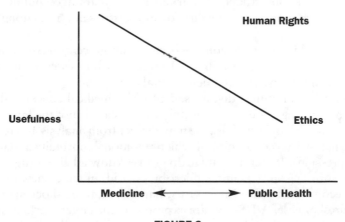

FIGURE 2

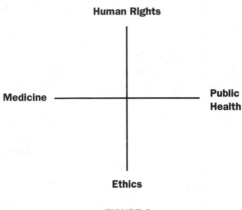

FIGURE 3

Where are the ethics of public health? In contrast to the important declarations of medical ethics such as the International Code of Medical Ethics of the World Medical Association and the Nuremberg Code, the world of public health does not have a reasonably explicit set of ethical guidelines. In part, this deficiency may stem from the broad diversity of professional identities within public health. Yet, curiously, many of the occupational groups central to public health (epidemiologists, policy analysts, social scientists, biostatisticians, nutritionists, health system managers) have not yet developed, or are only now developing, widely accepted ethical guidelines or statements of principle for their work in the public health context. Thus, while a public health physician may draw upon medical ethics for guidance, the ethics of a public health physician have yet to be clearly articulated.

The central problem is one of coherence and identity: public health cannot develop an ethics until it has achieved clarity about its own identity. Technical expertise and methodology are not substitutes for conceptual coherence. Or, as one student remarked a few years ago, public health spends too much time on the p values of biostatistics and not enough time on values.

To have an ethics, a profession needs clarity about central issues, including its major role and responsibilities. Two steps will be essential for public health to reach this analytic and definitional clarity.

First, public health must divest itself of its biomedical conceptual foundation. The language of disease, disability and death is not the language of well-being; the vocabulary of disease may detract from analysis and response to underlying societal conditions, of which traditional morbidity and mortality are expressions. It is clear that we do not yet know all about the universe of human suffering. Just as in the microbial world, in which new discoveries have become the norm—Ebola virus, hantavirus, toxic shock syndrome, Legionnaires' disease, AIDS—we are explorers in the larger world of human suffering and well-being. And our current maps of this universe, like world maps from sixteenth-century Europe, have some very well-defined, familiar coastlines and territories as well as large blank spaces, which beckon the explorer.

The language of biomedicine is cumbersome and ultimately is perhaps of little usefulness in exploring the impacts of violations of dignity on physical, mental, and social well-being. The definition of dignity itself is complex and thus far elusive and unsatisfying. While the Universal Declaration of Human Rights starts by placing dignity first, "all people are born equal in dignity and rights," we do not yet have a vocabulary or taxonomy, let alone an epidemiology, of dignity violations.

Yet it seems we all know when our dignity is violated or impugned. Perform the following experiment: recall, in detail, an incident from your own life in which your dignity was violated, for whatever reason. If you will immerse yourself in the memory, powerful feelings will likely arise—of anger, shame, powerlessness, despair. When you connect with the power of these feelings, it seems intuitively obvious that such feelings, particularly if evoked repetitively, could have deleterious impacts on health. Yet most of us are relatively privileged: we live in a generally dignity-affirming environment and suffer only the occasional lapse of indignity. However, many people live constantly in a dignity-impugning environment, in which affirmations of dignity may be the exceptional occurrence. An exploration of the meanings of dignity and the forms of its violation—and the impact on physical, mental, and social well-being—may help uncover a new universe of human suffering, for which the biomedical language may be inapt and even inept. After all, the power of naming, describing, and then measuring is truly enormous. Child abuse did not exist in meaningful societal terms until it was named and then measured; nor did domestic violence.

A second precondition for developing an ethics of public health is the adoption and application of a human rights framework for analyzing and responding to the societal determinants of health. The human rights framework can provide the coherence and clarity required for public health to identify and work with conscious attention to its roles and responsibilities. At that point, an ethics of public health, rather than the ethics of individual constituent disciplines within public health, can emerge.

Issues of respect for autonomy, beneficence, nonmaleficence, and justice can then be articulated from within the set of goals and responsibilities called for by seeking to improve public health through the combination of traditional approaches and those that strive concretely to promote realization of human rights. This is not to replace health education, information, and clinical service-based activities of public health with an exclusive focus on human rights and dignity. Both are necessary.

For example, the challenges for public health officials in balancing the goals of promoting and protecting public health and ensuring that human rights and dignity are not violated call urgently for ethical analysis. The official nature of much public health work places public health practitioners in a complex environment, in which work to promote rights inevitably challenges the state system within which the official is employed. Ethical dimensions are highly relevant to collecting, disseminating, and acting on information about the health impacts of the entire range of human rights violations. As public health seeks to ensure the conditions in which people can be healthy, and as those conditions are societal, to be engaged in public health necessarily involves a commitment to societal transformation. The difficulties in assessing human rights status and in developing useful and appropriate ways to promote human rights and dignity necessarily engage ethical considerations. For example, beyond accurate diagnosis, beyond efforts to cure and even beyond the ever-present responsibility for relief of pain, the physician agrees to accompany the patient, to stand by the patient through her suffering, even to the edge of life itself, even when the only thing the physician can offer is his or her presence. Is this not as relevant to public health? For public health must engage difficult issues even when no cure or effective instruments are yet available, and public health also must accompany, remain with, and not abandon vulnerable populations.

That this work—added to, not substituted for, the current approach of public health—will require major changes in public health reflection, analysis, action, and education, is clear. That it is urgently required, in order to confront the major health challenges of the modern world, is equally clear.

PHYSICIANS AND HUMAN RIGHTS

Finally, turning to the third issue raised by new challenges to the domains of public health, medicine, ethics and human rights: what about the human rights role and responsibilities of medicine and the medical professional? To what extent and in what ways are—or might, or should—medicine generally and physicians in particular be involved in human rights issues?

Physicians have developed important roles in the context of human rights work. This work generally started from a corporatist interest in the fate of fellow physicians suffering human rights abuses, and then expanded in four directions. First, physicians created the French doctors movement, providing medical assistance to populations in need, across borders. This dramatic and catalyzing work, including the concept of the right to assistance and the duty to intervene, expressed—in medical terms—the same transnational, universalist impulse as the modern human rights movement. Then groups such as Physicians for Human Rights applied medical methods and analysis to detect and document torture, executions and other similar human rights violations. In this manner, credible documentation, necessary also for redress and prosecution, has increasingly been made available. Meanwhile, Amnesty International has been concerned with the participation of physicians in human rights violations, usually in the context of torture and imprisonment under inhumane conditions. Finally, at a global level, physicians have articulated a role in seeking to prevent health catastrophes, exemplified by the

Nobel Peace Prize-winning organization International Physicians for Prevention of Nuclear War.

These historic and often courageous engagements with human rights issues have carried physicians to the frontiers of new challenges, exemplified by complex humanitarian emergencies, efforts to identify the full range of health consequences from human rights violations and further struggle with societal issues inextricably linked with the health dimensions of conflict, economic consumption and the degradation of the global environment. Increased physician participation and concern with these issues will inevitably blur preexisting boundaries between public health and medicine and create new interactive configurations between human rights and ethics.

Yet for individual medical practitioners, how is a human rights perspective relevant? Human rights and dignity will be engaged to the extent that the physician seeks to go beyond the usual, limited boundaries of medical care. Take two examples: a child with asthma, or a woman seeking emergency room care for injuries inflicted by her spouse. In each case, the limited medical perspective is vital. For the precipitating factors for asthma, and the likelihood of seeking early care as asthmatic attacks begin, lead directly to environmental conditions, economic issues, and discrimination. Similarly, domestic violence invokes, necessarily, societal issues in which the human rights framework will be useful, if not essential. Whether considering cancer, heart disease, lead poisoning, asthma, injuries, or infectious diseases, while the medical professional may start from a context dominated by individual relationships, a larger, societal set of issues will inevitably exist. The question then becomes: to what extent is the physician responsible for what happens outside the immediate context and setting of medical care? To what extent is a physician responsible for ensuring access to care for marginalized populations in the community, or helping the community understand the medical implications of public policy measures, or identifying, responding to and preventing discrimination occurring within medical institutions?

Where, that is, does the boundary of medicine end? This seems a uniquely rich context for ethical discussion, at the frontiers of human rights and public health.

Of course, for those interested in the human rights dimensions of medicine, many may accuse physicians of "meddling" in societal issues that go far beyond their scope or competence. Also, issues of human rights inherently and inevitably represent a challenge to power—and health professionals are often part of, or direct beneficiaries of, the societal or institutional status quo that is challenged by the claims of human rights and dignity.

In conclusion, there is more to modern health than new scientific discoveries, or development of new technologies, of emerging or reemerging diseases, or changes in patterns of morbidity and mortality around the world. For we are living at a time of paradigm shift in thinking about health, and therefore about medicine and public health. Health as well-being, despite the World Health Organization's definition, lacks more than rudimentary definition, especially regarding its mental and societal dimensions. The universe of human suffering and its alleviation is being more fully explored. Awareness of the limits of medicine and medical care, growing recognition of the health impacts of societal structure and function, globalization and consequent interdependence, and the sometimes active, sometimes ineffectual actions of nation-states all intersect to lead toward a new vision of health.

In the ongoing work on values and their articulation, we must acknowledge the provisional, untidy, and necessarily incomplete character of our understanding of the universe of health. In this context, medicine need not compete with public health, nor ethics with human rights. The search for meaning deserves to draw on all as new constellations emerge and new relationships evolve.

Yet at such times of profound change, another kind of value becomes all the more vital. To build bridges—between medicine and public health, and between ethics and human rights—the critical underlying question may be: do we believe that the world can change? Do we believe that the long chains of human suffering can be broken? Do we agree with Martin Luther King Jr. that "the arc of history is long, but it bends towards justice"? Bioethical pioneers at the frontier of human history, we affirm that the past does not inexorably determine the future—and that it is precisely through this historic effort to explore and promote values in the world for which we share responsibility, articulated in philosophy and in action, that we express confidence in our own lives, in our community, and in the future of our world.

REFERENCE

1. N. E. Adler et al. "Socioeconomic Status and Health: The Challenges of the Gradient." *American Psychologist* 49 (1994): 15–24.

Appendix A
Universal Declaration of Human Rights

Adopted and proclaimed by United Nations General Assembly
resolution 217 A (III) on 10 December 1948

PREAMBLE

Whereas recognition of the inherent dignity and of the equal and inalienable rights of all members of the human family is the foundation of freedom, justice and peace in the world,

Whereas disregard and contempt for human rights have resulted in barbarous acts which have outraged the conscience of mankind, and the advent of a world in which human beings shall enjoy freedom of speech and belief and freedom from fear and want has been proclaimed as the highest aspiration of the common people,

Whereas it is essential, if man is not to be compelled to have recourse, as a last resort, to rebellion against tyranny and oppression, that human rights should be protected by the rule of law,

Whereas it is essential to promote the development of friendly relations between nations,

Whereas the peoples of the United Nations have in the Charter reaffirmed their faith in fundamental human rights, in the dignity and worth of the human person and in the equal rights of men and women and have determined to promote social progress and better standards of life in larger freedom,

Whereas Member States have pledged themselves to achieve, in cooperation with the United Nations, the promotion of universal respect for and observance of human rights and fundamental freedoms,

Whereas a common understanding of these rights and freedoms is of the greatest importance for the full realisation of this pledge,

Now, therefore,
The General Assembly

Proclaims this Universal Declaration of Human Rights as a common standard of achievement for all peoples and all nations, to the end that every individual and every organ of society, keeping this Declaration constantly in mind, shall strive by teaching and education to promote respect for these rights and freedoms and by progressive measures, national and international, to secure their universal and effective recognition and observance, both among the peoples of Member States themselves and among the peoples of territories under their jurisdiction.

Article 1

All human beings are born free and equal in dignity and rights. They are endowed with reason and conscience and should act towards one another in a spirit of brotherhood.

Article 2

Everyone is entitled to all the rights and freedoms set forth in this Declaration, without distinction of any kind, such as race, colour, sex, language, religion, political or other opinion, national or social origin, property, birth or other status.

Furthermore, no distinction shall be made on the basis of the political, jurisdictional or international status of the country or territory to which a person belongs, whether it be independent, trust, non-self-governing or under any other limitation of sovereignty.

Article 3

Everyone has the right to life, liberty and security of person.

Article 4

No one shall be held in slavery or servitude; slavery and the slave trade shall be prohibited in all their forms.

Article 5

No one shall be subjected to torture or to cruel, inhuman or degrading treatment or punishment.

Article 6

Everyone has the right to recognition everywhere as a person before the law.

Article 7

All are equal before the law and are entitled without any discrimination to equal protection of the law. All are entitled to equal protection against any discrimination in violation of this Declaration and against any incitement to such discrimination.

Article 8

Everyone has the right to an effective remedy by the competent national tribunals for acts violating the fundamental rights granted him by the constitution or by law.

Article 9

No one shall be subjected to arbitrary arrest, detention or exile.

Article 10

Everyone is entitled in full equality to a fair and public hearing by an independent and impartial tribunal, in the determination of his rights and obligations and of any criminal charge against him.

Article 11

1. Everyone charged with a penal offence has the right to be presumed innocent until proved guilty according to law in a public trial at which he has had all the guarantees necessary for his defense.
2. No one shall be held guilty of any penal offence on account of any act or omission which did not constitute a penal offence, under national or international law, at the time when it was committed. Nor shall a heavier penalty be imposed than the one that was applicable at the time the penal offence was committed.

Article 12

No one shall be subjected to arbitrary interference with his privacy, family, home or correspondence, nor to attacks upon his honor and reputation. Everyone has the right to the protection of the law against such interference or attacks.

Article 13

1. Everyone has the right to freedom of movement and residence within the borders of each State.
2. Everyone has the right to leave any country, including his own, and to return to his country.

Article 14

1. Everyone has the right to seek and to enjoy in other countries asylum from persecution.
2. This right may not be invoked in the case of prosecutions genuinely arising from non-political crimes or from acts contrary to the purposes and principles of the United Nations.

Article 15

1. Everyone has the right to a nationality.
2. No one shall be arbitrarily deprived of his nationality nor denied the right to change his nationality.

Article 16

1. Men and women of full age, without any limitation due to race, nationality or religion, have the right to marry and to found a family. They are entitled to equal rights as to marriage, during marriage and at its dissolution.
2. Marriage shall be entered into only with the free and full consent of the intending spouses.
3. The family is the natural and fundamental group unit of society and is entitled to protection by society and the State.

Article 17

1. Everyone has the right to own property alone as well as in association with others.
2. No one shall be arbitrarily deprived of his property.

Article 18

Everyone has the right to freedom of thought, conscience and religion; this right includes freedom to change his religion or belief, and freedom, either alone or in community with others and in public or private, to manifest his religion or belief in teaching, practice, worship and observance.

Article 19

Everyone has the right to freedom of opinion and expression; this right includes freedom to hold opinions without interference and to seek, receive and impart information and ideas through any media and regardless of frontiers.

Article 20

1. Everyone has the right to freedom of peaceful assembly and association.
2. No one may be compelled to belong to an association.

Article 21

1. Everyone has the right to take part in the government of his country, directly or through freely chosen representatives.

2. Everyone has the right to equal access to public service in his country.
3. The will of the people shall be the basis of the authority of government; this will shall be expressed in periodic and genuine elections which shall be by universal and equal suffrage and shall be held by secret vote or by equivalent free voting procedures.

Article 22

Everyone, as a member of society, has the right to social security and is entitled to realization, through national effort and international cooperation and in accordance with the organization and resources of each State, of the economic, social and cultural rights indispensable for his dignity and the free development of his personality.

Article 23

1. Everyone has the right to work, to free choice of employment, to just and favourable conditions of work and to protection against unemployment.
2. Everyone, without any discrimination, has the right to equal pay for equal work.
3. Everyone who works has the right to just and favourable remuneration ensuring for himself and his family an existence worthy of human dignity, and supplemented, if necessary, by other means of social protection.
4. Everyone has the right to form and to join trade unions for the protection of his interests.

Article 24

Everyone has the right to rest and leisure, including reasonable limitation of working hours and periodic holidays with pay.

Article 25

1. Everyone has the right to a standard of living adequate for the health and well-being of himself and of his family, including food, clothing, housing and medical care and necessary social services, and the right to security in the event of unemployment, sickness, disability, widowhood, old age or other lack of livelihood in circumstances beyond his control.
2. Motherhood and childhood are entitled to special care and assistance. All children, whether born in or out of wedlock, shall enjoy the same social protection.

Article 26

1. Everyone has the right to education. Education shall be free, at least in the elementary and fundamental stages. Elementary education shall be compulsory. Technical and professional education shall be made generally available, and higher education shall be equally accessible to all on the basis of merit.
2. Education shall be directed to the full development of the human personality and to the strengthening of respect for human rights and fundamental freedoms. It shall promote understanding, tolerance and friendship among all nations, racial or religious groups, and shall further the activities of the United Nations for the maintenance of peace.
3. Parents have a prior right to choose the kind of education that shall be given to their children.

Article 27

1. Everyone has the right freely to participate in the cultural life of the community, to enjoy the arts and to share in scientific advancement and its benefits.

2. Everyone has the right to the protection of the moral and material interests resulting from any scientific, literary or artistic production of which he is the author.

Article 28

Everyone is entitled to a social and international order in which the rights and freedoms set forth in this Declaration can be fully realized.

Article 29

1. Everyone has duties to the community in which alone the free and full development of his personality is possible.
2. In the exercise of his rights and freedoms, everyone shall be subject only to such limitations as are determined by law solely for the purpose of securing due recognition and respect for the rights and freedoms of others and of meeting the just requirements of morality, public order and the general welfare in a democratic society.
3. These rights and freedoms may in no case be exercised contrary to the purposes and principles of the United Nations.

Article 30

Nothing in this Declaration may be interpreted as implying for any State, group or person any right to engage in any activity or to perform any act aimed at the destruction of any of the rights and freedoms set forth herein.

Appendix B

International Covenant on Economic, Social, and Cultural Rights

Adopted and opened for signature, ratification, and accession by United Nations General Assembly resolution 2200 A (XXI) on 16 December 1966. Entered into force on 3 January 1976 in accordance with article 27.

PREAMBLE

The States Parties to the present Covenant,

Considering that, in accordance with the principles proclaimed in the Charter of the United Nations, recognition of the inherent dignity and of the equal and inalienable rights of all members of the human family is the foundation of freedom, justice and peace in the world,

Recognizing that these rights derive from the inherent dignity of the human person,

Recognizing that, in accordance with the Universal Declaration of Human Rights, the ideal of free human beings enjoying freedom from fear and want can only be achieved if conditions are created whereby everyone may enjoy his economic, social and cultural rights, as well as his civil and political rights,

Considering the obligation of States under the Charter of the United Nations to promote universal respect for, and observance of, human rights and freedoms,

Realizing that the individual, having duties to other individuals and to the community to which he belongs, is under a responsibility to strive for the promotion and observance of the rights recognized in the present Covenant,

Agree upon the following articles:

PART I

Article 1

1. All peoples have the right of self-determination. By virtue of that right they freely determine their political status and freely pursue their economic, social and cultural development.
2. All peoples may, for their own ends, freely dispose of their natural wealth and resources without prejudice to any obligations arising out of international economic cooperation, based upon the principle of mutual benefit, and international law. In no case may a people be deprived of its own means of subsistence.
3. The States Parties to the present Covenant, including those having responsibility for the administration of Non-Self-Governing and Trust Territories, shall promote the realization of the right of self-determination, and shall respect that right, in conformity with the provisions of the Charter of the United Nations.

PART II

Article 2

1. Each State Party to the present Covenant undertakes to take steps, individually and through international assistance and cooperation, especially economic and technical, to the maximum of its available resources, with a view to achieving progressively the full realization of the rights recognized in the present Covenant by all appropriate means, including particularly the adoption of legislative measures.

2. The States Parties to the present Covenant undertake to guarantee that the rights enunciated in the present Covenant will be exercised without discrimination of any kind as to race, colour, sex, language, religion, political or other opinion, national or social origin, property, birth or other status.

3. Developing countries, with due regard to human rights and their national economy, may determine to what extent they would guarantee the economic rights recognized in the present Covenant to non-nationals.

Article 3

The States Parties to the present Covenant undertake to ensure the equal right of men and women to the enjoyment of all economic, social and cultural rights set forth in the present Covenant.

Article 4

The States Parties to the present Covenant recognize that, in the enjoyment of those rights provided by the State in conformity with the present Covenant, the State may subject such rights only to such limitations as are determined by law only insofar as this may be compatible with the nature of these rights and solely for the purpose of promoting the general welfare in a democratic society.

Article 5

1. Nothing in the present Covenant may be interpreted as implying for any State, group or person any right to engage in any activity or to perform any act aimed at the destruction of any of the rights or freedoms recognized herein, or at their limitation to a greater extent than is provided for in the present Covenant.

2. No restriction upon or derogation from any of the fundamental human rights recognized or existing in any country in virtue of law, conventions, regulations or custom shall be admitted on the pretext that the present Covenant does not recognize such rights or that it recognizes them to a lesser extent.

PART III

Article 6

1. The States Parties to the present Covenant recognize the right to work, which includes the right of everyone to the opportunity to gain his living by work which he freely chooses or accepts, and will take appropriate steps to safeguard this right.

2. The steps to be taken by a State Party to the present Covenant to achieve the full realization of this right shall include technical and vocational guidance and training programmes, policies and techniques to achieve steady economic, social and cultural development and full and productive employment under conditions safeguarding fundamental political and economic freedoms to the individual.

Article 7

The States Parties to the present Covenant recognize the right of everyone to the enjoyment of just and favourable conditions of work which ensure, in particular:

a. Remuneration which provides all workers, as a minimum, with:
  (i) Fair wages and equal remuneration for work of equal value without distinction of any kind, in particular women being guaranteed conditions of work not inferior to those enjoyed by men, with equal pay for equal work;
  (ii) A decent living for themselves and their families in accordance with the provisions of the present Covenant;
b. Safe and healthy working conditions;
c. Equal opportunity for everyone to be promoted in his employment to an appropriate higher level, subject to no considerations other than those of seniority and competence;
d. Rest, leisure and reasonable limitation of working hours and periodic holidays with pay, as well as remuneration for public holidays.

Article 8

1. The States Parties to the present Covenant undertake to ensure:
   a. The right of everyone to form trade unions and join the trade union of his choice, subject only to the rules of the organization concerned, for the promotion and protection of his economic and social interests. No restrictions may be placed on the exercise of this right other than those prescribed by law and which are necessary in a democratic society in the interests of national security or public order or for the protection of the rights and freedoms of others;
   b. The right of trade unions to establish national federations or confederations and the right of the latter to form or join international trade-union organizations;
   c. The right of trade unions to function freely subject to no limitations other than those prescribed by law and which are necessary in a democratic society in the interests of national security or public order or for the protection of the rights and freedoms of others;
   d. The right to strike, provided that it is exercised in conformity with the laws of the particular country.
2. This article shall not prevent the imposition of lawful restrictions on the exercise of these rights by members of the armed forces or of the police or of the administration of the State.
3. Nothing in this article shall authorize States Parties to the International Labor Organisation Convention of 1948 concerning Freedom of Association and Protection of the Right to Organize to take legislative measures which would prejudice, or apply the law in such a manner as would prejudice, the guarantees provided for in that Convention.

Article 9

The States Parties to the present Covenant recognize the right of everyone to social security, including social insurance.

Article 10

The States Parties to the present Covenant recognize that:
1. The widest possible protection and assistance should be accorded to the family, which is the natural and fundamental group unit of society, particularly for its establishment and while it is responsible for the care and education of dependent children. Marriage must be entered into with the free consent of the intending spouses.

2. Special protection should be accorded to mothers during a reasonable period before and after childbirth. During such period working mothers should be accorded paid leave or leave with adequate social security benefits.
3. Special measures of protection and assistance should be taken on behalf of all children and young persons without any discrimination for reasons of parentage or other conditions. Children and young persons should be protected from economic and social exploitation. Their employment in work harmful to their morals or health or dangerous to life or likely to hamper their normal development should be punishable by law. States should also set age limits below which the paid employment of child labour should be prohibited and punishable by law.

Article 11

1. The States Parties to the present Covenant recognize the right of everyone to an adequate standard of living for himself and his family, including adequate food, clothing and housing, and to the continuous improvement of living conditions. The States Parties will take appropriate steps to ensure the realization of this right, recognizing to this effect the essential importance of international cooperation based on free consent.
2. The States Parties to the present Covenant, recognizing the fundamental right of everyone to be free from hunger, shall take, individually and through international cooperation, the measures, including specific programmes, which are needed;
   a. To improve methods of production, conservation and distribution of food by making full use of technical and scientific knowledge, by disseminating knowledge of the principles of nutrition and by developing or reforming agrarian systems in such a way as to achieve the most efficient development and utilization of natural resources;
   b. Taking into account the problems of both food-importing and food-exporting countries, to ensure an equitable distribution of world food supplies in relation to need.

Article 12

1. The States Parties to the present Covenant recognize the right of everyone to the enjoyment of the highest attainable standard of physical and mental health.
2. The steps to be taken by the States Parties to the present Covenant to achieve the full realization of this right shall include those necessary for:
   a. The provision for the reduction of the stillbirth rate and of infant mortality and for the healthy development of the child;
   b. The improvement of all aspects of environmental and industrial hygiene;
   c. The prevention, treatment and control of epidemic, endemic, occupational and other diseases;
   d. The creation of conditions which would assure to all medical service and medical attention in the event of sickness.

Article 13

1. The States Parties to the present Covenant recognize the right of everyone to education. They agree that education shall be directed to the full development of the human personality and the sense of its dignity, and shall strengthen the respect for human rights and fundamental freedoms. They further agree that education shall enable all persons to participate effectively in a free society, promote understanding, tolerance and friendship among all nations and all racial, ethnic or religious groups, and further the activities of the United Nations for the maintenance of peace.

2. The States Parties to the present Covenant recognize that, with a view to achieving the full realization of this right:
   a. Primary education shall be compulsory and available free to all;
   b. Secondary education in its different forms, including technical and voca-
      tional secondary education, shall be made generally available and accessible
      to all by every appropriate means, and in particular by the progressive intro-
      duction of free education;
   c. Higher education shall be made equally accessible to all, on the basis of
      capacity, by every appropriate means, and in particular by the progressive
      introduction of free education;
   d. Fundamental education shall be encouraged or intensified as far as possible
      for those persons who have not received or completed the whole period of
      their primary education;
   e. The development of a system of schools at all levels shall be actively pursued,
      an adequate fellowship system shall be established, and the material condi-
      tions of teaching staff shall be continuously improved.
3. The States Parties to the present Covenant undertake to have respect for the
   liberty of parents and, when applicable, legal guardians to choose for their children schools other than those established by the public authorities, which
   conform to such minimum educational standards as may be laid down or
   approved by the State and to ensure the religious and moral education of their
   children in conformity with their own convictions.
4. No part of this article shall be construed so as to interfere with the liberty of
   individuals and bodies to establish and direct educational institutions, subject
   always to the observance of the principles set forth in paragraph 1 of this article and to the requirement that the education given in such institutions shall
   conform to such minimum standards as may be laid down by the State.

Article 14

Each State Party to the present Covenant which, at the time of becoming a Party, has
not been able to secure in its metropolitan territory or other territories under its jurisdiction compulsory primary education, free of charge, undertakes within two years
to work out and adopt a detailed plan of action for the progressive implementation,
within a reasonable number of years, to be fixed in the plan, of the principle of
compulsory education free of charge for all.

Article 15

1. The States Parties to the present Covenant recognize the right of everyone:
   a. To take part in cultural life;
   b. To enjoy the benefits of scientific progress and its applications;
   c. To benefit from the protection of the moral and material interests resulting
      from any scientific, literary or artistic production of which he is the author.
2. The steps to be taken by the States Parties to the present Covenant to achieve the
   full realization of this right shall include those necessary for the conservation, the
   development and the diffusion of science and culture.
3. The States Parties to the present Covenant undertake to respect the freedom
   indispensable for scientific research and creative activity.
4. The States Parties to the present Covenant recognize the benefits to be derived
   from the encouragement and development of international contacts and cooperation in the scientific and cultural fields.

PART IV

Article 16

1. The States Parties to the present Covenant undertake to submit in conformity with this part of the Covenant reports on the measures which they have adopted and the progress made in achieving the observance of the rights recognized herein.

2. a. All reports shall be submitted to the Secretary-General of the United Nations, who shall transmit copies to the Economic and Social Council for consideration in accordance with the provisions of the present Covenant;

   b. The Secretary-General of the United Nations shall also transmit to the specialized agencies copies of the reports, or any relevant parts therefrom, from States Parties to the present Covenant which are also members of these specialized agencies insofar as these reports, or parts therefrom, relate to any matters which fall within the responsibilities of the said agencies in accordance with their constitutional instruments.

Article 17

1. The States Parties to the present Covenant shall furnish their reports in stages, in accordance with a programme to be established by the Economic and Social Council within one year of the entry into force of the present Covenant after consultation with the States Parties and the specialized agencies concerned.

2. Reports may indicate factors and difficulties affecting the degree of fulfillment of obligations under the present Covenant.

3. Where relevant information has previously been furnished to the United Nations or to any specialized agency by any State Party to the present Covenant, it will not be necessary to reproduce that information, but a precise reference to the information so furnished will suffice.

Article 18

Pursuant to its responsibilities under the Charter of the United Nations in the field of human rights and fundamental freedoms, the Economic and Social Council may make arrangements with the specialized agencies in respect of their reporting to it on the progress made in achieving the observance of the provisions of the present Covenant falling within the scope of their activities. These reports may include particulars of decisions and recommendations on such implementation adopted by their competent organs.

Article 19

The Economic and Social Council may transmit to the Commission on Human Rights for study and general recommendation or, as appropriate, for information the reports concerning human rights submitted by States in accordance with articles 16 and 17, and those concerning human rights submitted by the specialized agencies in accordance with article 18.

Article 20

The States Parties to the present Covenant and the specialized agencies concerned may submit comments to the Economic and Social Council on any general recommendation under article 19 or reference to such general recommendation in any report of the Commission on Human Rights or any documentation referred to therein.

Article 21

The Economic and Social Council may submit from time to time to the General Assembly reports with recommendations of a general nature and a summary of the information received from the States Parties to the present Covenant and the specialized agencies on the measures taken and the progress made in achieving general observance of the rights recognized in the present Covenant.

Article 22

The Economic and Social Council may bring to the attention of other organs of the United Nations, their subsidiary organs and specialized agencies concerned with furnishing technical assistance any matters arising out of the reports referred to in this part of the present Covenant which may assist such bodies in deciding, each within its field of competence, on the advisability of international measures likely to contribute to the effective progressive implementation of the present Covenant.

Article 23

The States Parties to the present Covenant agree that international action for the achievement of the rights recognized in the present Covenant includes such methods as the conclusion of conventions, the adoption of recommendations, the furnishing of technical assistance and the holding of regional meetings and technical meetings for the purpose of consultation and study organized in conjunction with the Governments concerned.

Article 24

Nothing in the present Covenant shall be interpreted as impairing the provisions of the Charter of the United Nations and of the constitutions of the specialized agencies which define the respective responsibilities of the various organs of the United Nations and of the specialized agencies in regard to the matters dealt with in the present Covenant.

Article 25

Nothing in the present Covenant shall be interpreted as impairing the inherent right of all peoples to enjoy and utilize fully and freely their natural wealth and resources.

PART V
Article 26

1. The present Covenant is open for signature by any State Member of the United Nations or member of any of its specialized agencies, by any State Party to the Statute of the International Court of Justice, and by any other State which has been invited by the General Assembly of the United Nations to become a party to the present Covenant.
2. The present Covenant is subject to ratification. Instruments of ratification shall be deposited with the Secretary-General of the United Nations.
3. The present Covenant shall be open to accession by any State referred to in paragraph 1 of this article.
4. Accession shall be effected by the deposit of an instrument of accession with the Secretary-General of the United Nations.
5. The Secretary-General of the United Nations shall inform all States which have signed the present Covenant or acceded to it of the deposit of each instrument of ratification or accession.

Article 27

1. The present Covenant shall enter into force three months after the date of the deposit with the Secretary-General of the United Nations of the thirty-fifth instrument of ratification or instrument of accession.
2. For each State ratifying the present Covenant or acceding to it after the deposit of the thirty-fifth instrument of ratification or instrument of accession, the

present Covenant shall enter into force three months after the date of the deposit of its own instrument of ratification or instrument of accession.

Article 28

The provisions of the present Covenant shall extend to all parts of federal States without any limitations or exceptions.

Article 29

1. Any State Party to the present Covenant may propose an amendment and file it with the Secretary-General of the United Nations. The Secretary-General shall thereupon communicate any proposed amendments to the States Parties to the present Covenant with a request that they notify him whether they favour a conference of States Parties for the purpose of considering and voting upon the proposals.

   In the event that at least one third of the States Parties favours such a conference, the Secretary-General shall convene the conference under the auspices of the United Nations. Any amendment adopted by a majority of the States parties present and voting at the conference shall be submitted to the General Assembly of the United Nations for approval.
2. Amendments shall come into force when they have been approved by the General Assembly of the United Nations and accepted by a two-thirds majority of the States Parties to the present Covenant in accordance with their respective constitutional processes.
3. When amendments come into force they shall be binding on those States Parties which have accepted them, other States Parties still being bound by the provisions of the present Covenant and any earlier amendment which they have accepted.

Article 30

Irrespective of the notifications made under article 26, paragraph 5, the Secretary-General of the United Nations shall inform all States referred to in paragraph 1 of the same article of the following particulars:
   a. Signatures, ratifications and accessions under article 26;
   b. The date of the entry into force of the present Covenant under article 27 and the date of the entry into force of any amendments under article 29.

Article 31

1. The present Covenant, of which the Chinese, English, French, Russian and Spanish texts are equally authentic, shall be deposited in the archives of the United Nations.
2. The Secretary-General of the United Nations shall transmit certified copies of the present Covenant to all States referred to in article 26.

Appendix C

International Covenant on Civil and Political Rights

Adopted and opened for signature, ratification, and accession by United Nations General Assembly resolution 2200 A (XXI) on 16 December 1966. Entered into force on 23 March 1976 in accordance with article 49.

PREAMBLE

The States Parties to the present Covenant,

Considering that, in accordance with the principles proclaimed in the Charter of the United Nations, recognition of the inherent dignity and of the equal and inalienable rights of all members of the human family is the foundation of freedom, justice and peace in the world,

Recognizing that these rights derive from the inherent dignity of the human person,

Recognizing that, in accordance with the Universal Declaration of Human Rights, the ideal of free human beings enjoying civil and political freedom and freedom from fear and want can only be achieved if conditions are created whereby everyone may enjoy his civil and political rights, as well as his economic, social and cultural rights,

Considering the obligation of States under the Charter of the United Nations to promote universal respect for, and observance of, human rights and freedoms,

Realizing that the individual, having duties to other individuals and to the community to which he belongs, is under a responsibility to strive for the promotion and observance of the rights recognized in the present Covenant,

Agree upon the following articles:

PART I

Article 1

1. All peoples have the right of self-determination. By virtue of that right they freely determine their political status and freely pursue their economic, social and cultural development.
2. All peoples may, for their own ends, freely dispose of their natural wealth and resources without prejudice to any obligations arising out of international economic cooperation, based upon the principle of mutual benefit, and international law. In no case may a people be deprived of its own means of subsistence.
3. The States Parties to the present Covenant, including those having responsibility for the administration of Non-Self-Governing and Trust Territories, shall promote the realization of the right of self-determination, and shall respect that right, in conformity with the provisions of the Charter of the United Nations.

PART II
Article 2

1. Each State Party to the present Covenant undertakes to respect and to ensure to all individuals within its territory and subject to its jurisdiction the rights recognized in the present Covenant, without distinction of any kind, such as race, colour, sex, language, religion, political or other opinion, national or social origin, property, birth or other status.
2. Where not already provided for by existing legislative or other measures, each State Party to the present Covenant undertakes to take the necessary steps, in accordance with its constitutional processes and with the provisions of the present Covenant, to adopt such legislative or other measures as may be necessary to give effect to the rights recognized in the present Covenant.
3. Each State Party to the present Covenant undertakes:
   a. To ensure that any person whose rights or freedoms as herein recognized are violated shall have an effective remedy, notwithstanding that the violation has been committed by persons acting in an official capacity;
   b. To ensure that any person claiming such a remedy shall have his right thereto determined by competent judicial, administrative or legislative authorities, or by any other competent authority provided for by the legal system of the State, and to develop the possibilities of judicial remedy;
   c. To ensure that the competent authorities shall enforce such remedies when granted.

Article 3

The States Parties to the present Covenant undertake to ensure the equal right of men and women to the enjoyment of all civil and political rights set forth in the present Covenant.

Article 4

1. In time of public emergency which threatens the life of the nation and the existence of which is officially proclaimed, the States Parties to the present Covenant may take measures derogating from their obligations under the present Covenant to the extent strictly required by the exigencies of the situation, provided that such measures are not inconsistent with their other obligations under international law and do not involve discrimination solely on the ground of race, colour, sex, language, religion or social origin.
2. No derogation from articles 6, 7, 8 (paragraphs 1 and 2), 11, 15, 16 and 18 may be made under this provision.
3. Any State Party to the present Covenant availing itself of the right of derogation shall immediately inform the other States Parties to the present Covenant, through the intermediary of the Secretary-General of the United Nations, of the provisions from which it has derogated and of the reasons by which it was actuated. A further communication shall be made, through the same intermediary, on the date on which it terminates such derogation.

Article 5

1. Nothing in the present Covenant may be interpreted as implying for any State, group or person any right to engage in any activity or perform any act aimed at the destruction of any of the rights and freedoms recognized herein or at their limitation to a greater extent than is provided for in the present Covenant.
2. There shall be no restriction upon or derogation from any of the fundamental human rights recognized or existing in any State Party to the present Covenant

pursuant to law, conventions, regulations or custom on the pretext that the present Covenant does not recognize such rights or that it recognizes them to a lesser extent.

PART III

Article 6

1. Every human being has the inherent right to life. This right shall be protected by law. No one shall be arbitrarily deprived of his life.
2. In countries which have not abolished the death penalty, sentence of death may be imposed only for the most serious crimes in accordance with the law in force at the time of the commission of the crime and not contrary to the provisions of the present Covenant and to the Convention on the Prevention and Punishment of the Crime of Genocide. This penalty can only be carried out pursuant to a final judgement rendered by a competent court.
3. When deprivation of life constitutes the crime of genocide, it is understood that nothing in this article shall authorize any State Party to the present Covenant to derogate in any way from any obligation assumed under the provisions of the Convention on the Prevention and Punishment of the Crime of Genocide.
4. Anyone sentenced to death shall have the right to seek pardon or commutation of the sentence. Amnesty, pardon or commutation of the sentence of death may be granted in all cases.
5. Sentence of death shall not be imposed for crimes committed by persons below eighteen years of age and shall not be carried out on pregnant women.
6. Nothing in this article shall be invoked to delay or to prevent the abolition of capital punishment by any State Party to the present Covenant.

Article 7

No one shall be subjected to torture or to cruel, inhuman or degrading treatment or punishment. In particular, no one shall be subjected without his free consent to medical or scientific experimentation.

Article 8

1. No one shall be held in slavery; slavery and the slave trade in all their forms shall be prohibited.
2. No one shall be held in servitude.
3. a. No one shall be required to perform forced or compulsory labour;
   b. Paragraph 3 (a) shall not be held to preclude, in countries where imprisonment with hard labour may be imposed as a punishment for a crime, the performance of hard labour in pursuance of a sentence to such punishment by a competent court;
   c. For the purpose of this paragraph the term "forced or compulsory labour" shall not include:
      (i) Any work or service, not referred to in subparagraph (b), normally required of a person who is under detention in consequence of a lawful order of a court, or of a person during conditional release from such detention;
      (ii) Any service of a military character and, in countries where conscientious objection is recognized, any national service required by law of conscientious objectors;
      (iii) Any service exacted in cases of emergency or calamity threatening the life or well-being of the community;
      (iv) Any work or service which forms part of normal civil obligations.

Article 9

1. Everyone has the right to liberty and security of person. No one shall be subjected to arbitrary arrest or detention. No one shall be deprived of his liberty except on such grounds and in accordance with such procedure as are established by law.
2. Anyone who is arrested shall be informed, at the time of arrest, of the reasons for his arrest and shall be promptly informed of any charges against him.
3. Anyone arrested or detained on a criminal charge shall be brought promptly before a judge or other officer authorized by law to exercise judicial power and shall be entitled to trial within a reasonable time or to release. It shall not be the general rule that persons awaiting trial shall be detained in custody, but release may be subject to guarantees to appear for trial, at any other stage of the judicial proceedings, and, should occasion arise, for execution of the judgement.
4. Anyone who is deprived of his liberty by arrest or detention shall be entitled to take proceedings before a court, in order that that court may decide without delay on the lawfulness of his detention and order his release if the detention is not lawful.
5. Anyone who has been victim of unlawful arrest or detention shall have an enforceable right to compensation.

Article 10

1. All persons deprived of their liberty shall be treated with humanity and with respect for the inherent dignity of the human person.
2. a. Accused persons shall, save in exceptional circumstances, be segregated from convicted persons and shall be subject to separate treatment appropriate to their status as unconvicted persons;
   b. Accused juvenile persons shall be separated from adults and brought as speedily as possible for adjudication.
3. The penitentiary system shall comprise treatment of prisoners the essential aim of which shall be their reformation and social rehabilitation. Juvenile offenders shall be segregated from adults and be accorded treatment appropriate to their age and legal status.

Article 11

No one shall be imprisoned merely on the ground of inability to fulfil a contractual obligation.

Article 12

1. Everyone lawfully within the territory of a State shall, within that territory, have the right to liberty of movement and freedom to choose his residence.
2. Everyone shall be free to leave any country, including his own.
3. The above-mentioned rights shall not be subject to any restrictions except those which are provided by law, are necessary to protect national security, public order (*ordre public*), public health or morals or the rights and freedoms of others, and are consistent with the other rights recognized in the present Covenant.
4. No one shall be arbitrarily deprived of the right to enter his own country.

Article 13

An alien lawfully in the territory of a State Party to the present Covenant may be expelled therefrom only in pursuance of a decision reached in accordance with law and shall, except where compelling reasons of national security otherwise require, be allowed to submit the reasons against his expulsion and to have his case reviewed by, and be represented for the purpose before, the competent authority or a person or persons especially designated by the competent authority.

Article 14

1. All persons shall be equal before the courts and tribunals. In the determination of any criminal charge against him, or of his rights and obligations in a suit at law, everyone shall be entitled to a fair and public hearing by a competent, independent and impartial tribunal established by law. The Press and the public may be excluded from all or part of a trial for reasons of morals, public order (*ordre public*) or national security in a democratic society, or when the interest of the private lives of the Parties so requires, or to the extent strictly necessary in the opinion of the court in special circumstances where publicity would prejudice the interests of justice; but any judgement rendered in a criminal case or in a suit at law shall be made public except where the interest of juvenile persons otherwise requires or the proceedings concern matrimonial disputes or the guardianship of children.

2. Everyone charged with a criminal offence shall have the right to be presumed innocent until proved guilty according to law.

3. In the determination of any criminal charge against him, everyone shall be entitled to the following minimum guarantees, in full equality:

   a. To be informed promptly and in detail in a language which he understands of the nature and cause of the charge against him;
   b. To have adequate time and facilities for the preparation of his defence and to communicate with counsel of his own choosing;
   c. To be tried without undue delay;
   d. To be tried in his presence, and to defend himself in person or through legal assistance of his own choosing; to be informed, if he does not have legal assistance, of this right; and to have legal assistance assigned to him, in any case where the interests of justice so require, and without payment by him in any such case if he does not have sufficient means to pay for it;
   e. To examine, or have examined, the witnesses against him and to obtain the attendance and examination of witnesses on his behalf under the same conditions as witnesses against him;
   f. To have the free assistance of an interpreter if he cannot understand or speak the language used in court;
   g. Not to be compelled to testify against himself or to confess guilt.

4. In the case of juvenile persons, the procedure shall be such as will take account of their age and the desirability of promoting their rehabilitation.

5. Everyone convicted of a crime shall have the right to his conviction and sentence being reviewed by a higher tribunal according to law.

6. When a person has by a final decision been convicted of a criminal offence and when subsequently his conviction has been reversed or he has been pardoned on the ground that a new or newly discovered fact shows conclusively that there has been a miscarriage of justice, the person who has suffered punishment as a result of such conviction shall be compensated according to law, unless it is proved that the non-disclosure of the unknown fact in time is wholly or partly attributable to him.

7. No one shall be liable to be tried or punished again for an offence for which he has already been finally convicted or acquitted in accordance with the law and penal procedure of each country.

Article 15

1. No one shall be held guilty of any criminal offence on account of any act or omission which did not constitute a criminal offence, under national or inter-

national law, at the time when it was committed. Nor shall a heavier penalty be imposed than the one that was applicable at the time when the criminal offence was committed. If, subsequent to the commission of the offence, provision is made by law for the imposition of the lighter penalty, the offender shall benefit thereby.

2. Nothing in this article shall prejudice the trial and punishment of any person for any act or omission which, at the time when it was committed, was criminal according to the general principles of law recognized by the community of nations.

Article 16

Everyone shall have the right to recognition everywhere as a person before the law.

Article 17

1. No one shall be subjected to arbitrary or unlawful interference with his privacy, family, home or correspondence, nor to unlawful attacks on his honour and reputation.
2. Everyone has the right to the protection of the law against such interference or attacks.

Article 18

1. Everyone shall have the right to freedom of thought, conscience and religion. This right shall include freedom to have or to adopt a religion or belief of his choice, and freedom, either individually or in community with others and in public or private, to manifest his religion or belief in worship, observance, practice and teaching.
2. No one shall be subject to coercion which would impair his freedom to have or to adopt a religion or belief of his choice.
3. Freedom to manifest one's religion or beliefs may be subject only to such limitations as are prescribed by law and are necessary to protect public safety, order, health, or morals or the fundamental rights and freedoms of others.
4. The States Parties to the present Covenant undertake to have respect for the liberty of parents and, when applicable, legal guardians to ensure the religious and moral education of their children in conformity with their own convictions.

Article 19

1. Everyone shall have the right to hold opinions without interference.
2. Everyone shall have the right to freedom of expression; this right shall include freedom to seek, receive and impart information and ideas of all kinds, regardless of frontiers, either orally, in writing or in print, in the form of art, or through any other media of his choice.
3. The exercise of the rights provided for in paragraph 2 of this article carries with it special duties and responsibilities. It may therefore be subject to certain restrictions, but these shall only be such as are provided by law and are necessary:
   a. For respect of the rights or reputations of others;
   b. For the protection of national security or of public order (*ordre public*), or of public health or morals.

Article 20

1. Any propaganda for war shall be prohibited by law.
2. Any advocacy of national, racial or religious hatred that constitutes incitement to discrimination, hostility or violence shall be prohibited by law.

Article 21

The right of peaceful assembly shall be recognized. No restrictions may be placed on the exercise of this right other than those imposed in conformity with the law and which are necessary in a democratic society in the interests of national security or public safety, public order (*ordre public*), the protection of public health or morals or the protection of the rights and freedoms of others.

Article 22

1. Everyone shall have the right to freedom of association with others, including the right to form and join trade unions for the protection of his interests.
2. No restrictions may be placed on the exercise of this right other than those which are prescribed by law and which are necessary in a democratic society in the interests of national security or public safety, public order (*ordre public*), the protection of public health or morals or the protection of the rights and freedoms of others. This article shall not prevent the imposition of lawful restrictions on members of the armed forces and of the police in their exercise of this right.
3. Nothing in this article shall authorize States Parties to the International Labour Organisation Convention of 1948 concerning Freedom of Association and Protection of the Right to Organize to take legislative measures which would prejudice, or to apply the law in such a manner as to prejudice the guarantees provided for in that Convention.

Article 23

1. The family is the natural and fundamental group unit of society and is entitled to protection by society and the State.
2. The right of men and women of marriageable age to marry and to found a family shall be recognized.
3. No marriage shall be entered into without the free and full consent of the intending spouses.
4. States Parties to the present Covenant shall take appropriate steps to ensure equality of rights and responsibilities of spouses as to marriage, during marriage and at its dissolution. In the case of dissolution, provision shall be made for the necessary protection of any children.

Article 24

1. Every child shall have, without any discrimination as to race, colour, sex, language, religion, national or social origin, property or birth, the right to such measures of protection as are required by his status as a minor, on the part of his family, society and the State.
2. Every child shall be registered immediately after birth and shall have a name.
3. Every child has the right to acquire a nationality.

Article 25

Every citizen shall have the right and the opportunity, without any of the distinctions mentioned in article 2 and without unreasonable restrictions:

    a. To take part in the conduct of public affairs, directly or through freely chosen representatives;

    b. To vote and to be elected at genuine periodic elections which shall be by universal and equal suffrage and shall be held by secret ballot, guaranteeing the free expression of the will of the electors;

    c. To have access, on general terms of equality, to public service in his country.

Article 26

All persons are equal before the law and are entitled without any discrimination to the equal protection of the law. In this respect, the law shall prohibit any discrimination and guarantee to all persons equal and effective protection against discrimination on any ground such as race, colour, sex, language, religion, political or other opinion, national or social origin, property, birth or other status.

Article 27

In those States in which ethnic, religious or linguistic minorities exist, persons belonging to such minorities shall not be denied the right, in community with the other members of their group, to enjoy their own culture, to profess and practice their own religion, or to use their own language.

PART IV

Article 28

1. There shall be established a Human Rights Committee (hereafter referred to in the present Covenant as the Committee). It shall consist of eighteen members and shall carry out the functions hereinafter provided.
2. The Committee shall be composed of nationals of the States Parties to the present Covenant who shall be persons of high moral character and recognized competence in the field of human rights, consideration being given to the usefulness of the participation of some persons having legal experience.
3. The members of the Committee shall be elected and shall serve in their personal capacity.

Article 29

1. The members of the Committee shall be elected by secret ballot from a list of persons possessing the qualifications prescribed in article 28 and nominated for the purpose by the States Parties to the present Covenant.
2. Each State Party to the present Covenant may nominate not more than two persons. These persons shall be nationals of the nominating State.
3. A person shall be eligible for renomination.

Article 30

1. The initial election shall be held no later than six months after the date of the entry into force of the present Covenant.
2. At least four months before the date of each election to the Committee, other than an election to fill a vacancy declared in accordance with article 34, the Secretary-General of the United Nations shall address a written invitation to the States Parties to the present Covenant to submit their nominations for membership of the Committee within three months.
3. The Secretary-General of the United Nations shall prepare a list in alphabetical order of all the persons thus nominated, with an indication of the States Parties which have nominated them, and shall submit it to the States Parties to the present Covenant no later than one month before the date of each election.
4. Elections of the members of the Committee shall be held at a meeting of the States Parties to the present Covenant convened by the Secretary-General of the United Nations at the Headquarters of the United Nations. At that meeting, for which two-thirds of the States Parties to the present Covenant shall constitute a quorum, the persons elected to the Committee shall be those nominees who obtain the largest number of votes and an absolute majority of the votes of the representatives of States Parties present and voting.

Article 31

1. The Committee may not include more than one national of the same State.
2. In the election of the Committee, consideration shall be given to equitable geographical distribution of membership and to the representation of the different forms of civilization and of the principal legal systems.

Article 32

1. The members of the Committee shall be elected for a term of four years. They shall be eligible for re-election if renominated. However, the terms of nine of the members elected at the first election shall expire at the end of two years; immediately after the first election, the names of these nine members shall be chosen by lot by the Chairman of the meeting referred to in article 30, paragraph 4.
2. Elections at the expiry of office shall be held in accordance with the preceding articles of this part of the present Covenant.

Article 33

1. If, in the unanimous opinion of the other members, a member of the Committee has ceased to carry out his functions for any cause other than absence of a temporary character, the Chairman of the Committee shall notify the Secretary-General of the United Nations, who shall then declare the seat of that member to be vacant.
2. In the event of the death or the resignation of a member of the Committee, the Chairman shall immediately notify the Secretary-General of the United Nations, who shall declare the seat vacant from the date of death or the date on which the resignation takes effect.

Article 34

1. When a vacancy is declared in accordance with article 33 and if the term of office of the member to be replaced does not expire within six months of the declaration of the vacancy, the Secretary-General of the United Nations shall notify each of the States Parties to the present Covenant, which may within two months submit nominations in accordance with article 29 for the purpose of filling the vacancy.
2. The Secretary-General of the United Nations shall prepare a list in alphabetical order of the persons thus nominated and shall submit it to the States Parties to the present Covenant. The election to fill the vacancy shall then take place in accordance with the relevant provisions of this part of the present Covenant.
3. A member of the Committee elected to fill a vacancy declared in accordance with article 33 shall hold office for the remainder of the term of the member who vacated the seat on the Committee under the provisions of that article.

Article 35

The members of the Committee shall, with the approval of the General Assembly of the United Nations, receive emoluments from United Nations resources on such terms and conditions as the General Assembly may decide, having regard to the importance of the Committee's responsibilities.

Article 36

The Secretary-General of the United Nations shall provide the necessary staff and facilities for the effective performance of the functions of the Committee under the present Covenant.

Article 37

1. The Secretary-General of the United Nations shall convene the initial meeting of the Committee at the Headquarters of the United Nations.
2. After its initial meeting, the Committee shall meet at such times as shall be provided in its rules of procedure.
3. The Committee shall normally meet at the Headquarters of the United Nations or at the United Nations Office at Geneva.

Article 38

Every member of the Committee shall, before taking up his duties, make a solemn declaration in open committee that he will perform his functions impartially and conscientiously.

Article 39

1. The Committee shall elect its officers for a term of two years. They may be re-elected.
2. The Committee shall establish its own rules of procedure, but these rules shall provide, inter alia, that:
   a. Twelve members shall constitute a quorum;
   b. Decisions of the Committee shall be made by a majority vote of the members present.

Article 40

1. The States Parties to the present Covenant undertake to submit reports on the measures they have adopted which give effect to the rights recognized herein and on the progress made in the enjoyment of those rights:
   a. Within one year of the entry into force of the present Covenant for the States Parties concerned;
   b. Thereafter whenever the Committee so requests.
2. All reports shall be submitted to the Secretary-General of the United Nations, who shall transmit them to the Committee for consideration. Reports shall indicate the factors and difficulties, if any, affecting the implementation of the present Covenant.
3. The Secretary-General of the United Nations may, after consultation with the Committee, transmit to the specialized agencies concerned copies of such parts of the reports as may fall within their field of competence.
4. The Committee shall study the reports submitted by the States Parties to the present Covenant. It shall transmit its reports, and such general comments as it may consider appropriate, to the States Parties. The Committee may also transmit to the Economic and Social Council these comments along with the copies of the reports it has received from States Parties to the present Covenant.
5. The States Parties to the present Covenant may submit to the Committee observations on any comments that may be made in accordance with paragraph 4 of this article.

Article 41

1. A State Party to the present Covenant may at any time declare under this article that it recognizes the competence of the Committee to receive and consider communications to the effect that a State Party claims that another State Party is not fulfiling its obligations under the present Covenant. Communications under this article may be received and considered only if submitted by a State Party which has made a declaration recognizing in regard to itself the competence of the Committee. No communication shall be received by the Commit-

tee if it concerns a State Party which has not made such a declaration. Communications received under this article shall be dealt with in accordance with the following procedure:

a. If a State Party to the present Covenant considers that another State Party is not giving effect to the provisions of the present Covenant, it may, by written communication, bring the matter to the attention of that State Party. Within three months after the receipt of the communication the receiving State shall afford the State which sent the communication an explanation, or any other statement in writing clarifying the matter which should include, to the extent possible and pertinent, reference to domestic procedures and remedies taken, pending, or available in the matter;

b. If the matter is not adjusted to the satisfaction of both States Parties concerned within six months after the receipt by the receiving State of the initial communication, either State shall have the right to refer the matter to the Committee, by notice given to the Committee and to the other State;

c. The Committee shall deal with a matter referred to it only after it has ascertained that all available domestic remedies have been invoked and exhausted in the matter, in conformity with the generally recognized principles of international law. This shall not be the rule where the application of the remedies is unreasonably prolonged;

d. The Committee shall hold closed meetings when examining communications under this article;

e. Subject to the provisions of subparagraph (c), the Committee shall make available its good offices to the States Parties concerned with a view to a friendly solution of the matter on the basis of respect for human rights and fundamental freedoms as recognized in the present Covenant;

f. In any matter referred to it, the Committee may call upon the States Parties concerned, referred to in subparagraph (b), to supply any relevant information;

g. The States Parties concerned, referred to in subparagraph (b), shall have the right to be represented when the matter is being considered in the Committee and to make submissions orally and/or in writing;

h. The Committee shall, within twelve months after the date of receipt of notice under subparagraph (b), submit a report;

   (i)   If a solution within the terms of subparagraph (e) is reached, the Committee shall confine its report to a brief statement of the facts and of the solution reached;

   (ii) If a solution within the terms of subparagraph (e) is not reached, the Committee shall confine its report to a brief statement of the facts; the written submissions and record of the oral submissions made by the States Parties concerned shall be attached to the report. In every matter, the report shall be communicated to the States Parties concerned.

2. The provisions of this article shall come into force when ten States Parties to the present Covenant have made declarations under paragraph 1 of this article. Such declarations shall be deposited by the States Parties with the Secretary-General of the United Nations, who shall transmit copies thereof to the other States Parties. A declaration may be withdrawn at any time by notification to the Secretary-General. Such a withdrawal shall not prejudice the consideration of any matter which is the subject of a communication already transmitted under this article; no further communication by any State Party shall be received after the notification of withdrawal of the declaration has been received by the Secretary-General, unless the State Party concerned has made a new declaration.

Article 42

1. a. If a matter referred to the Committee in accordance with article 41 is not resolved to the satisfaction of the States Parties concerned, the Committee may, with the prior consent of the States Parties concerned, appoint an *ad hoc* Conciliation Commission (hereinafter referred to as the Commission). The good offices of the Commission shall be made available to the States Parties concerned with a view to an amicable solution of the matter on the basis of respect for the present Covenant;

    b. The Commission shall consist of five persons acceptable to the States Parties concerned. If the States Parties concerned fail to reach agreement within three months on all or part of the composition of the Commission, the members of the Commission concerning whom no agreement has been reached shall be elected by secret ballot by a two-thirds majority vote of the Committee from among its members.

2. The members of the Commission shall serve in their personal capacity. They shall not be nationals of the States Parties concerned, or of a State not Party to the present Covenant, or of a State Party which has not made a declaration under article 41.

3. The Commission shall elect its own Chairman and adopt its own rules of procedure.

4. The meetings of the Commission shall normally be held at the Headquarters of the United Nations or at the United Nations Office at Geneva. However, they may be held at such other convenient places as the Commission may determine in consultation with the Secretary-General of the United Nations and the States Parties concerned.

5. The secretariat provided in accordance with article 36 shall also service the commissions appointed under this article.

6. The information received and collated by the Committee shall be made available to the Commission, and the Commission may call upon the States Parties concerned to supply any other relevant information.

7. When the Commission has fully considered the matter, but in any event not later than twelve months after having been seized of the matter, it shall submit to the Chairman of the Committee a report for communication to the States Parties concerned:

    a. If the Commission is unable to complete its consideration of the matter within twelve months, it shall confine its report to a brief statement of the status of its consideration of the matter;

    b. If an amicable solution to the matter on the basis of respect for human rights as recognized in the present Covenant is reached, the Commission shall confine its report to a brief statement of the facts and of the solution reached;

    c. If a solution within the terms of subparagraph (b) is not reached, the Commission's report shall embody its findings on all questions of fact relevant to the issues between the States Parties concerned, and its views on the possibilities of an amicable solution of the matter. This report shall also contain the written submissions and a record of the oral submissions made by the States Parties concerned;

    d. If the Commission's report is submitted under subparagraph (c), the States Parties concerned shall, within three months of the receipt of the report, notify the Chairman of the Committee whether or not they accept the contents of the report of the Commission.

8. The provisions of this article are without prejudice to the responsibilities of the Committee under article 41.

9. The States Parties concerned shall share equally all the expenses of the members

of the Commission in accordance with estimates to be provided by the Secretary-General of the United Nations.

10. The Secretary-General of the United Nations shall be empowered to pay the expenses of the members of the Commission, if necessary, before reimbursement by the States Parties concerned, in accordance with paragraph 9 of this article.

Article 43

The members of the Committee, and of the ad hoc conciliation commissions which may be appointed under article 42, shall be entitled to the facilities, privileges and immunities of experts on mission for the United Nations as laid down in the relevant sections of the Convention on the Privileges and Immunities of the United Nations.

Article 44

The provisions for the implementation of the present Covenant shall apply without prejudice to the procedures prescribed in the field of human rights by or under the constituent instruments and the conventions of the United Nations and of the specialized agencies and shall not prevent the States Parties to the present Covenant from having recourse to other procedures for settling a dispute in accordance with general or special international agreements in force between them.

Article 45

The Committee shall submit to the General Assembly of the United Nations, through the Economic and Social Council, an annual report on its activities.

PART V
Article 46

Nothing in the present Covenant shall be interpreted as impairing the provisions of the Charter of the United Nations and of the constitutions of the specialized agencies which define the respective responsibilities of the various organs of the United Nations and of the specialized agencies in regard to the matters dealt with in the present Covenant.

Article 47

Nothing in the present Covenant shall be interpreted as impairing the inherent right of all peoples to enjoy and utilize fully and freely their natural wealth and resources.

PART VI
Article 48

1. The present Covenant is open for signature by any State Member of the United Nations or member of any of its specialized agencies, by any State Party to the Statute of the International Court of Justice, and by any other State which has been invited by the General Assembly of the United Nations to become a Party to the present Covenant.

2. The present Covenant is subject to ratification. Instruments of ratification shall be deposited with the Secretary-General of the United Nations.

3. The present Covenant shall be open to accession by any State referred to in paragraph 1 of this article.

4. Accession shall be effected by the deposit of an instrument of accession with the Secretary-General of the United Nations.

5. The Secretary-General of the United Nations shall inform all States which have signed this Covenant or acceded to it of the deposit of each instrument of ratification or accession.

Article 49

1. The present Covenant shall enter into force three months after the date of the deposit with the Secretary-General of the United Nations of the thirty-fifth instrument of ratification or instrument of accession.
2. For each State ratifying the present Covenant or acceding to it after the deposit of the thirty-fifth instrument of ratification or instrument of accession, the present Covenant shall enter into force three months after the date of the deposit of its own instrument of ratification or instrument of accession.

Article 50

The provisions of the present Covenant shall extend to all parts of federal States without any limitations or exceptions.

Article 51

1. Any State Party to the present Covenant may propose an amendment and file it with the Secretary-General of the United Nations. The Secretary-General of the United Nations shall thereupon communicate any proposed amendments to the States Parties to the present Covenant with a request that they notify him whether they favour a conference of States Parties for the purpose of considering and voting upon the proposals. In the event that at least one-third of the States Parties favours such a conference, the Secretary-General shall convene the conference under the auspices of the United Nations. Any amendment adopted by a majority of the States Parties present and voting at the conference shall be submitted to the General Assembly of the United Nations for approval.
2. Amendments shall come into force when they have been approved by the General Assembly of the United Nations and accepted by a two-thirds majority of the States Parties to the present Covenant in accordance with their respective constitutional processes.
3. When amendments come into force, they shall be binding on those States Parties which have accepted them, other States Parties still being bound by the provisions of the present Covenant and any earlier amendment which they have accepted.

Article 52

Irrespective of the notifications made under article 48, paragraph 5, the Secretary-General of the United Nations shall inform all States referred to in paragraph 1 of the same article of the following particulars:

a. Signatures, ratifications and accessions under article 48;
b. The date of the entry into force of the present Covenant under article 49 and the date of the entry into force of any amendments under article 51.

Article 53

1. The present Covenant, of which the Chinese, English, French, Russian and Spanish texts are equally authentic, shall be deposited in the archives of the United Nations.
2. The Secretary-General of the United Nations shall transmit certified copies of the present Covenant to all States referred to in article 48.

Appendix D

List of Additional
Selected Documents

INTERNATIONAL HUMAN RIGHTS INSTRUMENTS UNDER THE AUSPICES OF THE UNITED NATIONS

- Convention on the Prevention and Punishment of the Crime of Genocide (1948)
- Convention Relating to the Status of Refugees (1950)
- Standard Minimum Rules for the Treatment of Prisoners (1955)
- International Convention on the Elimination of All Forms of Racial Discrimination (1965)
- Protocol Relating to the Status of Refugees (1966)
- Convention on the Elimination of All Forms of Discrimination Against Women (1979)
- Declaration on the Elimination of All Forms of Intolerance and of Discrimination Based on Religion or Belief (1981)
- Convention Against Torture and Other Cruel, Inhuman or Degrading Treatment or Punishment (1984)
- ILO Convention Concerning Indigenous and Tribal Peoples in Independent Countries (1989)
- The Convention on the Rights of the Child (1989)

REGIONAL HUMAN RIGHTS INSTRUMENTS

- American Declaration of the Rights and Duties of Man (1948)
- European Convention for the Protection of Human Rights and Fundamental Freedoms, and its Nine Protocols (1959)
- European Social Charter (1961)
- American Convention on Human Rights (1969)
- Conference on Security and Cooperation in Europe: Final Act 1(a) (1975)
- The African (Banjul) Charter on Human and Peoples' Rights (1981)
- European Convention on the Prevention of Torture and Inhuman or Degrading Treatment (1987)
- The Cairo Declaration on Human Rights in Islam (1990)
- Charter of Paris for a New Europe: A New Era of Democracy, Peace and Unity (1990)

SEE ALSO

- Charter of the United Nations (1945)
- Declaration of Alma-Ata, Report of the International Conference on Primary Health Care, WHO and UNICEF (1978)
- Declaration on the Right to Development (1986)
- Vienna Declaration and Programme of Action, World Conference on Human Rights (1993). A/Conf. 157/23—12 July 1993.
- Programme of Action of the United Nations International Conference on Population and Development (Cairo) (1994). A/Conf. 171/13—18 October 1994.
- Beijing Declaration and Platform for Action Adopted by the Fourth World Conference on Women: Action for Equality, Development and Peace (1995). A Conf. 177/20—17 October 1995.

A good source for the texts of human rights documents is *Twenty-five Human Rights Documents* (New York: Center for the Study of Human Rights, Columbia University, 1994).

For human rights and health database, see the Global Lawyers and Physicians homepage: glphr.org.

Permission Acknowledgments

Ad Hoc Committee to Defend Health Care. *For Our Patients, Not For Profits: A Call to Action.* Reprinted from *JAMA* 1997; 278: 1733–34. Copyright 1997, American Medical Association. Reprinted with permission.

Adler, Nancy. Boyce, Thomas. Chesney, Margaret. Cohen, Sheldon. Folkman, Susan. Kahn, Robert. Syme, S. Leonard. *Socioeconomic Status and Health: The Challenge of the Gradient.* Reprinted from *American Psychologist*, 1994. Copyright © 1994 by American Psychological Association Reprinted with permission.

Annas, Catherine. *Irreversible Error: The Power and Prejudice of Female Genital Mutilation.* Reprinted from *Journal of Contemporary Health Law and Policy*, 1996, with permission.

Annas, George. *Health Policies and Human Rights: AIDS and TB Control.* Reprinted from *New England Journal of Medicine*, 1993. Copyright © 1993 by George J. Annas.

Annas, George. *Questing for Grails: Duplicity, Betrayal and Self-Deception in Postmodern Medical Research.* Reprinted from *Journal of Contemporary Health Law and Policy.* Copyright © 1993 by George J. Annas.

Annas, George. Grodin, Michael. *Human Rights and Maternal-Fetal HIV Transmission Prevention Trials in Africa.* Reprinted from *American Journal of Public Health*, © 1998 by American Public Health Association. Reprinted with permission.

Annas, George. Grodin, Michael. *Medicine and Human Rights: Reflections on the Fiftieth Anniversary of the Doctors' Trial.* Reprinted from *Health and Human Rights* 2 (1), with permission from the François-Xavier Bagnoud Center for Health and Human Rights, Harvard School of Public Health. Copyright © 1996 by the President and Fellows of Harvard College.

Center for Economic and Social Rights. *Rights Violations in the Ecuadorian Amazon: The Human Consequences of Oil Development.* Reprinted from *Health and Human Rights* 1 (1), with permission from the François-Xavier Bagnoud Center for Health and Human Rights, Harvard School of Public Health. Copyright © 1994 by the President and Fellows of Harvard College.

Committee on Human Genetic Diversity, National Research Council. *Evaluating Human Genetic Diversity.* Reprinted with permission of National Academy Press, Copyright 1997.

Cook, Rebecca. *Gender, Health and Human Rights.* Reprinted from *Health and Human Rights* 1 (4), with permission from the François-Xavier Bagnoud Center for Health and Human Rights, Harvard School of Public Health. Copyright © 1995 by the President and Fellows of Harvard College.

International Federation of Red Cross and Red Crescent Societies and François-Xavier Bagnoud Center for Health and Human Rights. *The Public Health—Human Rights Dialogue.* Reprinted from *AIDS, Health and Human Rights: An Explanatory Manual,* with permission from the organizations. Copyright © 1995.

Mann, Jonathan. *Human Rights and AIDS: The Future of the Pandemic.* Reprinted from *The John Marshall Law Review,* 1996. Reprinted with permission.

Mann, Jonathan. *Medicine and Public Health, Ethics and Human Rights.* Reprinted from *Hastings Center Report,* reprinted with permission. Copyright 1997 by Hastings Center.

Mann, Jonathan. Gostin, Lawrence. Gruskin, Sofia. Brennan, Troyen. Lazzarini, Zita. Fineberg, Harvey. *Health and Human Rights.* Reprinted from *Health and Human Rights* 1 (1), with permission from the François-Xavier Bagnoud Center for Health and Human Rights, Harvard School of Public Health. Copyright © 1994 by the President and Fellows of Harvard College.

Marks, Stephen. *Common Strategies for Health and Human Rights: From Theory to Practice.* Reprinted from *Health and Human Rights* 2 (3), with permission from the François-Xavier Bagnoud Center for Health and Human Rights, Harvard School of Public Health. Copyright © 1997 by the President and Fellows of Harvard College.

Marotte, Cécile. Razafimbahiny, Hervé Rakoto. *Haiti: 1991–1994: The International Civilian Mission's Medical Unit.* Reprinted from *Health and Human Rights* 2 (2), with permission from the François-Xavier Bagnoud Center for Health and Human Rights, Harvard School of Public Health. Copyright © 1997 by the President and Fellows of Harvard College.

Miller, Alice M. Rosga, AnnJanette. Satterthwaite, Meg. *Health, Human Rights, and Lesbian Existence.* Reprinted from *Health and Human Rights* 1 (4), with permission from the François-Xavier Bagnoud Center for Health and Human Rights, Harvard School of Public Health. Copyright © 1995 by the President and Fellows of Harvard College.

Yamin, Alicia Ely. *Ethnic Cleansing and Other Lies: Combining Health and Human Rights in the Search for Truth and Justice in the Former Yugoslavia.* Reprinted from *Health and Human Rights* 2 (1), with permission from the François-Xavier Bagnoud Center for Health and Human Rights, Harvard School of Public Health. Copyright © 1996 by the President and Fellows of Harvard College.

About the Contributors

Ad Hoc Committee to Defend Health Care, Boston, MA, USA

Nancy Adler, PhD, Professor of Medical Psychology, Department of Psychiatry and Pediatrics, Director, Health Psychology Program, University of California, San Francisco, CA, USA

Catherine L. Annas, JD, Analyst, Joint Committee on Health Care, Senate and House of Representatives, Commonwealth of Massachusetts, Boston, MA, USA

George J. Annas, JD, MPH, Edward R. Utley Professor and Chair, Health Law Department, Boston University School of Public Health, Boston, MA, USA

W. Thomas Boyce, MD, Professor of Pediatrics, School of Medicine, University of California, San Francisco, CA, USA

Troyen A. Brennan, MA, JD, MD, MPH, Professor of Medicine, Professor of Law and Public Health in the Faculty of Public Health, Harvard School of Public Health, Boston, MA, USA

Center for Economic and Social Rights, New York, NY, USA

Margaret A. Chesney, MD, PhD, Professor of Medicine and Epidemiology, School of Medicine, University of California, San Francisco, CA, USA

Sheldon Cohen, MD, PhD, Professor of Psychology, Carnegie-Mellon University, Pittsburgh, PA, USA

Committee on Human Genetic Diversity, National Research Council, Washington, DC, USA

Rebecca J. Cook, MPA, JD, JSD, Professor in the Faculty of Law and in the Faculty of Medicine, University of Toronto, Canada

Alain Destexhe, MD, Senator, Belgian Parliament, Brussels, Belgium

Ruth Faden, PhD, MPH, Professor of Health Policy and Management, Johns Hopkins University School of Hygiene and Public Health, Baltimore, MD

Harvey V. Fineberg, MD, PhD, Professor of Health Policy and Management in the Faculty of Public Health, Provost, Harvard University, Cambridge, MA, USA

Susan Folkman, PhD, Professor of Medicine, Center for AIDS Prevention Studies, University of California, San Francisco, CA, USA

Renée Fox, PhD, Annenberg Professor of the Social Sciences, Department of Sociology, University of Pennsylvania, Philadelphia, PA, USA

François-Xavier Bagnoud Center for Health and Human Rights, Harvard School of Public Health, Boston, MA, USA

Lynn P. Freedman, JD, MPH, Associate Professor of Clinical Public Health, Columbia University School of Public Health, New York, NY, USA

Lawrence O. Gostin, JD, Professor of Law, Georgetown University Law Center, Adjunct Professor of Public Health, Johns Hopkins University, Co-Director, Georgetown–Johns Hopkins Program on Law and Public Health, Washington, DC, USA

Michael A. Grodin, MD, FAAP, Director, Law, Medicine and Ethics Program, and Professor, Health Law Department, Boston University Schools of Medicine and Public Health, Boston, MA, USA

Sofia Gruskin, JD, MIA, Director, Human Rights Program, François-Xavier Bagnoud Center for Health and Human Rights, Lecturer in the Department of Population and International Health, Harvard School of Public Health, Boston, MA, USA

Jacques du Guerny, Chief, Population Program Service, Division of Women and Population, Food and Agriculture Organization of the United Nations, Rome, Italy

Kari Hannibal, MA, National Program Coordinator, The Albert Schweitzer Fellowship, Boston, MA, USA

Aart Hendriks, LLM, MA, Research Associate, Netherlands Institute of Human Rights, Utrecht, The Netherlands

Carel Ijsselmuiden, MD, MPH, Medical University of Southern Africa, Medunsa, South Africa

International Federation of Red Cross and Red Crescent Societies, Geneva, Switzerland

Robert L. Kahn, Institute for Social Research, University of Michigan, Ann Arbor, USA

Robert Lawrence, MD, Associate Dean for Professional Education and Programs, Professor of Health Policy, Johns Hopkins University, Baltimore, MD, USA

Zita Lazzarini, JD, MPH, Adjunct Lecturer on Law and Public Health in the

Faculty of Public Health, Department of Health Policy and Management, Harvard School of Public Health, Boston, MA, USA

Jonathan M. Mann, MD, MPH, Dean, School of Public Health, Allegheny University of the Health Sciences, Philadelphia, PA, USA. (deceased)

Stephen Marks, PhD, Director of United Nations Studies Program, Columbia University, New York, NY, USA

Cécile Marotte, PhD, Consultant, Human Rights Fund, Port-au-Prince, Haiti

Alice M. Miller, JD, Director, Women's Rights Advocacy Program, International Human Rights Law Group, Washington, DC, USA

Hervé Rakoto Razafimbahiny, MD, Consultant, Human Rights Fund, Port-au-Prince, Haiti

AnnJanette Rosga, Assistant Professor of Sociology and Anthropology, Knox College, Galesburg, IL, USA

Meg Satterthwaite, MA, law student, New York University School of Law ('99).

Elisabeth Sjöberg, MA, Administrative Coordinator, Programme for Research and Documentation of a Sustainable Society (Prosus), The Research Council of Norway, Norway.

S. Leonard Syme, PhD, Professor Emeritus of Epidemiology, University of California—Berkeley, USA

Telford Taylor, LLD, LHD, LCD, Nash Professor Emeritus of Law, Columbia University School of Law, Professor of Constitutional Law, Benjamin N. Cardozo School of Law, New York, NY, USA (deceased)

Alicia Ely Yamin, JD, MPH, Assistant Professor of Clinical Public Health, Columbia University School of Public Health, New York, NY, USA

About the Editors

Jonathan M. Mann, MD, MPH, was the first François-Xavier Bagnoud Professor of Health and Human Rights and founding director of the François-Xavier Bagnoud Center for Health and Human Rights at the Harvard School of Public Health. From 1986–1990, Mann was founding director of the World Health Organization's Global Program on AIDS, based in Geneva. He is the author and editor of many books and articles, including coeditor of *AIDS in the World* and *AIDS in the World II*.

Sofia Gruskin, JD, MIA, is the Director of the Human Rights Program at the François-Xavier Bagnoud Center for Health and Human Rights and a lecturer in Population and International Health at the Harvard School of Public Health. Gruskin has extensive experience working with United Nations agencies and nongovernmental orgaizations, and has authored numerous chapters and articles on health and human rights related issues. She is a member of the Board of Directors of Amnesty International, USA.

Michael A. Grodin, MD, FAAP, is Director of the Law, Medicine, and Ethics Program and Professor of Health Law, Health Law Department, Boston University Schools of Public Health and Medicine. His books include *The Nazi Doctors and the Nuremberg Code: Human Rights in Human Experimentation, Children as Research Subjects: Science, Ethics and Law* and *Meta Medical Ethics: The Philosophical Foundation of Bioethics*. He is the co-founder of Global Lawyers and Physicians.

George J. Annas, JD, MPH, is the Edward R. Utley Professor and Chair, Health Law Department, Boston University School of Public Health. He is the author or editor of a dozen books on health law and ethics, including *The Rights of Patients, Judging Medicine, Standard of Care*, and *Some Choice*, and is the legal feature writer for the *New England Journal of Medicine* and co-founder of Global Lawyers and Physicians.

The **François-Xavier Bagnoud Center for Health and Human Rights** was founded in 1993 at the Harvard School of Public Health to promote and catalyze the health and human rights movement; to influence policies and practices in health and human rights; and to expand the knowledge about linkages between health and human rights in specific contexts such as HIV/AIDS, children's rights and health, and women's health and rights. The Center has developed and conducts a variety of academic and professional training courses on health and human rights. Current research and thinking in health and human rights is published in the Center's journal, *Health and Human Rights*, and in additional publications. The Center seeks to influence policy and programs through its collaboration with various UN agencies and in partnership with NGOs, international agencies, and governments worldwide (www.hri.ca/partners/fxbcenter).

Global Lawyers and Physicians (GLP)'s mission is to work collaboratively toward the global implementation of the health-related provisions of the Universal Declaration of Human Rights and the Covenants on Civil and Political Rights and Economic, Social and Cultural Rights, with a focus on health-care ethics, patients' rights, and human experimentation. GLP was founded in 1996 at an international symposium held at the United States Holocaust Memorial Museum to commemorate the fiftieth anniversary of the Nuremberg Doctors' Trial. GLP was formed to reinvigorate the collaboration of legal and medical/public health professionals to protect the human rights and dignity of all persons (www.glphr.org).

Index

I